Donovan

VASCULAR SURGICAL EMERGENCIES

VASCULAR SURGICAL EMERGENCIES

Edited by

John J. Bergan, M.D., F.A.C.S., Hon. F.R.C.S. (Eng.)
Margerstadt Professor of Surgery
Chief, Division of Vascular Surgery
Northwestern University Medical School
Chicago, Illinois

James S.T. Yao, M.D., Ph.D., F.A.C.S.
Professor of Surgery
Director, Blood Flow Laboratory
Northwestern University Medical School
Chicago, Illinois

Grune & Stratton, Inc.
Harcourt Brace Jovanovich, Publishers
Orlando   New York   San Diego   London
San Francisco   Tokyo   Sydney   Toronto

Library of Congress Cataloging-in-Publication Data
Vascular surgical emergencies.

   Includes bibliographies and index.
1. Blood-vessels—Surgery.   2. Surgical
emergencies.   I. Bergan, John J., 1927–
II. Yao, James S. T.   [DNLM: 1. Emergencies.
2. Vascular Surgery.   WG 170 V33175]
RD598.5.V397   1987   617′.413026   86-19496
ISBN 0-8089-1843-5

   Grune & Stratton, Inc.
   Orlando, Florida 32887

   Distributed in the United Kingdom by
   Grune & Stratton, Ltd.
   24/28 Oval Road, London NW 1

Library of Congress Catalog Number 86-19496
International Standard Book Number 0-8089-1843-5

Printed in the United States of America
87 88 89 90   10 9 8 7 6 5 4 3 2 1

Contents

PART VI: EMERGENCY SURGERY IN ARTERIAL ANEURYSM

PART VII: EMERGENCY AORTIC SURGERY

PART VIII: VISCERAL ARTERIES

PART IX: IATROGENIC VASCULAR EMERGENCIES

PART X: VENOUS EMERGENCIES

Foreword

As the table of contents demonstrates, there is a surprisingly long list of emergency situations that may be encountered by general and vascular surgeons. The breadth of knowledge necessary to deal with this diverse array of emergencies is equally impressive. The complexity of the information needed to manage vascular trauma alone is staggering; for example, a retrophepatic vena caval injury may be associated with major hepatic or colon injury and spinal cord damage with paraplegia. Management of the associated injuries is a formidable task, and repair of the vena caval injury itself is one of the most challenging technical feats in all of surgery, requiring the insertion of a temporary shunt to sustain life, extensive knowledge of anatomy to gain exposure of the injury, and outstanding technical skill to repair the wound rapidly. Superb preoperative and postoperative care is crucial to a successful outcome, requiring the application of basic science to the management of shock, sepsis, coagulation disorders and organ failure, to name only a few of the problems encountered. Most vascular emergencies require equally extensive knowlege, and this book provides it through succinct presentations written by internationally recognized experts.

Perusal of the table of contents also will impress the reader with the need for broadly based, in-depth training experience for the young surgeons who will care for these patients in the future. The recent formalization of general vascular surgical residences will stimulate additional research and education in the management of these catastrophic events. The complex knowledge needed to manage them successfully underscores the wisdom of requiring the broadly based training of a residency in general surgery prior to more specialized training in vascular surgery. General surgeons should also be trained in vascular surgery, because in vascular emergencies the time required to transport patients to a specialized surgeon may be too long to save life or limb.

This book should also serve to foster an interdisciplinary approach to emergency vascular problems. Successful treatment of many of the conditions discussed requires close working relationships with neurologists, neurosurgeons, anesthesiologists, orthopedic and cardiac surgeons, as well as radiologists and emergency medicine physicians. The crucial importance of expert and easily available nurses and technical personnel for provision of extracorporeal circulation, collection and reinfusion of shed blood, and the newer forms of respiratory support such as jet ventilation cannot be overlooked. Truly, the surgeon responsible for vascular emergencies needs to be an organizer and a teacher. The framework for his task may be found in this book.

David L. Nahrwold, M.D.
Loyal and Edith Davis Professor
and Chairman
Department of Surgery
Northwestern University Medical School
Chicago, Illinois

Introduction

Descriptions of care of vascular surgical emergencies punctuate the recorded history of surgery. These include detailed depictions of care of injuries obtained by gladiators and soldiers as shown in the frescoes of Pompeii and bas relief at Herculaneum, amputations for vascular and soft tissue injury as cared for by Ambroise Paré, thigh wounds and those to the femoral artery in toreadors in Madrid, and even iatrogenic injuries occurring during blundered venesection as described by Hippocrates and Matthaeus Purmann.

Care of vascular surgical emergencies varies with the times. It is timely now to review such care. The objective here has been to accumulate current information in an easily referred to source so that those who treat vascular emergencies can proceed in an orderly yet urgent fashion, applying the most modern techniques available as described in a single reference resource.

With this in mind, it has been appropriate to include in this volume a section on general considerations that describes current theories of shock and resuscitation, as accomplished by Charles Rice; the complex metabolic disorders induced by ischemia of limb musculature, thoroughly elucidated by Bernard Nachbur's group from Bern, Switzerland; and the complex problems of shifting tides of mesenteric blood flow, as researched by Gregory Bulkley and his associates.

Litigation is a fact of life in surgery today, and therefore, the subject of litigation after vascular emergencies has been included in this section on general considerations and is written by John Bergan.

Vascular emergencies as obtained in the Colliseum by gladiators and from the bull's charging horn in the corrida were in the past largely assessed by the five senses of the attending surgeon. In our modern era, we have available both invasive and noninvasive techniques, and the question is, when should they be used and how should they not be misused. These subjects are described in detail: that of angiographic examination by Jonathan Towne and his coworkers, who have accumulated a large experience; that of the Northwestern group by Robert Vogelzang and Madeleine Fisher, authorities on computed tomography and magnetic resonance imaging; and the use of noninvasive testing in vascular emergencies by Eugene Strandness, who introduced the era of nonivasive testing and made these examinations available to interested surgeons. Vascular physiology includes more than the simple interactions of blood vessel wall with rheology. It now includes the ebb and flow of coagulation factors in response to daily activity. Hematological assessments in vascular emergencies, therefore, have become an important consideration, and this is discussed in this volume by Donald Silver and Ricardo Rao.

Cerebrovascular emergencies once described only the management of cartoid trauma. In fact, this subject is described very well here from the large Parkland Hospital experience by William Fry and his son, Richard. However, increased sophistication in knowledge of cerebral blood supply has brought up other, formerly little recognized topics, such as the management of cartoid artery dissection, as described by Ronald Stoney and Steven Okuhn in this volume, and the consideration of emergency cartoid endarterectomy, a subject which has been of great interest to Roger Greenhalgh and his coworkers at Charing Cross Hospital in London.

Naturally, vascular injuries, both arterial and venous, are important considerations in discussion of vascular emergencies. One would expect that these would form the backbone of the skeleton of knowledge comprising this subject. Therefore, large sections are devoted to these topics in this volume. With regard to arterial injuries, Malcolm Perry has provided an insightful discussion of the management of penetrating injuries; Robert McCready and Gordon Hyde of Lexington have explored the limitations in use of autogenous tissue revascularization; while David Feliciano has described the Houston group's very large experience with prostheses in treatment of arterial injuries.

Compartment syndromes are of great interest to orthopaedic surgeons but not any less so to vascular surgeons. This topic is thoroughly discussed by William Russell and Phillip Burns, who have made important observations from their own experience. Pediatric vascular surgery cannot be considered as merely the repair of blood vessels in small adults, and therefore, the topic of pediatric vascular emergencies has been selected for presentation by Preston Flanigan and James Schuler, utilizing the large experience of the Univerity of Illinois Medical Center in Chicago. In a double contribution, they have also described repair of vascular injuries deriving from orthopaedic surgery of the spine and joints. Ultimately, the most definitive form of vascular injury is severance of a limb. In Munich, Peter Maurer's group has accumulated an experience with upper and lower limb replantation that is summarized here and makes important observations for future use, as well as future investigations.

No one in vascular surgery today has made more fundamental contributions to management of venous injuries than William Blaisdell, who describes the management of vena cava and portal vein injury here, and Norman Rich, who with his colleagues at the Uniformed Services University of the Health Sciences, has accumulated a registry of venous injuries which continues to document the natural history of repair of these injuries.

In general, vascular emergencies can be divided into those occurring during trauma, those which arise from degenerative diseases and their treatment, and iatrogenic vascular injuries. These three subjects are thoroughly covered in this volume. Emergency surgery in arterial aneurysm is summarized by Jesse Thompson and John Bergan for the ruptured abdominal aortic aneurysm; the anastomotic aneurysm by Walter McCarthy of the Northwestern group; thoracic surgical emergencies, including dissections by Craig Miller of Stanford, those of decelerating aortic injury by Kenneth Mattox, who is well known for his contributions to management of vascular trauma; and the management of aortoenteric erosions and aortocaval fistula by Calvin Ernst and Alexander Shepard from the Henry Ford Hospital.

Other vascular emergencies arising from degenerative disease include acute renal artery occlusion, which is given a thorough treatment by Richard Dean and his group from Vanderbilt University; the problems of ruptured splanchnic artery aneurysms as described by James Stanley and the University of Michigan group, long known for its knowledge of the natural history of splanchnic artery aneurysms; and acute mesenteric ischemia occurring from thrombosis, emoblization, and nonocclusive causes by John Bergan and the Northwestern group.

Somewhere between the care of degenerative vascular emergencies and iatrogenic vascular emergencies lies the subject of self-inflicted injuries acquired from intravascular injection of drugs. This topic, important in modern vascular surgery, is thoroughly discussed by Ramon Berguer and Pamela Benitez of Detroit. With regard to iatrogenic vascular emergencies, these are discussed by Robert Rutherford and William Pearce, while the little-discussed topic of vascular complications of intraaortic balloon pumping is covered by Giacomo DeLaria from the very experienced group of cardiovascular surgeons at the Rush-Presbyterian-St. Lukes's Medical Center in Chicago.

Sudden occlusions of veins and arteries arise from many causes and produce different manifestations in the various regional anatomies of the body. The problem of venous gangrene, for example, is a very real one, arising as it does from phlegmasia cerulea dolens. This topic has been of interest to, and is described here by Andrew Dale of Nashville. The problems of pulmonary embolectomy and its prevention have been of great interest to Lazar Greenfield, who provides us with a very objective analysis of these difficulties. The subject of emergency management of superficial venous problems has not been described elsewhere in modern times. This subject has attracted the attention of James Yao and William Flinn, who present several new and very interesting observations in a detailed chapter on this subject.

Acute extremity ischemia historically has occupied the attention of many vascular surgeons. Its management today is clouded by misconceptions regarding anticoagulant therapy and misapplication of surgical revascularization procedures. The topic of upper extremity ischemia is discussed here by James Yao and William Flinn, and that of lower extremity ischemia by John Cranley, whose group with Tom Fogarty made the original contribution of the Fogarty catheter to the armamentarium of vascular surgeons. Acute extremity arterial thrombosis can occur as a result of degenerative disease, and this is discussed by David Brewster and George Meier of the Massachusetts General Hospital group, and also occurs as a result of acute occlusion of vascular reconstructions, a subject that Frank Veith and his group at the Montefiore Medical Center in New York have elucidated for us in this volume. Finally, on occasion no reconstruction is possible, and an emergency amputation must be done to save life. This subject is described for us by Wesley Moore and William Cole of Los Angeles.

As detailed above, emergency vascular surgery combines the study of many elements including basic physiology at an intellectual level, and rapid action at its most pragmatic. Socially, the management of vascular emergencies can be rewarding as life and limb are saved or devastating when they are lost. Discussions of relevant topics are brought together in this volume for use by surgeons interested in improving care of vascular emergencies in the hope that more lives will be saved, more limbs made useful, and that vascular surgery can remain a very important part of the emergency care of the injured patient.

John J. Bergan, M.D., F.A.C.S., Hon. F.R.C.S. (Eng.)
James S. T. Yao, M.D., Ph.D., F.A.C.S.

Contributors

ENRICO ASCER, M.D.
   Assistant Professor of Surgery and
   Head, Vascular Surgery Research
   Laboratory, Albert Einstein College of
   Medicine—Montefiore Medical
   Center, New York, New York

PAMELA BENITEZ, M.D.
   Assistant Professor of Surgery, Wayne
   State University School of Medicine,
   Detroit, Michigan

JOHN J. BERGAN, M.D., F.A.C.S.,
HON. F.R.C.S. (ENG.)
   Magerstadt Professor of Surgery and
   Chief, Division of Vascular Surgery,
   Northwestern University Medical
   School, Chicago, Illinois

RAMON BERGUER, M.D., PH.D.
   Professor of Surgery and Chief of
   Vascular Surgery, Wayne State
   University School of Medicine,
   Detroit, Michigan

F. WILLIAM BLAISDELL, M.D.
   Professor and Chairman, Department of
   Surgery, University of California,
   Davis, School of Medicine,
   Sacramento, California

DAVID C. BREWSTER, M.D.
   Associate Clinical Professor of Surgery,
   Harvard Medical School
   —Massachusetts General Hospital,
   Boston, Massachusetts

B. M. BOURKE, F.R.A.C.S.
   Senior Registrar, Department of Surgery,
   Charing Cross Hospital, London,
   England

GREGORY B. BULKLEY, M.D.,
F.A.C.S.
   Associate Professor of Surgery and
   Director of Surgical Research, The
   Johns Hopkins Medical Institutions,
   Baltimore, Maryland

WILFRIED BURMEISTER, M.D.
   Department of Vascular Surgery,
   Technical University of Munich
   Medical School, Rechts der Isar
   Medical Center, Munich, West
   Germany

R. PHILLIP BURNS, M.D., F.A.C.S.
   Professor and Chairman, Department of
   Surgery, University of Tennessee
   College of Medicine, Chattanooga,
   Tennessee

C. WILLIAM COLE, M.D.
  Assistant Professor of Surgery, Ottawa
  Civic Hospital, Ottawa, Ontario,
  Canada

PAUL COLLIER, M.D.
  Fellow in Vascular Surgery and
  Instructor in Surgery, Albert Einstein
  College of Medicine—Montefiore
  Medical Center, New York, New York

JOHN J. CRANLEY, M.D.
  Professor of Surgery, University of
  Cincinnati College of Medicine;
  Director Emeritus, Department of
  Surgery and Director, Vascular
  Laboratory, Good Samaritan Hospital,
  Cincinnati, Ohio

RACHEL DAIN, S.R.N.
  Research Medical Laboratory Scientific
  Officer, Department of Surgery,
  Charing Cross Hospital, London,
  England

W. ANDREW DALE, M.D.
  Clinical Professor of Surgery, Vanderbilt
  University School of Medicine,
  Nashville, Tennessee

RICHARD H. DEAN, M.D.
  Professor of Surgery and Head, Division
  of Vascular Surgery, Vanderbilt
  University School of Medicine,
  Nashville, Tennessee

GIACOMO A. DELARIA, M.D.
  Assistant Professor of Surgery, Rush
  Medical College; Associate
  Attending, Cardiovascular-Thoracic
  Surgery, Rush-Presbyterian-St. Luke's
  Medical Center, Chicago, Illinois

JOACHIM DOERRLER, M.D.
  Assistant Professor of Surgery,
  Department of Vascular Surgery,
  Technical University of Munich
  Medical School, Rechts der Isar
  Medical Center, Munich, West
  Germany

CALVIN B. ERNST, M.D.
  Clinical Professor of Surgery, University
  of Michigan, Ann Arbor, Michigan;
  Head, Division of Vascular Surgery,
  Henry Ford Hospital, Detroit,
  Michigan

DAVID V. FELICIANO, M.D.
  Associate Professor of Surgery, Baylor
  College of Medicine; Director,
  Surgical Intensive Care Unit, Ben
  Taub General Hospital, Houston,
  Texas

MADELEINE R. FISHER, M.D.
  Assistant Professor of Radiology,
  Northwestern University Medical
  School; Director, Magnetic
  Resonance, Department of Diagnostic
  Radiology, Northwestern Memorial
  Hospital, Chicago, Illinois

D. PRESTON FLANIGAN, M.D.
  Associate Professor of Surgery and
  Chief, Division of Vascular Surgery,
  University of Illinois College of
  Medicine at Chicago, Chicago,
  Illinois

WILLIAM R. FLINN, M.D.
  Associate Professor of Surgery, Division
  of Vascular Surgery, Northwestern
  University Medical School, Chicago,
  Illinois

RICHARD E. FRY, M.D.
  Assistant Professor, Department of
  Surgery, University of Texas
  Southwestern Medical School Health
  Sciences Center, Dallas, Texas

WILLIAM J. FRY. M.D.
  Professor and Chairman, Department of
  Surgery, University of Texas
  Southwestern Medical School Health
  Sciences Center, Dallas, Texas

EDWARD R. GOMEZ, M.D., MAJ,
M.C., U.S.A.
  Instructor of Surgery, F. Edward Hébert
  School of Medicine, Uniformed

Services University of the Health
Sciences, Bethesda, Maryland;
Fellow, Peripheral Vascular Surgery
Service, Walter Reed Army Medical
Center, Washington, D.C.

LINDA M. GRAHAM, M.D.
Assistant Professor, Division of
Peripheral Vascular Surgery,
University of Michigan Medical
School; 2nd Chief, Peripheral
Vascular Surgery Service, Veterans
Administration Hospital, Ann Arbor,
Michigan

LAZAR J. GREENFIELD, M.D.
Stuart McGuire Professor of Surgery and
Chairman, Department of Surgery,
Medical College of Virginia, Virginia
Commonwealth University,
Richmond, Virginia

ROGER M. GREENHALGH, M.A.,
M.D., M.CHIR., F.R.C.S.
Professor of Surgery, Department of
Surgery, Charing Cross Hospital,
London, England

SUSHIL K. GUPTA, M.D.
Associate Professor of Surgery,
Associate Chief of Vascular Surgical
Services, and Director, Vascular
Registry, Albert Einstein College of
Medicine—Montefiore Medical
Center, New York, New York

ULF H. HAGLUND, M.D., PH.D.
Associate Professor of Surgery,
University of Lund Mälmo General
Hospital, Mälmo, Sweden; Visiting
Assistant Professor of Surgery, The
Johns Hopkins Medical Institutions,
Baltimore, Maryland

JOHANNES HEISS, M.D.
Department of Vascular Surgery,
Technical University of Munich
Medical School, Rechts der Isar
Medical Center, Munich, West
Germany

FRITZ HORBER, M.D.
Chief Resident, Medical Policlinic,
University of Berne, Berne,
Switzerland

GORDON L. HYDE, M.D.
Professor of Surgery, University of
Kentucky Medical Center, Lexington,
Kentucky

HERMANN W. KAEBNICK, M.D.
Fellow, Department of Vascular
Surgery, Medical College of
Wisconsin, Milwaukee, Wisconsin

RICHARD G. KILFOLYE, M.D., MAJ,
M.C., U.S.A.
Instructor of Surgery, F. Edward Hébert
School of Medicine, Uniformed
Services University of the Health
Sciences, Bethesda, Maryland;
Fellow, Peripheral Vascular Surgery
Service, Walter Reed Army Medical
Center, Washington, D.C.

ELLIOT O. LIPCHIK, M.D.
Professor of Radiology and Chief,
Section of Angiography, Medical
College of Wisconsin, Milwaukee,
Wisconsin

KENNETH L. MATTOX, M.D.
Professor of Surgery, Baylor College of
Medicine; Chief of Surgery and
Director of Emergency Services, Ben
Taub General Hospital, Houston,
Texas

PETER CARL MAURER, M.D.,
F.A.C.S.
Professor of Surgery and Head,
Department of Vascular Surgery,
Technical University of Munich
Medical School, Rechts der Isar
Medical Center, Munich, West
Germany

WALTER J. McCARTHY, III, M.D.
Associate in Surgery, Division of
Vascular Surgery, Northwestern
University Medical School; Director,

Vascular Laboratory, V.A. Lakeside
Medical Center, Chicago, Illinois

CHARLES N. McCOLLUM, M.D.
F.R.C.S.
Senior Lecturer, Department of Surgery,
Charing Cross Hospital, London,
England

ROBERT A. McCREADY, M.D.
Assistant Professor of Surgery,
University of Kentucky Medical
Center, Lexington, Kentucky

PATRICK W. MEACHAM, M.D.
Assistant Professor of Surgery,
Vanderbilt University School of
Medicine, Nashville, Tennessee

GEORGE H. MEIER, M.D.
Resident in General Vascular Surgery,
Harvard Medical
School—Massachusetts General
Hospital, Boston, Massachusetts

D. CRAIG MILLER, M.D.
Associate Professor of Cardiovascular
Surgery, Director, Cardiovascular
Surgical Research Laboratories, Head,
Division of Peripheral Vascular
Surgery, and Program Director,
General Vascular Surgery Residency
Program, Stanford University School
of Medicine, Stanford, California;
Chief, Cardiac Surgery Section, V.A.
Medical Center, Palo Alto, California

WESLEY S. MOORE, M.D.
Professor of Surgery and Chief, Section
of Vascular Surgery, University of
California, Los Angeles School of
Medicine, Center for the Health
Sciences, Los Angeles, California

JON B. MORRIS, M.D.
Fellow in Surgery, The Johns Hopkins
Hospital, Baltimore, Maryland

BERNARD H. NACHBUR, M.D.
Professor of Surgery and Head,
Department of Thoracic and

Cardiovascular Surgery, University of
Berne, Berne, Switzerland

ANSELMO A. NUNEZ, M.D.
Fellow in Vascular Surgery and
Instructor in Surgery, Albert Einstein
College of Medicine—Montefiore
Medical Center, New York, New York

STEVEN P. OKUHN, M.D.
Vascular Research Resident, University
of California, San Francisco School of
Medicine, San Francisco, California

PAUL M. ORECCHIA, M.D., LTC,
M.C., U.S.A.
Assistant Professor of Surgery, F.
Edward Hébert School of Medicine,
Uniformed Services University of the
Health Sciences, Bethesda, Maryland;
Assistant Chief, Peripheral Vascular
Surgery Service, Walter Reed Army
Medical Center, Washington, D.C.

WILLIAM H. PEARCE, M.D.
Assistant Professor of Surgery, Vascular
Surgery Section, University of
Colorado Health Sciences Center,
Denver, Colorado

G. D. PERKIN, F.R.C.P.
Consultant Neurologist, Regional
Neurosciences Unit, Charing Cross
Hospital, London, England

MALCOLM O. PERRY, M.D.
Professor of Surgery, Cornell University
Medical College; Chief, Division of
Vascular Surgery, New York
Hospital-Cornell Medical Center,
New York, New York

RICARDO RAO, B.A.
Department of Surgery, University of
Missouri-Columbia Health Sciences
Center, Columbia, Missouri

CHARLES L. RICE, M.D.
Professor and Vice-Chairman,
Department of Surgery, University of
Washington School of Medicine;

Surgeon-in-Chief, Harborview
Medical Center, Seattle, Washington

NORMAN M. RICH, M.D., F.A.C.S.
Professor and Chairman, Department of
Surgery and Chief, Division of
Vascular Surgery, F. Edward Hébert
School of Medicine, Uniformed
Services University of the Health
Sciences, Bethesda, Maryland;
Co-Director, Vascular Fellowship
Program, Walter Reed Army Medical
Center, Washington, D.C.

F. CLIFFORD ROSE, F.R.C.P.
Consultant Neurologist, Regional
Neurosciences Unit, Charing Cross
Hospital, London, England

WILLIAM L. RUSSELL, M.D., F.A.C.S.
Associate Professor and Vice Chairman,
Department of Surgery, University of
Tennessee College of Medicine,
Chattanooga, Tennessee

ROBERT B. RUTHERFORD, M.D.
Professor of Surgery, Vascular Surgery
Section, University of Colorado
Health Sciences Center, Denver,
Colorado

JAMES M. SALANDER, M.D., COL,
M.C., U.S.A.
Associate Professor of Surgery, F.
Edward Hébert School of Medicine,
Uniformed Services University of the
Health Sciences, Bethesda, Maryland;
Chief, Peripheral Vascular Surgery
Service, Walter Reed Army Medical
Center, Washington, D.C.

JAMES J. SCHULER, M.D.
Associate Professor of Surgery, Division
of Vascular Surgery, University of
Illinois College of Medicine at
Chicago, Chicago, Illinois

ALEXANDER D. SHEPARD, M.D.
Medical Director, Non-Invasive
Laboratory, Division of Vascular

Surgery, Henry Ford Hospital,
Detroit, Michigan

STEFAN SIGRIST, M.D.
Fellow in Vascular Surgery, Department
of Thoracic and Cardiovascular
Surgery, University of Berne, Berne,
Switzerland

DONALD SILVER, M.D.
Professor and Chairman, Department of
Surgery, University of
Missouri-Columbia Health Sciences
Center, Columbia, Missouri

JAMES C. STANLEY, M.D.
Professor of Surgery and Head, Division
of Peripheral Vascular Surgery,
University of Michigan Medical
School, Ann Arbor, Michigan

RONALD J. STONEY, M.D.
Professor of Surgery and Co-Chief,
Division of Vascular Surgery,
University of California, San
Francisco School of Medicine, San
Francisco, California

D. EUGENE STRANDNESS, JR., M.D.
Professor of Surgery, University of
Washington School of Medicine,
Seattle, Washington

JESSE E. THOMPSON, M.D.
Clinical Professor of Surgery, University
of Texas Southwestern Medical
School; Chief of Surgery and Chief of
Vascular Surgery, Baylor University
Medical Center, Dallas, Texas

JONATHAN B. TOWNE, M.D.
Professor of Surgery and Head,
Department of Vascular Surgery,
Medical College of Wisconsin,
Milwaukee, Wisconsin

FRANK J. VEITH, M.D.
Professor of Surgery and Chief of
Vascular Surgical Services, Albert
Einstein College of Medicine–

Montefiore Medical Center, New
York, New York

J. LEONEL VILLAVICENCIO, M.D.,
F.A.C.S.
Professor of Surgery, F. Edward Hébert
School of Medicine, Uniformed
Services University of the Health
Sciences, Bethesda, Maryland; Chief,
Vein Clinic, Walter Reed Army
Medical Center, Washington, D.C.

ROBERT L. VOGELZANG, M.D.
Assistant Professor of Radiology,
Northwestern University Medical
School; Director, Angiography and
Interventional Radiology and
Co-Director, Computed Body
Tomography, Department of
Diagnostic Radiology, Northwestern
Memorial Hospital, Chicago, Illinois

THOMAS W. WAKEFIELD, M.D.
Assistant Professor, Division of
Peripheral Vascular Surgery,

University of Michigan Medical
School, Ann Arbor, Michigan

FRED A. WEAVER, M.D.
Fellow in Vascular Surgery, Vanderbilt
University School of Medicine,
Nashville, Tennessee

JAMES S. T. YAO, M.D., PH.D.,
F.A.C.S.
Professor of Surgery and Director,
Vascular Fellowship Program,
Northwestern University Medical
School; Director, Blood Flow
Laboratory, Northwestern Memorial
Hospital, Chicago, Illinois

GERALD B. ZELENOCK, M.D.
Associate Professor, Division of
Peripheral Vascular Surgery,
University of Michigan Medical
School, Ann Arbor, Michigan

VASCULAR
SURGICAL
EMERGENCIES

PART I

General Considerations

Charles L. Rice

Shock and Resuscitation

SHOCK

Of the urgent situations that may confront the vascular surgeon, few are more anxiety producing than the hypotensive patient. This chapter will review the causes of hypotension, their physiologic consequences, and outline an approach to management.

HISTORY

The complex of symptoms and physical findings that we term *shock* was known to Hippocrates, who commented "when there is some large nerve, vein or artery injured, the convulsion and flow of escaping blood prostrates the wounded one and exhausts his strength."[1] Ambroise Paré, the celebrated 16th century French military surgeon characterized shock as "syncope and heart failure." John Hunter described shock quite well in his work *Blood, Inflammation, and Gunshot Wounds* (1793), and clearly recognized the danger of a reduction in blood volume, but, paradoxically, recommended bleeding as therapy for it. In 1872, Gross depicted shock as "the rude unhinging of the machinery of life"—a poetic, but physiologically unhelpful description. In 1940, Alfred Blalock defined shock as "a peripheral circulatory failure, resulting from a discrepancy in the size of the vascular bed and the volume of the intravascular fluid."[2] Other authors have emphasized the central importance of inadequacy of tissue perfusion in the pathophysiology of shock.

The physiologic classification proposed by Blalock in 1937[3] is still useful a half-century later. The four categories that he proposed are:

    I.   Hematogenic (oligemia)
   II. Neurogenic (caused primarily by neural influences)
  III. Vasogenic (decreased vascular resistance with increased capacitance)
  IV. Cardiogenic (failure of the heart as a pump)

Vascular Surgical Emergencies
ISBN 0-8089-1843-5

Surgeons concerned with vascular emergencies are concerned mainly with oligemric shock but each of the other categories is also important.

A clinically useful analogy may be drawn with Ohm's Law:

$$E = IR$$

where E refers to voltage, I to current, and R to resistance. In the hemodynamic setting, voltage (driving force) would be analogous to Mean Arterial Pressure, current (flow) to cardiac output, and electrical resistance to systemic vascular (or peripheral vascular) resistance. We may thus rewrite Ohm's Law (at the risk of offending the electrical engineering community) as

$$MAP = C.O. \times SVR$$

When confronted with a hypotensive patient, therefore, it is convenient to refine further terms and recall that cardiac output is the product of heart rate and stroke volume. In general, if intravascular volume is adequate, heart rates of from 50 to 150 are accompanied by corresponding changes in stroke volume, so that net cardiac output is not changed. Therefore, changes in the cardiac output term of our "Ohm's Law" are usually attributable to changes in stroke volume. Stroke volume is primarily determined by preload (venous return), contractility, and afterload. It will be apparent that this is simply another way of expressing Blalock's classification scheme.

Hematogenic shock, seen in vascular emergencies, is now more commonly referred to as *hemorrhagic* or *hypovolemic*. *Neurogenic* shock is caused primarily by sudden loss of vasoregulatory control (as in spinal cord injury), which results in venous pooling and a decreased venous return to the heart. It may be functionally considered as a special case of hypovolemic shock. *Vasogenic* shock includes shock that occurs in sepsis, anaphylaxis, and other factors that result in decreased peripheral vascular resistance. Finally, *cardiogenic* shock is that in which absolute intravascular volume is adequate, but in which the heart is incapable of effectively pumping that volume. This phenomenon most frequently occurs in the setting of an acute myocardial ischemic event, but may also be the terminal expression of cardiomyopathy.

HEMORRHAGIC SHOCK

Hypovolemic or hemorrhagic shock is the most easily understood and most readily treated form of shock, and it is the form that will be encountered most often by the vascular surgeon. It results from the reduction of circulating intravascular volume beyond the compensatory ability of normal homeostatic mechanisms. This reduction may occur because of the loss of *whole blood* from a penetrating injury to a great vessel; of *plasma* in a patient with a large burn injury; or of *extracellular fluid* in a patient with gastrointestinal losses or so-called third space sequestration after pancreatitis or retroperitoneal surgery.

The description of the patient with hypovolemic shock is as ancient as the Greeks and Egyptians: pale, clammy, apathetic, and glassy-eyed. It has been relatively recently that the critical regulatory phenomena that account for this condition have been elucidated. As intravascular volume is lost, the patient is initially able to maintain blood pressure by a neuroendocrine-mediated increase in peripheral vascular resistance. This increase in resistance is the result of intense vasoconstriction in skin, muscle, renal, and (to a lesser extent in man) splanchnic arteriolar beds. The remaining intravascular volume is distributed primarily to heart and brain. It is important to realize that so efficient is this compensation in a young, previously healthy adult, as much as 40 percent of blood volume may be lost before there is a noticeable decline in blood pressure.

Heart rate is virtually universally elevated with declining intravascular volume. Although cardiac output is defined as the product of heart rate and stroke volume, the increase in heart rate occurs as a result of declining stroke volume, and thus does not result in an increase in cardiac output. The decline in stroke volume occurs because venous return is decreased, right and left atrial pressures are lower, and, to a lesser extent, the diastolic filling time is reduced.

With the decline in cardiac output and the accompanying increase in peripheral vascular resistance, renal blood flow, glomerular filtration rate, and, thus, urine output all decline. The secretion of aldosterone results in the avid reclamation of sodium in the proximal renal tubule, with further reduction in urine volume. With continuing reduction of intravascular volume, peripheral compensatory mechanisms begin to fail, and blood pressure falls. With the fall in blood pressure, cerebral autoregulation is unable to sustain adequate flow, and the patient's level of consciousness deteriorates from apathy to unconsciousness.

Another hallmark of severe volume loss is lactic acidosis, which occurs with the shift from aerobic to anaerobic metabolism. Compounding this increase in lactic acid production is a decrease in lactic acid metabolism, which is the direct result of decreasing hepatic blood flow. Weil related the level of lactic acidosis to survival in patients with hemorrhagic shock and found that no patient with a lactic acid level in excess of 8 mM/L survived.[4]

Static measurements of blood volume have not been widely employed in patients in hemorrhagic shock because of the difficulty in obtaining reliable data in the rapidly changing clinical situation and because of the wide disparity of normal blood volumes among individuals. Moreover, work by Shires has clearly demonstrated that successful management of the victim of hemorrhagic shock depends on restoration not only of the blood volume lost, but on the repletion of extracellular fluid loss as well.[5]

CARDIOGENIC SHOCK

Some degree of myocardial dysfunction is a frequent accompaniment to myocardial infarction, but overt shock is relatively uncommon, usually occurring in less than 15 percent of patients admitted to coronary care units.[6] Many of the clinical features already described in hemorrhagic shock are also present in cardiogenic shock: pallor, restlessness, diaphoresis, hypotension, and oliguria. Cardiac index is generally less than 1.8 L/min/ m^2, and systemic vascular resistance is greater than 2000 dyne-cm-sec^{-5}. Pulmonary capillary wedge pressure is usually in excess of 18 torr. The vast majority of patients with cardiogenic shock are those with severe myocardial dysfunction, caused by a severe reduction in left ventricular contractile mass. Although there are some promising early results from the use of balloon left-ventricular assist devices, the probability of survival remains quite low. Temporary use of balloon assist can tide a patient over a cardiac event following aortic surgery. On the other hand, if the patient has sustained a mechanical event such as a rupture of the intraventricular septum or of the papillary muscle, surgical correction of the precipitating factor dramatically increases the probability of survival.

Physiologically, most of the effects that occur in hemorrhagic shock can also be identified in cardiogenic shock, for largely the same underlying reason: inadequate perfusion. Hence, one should expect marked decreases in hepatic, renal, and cerebral function.

SEPTIC SHOCK

The profound vascular collapse associated with overwhelming infection was recognized by Laënnec. As the microbial etiology came to be recognized, the phrases "bacterial shock," "endotoxin shock," and "gram-negative shock" were used interchangeably to describe the syndrome. Most bacteria, including *E. coli, Staphylococcus aureus,* and *Pseudomonas,* and fungi, especially *Candida,* have been isolated from patients with septic shock. It is now clear that while endotoxin from microbial cell membranes is an important etiologic factor in the development of the syndrome, it is by no means the only one.[7]

Septic shock is an extremely complex sequence of events and has been the subject of much investigation. It may occur after revascularization of extremity gangrene or manipulation of an infected graft. A number of important questions remain unanswered in septic shock, but there is general agreement on the most prominent features of its pathophysiology. First, it is evident that microbial toxins activate Factor XII (Hageman factor), initiating intravascular clotting and fibrinolysis alike, as well as complement. Additionally, vasoactive peptides, such as bradykinin and histamine, are released, which produce peripheral vasodilation and increased capillary permeability.[8] These phenomena produce inadequate oxygen delivery by a loss of intravascular volume (as a result of trans-capillary fluid loss), and peripheral vasodilation reduces venous return. Hence there is an initial decrease in cardiac output in septic shock.

A more complex series of events occurs at the cellular level in sepsis, leading to inefficiency in offloading of oxygen in the periphery or an inefficiency in utilization by the mitochondria, or both. This sequence, untreated, leads to the cellular anoxia, which septic shock shares with other forms of shock as the ultimate terminal event.

CLINICAL MANAGEMENT

Unfortunately, patients may not present neatly labeled with the classification of which type of shock from which they suffer. The clinician is simply confronted with a hypotensive patient, or, at least, one who has the other manifestations of hypoperfusion outlined above. Obviously, if there is a bleeding vessel clearly evident, the situation is not terribly mysterious. More often, however, one may be presented in the emergency room or on the hospital ward with a patient who is hypotensive and who may have any of the three major categories as the explanation for his hypotension.

The initial response to the hypotensive patient must always be *volume restoration.* If the patient is suffering from hypovolemic shock, volume is the mainstay of management, and should rapidly begin to reverse the adverse physiologic consequences of hypovolemia. The only task left then will be to identify the source of volume loss and, if possible (or necessary), correct it.

If the patient has sustained cardiogenic shock, the administration of volume may seem paradoxical, but is, in fact, frequently useful, at least transiently. Two factors may make further increase of left ventricular filling pressure beneficial: first the normal relationship between left ventricular end-diastolic *volume* and left ventricular end-diastolic *pressure* may be distorted, principally because of decreased ventricular compliance in ischemia. Second, acute mitral regurgitation may produce a pulmonary capillary wedge pressure that appears high, while left ventricular end-diastolic volume is, in fact, low. In either case, if there is relative hypovolemia, cautious administration of volume may help take advantage of the Frank-Starling mechanism by increasing left ventricular end-diastolic volume, and, hence, cardiac output.[9]

If the patient has sustained septic shock, fluid administration will help compensate for the increase in venous capacitance and the profound peripheral vasodilatation that has occurred. If the patient does not have underlying coronary artery disease, cardiac output will rise rapidly with volume administration, and perfusion of brain and kidneys will be restored, although the patient's blood pressure may not return to normal.

The first step in all three kinds of shock, is, therefore, the administration of fluid. The next step is to evaluate the response. If the patient's problem is that of hypovolemia, he should be substantially improved (unless volume loss is continuing). If the patient is in cardiogenic shock, small amounts of fluid may result in marginal clinical improvement, but it is likely that further therapy will be indicated, as evidenced by failure to restore organ perfusion to normal. If the problem is septic shock, organ perfusion may be restored, but the patient will continue to be relatively hypotensive.

RESUSCITATION

Hemorrhagic Shock

It should be self-evident that the proper therapy for hypovolemia is volume replacement. Which fluid to choose to restore volume has been the subject of intense debate. While it might seem that the best replacement for lost whole blood would be whole blood, in fact patients do not die acutely of red cell loss, but rather of volume loss. Therefore, immediate institution of asanguinous fluid is mandatory, and administration of red cells, either in the form of whole blood or packed red cells, can await determination of need.

There has been considerable debate regarding whether to use a colloid-containing fluid or simply a balanced salt solution for volume replacement. Advocates of the former point to the Starling equation of fluid movement across capillary membranes[10]:

$$Q_f = K_f[(P_{mv} - P_{pmv}) - \sigma_f(P_{mv} - P_{pmv})]$$

where Q_f = net transvascular flow of fluid; K_f = apparent fluid filtration coefficient; P_{mv} = microvascular hydrostatic pressure; P_{pmv} = perimicrovascular interstitial hydrostatic pressure; σ_f = apparent reflection coefficient; P_{mv} = plasma protein oncotic pressure; and P_{pmv} = perimicrovascular protein oncotic pressure. This equation holds that fluid movement across the capillary is equal to the differences in the hydrostatic and oncotic pressures on either side of the capillary membrane, and that the pressures are modified by two coefficients. The first is K, the filtration coefficient, which represents the rate of fluid movement across the capillary per unit of pressure gradient, per unit time, per unit of tissue mass. The second, σ, is the reflection coefficient, which describes the permeability state of the membrane. Starling assumed that $\sigma = 1$, meaning that all protein within the capillary would remain inside the capillary, and all that were outside would remain outside. As the reflection coefficient falls, the effective oncotic pressure gradient becomes less and less important in affecting transvascular flow.

It has been argued that resuscitation with salt solutions decreases oncotic pressure, and therefore must result in an increase in lung water. Guyton and Lindsey[11] raised left atrial pressure in dogs and measured lung water. They found that lung water began to increase in normal dogs at left atrial pressures in excess of 25 torr, but when oncotic pressure was reduced, only 12 torr were required to produce an increase in lung water. Below 12 torr left atrial pressure, lung water was not increased. Zarins et al[12] collected pulmonary lymph in baboons and lowered colloid oncotic pressure to near zero while keeping left atrial pressure constant near 8 torr. Although the animals developed marked peripheral edema, there was no increase in lung water. These two studies argue that oncotic pressure is important only to the extent to which it allows for increases in hydrostatic pressure without producing pulmonary edema. If hydrostatic pressure is kept at normal levels, pulmonary edema does not occur even with extremely low oncotic pressure.

The first human trial examining the effects of colloid resuscitation vs. noncolloid resuscitation was reported by Skillman.[13] Sixteen patients undergoing elective abdominal aortic surgery were studied, and received either 500 ml Ringer's lactate per hour or a bolus of albumin followed by 1 liter of 5 percent albumin. Blood loss was replaced with an average of 3 liters of whole blood in both groups. The authors reported a significant difference in colloid oncotic pressure between the two groups, but there was no difference in lung function.

A similar group of patients was studied by Virgilio et al.[14] Twenty-nine patients undergoing elective aortic reconstruction (for aneurysm or aortoiliac occlusive disease) were randomized to receive either Ringer's lactate solution (14 patients) or 5 percent albumin solution (15 patients) to maintain intravascular volume, and packed red cells were administered to maintain hematocrit at 30 percent. An average of 11 liters was required in the group given Ringer's lactate, while the albumin group received 6 liters. No differences were detected in pulmonary function between the groups. Two patients in the colloid group did develop pulmonary edema, and underscore the cardinal role of hydrostatic pressure in the pathophysiology of pulmonary edema: both had abrupt increases in pulmonary capillary wedge pressures. This study concluded that patients undergoing aortic reconstruction could be safely resuscitated without albumin. Other studies in similar patients have confirmed these observations, and there is no convincing evidence in either laboratory or clinical models to support the use of oncotically active solutions.

The changes described above, which occur in hemorrhagic shock, provide the clinician with endpoints to gauge volume replenishment. The most commonly employed "clinical criteria" are heart rate, blood pressure, urine output, acid-base status, and mental status. These all share the characteristic of being relatively sensitive, but not particularly specific. That is, if all of these variables are normal, it is safe to conclude that the patient's intravascular volume has been adequately restored. None of them is specific, however, and there may be a multitude of other explanations why any of them may be abnormal in spite of normal intravascular volume. Measurements that are extremely useful, especially in the setting of underlying heart or lung disease (common to many patients with atherosclerotic peripheral vascular disease), include cardiac filling pressures (central venous pressure and pulmonary capillary wedge pressure), cardiac output, and mixed venous oxygen tension.

Cardiogenic Shock

As mentioned above, cautious administration of fluid to the victim of cardiogenic shock is not inappropriate and may be beneficial. Other supportive therapy that may be required consists of inotropic support and afterload reduction. Inotropic agents that are available include dopamine, dobutamine, and, of course, digoxin. Dobutamine is our preference, since it is a virtually pure β_1 agonist, and does not produce either peripheral vasoconstriction or tachycardia. As described above, however, unless a surgically treatable lesion is present, the mortality rate for cardiogenic shock remains quite high because of the large amount of myocardium that has been irreparably damaged.

Septic Shock

Survival from septic shock is primarily dependent on the identification and eradication of the source of the sepsis. Although antibiotics effective against the causative organisms are important as adjunctive therapy, drainage of the septic source is essential for successful management. Other agents, including steroids, have been employed, but their overall contribution to survival remains uncertain.[15]

RED CELL REPLACEMENT

As pointed out above, virtually all patients with hemorrhagic, septic, or cardiogenic shock will require fluid resuscitation. The question of when to administer red cells remains. A young, previously healthy patient with a normal heart can easily tolerate at least a 30 percent loss of red cell mass, and losses of half baseline red cell mass are well within the compensatory capabilities of such a patient. Rather than define an arbitrary hematocrit (or hemoglobin concentration), it is preferable to consider the determinants of oxygen delivery:

$$\text{Oxygen delivery} = \text{Cardiac output} \times \text{arterial oxygen content}$$
$$\text{Arterial oxygen content} = [\text{Hb}] \times 1.38 \times \% \text{ saturation} + \text{PaO}_2 \times .0031$$

Our previous discussion has centered on restoration of cardiac output. Increases in cardiac output can compensate for a decline in arterial oxygen content up to a certain point, but only if intravascular volume has been maintained with asanguinous fluid. Since under ordinary circumstances arterial oxygen saturation is near 100 percent, and since the dissolved oxygen in plasma is such a small fraction of the total, it is clear that the two variables that can most easily be manipulated to maintain oxygen delivery are cardiac output and hemoglobin concentration. For patients whose cardiac output cannot be increased, either as a result of valvular heart disease or coronary artery disease, replacement of red cells beyond the usual 30 percent hematocrit may be beneficial. Determination of the physiologic need for that requires the measurement of cardiac output and the calculation of oxygen delivery and oxygen consumption.

SUMMARY

The patient in shock represents an acute crisis for those managing him or her. The first priority in management is an aggressive approach to restoration of adequate tissue oxygen delivery by the administration of balanced salt solution. Only after that step has been taken is it necessary to determine whether the shock is due to hypovolemia, myocardial failure, or sepsis. If it is due to hypovolemia, volume restoration is the mainstay of therapy, and it only remains to determine the source of the loss. If the problem is one of myocardial performance, fluid administration will have only a modestly beneficial effect, and inotropic support will be required, although it must be recognized that the prognosis is grave. And last, if the problem is due to sepsis, volume infusion will restore the clinical markers of adequate circulation (although not necessarily blood pressure), affording time for the identification and eradication of the septic focus.

REFERENCES

1. Meade RH: An Introduction to the History of General Surgery. Philadelphia, W.B. Saunders Co., 1968
2. Blalock A: Principles of Surgical Care, Shock and Other Problems. St. Louis, C.V. Mosby Co., 1940
3. Blalock A: Shock: Further studies with particular reference to the effects of hemorrhage. Arch Surg 29:837, 1937
4. Weil MH, Afifi AA: Experimental and clinical studies on lactate and pyruvate as indicators of the severity of acute circulatory failure (shock). Circulation 41:989, 1970
5. Shires GT, Coln D, Carrico CJ, et al: Fluid therapy in hemorrhagic shock. Arch Surg 88:688, 1964
6. Rackley CE, Russell RK, Mantle RD, et al: Cardiogenic shock: recognition and management. Cardiovasc Clin 7:251, 1975
7. Young LS, Martin WJ, Meyer RD, et al: Gram-negative rod bacteremia: microbiologic, immunologic, and therapeutic considerations. Ann Intern Med 86:456, 1977
8. O'Donnell TF, Clowes GH, Talamo RC, et al: Kinin activation in the blood of patients with sepsis. Surg Gynecol Obstet 143:539, 1976
9. Russell RO, Rackley CE, Pombo J, et al: Effects of increasing left ventricular filling pressures in patients with acute myocardial infarction. J Clin Invest 49:1539, 1970
10. Starling EH: On the absorption of fluids from the connective tissue spaces. J Physiol Lond 19:312, 1895
11. Guyton AC, Lindsey AW: Effect of left atrial pressure and decreased plasma protein concentration on the development of pulmonary edema. Circ Res 7:649, 1959
12. Zarins CK, Rice CL, Peters RM, et al: Lymph and pulmonary response to isobaric reduction in plasma oncotic pressure in baboons. Circ Res 43:925, 1978
13. Skillman JJ, Restall S, Salzman EW: Randomized trial of albumin vs electrolyte solutions during abdominal aortic operations. Surgery 78:219, 1975
14. Virgilio RW, Rice CL, Smith DE, et al: Crystalloid vs colloid resuscitation: is one better? Surgery 85:129, 1979
15. Sprung CL, Caralis PV, Marcial EH: The effects of high-dose corticosteroids in patients with septic shock: a prospective, controlled study. N Engl J Med 312:1142, 1984

Bernard H. Nachbur
Fritz Horber
Stefan Sigrist

Metabolic Disorders in Acute Limb Ischemia

Every vascular surgeon is familiar with examples of fatal outcome in patients subjected to hemodynamically successful arterial reconstruction. This is especially well-known in elderly patients treated for embolic occlusion of the aortic bifurcation with clinical signs of complete ischemia of the lower extremities extending bilaterally right up to the groin. Following successful embolectomy it is not unusual to see these patients die within a few hours, the cause of death being attributed to a combination of acidosis and the release of toxic products of anaerobic metabolism from revascularized muscle tissue. Similar clinical courses can be associated with delayed arterial reconstruction in extensive ischemia of a single extremity or following arterial occlusion caused by traumatic laceration. When younger individuals are affected the clinical course is usually milder, the outcome being apparently age-related and closely dependent upon individual tolerance of metabolic disorders.

This chapter deals with the manifold sequence of events due to metabolic derangements that appear to follow a clear-cut pattern. Some of the threats to life and limb such as acidosis, hyperkalemia, and uremia associated with acute renal failure (ARF) and the closed compartment syndrome are familiar to most physicians. Stress will therefore be laid on aspects that have hitherto attracted less attention in the literature, such as the rapid onset of hyperkalemia and the dangerous hypercalcemia syndrome in the polyuric phase following ARF.

HISTORICAL CONSIDERATIONS

The clinical picture of severe metabolic disorder brought on by tissue anoxia was first described in detail by Bywaters,[1] who observed many cases of ARF following large-scale injury to muscle tissue sustained by Londoners exposed to the German "Blitz" in 1941. The victims were usually rescued from the rubble of collapsed buildings; thus the term *crush-syndrome* was coined. Pathophysiologically muscle damage associated with massive release of myoglobin leading to myoglobinuria was considered the decisive mecha-

Vascular Surgical Emergencies
ISBN 0-8089-1843-5

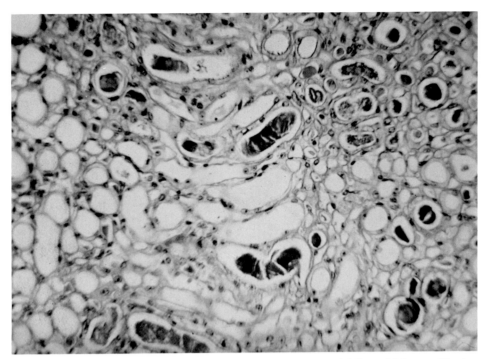

Fig. 1. Histological specimen from a kidney biopsied in acute renal failure. High magnification reveals numerous myoglobin cylinders and casts in the tubules.

nism of ARF. The histomorphological changes occurring in damaged muscles closely resembled what in later years has been called *rhabdomyolysis*. Renal failure on the other hand is attributed to the presence of myoglobinuric cylinders and casts occluding the renal tubules. Figure 1 shows the histological aspect of myoglobin casts in the kidney.

ETIOLOGY OF RHABDOMYOLYSIS

Rhabdomyolysis has been extensively described in nontraumatic cases[2] in which various etiological factors were involved. Gabow et al[3] consider the term *rhabdomyolysis* preferable to *myoglobinuria* as a general description of the syndrome because rhabdomyolysis may or may not result in visible myoglobinuria. The signs of myoglobinuria are: dark red ortholidine positive urine, pigmented granular casts in the urine sediment, and marked elevation of serum creatine phosphokinase (CK). Also, the calcium deposits showing up in the damaged muscle during the oliguric phase of imminent ARF are evidence of dystrophic alterations attending rhabdomyolysis. These are readily detected and picked up by a technetium 99m diphosphonate (TcDP) scan.[4,5] TcDP scans are the most sensitive method of detecting calcium deposits in these patients. Figure 2 shows an example of bilateral calcification in vastus muscles of the thigh following strenuous exercise.

Various causes for rhabdomyolysis have been reported. They can be grouped as follows: (1) excessive muscular activity (as demonstrated in Fig. 2), (2) direct muscular

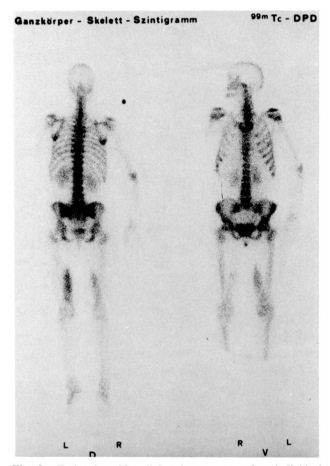

Fig. 2. Technetium 99m diphosphonate scan of an individual with bilateral calcification of M. vastus medialis following strenuous exercise.

injury, as in the crush-syndrome, (3) ischemia, (4) immunological diseases, and (5) prolonged coma due to intoxication by heroin, amphetamines, barbiturates, methadone, LSD, etc. Other causes are (6) infectious diseases, especially of viral origin, (7) hyper- or hypothermia, and (8) seizures. The common denominator of most if not all of these etiological factors is most likely prolonged muscle ischemia. For instance, in rhabdomyolysis following drug-intoxication muscle ischemia is caused by long lasting immobilization in frequently unnatural positions. In normal sleep the body position is unconsciously changed at regular intervals.[6]

In addition to the common concept of rhabdomyolysis due to ischemia other factors may play a role. For instance in alcohol-related rhabdomyolysis the following factors have been shown to have an influence: direct toxic effect of ethanol, starvation, refeeding, hypokalemia, hypophosphatemia.[5] Histomorphologically rhabdomyolysis is characterized by partial necrosis of muscle fibers, one of the first signs thereof being the loss of muscular striae, as demonstrated in Figure 3.

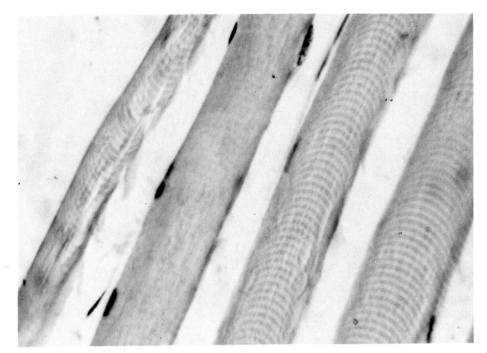

Fig. 3. Histological specimen of muscle fibers in rhabdomyolysis. There are signs of partial necrosis in one of the fibers with loss of striae.

THE SEQUENCE OF EVENTS IN SEVERE RHABDOMYOLYSIS

In the United States Haimovici[7] has named the association of rhabdomyolysis with renal failure the *myo-nephropathic-metabolic* syndrome. In this term the importance of metabolic disorder is invoked. He and others such as Cormier[8] differentiate between an ischemic phase and a revascularization phase, the former being capable of heralding the myo-nephropathic-metabolic syndrome, such cases being characteristically defined by rigor mortis. This symptom marks critical delay and if it is of rapid onset the alternative is either early primary amputation or revascularization with or without delayed amputation, in which case one must brace for a series of complicated life-threatening metabolic derangements exacting intensive medical care.

To some degree large scale ischemia of the lower extremities can be likened to cardiac arrest. In cardiac arrest the immediate consequences of anaerobic metabolism must be offset. During cardiac resuscitation and following restoration of autonomous cardiac activity the circulation is flooded with acid metabolites (lactate, pyruvate) due to oxygen deprivation of muscle tissue associated with the decrease of pO_2 and the increase of pCO_2. pH of capillary blood may fall to 7.1 or lower with base excess values dropping to minus 10–15 mmol/liter. Levels of creatine phosphokinase (CK), lactate dehydrogenase (LDH), and transaminase (SGOT) are increased. The influx of acid metabolites can be countered by early infusion of buffer substances such as THAM (Tris-hydroxymethylaminomethane) or bicarbonates, as advocated by Esato[9] and others.

However, the analogy of large-scale lower extremity ischemia to cardiac arrest ends here. Successful cardiac resuscitation is for instance rarely, if ever, associated with rhabdomyolysis, myoglobinuria, and ARF. Life-threatening metabolic disorders caused by cardiac arrest are limited to acidosis and varying degrees of hyperkalemia.

Following delayed arterial reconstruction for severe limb ischemia, however, the ensuing metabolic disorders are of a quite different order of magnitude. These are: acidosis and unrelenting hyperkalemia in conjunction with ARF, the closed compartment or tourniquet syndrome, hypocalcemia and hyperphosphatemia and eventually, following recovery of renal function, the hypercalcemia syndrome. ARF caused by myoglobinuria often displays laboratory findings that are exaggerations of those usually found in ARF of other causes. Aggressive countermeasures are therefore mandatory and are listed here in the order of succession of their appearance.

Acidosis

This condition has already been dealt with in connection with the analogy to cardiac arrest. The importance of early administration of THAM or bicarbonates has been mentioned in order to correct a negative base excess. Furthermore, following vascular reconstruction it would be desirable to wash out the ischemic limb with saline or lactated Ringer's solution immediately before release of the occluding clamp[9] in order to reduce the influx of acid metabolites.

The Closed Compartment Syndrome

Following delayed revascularization there is muscular swelling due to increased capillary permeability. In order to avoid strangulation and secondary muscle necrosis, immediate and generous fasciotomy involving the anterior tibial muscle, the peroneal muscles, and the deep and superficial flexor compartment is of vital importance for restoration of limb function. Should there be any doubt in regard to the indication for fasciotomy subfascial pressure recordings will be helpful. Pressure readings exceeding 30 mmHg cannot be tolerated by muscle tissue and make fasciotomy mandatory. Figure 4 shows schematically the proposed route of access for fasciotomy of all four compartments of the calf.

Hyperkalemia

Hyperkalemia, very early in the disease and repeatedly at life-threatening levels is often observed in patients with this form of rhabdomyolysis. The rapid increase of serum potassium levels seen in these patients probably catches many surgeons by surprise and is due to rupture of muscle-cell membranes and release of large amounts of intracellular potassium.[10] In one of our patients, whose case history will be reported in detail, hemodialysis had to be performed for this reason alone 20 hours after hospital admittance, 16 hours after surgical revascularization, and then almost daily for a week (Fig. 5), merely to keep serum potassium at acceptable levels. Use of resins administered rectally or through a gastric tube is not contraindicated but will not suffice.

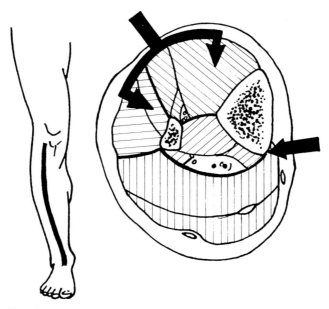

Fig. 4. Schematic demonstration of access to all four compartments of the calf in fasciotomy.

Serum Creatinine

Another characteristic of ARF in rhabdomyolysis with delayed vascular reconstruction is the rapid increment of serum creatinine—probably also due to the release of preformed intracellular creatinine into the intracellular fluid through damaged muscle cell membranes.[10] Thus we needed, in the case mentioned above, 13 hemodialyses in 20 days, which is well above the average necessary in ordinary cases of ARF.

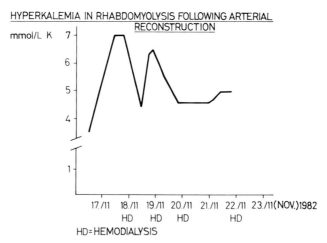

Fig. 5. Showing the rapid increment of serum potassium and repeated hyperkalemia necessitating daily hemodialysis in a case of rhabdomyolysis associated with ARF.

Table 1

Hypercalcemia Syndrome

Metastatic calcifications in sites of acidosis
Gastric atony → loss of appetite
Loss of neuromuscular excitability
  short systole
  muscular atony
Apathy, lethargy, coma
Nausea, vomiting (brain stem?)
In chronic cases: nephrocalcinosis

Serum Creatine Phosphokinase (CK)

CK serum levels reach maximum values of 30–60,000 IU/l within the first 2–3 days following soft tissue injury (see Table 2) and usually return to normal within 10–14 days. CK determinations in the very first days following vascular reconstruction in severe cases of limb ischemia offer important clues regarding the amount of damage afflicted to muscle tissue and are hence predictive factors of potentially prognostic importance with regard to the development of ARF.

Uremia

Blood urea nitrogen (BUN) roughly parallels global renal function and shows increments in relation to the extent of oliguria or anuria. Following restoration of renal function BUN fairly rapidly returns to normal. The consequences of severe uremia, pericarditis, bleeding complications, gastrointestinal disorders, and frank tetany necessitate repeated hemodialysis, as is well recognized.

Hyperphosphatemia and Hypocalcemia

ARF is commonly associated with a rapid increase of inorganic phosphate and correspondingly with hypocalcemia (see also Fig. 10). Calcium deposits rapidly form in areas of acidosis in dystrophic muscle tissue following rhabdomyolysis as is readily detected by a TcDP scan (Fig. 2) and an elastin stain (von Kossa coloration) of biopsied calcified muscle tissue (Fig. 6). Most myocytes are of normal color, a few show higher density and are on the verge of necrosis, and other fibers are totally replaced by calcification. After restoration of renal function, when the kidney has regained its capacity to convert 25-hydroxycholecalciferol (the precursor of vitamin D) to $1,25 (OH)_2D$, in the early polyuric phase, there is reversal of the relationship between phosphorus and calcium. In the oliguric or anuric phase of ARF bones and calcium deposits are probably resistant to the calcemic action of increased levels of parathyroid hormone which may be the reason for hypocalcemia during ARF.[11] The reversal of the phosphorus/calcium relation is paralleled by a loss of skeletal resistance to the calcemic action of parathyroid hormone. Calcium is now mobilized either from the skeleton or from calcifications in areas of muscular dystrophy and hypercalcemia might ensue. This phenomenon can lead to the life-threatening hypercalcemia syndrome that will be discussed next.

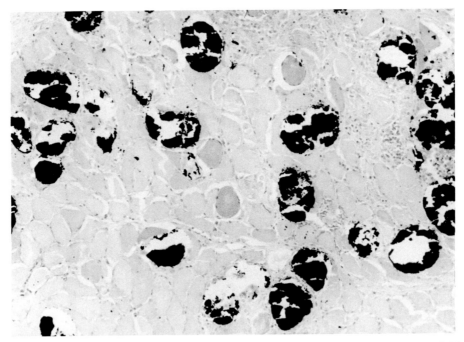

Fig. 6. Histological specimen of muscle tissue in rhabdomyolysis with partial necrosis and calcification. High magnification x200. Kossa coloration.

The Hypercalcemia Syndrome

Posttraumatic localized muscle necrosis with calcification is occasionally observed by surgeons in traumatology. Calcification in these cases tends to progress irreversibly to the well-known clinical or radiological image of myositis ossificans. Bütikofer and Molleyres[12] were probably among the very first to report in 1968 on a case of massive reversible calcification in partially necrotic muscle tissue (rhabdomyolysis) following local ischemia and simultaneous ARF. Severe hypocalcemia was observed initially, but after 3 weeks rapid absorption of the muscle calcifications occurred, accompanied by life-threatening hypercalcemia requiring treatment with phosphate infusions. After completion of the absorptive process and restoration of kidney function all serum values returned to normal.

The hypercalcemia syndrome is characterized by the features listed in Table 1.

PERSONAL EXPERIENCE

In the past 3 years we have observed 6 documented cases of clinically significant rhabdomyolysis following delayed vascular reconstruction for profound ischemia. They are listed in Table 2.

The 72-year old male patient who had been suffering from disabling claudication had an angiogram performed that showed aneurysmal disease of the iliac artery and occlusion of the superficial femoral artery on the right side. Immediately after completion of the

Table 2
Patients with Significant Rhabdomyolysis

Patient Age (yrs)	Affected Limb	Creatine Phosphokinase (IU/l)	Duration of Renal Failure
1. 47♀	left leg	1,800	clinically not detectable
2. 53♂	both legs	26,600	1 week
3.†72♂	right leg	34,400	3½ weeks
4. 68♂	both legs	19,000*	4 weeks
5. 65♂	right leg	8,600	3 days
6. 64♂	both legs	64,400	+ 3 days (heart failure with electromechanical dissociation)

*right kidney nephrectomized for tuberculosis
†Case 3 (encircled) is a showcase for all biochemical and metabolic disorders that are known in association with severe rhabdomyolysis.

angiograms the patient developed total ischemia of the entire right leg and was urgently referred to our service for treatment. At the time of operation 7 hours later rigor mortis of the calf muscles was so well pronounced that all movements in the ankle were totally blocked; the calf muscles themselves were stone hard. There was widespread patchy cyanosis. Thrombectomy of the recently occluded iliac segment failed and had to be followed by a hastily implanted femorofemoral cross-over bypass. Upon completion of this shunt the thigh muscles had in turn also become stiff and hard, and the knee-joint could no longer be flexed or bent, not even in general relaxation anesthesia. A second PTFE shunt extending from the groin down to the middle popliteal segment was rapidly sewn in under difficult circumstances, the knee-joint being in unsurmountable extension (Fig. 7). A few hours after vascular reconstruction and appropriate fasciotomy total renal shutdown occurred following a short phase of oliguria with dark red urine.

Hyperkalemia, very early in the disease and repeatedly at life-threatening levels, was found as the patient gradually drifted into a state of shock. Hemodialysis had to be performed urgently 20 hours after hospital admittance and repeated almost daily for a week (see Fig. 5) merely to keep the serum potassium at acceptable levels. Above-knee amputation was envisaged on the first postoperative day but was postponed after the first hemodialysis and then cancelled completely.

The rapid increment of serum creatinine described earlier was observed in this case. Thus we needed 13 hemodialyses in 20 days, which is much more than the average necessary in ordinary cases of ARF. The course of creatine phosphokinase levels, of serum creatinine and daily urine output is displayed in Figure 8. Once the dangers of hyperkalemia, acidosis, uremia, hypocalcemia, and hyperphosphatemia had been overcome we were next confronted with the equally life-threatening hypercalcemia syndrome, a specific feature of ARF in rhabdomyolysis of this kind, the signs and symptoms of which have been described in this chapter. Among other symptoms (see Table 1) muscular atony with the potential danger to the gut and to cardiac activity is noteworthy. The hypercalcemia syndrome therefore needed urgent treatment. Figure 9 describes how this was attempted. Serum calcium rose to highly pathological levels (13 mg%) that were aggressively treated initially with three sessions of hemodialysis with merely temporary effect, then with orthophosphates to increase solubility of calcium in the urine and also with calcitonin, an antagonist of parathyroid hormone. By far the best effect was obtained by forced diuresis, brought about by high doses of furosemid and massive crystalline

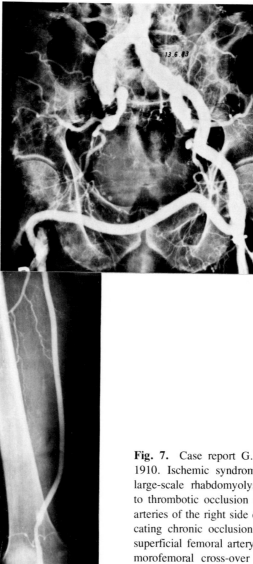

Fig. 7. Case report G.E., ♂, 1910. Ischemic syndrome with large-scale rhabdomyolysis due to thrombotic occlusion of iliac arteries of the right side complicating chronic occlusion of the superficial femoral artery. A femorofemoral cross-over bypass and a femoropopliteal PTFE shunt had to be hastily performed in the face of extensive rigor mortis. A long sequence of metabolic disorders was followed by uneventful recovery.

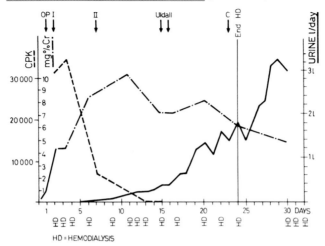

RHABDOMYOLYSIS WITH ACUTE RENAL FAILURE (Pat.G.E.1910)

HD = HEMODIALYSIS

Fig. 8. Case report G.E., ♂, 1910. Because of the rapid increment of serum creatinine probably due to the release of preformed intracellular creatinine 13 hemodialyses were necessary within 20 days. The course of creatine phosphokinase (CK) levels, of serum creatinine and daily urine output is displayed. CK levels return to normal within 10–14 days. Following the early polyuric phase after 25 days another series of hemodialyses was tried to combat hypercalcemia.

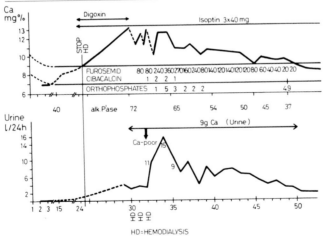

HYPERCALCEMIA IN THE POLYURIC PHASE OF ARF IN RHABDOMYOLYSIS

HD = HEMODIALYSIS

Fig. 9. Display of serum calcium levels in the polyuric phase of ARF. Treatment consisted of hemodialysis with temporary effect, forced diuresis with furosemid and massive crystalline infusions, orthophosphates and cibacalcin (calcitonin), an antagonist of parathyroid hormone. The lower tracing shows the daily urine output which enabled recovery of 9 grams of calcium.

21

infusions (see Fig. 9). Urinary output rose to 15 L/day and within 10 days 9 grams of calcium were collected in the urine. The patient's long ordeal lasted 50 days after which time he made an uneventful recovery. To this day he is well and without claudication.

DISCUSSION

Rhabdomyolysis may be caused by a number of widely varying etiological factors such as alcohol, mechanical compression and seizures, direct trauma, drug abuse,[2,3] metabolic derangement, hypothermia, sepsis, and influenza-like illness. Reports of severe rhabdomyolysis in acute ischemic disease are comparatively scarce,[3,7] which is surprising when the frequency of delayed vascular repair in acute ischemic disease is taken into account. In many cases the severe sequelae of massive rhabdomyolysis in vascular occlusion are avoided by major amputation. The mainly cardiotoxic biochemical and metabolic threats of massive rhabdomyolysis following delayed vascular repair for the acute ischemic syndrome are the following: acidosis, hyperkalemia, acute renal failure with anuria,

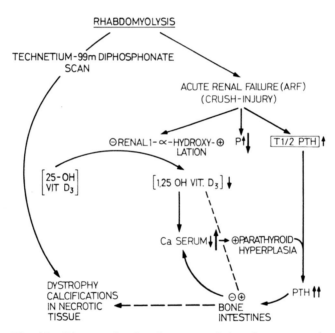

Fig. 10. Diagram showing the many relations between renal malfunction and the mobilization of calcium following restoration of renal function. 25-OH Vit D_3, the precursor of vitamin D, is produced in the liver. In order to become active it must be converted in the kidney to 1, 25 $(OH)_2$ Vit D. In the absence of this active form of vitamin D during ARF increased levels of parathyroid hormone lose their calcemic activity. With the restoration of kidney function sinking phosphorus levels, reappearing active Vit D and increased levels of parathyroid hormone may all three combine to mobilize calcium either from calcification deposits or from bone or gut.

and hypocalcemia in the oliguric or anuric phase; finally hypercalcemia in the polyuric phase. The laboratory abnormalities associated with the myoglobinuric form of acute renal failure are exaggerations of those usually found in ARF of other causes and are characterized by an unusually rapid increment of serum potassium and serum creatinine probably due to the release of those substances through damaged muscle cell membranes.[10] The interrelations involved in the hypercalcemia syndrome are complex. In Figure 10 an effort is made to show some mechanisms schematically: rhabdomyolysis causes muscle swelling and muscle calcification that is readily picked up by radioscan.[4,5] It can also cause acute renal failure with increase of the half life of parathyroid hormone, increase of serum phosphorus, hypocalcemia, and a diminished α-1-hydroxylation of 25-hydrocholecalciferol, the precursor of Vit D_3, to 1,25 dihydroxycholecalciferol, the active form of Vit D_3 that regulates serum calcium levels. This mechanism is reversed in the early polyuric phase, as indicated in Figure 10 by the inversed direction of arrows and changes of signs. The kidney recovers its ability to perform the α-1-hydroxylation of inactive Vit D_3, which, coupled with the elevated parathyroid hormone levels, results in an increase of active vitamin D_3. More calcium is resorbed either from calcified depots[12,15] or absorbed from bone and gut, probably resulting in hypercalcemia, as suggested by Llack et al.[11] For the same reason it might therefore be logical to administer Vit D early on, at the beginning of the oliguric phase.

Not all cases of severe rhabdomyolysis are followed by ARF. From the literature[16] and the presentation of our own 6 cases it appears that ARF is more likely in the elderly patients with preexisting atherosclerotic kidney damage and seems also roughly correlated with serum creatine phosphokinin levels.

The percutaneous muscle surface pH (pH_m) monitoring has been shown to correlate directly with Doppler ankle pressure and segmental plethysmography amplitude, but is not recommended in the routine assessment of the patient with acute arterial occlusive disease. In doubtful cases in which the indication for operative treatment is not clear on the basis of noninvasive examinations and clinical evaluation, pH_m may be helpful.[13,14]

SUMMARY

The biochemical disorders caused by severe rhabdomyolysis following delayed vascular reconstruction for widespread muscle ischemia are presented. Rhabdomyolysis is frequently associated with ARF in these cases and is highlighted by immediate and sustained hyperkalemia with acidosis in the oliguric and anuric phase, not infrequently followed by hypercalcemia in the ensuing polyuric phase. In analogy to the management of hyperkalemia and acidosis, treatment of the cardiotoxic hypercalcemia syndrome might also comprise hemodialysis or peritoneal dialysis. Acute hypercalcemia is however more effectively treated by forced diuresis in combination with complementary medication resulting in an increase of intrarenal calcium solubility with orthophosphates and by diminishing the uptake of calcium from the gut, bone, and calcified muscle tissue by giving calcitonin.

Perhaps the hypercalcemia syndrome might be avoided by administering the active form of vitamine D in the early oliguric phase in order to head off calcification of dystrophic muscle tissue and subsequent mobilization of calcium from these depots in the polyuric phase. It is understood that prior to these outlined steps, fasciotomy of all involved muscle compartments must be performed if vascular reconstruction and revascularization are followed by any degree of muscular swelling.

Knowledgeable awareness of the succession of biochemical threats endangering the life of patients with massive rhabdomyolysis following delayed revascularization is essential when evaluating the therapeutic options. The alternative to the costly and highly intensive treatment modality outlined here, major limb amputation, may be downright unacceptable to the patient.

REFERENCES

1. Bywaters EGL, Beall C: Crush injuries with impairment of renal function. Br Med J 1:427, 1941
2. Koltai E, Blumberg A: Akutes Nierenversagen infolge nicht-traumatischer Rhabdomyolyse. Schw Med Wschr 111:1041, 1981
3. Gabow PA, Kachny WD, Kelleher SP: The spectrum of rhabdomyolysis. Medicine 61:141, 1982
4. Höflin F, Ell PJ, Rösler H, et al: Acute muscular pain and positive bone scan. Nuclear Med Communic 3:30, 1982
5. Akmal M, Goldstein DA, Telfer N, et al: Resolution of muscle calcification in rhabdomyolysis and acute renal failure. Ann Internat Med 89:928, 1978
6. Dupont E, Tellerman-Toppet N: Insuffisance rénale aiguë et neuromyopathie ischémique au décours de comas toxiques: à propos de deux observations. J Urol Nephrol 81:306, 1975
7. Haimovici H: Metabolic complications of acute arterial occlusions. J Cardiovasc Surg 20:349, 1979
8. Cormier JM: Le syndrome ischémique aiguë; physio-pathologie. Rev Chir Orthoped 60:(Supp. 2) 50, 1974
9. Esato K, Nakano H, Ohara M, et al: Methods of suppression of myonephropathic metabolic syndrome. J Cardiovasc Surg 26:473, 1985
10. Grossman RA, Hamilton RW, Morse BM, et al: Nontraumatic rhabdomyolysis and acute renal failure. N Engl J Med 291:807, 1974
11. Llach F, Felsenfeld AJ, Haussler MR: The pathophysiology of altered calcium metabolism in rhabdomyolysis–induced acute renal failure. N Eng J Med 305:117, 1981
12. Bütikofer E, Molleyres J: Akute ischämische Muskelnekrosen, reversible Muskelverkalkungen und sekundäre Hypercalcämie bei akuter Anurie. Schweiz Med Wschr 98:961, 1968
13. Laks H, Dmachowski JR, Couch NP: The relationship between muscle surface pH and oxygen transport. Ann Surg 183:193, 1976
14. O'Donnell TF Jr, Raines JK, Darling RL: Relationship of muscle surface pH to noninvasive hemodynamic studies. Arch Surg 114:600, 1979
15. De Torrente A, Berl T, Cohn PD, et al: Hypercalcemia of acute renal failure. Am J Med 61:119, 1976
16. Famos M, Radü EW, Harder F: Rhabdomyolyse und Kompartmentsyndrom bei Heroinabusus. Helv Chir Acta 50:745, 1983

Gregory B. Bulkley
Ulf H. Haglund
Jon B. Morris

Mesenteric Blood Flow and the Pathophysiology of Intestinal Ischemia

Under normal conditions, the splanchnic circulation accounts for about 29 percent of cardiac output, and at any one time contains over 30 percent of the circulating blood volume.[1] This reflects not only the substantial requirements for nutrient maintenance of the gastrointestinal organs, but also a substantial influence on systemic hemodynamics as well. This chapter will discuss both local and systemic aspects of the splanchnic circulation. However, it will focus on those principles that impact directly upon patients with intestinal vascular disease. Consequently, it will deal primarily with the pathophysiology of splanchnic ischemia.

FUNDAMENTAL CAUSES OF INTESTINAL ISCHEMIA

Rather than classify mesenteric ischemia on the basis of clinical presentation, it is more useful here to outline briefly the spectrum of disease from the standpoint of fundamental etiology (Table 1).

Occlusive mesenteric ischemia is usually arterial, but the site of occlusion may range from a primary plaque at the origin of the superior mesenteric artery (SMA) to an embolic occlusion of a distal segmental branch. In this sense, mesenteric ischemia, like myocardial ischemia, can be global or regional. The effect(s) of occlusion on both the systemic and the regional circulatory beds will be very much dependent on the site of occlusion, relative to the status of the collateral circulation. It is important to remember that most instances of primary mesenteric vascular disease never manifest themselves clinically because of the adequacy of this collateral circulation, and of intrinsic intestinal compensating mechanisms, both of which are discussed below. *Mesenteric angina* is a very uncommon condition that is virtually always indicative of subacute global ischemia. This condition represents a borderline state in which the compensatory mechanisms are taxed to their utmost, barely adequate at rest, but insufficient under postprandial conditions of increased metabolic demand. *Venous occlusion* is also uncommon. Usually global when

Table 1
Fundamental Causes of Mesenteric Ischemia

I. Occlusive
   A. Arterial
     1. Acute
       a. Global (Thrombotic or Embolic)
       b. Segmental (Usually Embolic)
     2. Subacute/Chronic—Intestinal Angina
   B. Venous (Acute, Thrombotic)
   C. Strangulation (Segmental, Predominately Venous,
      Secondarily Thrombotic)
II. Nonocclusive
   A. Adult nonocclusive mesenteric ischemia
   B. Neonatal necrotizing enterocolitis

recognized clinically, this situation is intrinsically far more damaging to the intestine itself, and is necessarily accompanied by more severe fluid shifts and consequent systemic hemodynamic instability as well. *Intestinal strangulation* represents the most common form of mesenteric ischemia. Although this condition entails segmental occlusion of both the artery and the vein, the venous component predominates, at least initially.

Although the term *nonocclusive mesenteric ischemia* (NOMI) implies a diagnosis made largely by exclusion, this is in fact a well-defined pathologic entity, the primary cause of which is mesenteric vasospasm.[2] Although in the adult this condition is often associated with partial anatomic occlusion near the origin of the SMA, and diagnosed by the angiographic demonstration of macrovascular vasospasm, the fundamental site of vasoconstriction is in the microvasculature.[3] In the infant, this condition is probably manifest as *neonatal necrotizing enterocolitis* (NEC), a complex, and poorly understood condition seen in premature infants under conditions of severe stress. Although the etiology is multifactoral, vasospastic intestinal ischemia appears to play a prominent role in the pathophysiology of this disease as well.[4]

These conditions are all superimposed upon the mesenteric vascular bed, an entity with unique anatomic and physiologic characteristics, particularly with regard to its response to ischemia.

BASIC STRUCTURAL AND FUNCTIONAL CONSIDERATIONS

The intestinal vascular bed consists of several circuits coupled in parallel. These circuits supply the muscular, the submucosal, the deeper (crypt), and the superficial (villous) mucosal layers, respectively. Each of these circuits is itself composed of five components, coupled linearly in series: the resistance component (primarily arterioles), the precapillary sphincters, the capillaries, the postcapillary sphincters, and the venous capacitance vessels (Fig. 1).[5] The resistance vessels determine the overall resistance to blood flow and thereby regulate blood flow distribution through the intestine as a whole, as well as through each parallel circuit. The precapillary sphincters, which contribute quantitatively little to total vascular resistance, determine which of the capillary beds is perfused at any given time. The capillaries constitute the essential circuit component

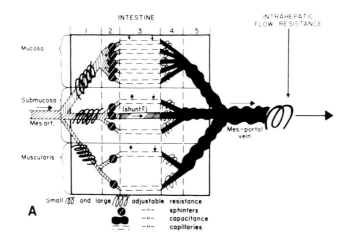

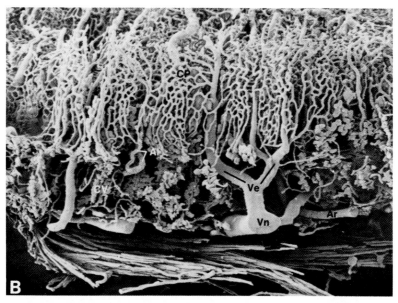

Fig. 1. Functional Anatomy of the Intestinal Vascular Bed. (A) The fundamental anatomic arrangement of the intestinal microvasculture is in three parallel circuits. Blood flow distribution between the three corresponding primary tissue layers is controlled by the relative resistances of the precapillary arterioles (zone 1). Distal to this, the precapillary sphincters (zone 2) control the actual number of capillary beds perfused. Zone 3 represents the capillary exchange vessels. The vascular tone of the postcapillary venules (zone 4) and collecting veins (zone 5) has little direct influence on nutrient intestinal flow, but controls the venous capacitance of the splanchnic bed. Therefore within each parallel circuit component, the five subcomponents are series-coupled. (Reprinted from Folkow B: Regional adjustments of intestinal blood flow. Gastroenterology 52:423–432, 1967. With permission.) (B) This is a scanning electron micrograph of a methacrylate-injected, digested specimen of the rat jejunum. Although oriented at 90° from the diagram in A, the anatomic basis for the above circuit arrangement is evident. (Reprinted from Kessek RG, Kardon RH: Tissues and Organs: A Text Atlas of Scanning Electron Microscopy. San Francisco, Freeman, 1979, p 175. With permission.)

wherein the interchange takes place between blood and tissue. The postcapillary sphincters do not substantially affect total vascular resistance. However, even very small
changes in their sphincter tone greatly influence the ratio of postcapillary to precapillary
resistance. This ratio determines the mean hydrostatic capillary pressure and thus strongly
influences the direction and magnitude of net fluid flux across the capillary wall. The
venous capacitance component, composed primarily of the small venules, primarily determines the regional tissue blood volume. In the splanchnic bed this volume is proportion-
ately quite large, comprising about 7 percent of the tissue volume.[6] In the adult human this
comprises a total volume of about 1400 ml, or roughly 30 percent of the total circulating
blood volume.

The endothelial layer lining the intestinal capillaries is continuous within the muscularis propria and fenestrated within the submucosal and mucosal layers. The pore radius of
the fenestrated capillaries is approximately 60 Å. The capillary permeability-surface area
product (ps product) for inulin is about 20 times larger in the small intestine than that
observed in the skeletal muscle,[7] and the capillary filtration coefficient ($K_{f,c}$), which
reflects both the available capillary surface area and its permeability, is more than ten
times larger.[7] The capillary surface area itself is about four times larger, indicating that the

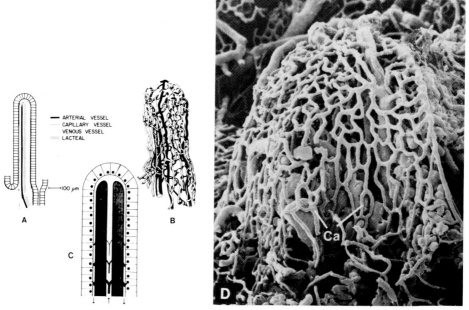

Fig. 2. Villus Microvascular Anatomy. (A & B) The villus is basically a longitudinal structure,
containing a central arteriole running its length from base to tip, where it arborizes to surface
capillaries. Blood draining from these capillaries is collected into a central venule. (C) The above
anatomic arrangement places the afferent arteriole parallel to the efferent venule, which allows the
passage of rapidly diffusable substances, such as oxygen, directly from arteriole to venule, short
circuiting the villus tip. This is the essential arrangement of a countercurrent diffusion phenomenon.
(A, B, and C reprinted from Lundgren O: Studies on blood flow distribution and countercurrent
exchange in the small intestine. Acta Physiol Scand (Suppl) 303:1–42, 1967. With permission.) (D)
Injection specimen of the rat villus prepared as in Figure 1B. The central arteriole, central collecting
venule, and surface capillaries (Ca) can be seen. (Reprinted from Kardon RG, Kardon RH. Tissues
and Organs: A Text Atlas of Scanning Electron Microscopy. San Francisco, Freeman, 1979, p 174.
With permission.)

fenestrated capillaries of the small intestine are themselves about five times more permeable to small solutes than are the continuous capillaries of skeletal muscle.[6]

The small intestine receives 1.5–2.0 times more blood flow per unit weight than the colon or the stomach or about 20–50 ml/min $\times$100g. The mucosal-submucosal region receives approximately 70 percent of this. Within the mucosa, the superficial villous region, comprising the primary absorptive site, receives about half the mucosal blood flow or about a third of the total intestinal blood flow.[8,9]

The villus vascular architecture is of particular interest, since it provides the anatomic basis for the villous countercurrent exchange mechanism.[10-12] In most mammalian species, including man, the villus is supplied by a single, unbranched arterial vessel, which arborizes at the tip into a network of capillaries and venules, which run subepithelially back down the villus (Fig. 2). The distances between these 2 sets of vessels, with predominantly opposite direction of flow, is less than 20 μ. This distance allows an equilibrium to be established for rapidly diffusible substances, within the time period of transit of blood through the villus vascular bed. Direct evidence supporting the existence of villous countercurrent exchange in the small intestine is substantial,[12] and the concept has recently been reconfirmed.[13]

THE LOCAL HEMODYNAMIC RESPONSE TO ISCHEMIA

When blood flow to the intestine is reduced acutely, there is a differential effect on flow to different tissue layers, and this differential is variable, depending upon the cause of the reduced flow. Acute reductions in perfusion pressure, as might be seen with an acute mesenteric embolus, are compensated by local regulatory mechanisms such that the reduction in flow is less than what would be proportional to the drop in perfusion pressure (Fig. 3A).[5] This capacity to autoregulate blood flow is also reflected in the phenomenon of autoregulatory escape, where the degree of blood flow reduction seen initially in response to a fixed partial arterial occlusion becomes substantially ameliorated over the next few minutes (Fig. 3B).[5] Autoregulation is due to the vasodilatory response of the resistance vessels downstream from the occlusion, largely in response to the release of local metabolites from the partially ischemic tissue (metabolic response). Some of this response is due also to the inherent properties of vascular smooth muscle, which are manifest as relaxation (vasodilation) in response to decreased perfusion pressure (myogenic response). This phenomenon of autoregulation is much more striking in response to vasoconstriction caused by sympathetic nerve stimulation, perhaps due somewhat to fatigue of the nerve terminals in the smooth muscle of the resistance vessels.[5] On the other hand, autoregulation of blood flow is minimal in denervated preparations, and also when the stimulus for ischemia is *systemic hypotension*.[14] In the latter case, the primary cause of the ischemia is a hyperresponsiveness of the splanchnic resistance vasculature to circulating levels of angiotensin II, which are generated as the result of renin release from the hypotensive kidney.[15-17] (This response to shock is discussed more fully below). This suggests that the local effects of ischemic metabolites are unable to override the direct effects of circulating angiotensin II on the vascular smooth muscle. Autoregulation is also lost even in response to partial arterial occlusion when perfusion pressures fall below 60 mmHg. Presumably this reflects the fact that the compensatory vasodilatory capability of the resistance vasculature downstream from the occlusion has been exceeded.

The intestine also responds to reductions in blood flow by redistributing flow to the

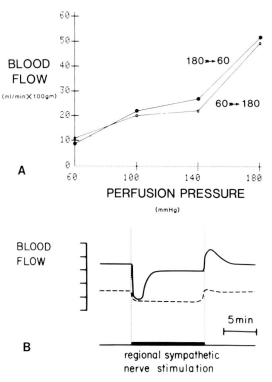

Fig. 3. Autoregulation of Blood Flow. (A) Pressure-Flow Autoregulation. As perfusion pressure is varied independently in an isolated loop of dog small intestine, the commensurate changes in blood flow are disproportionately smaller than would be seen in a passive system of rigid conduits. This reflects a reciprocal response of the resistance arterioles downstream from the point of arterial occlusion. (Reprinted from Shepherd AP, Granger DN: Metabolic Regulation of the Intestinal Circulation, in Shepherd AP and Granger DN (eds.): Physiology of the Splanchnic Circulation. New York, Raven Press, 1984, p. 38. With permission.) (B) Autoregulatory Escape. When blood flow is reduced suddenly by regional sympathetic nerve stimulation, the initial ischemia is rapidly ameliorated by vasodilatation in response to the sudden decrease in perfusion pressure (myogenic response) and the accumulation of local ischemic metabolites (metabolic response). Note also the reactive hyperemia following discontinuation of the stimulation.

various layers. In general, the intramural blood flow distribution changes in regional ischemia favor blood flow to the mucosa and above all to the superficial part of the mucosa.[9,18,19] For example, when perfusion pressure is reduced to 40 mmHg, villous plasma flow remains essentially unchanged,[19] while blood flow to the muscularis is disproportionately decreased.[20] In shock induced by live *E. coli* infusion, the superficial mucosal layer maintains its blood flow within the preseptic range, while total intestinal blood flow is reduced.[21] This redistribution is effected by changes in the relative resistances in the previously described parallel circuits. This phenomenon of flow redistribution should be distinguished from true arteriovenous shunting. Despite frequent postulations of such shunting in the older literature, there is good evidence that anatomic shunting through the small intestine is less than 1 percent of total mesenteric blood flow and therefore of negligible importance.[22]

Further protection from mesenteric ischemia is provided by the homeostatic autoregu-

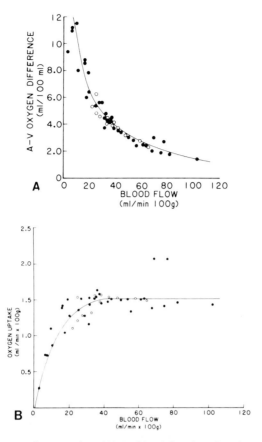

Fig. 4. Control of Oxygen Consumption. (A) As blood flow is reduced, oxygen extraction (A-V oxygen difference) increases in a reciprocal relationship. (B) As a consequence of the relationship shown in A, oxygen consumption (uptake) is maintained constant over a wide range of blood flows. Only when flow falls below about 25 ml/min ×100 g does oxygen consumption fall, reflecting the fact that this homeostatic capability has been exceeded. (A and B reprinted from Bulkley GB, et. al: Effects of cardiac tamponade on colonic hemodynamics and oxygen uptake. Am J Physiol 244:G605–G612, 1983. With permission.)

lation of oxygen consumption. When intestinal blood flow is reduced, tissue oxygen extraction is increased reciprocally, such that oxygen consumption is maintained constant over a wide range of blood flows (Fig.4).[23] However, when flow falls below a certain critical level (about 25 ml/min ×100g in the dog and cat intestine), the capacity to further increase oxygen extraction is exceeded and oxygen consumption then falls percipitously. This phenomenon is also seen in the stomach,[24] colon,[14] liver,[25] and pancreas.[26] This effect is mediated largely by the opening of unperfused capillary beds as total blood flow is reduced,[27] and therefore can be thought of as an extension of the blood flow autoregulatory response. This phenomenon appears to be quite important for the protection of the bowel during periods of hypoperfusion. We have found that the intestine is protected from even fairly subtle forms of mucosal injury for ischemic periods of at least 2 hours as long as oxygen consumption is maintained at or above 50 percent of control levels (Fig.5).[28]

The capacitance vessels are also constricted during ischemia and/or shock. The blood

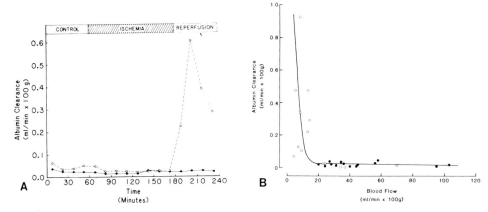

Fig. 5. Protection from Ischemic Injury by the Maintenance of Oxygen Consumption. In these experiments in the canine jejunum, we used the clearance of ^{125}I-albumin from the interstitium into the lumen to measure mucosal permeability as an index of mucosal injury. (Reprinted from Bulkley GB, et. al: Relationship of blood flow and oxygen consumption to ischemic injury in the canine small intestine. Gastroenterology 89:852–857, 1985. With permission.) (A) Transmucosal albumin clearance before, during, and after 2 hours of partial arterial occlusion. In one loop (broken line) blood flow was reduced very low, beyond the capability of the intestine to compensate by maintaining oxygen consumption. This loop showed evidence of injury (mucosal permeability) at reperfusion. The other loop sustained a lesser degree of ischemia, such that oxygen consumption was maintained (solid line). In this case, there was no evidence of injury afterwards. (B) When a large series of experiments, like that described in A, are plotted on a single figure, in which the level of blood flow reduction is graphed against the degree of injury, it is evident that there is no injury whatsoever unless blood flow has been reduced below 20 mg/min ×100 g. If this figure is compared to Figure 4B, it is evident that this threshold is below that at which oxygen consumption starts to decline. Actually, oxygen consumption must fall to about half its normal value before injury is seen.

volume thus mobilized from the splanchnic region is estimated to be in the order of 4 ml/ 100 g or approximately 400 ml of blood in a 70 kg man. If the ischemia persists, this venous vasoconstriction subsides somewhat, despite continuous nervous vasoconstrictor stimulation, probably due to the accumulation of metabolic products. Therefore, with the passage of time, most of this blood, which was mobilized initially from the splanchnic bed, is eventually returned to the splanchnic region and thereafter pooled in the splanchnic venous capacitance system. Although changes in the post to precapillary resistance ratio have also been demonstrated,[29,30] there is little evidence that this results in substantial levels of fluid sequestration in most cases of intestinal ischemia. The exceptions to this are strangulation obstruction and mesenteric venous thrombosis, where the predominant venous obstructive component results in the net filtration of relatively large volumes of fluid into the bowel wall and lumen, and even into the peritoneal cavity. Under these circumstances, the systemic hemodynamic effects of this loss of fluid from the intravascular space can be consequential.

Like most organs, the intestine also manifests reactive hyperemia following release of mechanical arterial occlusion (Fig. 6). This is a reflection of the persistence of the local metabolite-induced dilation of the splanchnic resistance vasculature.[30] It can result in a profound and sudden reduction in overall systemic afterload. This can contribute substantially to systemic hypotension, particularly when this effect is combined with that of circulating metabolic products from the ischemic bowel.

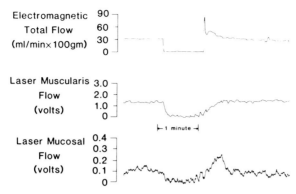

Fig. 6. Reactive Hyperemia. When total blood flow, muscularis blood flow, and mucosal blood flow are all measured simultaneously in an isolated loop of canine intestine, occlusion of the mesenteric artery for one minute is followed by reactive hyperemia. Note that although this response is reflected in the total blood flow tracing, it is limited to the mucosal layer. (Reprinted from Shepherd AP, Granger DN: Metabolic Regulation of the Intestinal Circulation, in Shepherd AP and Granger DN (eds.): Physiology of the Intestinal Circulation. New York: Raven Press, 1984, p. 36. With permission.)

SPLANCHNIC VASOCONSTRICTION

In addition to mechanical occlusion of the large and medium-sized splanchnic vessels, intestinal ischemia can result also from splanchnic vasoconstriction at the level of the resistance vessels.[32] This can be seen in response to alpha adrenergic stimulation, whether by circulating catecholamines or by the local release of norepinephrine from intestinal nerve terminals as a result of sympathetic nerve activity. In general, the splanchnic vascular response to adrenergic stimulation, although substantial, is proportionate to that of the body as a whole. While the sympathetic nervous system is important for the maintenance of the resting arteriolar tone, it does not appear to be a major mediator of the disproportionate splanchnic vasospasm seen in response to shock. The major effect of sympathetic stimulation is seen in the splanchnic capacitance vasculature, which is primarily under alpha adrenergic control.[33] Changes in tone of these vessels do not affect nutrient intestinal perfusion but have large effects on the functional circulating blood volume ("preload").

The vasoconstrictor peptide *vasopressin* affects primarily the splanchnic resistance vasculature, and this response is disproportionately greater than that of the systemic resistance vessels.[34] This differential is exploited in the use of vasopressin for the therapeutic control of gastrointestinal hemorrhage.

In the case of the renin-angiotensin axis, a differential vasoconstriction is also seen, probably due to an increased number of angiotensin II receptors in the splanchnic vascular smooth muscle.[35] This is important clinically, as the splanchnic hypersensitivity to angiotensin II generated by renin released from the hypotensive kidney during shock appears to be the fundamental mechanism underlying nonocclusive mesenteric ischemia. In pigs and dogs subjected to cardiogenic shock via pericardial tamponade, we found profound, disproportionate mesenteric ischemia due to severe, selective splanchnic vasospasm.[14-16,36] This response is unaffected by blockade of the sympathetic nervous system, but abolished by ablation of the renin-angiotensin axis. Furthermore, these hemodynamic changes correlate closely with plasma renin levels and can be mimicked, in the absence of shock, by central intravenous infusion of angiotensin II. Moreover, when the shock is sustained for a 4-hour period, and the pig subsequently resuscitated for 2 hours, the intestinal mucosa manifests severe hemorrhagic, necrotic lesions, characteristic of nonocclusive mesenteric ischemia.[16] These lesions are also prevented by renin-angiotensin ablation, but unaffected by alpha adrenergic blockade. A similar hemodynamic pattern has been described in response to hemorrhage in cats, with a similar primary role for mediation by the renin-angiotensin axis, not the sympathetic nervous system.[37] In these experiments, vasopressin also appeared to play an important role. In broader terms, it appears that nonocclusive small bowel ischemia, stress ulceration of the stomach,[17] ischemic colitis,[14,38] centrilobular liver necrosis,[15,39] and perhaps even ischemic pancreatitis, as well as some forms of acalculous cholecystitis, are all manifestations of the selective splanchnic vasoconstrictive response to the renin-angiotensin axis during shock states. The splanchnic vasoconstrictor effect of the digitalis glycosides may also contribute in some cases.[40]

COLLATERAL BLOOD FLOW

Numerous channels for collateral blood flow exist at every anatomic level in the splanchnic circulation. Systemic to splanchnic channels are provided between the esophageal arteries in the mediastinum and the gastric cardia, and from the middle to the superior hemorrhoidal arteries in the rectum. The celiac circulation communicates with the superior mesenteric bed primarily via the pancreaticoduodenal arcade. The superior mesenteric circulation communicates with the inferior mesenteric bed primarily via the marginal colonic artery at the splenic flexure, termed the *arch of Riolan,* or in chronic mesenteric ischemia, via the meandering artery of Drummond. Numerous collateral channels also exist between distal mesenteric branches, but the most important of these is the marginal artery itself, especially in the duodenum, jejunum, and colon.[41] Although intramural channels exist, primarily at the submucosal level, these contribute minimally to collateral flow,[41] and will only serve to sustain viability for a millimeter or two beyond the point of devascularization.[42] On the other hand, collateral flow through the marginal artery is substantial. It can maintain blood flow in an adjacent ischemic segment at about 60 percent of control levels, thereby maintaining oxygen consumption at normal levels,[41] and thus sustaining viability for a considerable distance beyond the point of devascularization.[42] This level of collateral blood flow is provided from the adjacent, nonischemic segment at no expense to itself, and with no effect on its perfusion pressure or upon its nutrient vascular resistance.[40] The driving force for collateral flow is solely the reduced resistance of the ischemic segment due to vasodilation that is isolated to that segment.[41] There is neither constriction nor dilation in the resistance bed of the adjacent nonischemic segments.[41] Moreover, collateral blood flow appears to be optimal in the absence of exogenous vasoactive agents.[43] Vasoconstrictors reduce collateral flow by producing vasoconstriction of the ischemic bed. Vasodilators also reduce collateral flow, at least in the acute situation, by preferentially dilating the (not previously dilated) adjacent nonischemic bed, and thereby generating a steal phenomenon.[43] Therefore, there seems to be little rationale for the administration of vasodilators to patients with anatomic mesenteric occlusion, unless the physician also sees evidence of nonocclusive ischemia superimposed upon this picture, possibly as a late response to sepsis.

THE LOCAL RESPONSE TO ISCHEMIA

The small intestine seems to be able to protect itself from ischemic injury when faced with lowered perfusion pressure by decreasing vascular resistance and further by increasing oxygen extraction when blood flow is decreased, as discussed at some length above. However, the mucosa and especially the villous layer seems affected when the perfusion pressure falls below a certain level, and this component of the intestinal wall is especially vulnerable to ischemic injury. Reduction of blood flow to a third or less of control levels for one to 2 hours reproducibly induces a characteristic histologic villus injury in most species, including man.[31,44] The villus tip has a very low pO_2, even under normotensive conditions. During ischemia, this hypoxia is worse due to the arteriovenous shunting of oxygen by diffusion via the countercurrent exchange.[10–12,18] During ischemia, villus blood flow velocity is reduced. The consequent increase in the mean blood transit time allows increased time for diffusion and thereby substantially amplifies the effectiveness of this countercurrent exchange mechanism.

The *histologic consequences* of short periods of partial or total vascular occlusion or of hypotensive shock is characterized initially by patchy lesions confined to the villi (Fig. 7). This layer can be totally destroyed while the remainder of the small intestine remains normal to microscopic examination. The villus lesion starts at the tip, and is manifest as epithelial lifting. Following prolonged, severe ischemia, the villi lose their epithelial lining. In still more severe ischemic injury, the entire villous layer disintegrates.[44,45] After more prolonged ischemia, the remainder of the mucosa and then still deeper layers of the intestinal wall are affected. In experiments using an obstructing strangulation model, the muscular layer became necrotic in about half of the rats after 8 hours of complete ischemia and in all animals after 12 hours. If the blood flow was restored before transmural necrosis had taken place, the regeneration process restored the intestinal wall remarkably rapidly. Even when the mucosa appeared to be completely destroyed, as long as a circumferential component of the muscularis remained viable, the mucosa was seen to regenerate an intact, albeit histologically somewhat abnormally proportioned, epithelial layer.[46] Such regeneration has been described to cause stenotic areas, and even less frequently, malabsorption, but the incidence of such sequelae is probably quite low.

The fundamental mechanism of intestinal ischemic injury is still not entirely understood, but an important component of the villus mucosal injury described above is not sustained during the period of ischemia, but is caused by toxic metabolites of oxygen termed *oxygen free radicals,* which are generated at reperfusion from xanthine oxidase, which is activated by ischemia.[46,47] This injury can be prevented by the administration of free radical scavengers such as superoxide dismutase at the end of the ischemic period, but prior to reperfusion. After more prolonged periods of ischemia, other factors appear to be more important. For example, we have found that the loss of *microvascular patency* due to microvascular thrombosis appears to be the primary factor limiting recovery from more severe degrees of ischemia.[46] Heparin pretreatment enhances survival of rat intestinal segments subjected to 8 and 12 hour periods of total vascular occlusion while superoxide dismutase has no effect. This principle is exploited by the use of intravenous fluorescein to assess *intestinal viability* following release of the underlying cause of ischemia. Since the fluorescein is carried by the circulating blood, its distribution is an indication of the

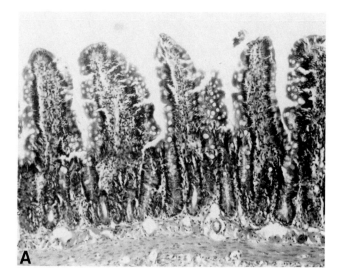

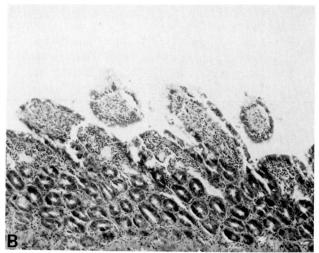

Fig. 7. The Spectrum of Ischemic Injury in the Intestinal Mucosa. Hemotoxylin and eosin sections of the rat small intestine (A) Normal (B) Villus tip injury

level of reperfusion. This technique has proven superior to others in the only controlled clinical trial of viability assessment techniques that has been reported to date.[49] Free radical-mediated reperfusion injury may be of greater clinical importance in neonatal necrotizing enterocolitis, where the free radical-mediated superficial mucosal injury can progress to transmural infarction.[4]

SYSTEMIC EFFECTS OF INTESTINAL ISCHEMIA

Partial intestinal vascular occlusion is not likely to cause a detectable increase in peripheral vascular resistance, especially if only a segment of the intestine is involved in

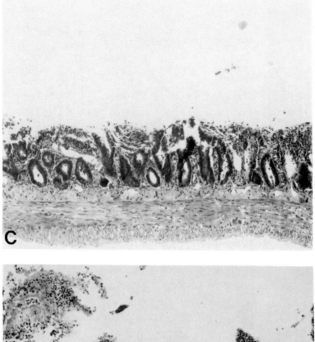

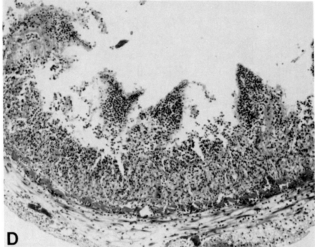

Fig. 7. (Continued) (C) Complete villus loss with some extension into the crypt layer (D) Transmucosal necrosis with extension of injury into the muscularis layer. Note, however, that a few viable myocytes remain. This loop would have survived, with regeneration of an intact mucosal epithelium, had the animal been supported over the next 5–7 days.

the ischemic process. On the other hand, a sudden, complete obstruction of the superior mesenteric artery is likely to be reflected as an increase in cardiac afterload. If surgical release of the obstruction is possible, the consequent reactive hyperemia will be manifest as reduced peripheral resistance and, if cardiac output does not increase to compensate, reduced arterial blood pressure.

If the ischemic situation has been present long enough to cause transmural intestinal necrosis and perforation, the resulting peritonitis and sepsis will significantly influence

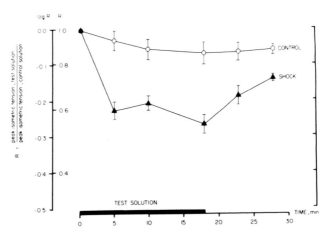

Fig. 8. Myocardial Depressant Factor. Myocardial contractility assayed in the isolated rat papillary muscle. When plasma taken from a cat following release of partial intestinal occlusion (shock) is added to the organ bath, a substantial depression in myocardial contractility is evident that is not seen in the control preparation.

cardiovascular performance. Once it has progressed to this state, intestinal ischemic disease is usually lethal, unless the lesion is limited and can be rapidly resected. However, intestinal ischemia can also exert systemic effects by other means, and prior to the appearance of transmural infarction. Mainly, two principle mechanisms have attracted attention in this respect: release of bacterial products (endotoxin) and release of cardiotoxic factors.

Endotoxin as a shock factor was initially proposed by Fine and his coworkers more than 30 years ago.[50] Unfortunately, endotoxin was proposed as the universal cause of mortality in all kinds of shock, and this concept has not withstood the test of time.[51] However, in cases of intestinal ischemia, the portal venous invasion of bacteria and endotoxins, combined with a decreased capacity of the liver to clear the blood, plays a prominent role in the systemic response to the primary lesion.

Experimentally, there is also an abundance of support for the release of cardiotoxic factors other than endotoxin from the ischemic splanchnic area into the systemic circulation via the portal venous blood or the thoracic duct lymph.[31,50] The release of these so-called *myocardial depressant factors* from the small intestine is closely correlated to the development of intestinal mucosal damage (Fig.8). The chemical identity of these substances has not yet been fully elucidated. It seems, however, that the cardiotoxic effect is not exerted by a single substance, but rather by substances of different sizes and solubility characteristics.

ACKNOWLEDGMENT

Supported by NIH Grant #AM31764.
Dr. Morris is a recipient of a Dudley P. Allen fellowship from the Department of Surgery, Case Western Reserve University, Cleveland, Ohio.

REFERENCES

1. Guyton AC: Textbook of Medical Physiology, 6th Edition. Philadelphia, W.B. Saunders, 1981, p 349
2. Fogarty TJ, Fletcher WS: Genesis of nonocclusive mesenteric ischemia. Am J Surg 111:130, 1966
3. Boley SJ, Sprayregen S, Siegelman SS, et al: Initial results from an aggressive roentgenological and surgical approach to acute mesenteric ischemia. Surgery 82:848, 1977
4. Bailey RW, Bulkley GB: Role of the circulation in neonatal necrotizing enterocolitis, in Kvietys PR, Granger DN, Barrowman JA (eds.): Pathophysiology of the Splanchnic Circulation. Boca Baton, Florida: CRC Press, Inc., in press
5. Folkow B: Regional adjustments of intestinal blood flow. Gastroenterology 52:423, 1967
6. Perry MA, Granger DN: Permeability characteristics of intestinal capillaries, in Shepherd AP and Granger DN (eds.): Physiology of the Intestinal Circulation. New York: Raven Press, 1984, pp 233–248
7. Folkow B, Lundgren O, Wallentin I: Studies on the relationship between flow resistance capillary filtration coefficient and regional blood volume in the intestine of the cat. Acta Physiol Scand 57:270, 1963
8. Hulten L, Jodal M, Lindhagen J, et al: Blood flow in the small intestine of the cat and man as analyzed by an inert gas washout technique. Gastroenterology 70:45, 1976
9. Redfors S, Hallback DA, Haglund U, et al: Blood flow distribution, villous tissue osmolality and fluid and electrolyte transport in the cat small intestine during regional hypotension. Acta Physiol Scand 121:193, 1984
10. Lundgren O: Studies on blood flow distribution and countercurrent exchange in the small intestine. Acta Physiol Scand (Suppl) 303:1, 1967
11. Lundgren O, Haglund U: The pathophysiology of the intestinal countercurrent exchanges. Life Sci 23:1411, 1978
12. Jodal M, Haglund U, Lundgren O: Countercurrent exchange mechanisms in the small intestine, in Shepherd AP and Granger DN (eds.): Physiology of the Intestinal Circulation. New York: Raven Press, 1984, p 83–97
13. Ryu KH, Grim E: Countercurrent exchange of water in canine jejunum. Am J Physiol 249:G377, 1985
14. Bulkley GB, Kvietys PR, Perry MA, et al: Effects of cardiac tamponade on colonic hemodynamics and oxygen uptake. Am J Physiol 244:G604, 1983
15. Bulkley GB, Oshima A, Bailey RW: Pathophysiology of hepatic ischemia in cardiogenic shock. Am J Surg 151:87, 1986
16. Bailey RW, Bulkley GB, Hamilton SR, et al: Protection of the small intestine from nonocclusive mesenteric ischemic injury due to cardiogenic shock. Am J Surg, in press
17. Bulkley GB, Oshima A, Bailey RW, et al: Control of gastric vascular resistance in cardiogenic shock. Surgery 98:213, 1985
18. Bond JH, Levitt DG, Levitt MD: Quantitation of countercurrent exchange during passive absorption from the dog small intestine. Evidence for marked species differences in the efficiency of exchange. J Clin Invest 59:308, 1977
19. Lundgren O, Svanvik J: Mucosal hemodynamics in the small intestine of the cat during reduced perfusion pressure. Acta Physiol Scand 88:551, 1973
20. Cassuto J, Cedgard S, Haglund U, et al: Intramural blood flows and flow distribution in the feline small bowel during arterial hypotension. Acta Physiol Scand 106:335, 1979
21. Falk A, Redfors S, Myrvold H, et al: Small intestinal lesions in feline septic shock: A study on the pathogenesis. Circ Shock 17:327, 1985
22. Delaney JP: Arteriovenous anastomotic blood flow in the mesenteric organs. Am J Physiol 216:1556, 1969

23. Kvietys PR, Granger DN: Relation between intestinal blood flow and oxygen uptake. Am J Physiol 242:G202, 1982

24. Perry MA, Bulkley GB, Kvietys PR, et al: Regulation of oxygen uptake in resting and pentagastrin-stimulated canine stomach. Am J Physiol 242:G565, 1982

25. Lutz JH, Henrich H, Bauereisen E: Oxygen supply and uptake in the liver and the intestine. Pfuegers Arch 360:7, 1975

26. Kvietys PR, McLendon JM, Bulkley GB, et al: Pancreatic circulation: Intrinsic regulation. Am J Physiol 242:G596, 1982

27. Granger DN, Kvietys PR, Perry MA: Role of exchange vessels in the regulation of intestinal oxygenation. Am J Physiol 242:G570, 1982

28. Bulkley GB, Kvietys PR, Parks DA, et al: Relationship of blood flow and oxygen consumption to ischemic injury in the canine small intestine. Gastroenterology 89:852, 1985

29. Lewis DH, Mellander S: Competitive effects of sympathetic control and tissue metabolites on resistance and capacitance vessels and capillary filtration in skeletal muscle. Acta Physiol Scand 56:162, 1962

30. Haglund U, Lundgren O: Reactions within consecutive vascular sections of the small intestine of the cat during prolonged hypotension. Acta Physiol Scand 844:151, 1972

31. Haglund U, Jodal M, Lundgren O: The small bowel in arterial hypotension and shock, in Shepherd AP and Granger DN (eds.): Physiology of the Intestinal Circulation. New York: Raven Press, 1984, pp 305–319

32. Banks RO, Gallavan RH, Zinner MJ, et al: Vasoactive agents in control of the mesenteric circulation. Fed Proc 44:2743, 1985

33. Rothe CF: Reflex control of veins and vascular capacitance. Physiol Reviews 63:1285, 1983

34. Said SI: Vasoactive peptides: State of the art review. Hypertension 5 (Suppl 1):17, 1983

35. Gunther S, Gimbrone MA Jr, Alexander RW: Identification and characterization of the high affinity vascular angiotensin II receptor in rat mesenteric artery. Circ Res 47:278, 1980

36. Bailey RW, Bulkley GB, Levy LI, et al: Pathogenesis of nonocclusive mesenteric ischemia: Studies in a porcine model induced by pericardial tamponade. Surg Forum 33:194, 1982

37. McNeill JR, Stark RD, Greenway CV: Intestinal vasoconstriction after hemorrhage: Roles of vasopressin and angiotensin. Am J Physiol 219:1342, 1970

38. Bailey RW, Bulkley GB, Hamilton SR, et al: Pathogenesis of nonocclusive ischemic colitis. Ann Surg 203:590, 1986

39. Bailey RW, Bulkley GB, Hamilton SR, et al: Protection of the liver from ischemic injury due to cardiogenic shock. Gastroenterology 90:1708, 1986

40. Gazes PC, Holmes CR, Moseley V, et al: Acute hemorrhage and necrosis of the intestines associated with digitalization. Circulation 23:358, 1961

41. Bulkley GB, Womack WA, Downey JM, et al: Characterization of segmental collateral blood flow in the small intestine. Am J Physiol 12:G228, 1985

42. Lee WPA, Weiss APC, Bulkley GB: Effect of collateral circulation on intestinal viability following segmental devascularization in the rat. Am Surg, in press

43. Bulkley GB, Womack WA, Downey J, Kvietys PR, Granger DN: Collateral blood flow in segmental intestinal ischemia: effects of vasoactive agents. Surgery, in press

44. Chiu CJ, McArdle AH, Brown R, et al: Intestinal mucosal lesions in low-flow states. Arch Surg 101:478, 1970

45. Ahren C, Haglund U: Mucosal lesions in the small intestine of the cat during low flow. Acta Physiol Scand 88:541, 1973

46. Amano H, Bulkley GB, Haglund U, et al: Pathophysiology of local injury and recovery following acute intestinal ischemia: The central role of microvascular reperfusion. Submitted for publication.

47. Parks DA, Bulkley GB, Granger DN, et al: Ischemic injury to the cat small intestine: Role of superoxide radicals. Gastroenterology 82:4, 1982

48. Parks DA, Bulkley GB, Granger DN: Role of oxygen-derived free radicals in digestive tract diseases. Surgery 94:415, 1983
49. Bulkley GB, Zuidema GD, O'Mara CS, et al: Intraoperative determination of intestinal viability following ischemic injury: A prospective, controlled trial of adjuvant methods (Doppler and fluorescein) compared to standard clinical judgment. Ann Surg 193:628, 1981
50. Fine J: The intestinal circulation in shock. Gastroenterology 52:454, 1967
51. Haglund U: Shock toxins, in Altura BM (ed.): Handbook of Shock and Trauma, Volume I: Basic Science. New York: Raven Press, 1983, pp 377–390

John J. Bergan

Litigation after Acute Vascular Emergencies

De minimus non curat lex. The law cannot be concerned with trifles.

Complications in surgery are common, and it is good practice to discuss them openly, looking for means of preventing them in future experience. It has become a fact of life that litigation in surgery is also common, yet there is a reluctance to discuss problems of litigation. Therefore, it becomes difficult to learn means of preventing law suits and their unfortunate consequences.

With regard to litigation, vascular surgery is one of the high-risk surgical subspecialties. This is because complications and unfortunate results in vascular surgery are not trivial occurrences, and the legal profession becomes concerned with such events.

In the emergency situation, decisions are made and acted upon in many instances from inadequate data because waiting for additional information is precluded by the nature of the emergency itself. In the emergency situation, it would be expected that litigation might develop, simply because communication between surgeon and patient or family is minimized, there is little opportunity to obtain adequate informed consent, and the intervention must be performed swiftly, with decision after decision being made without time for contemplation. The present study was undertaken in order to identify within the small field of emergency vascular surgery the types of cases that appear most commonly in law suits, the factors in those cases that led to the litigation, and the elements in those cases that might allow prevention of litigation.

MATERIALS AND METHODS

Over a three-year period ending March 1, 1986, the medical records of 114 patients involved in 116 legal events were reviewed. All cases were received from attorneys who had been consulted by patients or by their families. When received from defense attorneys, the cases had been filed for suit. Plaintiffs' lawyers in most instances sought clarification of the case and advice regarding whether to drop the case or file suit. Within those cases were 49 vascular emergencies occurring in 47 patients. Only those cases

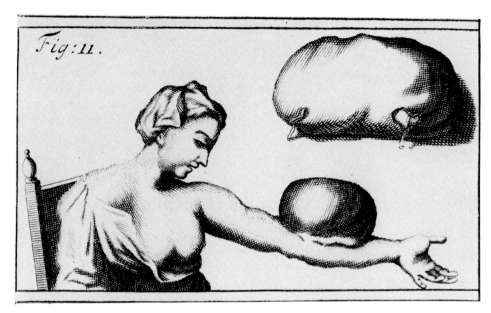

Fig. 1. This diagram, kindly provided by David Schechter, M.D. of New York City, illustrates a brachial artery aneurysm caused by iatrogenic injury during venesection. The illustration is from Matthaeus Purmann's book, *Chirurgia Curiosa,* London, D. Browne Publisher, 1706, and shows the case that he treated by aneurysmectomy in 1680. The case not only illustrates his treatment by excision but also illustrates the fact that iatrogenic vascular injury is as old as the art of surgery itself.

containing a major, crucial vascular component were reviewed, and only those situations in which emergency management was required were included. After collection of data from the case review, the cases were categorized and individual studies within each category undertaken. It should be noted that fatal pulmonary embolism was specifically excluded from this review. It is a frequent cause of litigation but originates in a chronic process.

RESULTS

Situations leading to litigation in vascular surgery could be categorized as follows: (1) iatrogenic vascular emergencies (Fig. 1), (2) failed recognition or treatment of acute arterial occlusion, (3) popliteal artery injuries, (4) aneurysm-related emergencies, and (5) a miscellaneous category including compartment syndromes, laceration repairs, and other problems (Table 1).

Table 1
Categories of Emergency Vascular Problems
Causing Litigation

Iatrogenic emergency	12 cases
Failed recognition of arterial occlusion	15 cases
Aneurysm-related	7 cases
Popliteal artery injury	7 cases
Miscellaneous	8 cases

Table 2

Iatrogenic Vascular Emergencies

Age	Sex	Procedure	Problem	Result
22	F	Internal iliac artery ligation	Damaged external iliac artery	Prosthetic graft
58	M	Splenectomy	Renovascular hypertension	Nephrectomy
77	M	Aortogram	Knotted catheter	Multiple operations
29	M	Gianturco coil	Occluded popliteal artery	Amputation
52	F	Aortogram	Distal thromboembolism	Bilateral amputation
50	M	Aortogram	Graft limb thrombosis	Amputation
36	F	Cardiac catheterization	Iliac artery thrombosis	Multiple operations
47	F	Cardiac catheterization	Arterial embolus*	Arm amputation
58	F	Cardiac catheterization	Transection of artery	Persistent neuropathy
42	M	Aortogram	Brachial hematoma	Persistent neuropathy
38	F	Laparoscopy	Iliac artery and vein injury	Successful operation
50	M	Cardiac catheterization	Aortic thrombosis	Bilateral amputation

*Also listed in the category of white clot syndrome

Iatrogenic Vascular Emergencies

Twelve patients were involved in litigation arising from iatrogenic events. There were 6 men and 6 women, ranging in age from 22 years through 77 years. The men were somewhat older (29 to 77 years, with an average age of 51.2 years), while the women ranged in age from 22 to 58 years (average, 42.2 years). This difference could be partially explained by the inclusion of two of six women who had obstetric or gynecologic-related events.

A review of Table 2 shows the severity of loss or disability suffered by those patients undergoing amputation, multiple operations, or sustaining persistent neuropathy. Failed treatment, especially leading to amputation, would be expected to precede litigation, but surprisingly, there were several successful procedures that led to suit in this category. Among these were the repair of the iliac artery and vein injured during laparoscopy, the successful grafting of an external iliac artery damaged during internal iliac artery ligation to control uterine hemorrhage following delivery, and successful repair of brachial artery trauma after arteriography.

Sustained neuropathy following transaxillary or transbrachial aortography or cardiac catheterization was identified as a singular problem. The neuropathy was often subjective rather than objective. In fact, the neuropathy may have been induced by injection of local anesthetics, brachial artery manipulation, or local trauma unrelated to distal ischemia.

Ironically, the patient sustaining a thrombosed aortofemoral graft limb during aortography had been managed successfully through graft placement, ischemic necrosis of the colon, and surgical excision of necrotic bowel without graft infection. The diagnostic intervention months later led to litigation.

Macroembolic Events

Although acute arterial occlusion is a special category of events leading to litigation, it is informative to divide this into subsections. The macroembolic events were distinctly different from acute thrombotic cases.

Table 3
Macroemboli

Age	Sex	Type of Embolus	Problem	Result
41	F	Cardiogenic	Multiple embolectomies	Amputation
67	F	Cardiogenic	Failed embolectomy	Amputation
58	F	Cardiogenic	Myoglobulinemia, multiple fasciotomies	Death
49	M	Cardiogenic	Missed diagnosis	Amputation
51	F	Atheroembolism	Failed bypass graft	Amputation
37	F	White clot	Failed lytic therapy and surgery	Amputation
64	M	White clot	Bilateral lower extremity ischemia	Bilateral amputation
37	F	White clot	Failed urokinase therapy	Amputation
47	F	White clot*	Failed embolectomy	Arm amputation
53	M	White clot	Missed arterial occlusion	Amputation

*Also listed in the category of iatrogenic vascular emergencies

Table 3 displays the range of conditions that led to litigation when patients were treated for acute arterial occlusion due to large emboli. In this category of patients, only 3 of 10 were men, and they were 64, 53, and 49 years of age. The 7 women ranged in age from 37 to 67 years and averaged 48 years. Clearly, the major problem in this category of events was the heparin-induced thrombocytopenia syndrome, with platelet emboli producing severe ischemia, leading to unilateral or bilateral amputation of lower or upper extremities. Of interest is the fact that two cases failed to respond to lytic therapy, one with streptokinase and one with urokinase.

Missed Acute Arterial Occlusion

In five cases, the diagnosis of acute arterial occlusion was missed, and therapy was delayed. In one case, a 19-year-old man with a gunshot wound of the femoral artery, the diagnosis was missed until the patient appeared in another emergency room, where the laceration was repaired successfully. In the four other patients, lower extremity amputations occurred unilaterally in three and bilaterally in one. This was a 43-year-old woman with a missed acute aortic thrombosis, delayed aortic repair, irreversible extremity ischemia, and compartmental hypertension.

Popliteal Artery Injury

Seven patients, all men, ranging in age from 22 to 62 years, sustained acute popliteal artery injury. Knee dislocation, either anterior or posterior, produced the injury on six occasions in five patients. A tibial plateau fracture accounted for a popliteal artery injury in one patient (Fig. 2), and a distal fracture of the femur accounted for the other. In the patient with the tibial plateau fracture, the repair was delayed but was ultimately successful. The patient suffered persistent ischemic neuropathy but retained his extremity. In each of the other instances, a lower-extremity amputation was required, either above-knee or below, and in one patient, a below-knee and an above-knee amputation were required.

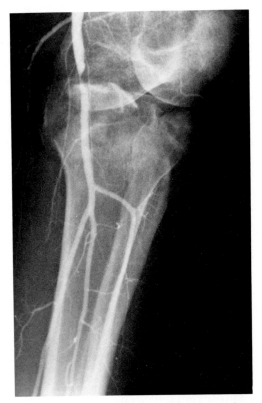

Fig. 2. This arteriogram, taken as treatment was begun for a patient with a tibial plateau fracture, shows the exact site of popliteal artery injury occurring with such a lesion. This is also the exact site of trauma to the popliteal artery during anterior and posterior knee dislocation.

Aneurysm-Related Emergencies

Table 4 displays the problems that led to litigation surrounding treatment of various forms of aneurysm. It would be expected that late recognition of a rupturing abdominal aortic aneurysm (AAA) could lead to litigation. In each of these three cases, the patient was hospitalized and under observation for a period of time that would have allowed

Table 4
Aneurysm-Related Emergencies

Age	Sex	Problem	Result
70	M	Missed diagnosis, rupturing AAA	Death
62	M	Missed diagnosis, rupturing AAA	Death
68	M	Late recognition, aortocaval fistula	Death
57	M	Missed recognition, colon ischemia after AAA resection	Death
17	F	Missed diagnosis, aortic dissection	Death
33	M	Missed diagnosis, femoral mycotic false aneurysm	Amputation
29	M	Missed diagnosis, gunshot wound false aneurysm	Amputation

aneurysm repair, had the diagnosis been entertained by the admitting physician. In all three instances, sufficient testing had been completed to establish the diagnosis of abdominal aortic aneurysm, and yet the surgical event was delayed sufficiently that the patient could not be salvaged.

The problem of recognition of colon ischemia after successful resection of an abdominal aortic aneurysm should be well known in vascular surgery. The syndrome of abdominal distension, diarrhea, fever, and leukocytosis in this instance was so clearly described in the nursing notes that the diagnosis could have been made from the chart.

In the instance of missed mycotic femoral false aneurysm, an arteriogram had been successfully accomplished and the patient admitted to the hospital for observation. The syndrome was obviously known by hospital personnel. Clearly, the arteriogram was not interpreted correctly, and a delay in treatment allowed the aneurysm to rupture, which ultimately necessitated amputation. Similarly, in the case of the gunshot wound producing a false aneurysm, the diagnosis was missed when an arteriogram was not done in the situation of penetrating injury in the region of a major neurovascular trunk. Therefore, a late diagnosis resulted, and ultimate treatment failed.

Miscellaneous Problems

In two instances, compartment syndrome led to loss of an extremity. In one instance, a 33-year-old man experienced compartment syndrome of the leg after ligament repair in the knee. Delayed recognition of the compartment syndrome led to above-knee amputation. In another instance, a 23-year-old man sustained a fall on an outstretched hand, and late recognition of forearm compartment syndrome led to disability rather than amputation (Fig. 3). In 2 instances, a 19-year-old man and a 17-year-old man sustained a popliteal or femoral artery laceration that was either poorly repaired and/or repaired late. In both instances, lower-extremity amputation was required.

In four other instances, miscellaneous occurrences developed. In 1 case, a 19-year-old woman sustained a motor-vehicle accident with thoracic transection that was successfully repaired. A graft infection developed postoperatively, and the patient ultimately died of complications resulting from treatment of the graft infection. In another instance, a 15-year-old boy with Ehlers Danlos syndrome experienced mesenteric artery rupture. The resultant mesenteric artery ligation produced massive intestinal necrosis, and the patient experienced short bowel syndrome requiring long-term parenteral alimentation. The treatment was prompt, the vascular condition recognized and expertly managed, all well above the standard of care expected for treatment of this rare condition. In another case, a 42-year-old man required axillary-bifemoral bypass because of aortic graft infection. In that instance, the internal iliac arteries and the profunda femoris artery had been closed by atherosclerotic occlusive disease; therefore, sacral plexus ischemia and massive myonecrosis developed, requiring a bilateral high-thigh amputation.* In a fourth case, a 53-year-old woman experienced mesenteric venous thrombosis that was recognized late and was unsuccessfully operated upon, resulting in death.

---

*Case also listed as brachial neuropraxia following iatrogenic brachial hematoma.

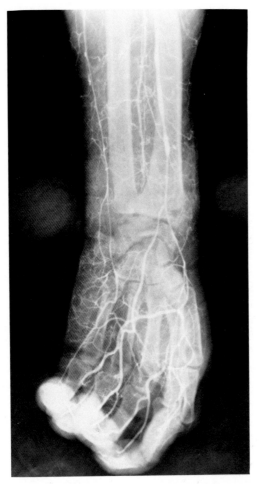

Fig. 3. Compartment syndrome of the forearm occurs after blunt and penetrating trauma and is characterized by marked spasm of the main arteries, as well as sharp cut-offs of branch vessels. Spasm is indicated by symmetrical segments of vasoconstriction, as well as tubular linear stenoses.

DISCUSSION

Vascular surgeons and general surgeons interested in vascular repair are involved with accidents, amputations, and the diagnostic injuries that make up three of the five most frequent categories of suits filed in this county in Illinois. As indicated in Table 5, diagnostic injuries and amputations are of extreme importance in the filing of cases in medical malpractice during the time encompassed by this study. Those are broad categories, but one of the objects of this review was to identify the specific areas of high risk to surgeons interested in emergency vascular surgery. This has been done, and it is appalling to note that iatrogenic vascular injury leads the list. Usually, iatrogenic injuries comprise a relatively small percentage of all vascular trauma. In 1963, Smith, Szilagyi, and Pfeifer

Table 5
Categories of Suits Filed in
Cook County, Illinois*

Category	1984	1985
Birth injury	127	231
Accidents	107	159
Failed diagnosis of cancer	78	103
Amputations	24	46
Diagnostic injuries	21	37†

*Two-thirds of malpractice cases in Illinois are filed in
Cook County.
†Nine angiograms included.

reported that 13 percent of arterial injuries in their review were iatrogenic.[1] In Orcutt et al's report from San Antonio in 1985, a 10 percent incidence of iatrogenic vascular injuries were treated in their institution, the University of Texas Health Science Center.[2] In the comprehensive review of iatrogenic vascular trauma from the Walter Reed Army Medical Center, Youkey et al reported that cardiac catheterization, angiography, and surgical procedures accounted for 29 percent, 34 percent, and 29 percent, respectively, of hospital-incurred vascular trauma.[3] Over the years, an increasing number of cases have resulted from angiographic procedures,[4] much as has been shown by the present review.

Intraaortic balloon counterpulsation is an important mechanism for production of vascular injury in most tertiary care hospitals. However, this was not a source of litigation in the cases reviewed here. Delay is one of the most important factors in failure of arterial repair. Indeed, that was noted in the cases reviewed in the present study.

Unfortunately, even in situations of successful repair of the vascular injury, residual neuropathy (actual or alleged) was an important cause of litigation. Robbs and Naidoo have reported experience with 17 patients with delayed onset of compression neuropraxia due to hemorrhage following penetrating arterial injuries,[5] an occurrence similar to the 2 present cases.

The review of cases of failed embolectomy is most revealing, showing as it does the importance of heparin-induced thrombocytopenia. The incidence of such heparin-induced thrombocytopenia varies widely in publications on this subject, and an immune mechanism has been demonstrated in many cases.[6-8] The absence of an immunologically-demonstrable mediation is possibly explained by the heparin itself. Salzman et al have shown that a direct platelet-aggregating activity of heparin can be related to the molecular weight of the substance, as well as its affinity for antithrombin III.[9] Heparin fractions of high molecular weight and low affinity for antithrombin are more effective mediators of platelet aggregation. The current hypothesis suggests that heparin-associated thrombocytopenia antibody is directed to heparin-platelet complexes, or that heparin induces conformational change of antigenic sites on the platelet membrane.[10,11]

Heparin-associated thrombocytopenia usually develops after 2–3 days of heparin therapy. It may be transient, mild, or clinically silent, but in the cases reviewed here, the thrombocytopenia was severe and the emboli produced acute arterial occlusion symptoms. It is of some interest to note the failure of lytic therapy in these cases. This confirms the logical hypothesis that lytic therapy should not dissolve pure platelet thrombi. Monitoring platelet counts during heparin therapy is an important factor in recognizing this syndrome, and recognition is the first step in effective treatment.

In failure of treatment of cardiogenic emboli, late embolectomy was characteristic, with late fasciotomy and myoglobulinemia being important in the single death in this group of patients. Blaisdell, Steele, and Allen's comprehensive review in 1978 showed a 25 percent mortality and 40 percent amputation rate in management of arterial emboli.[12] Yet, in this group of litigation cases, death occurred in only one case, while amputation was the eventual outcome in the nine survivors. This suggests that any therapy for acute embolic arterial occlusion that results in amputation raises risk of litigation. In the single case of atheroembolism, it was apparent that the surgeon did not recognize the syndrome and used an arterial reconstruction that failed to remove the embolic site from the arterial stream.

Since a bad outcome is characteristic in litigation for failed embolectomy, it is important to keep in mind that the best results of this surgery are achieved in cases where the diagnosis is clear, an early embolectomy is possible, and amputation is avoided.[13-15] The outcome is the worst in those cases with an unrecognized arterial occlusion or when protracted intraarterial manipulation is done before a full-scale vascular reconstruction is accomplished.

Similar to the problem of failed embolectomy are the problems of nonrecognition of acute arterial occlusion when thrombosis rather than embolus is the cause of the problem. In this category, the only successful arterial reconstruction resulted in litigation when there was a failure of recognition of the arterial occlusion caused by a gunshot wound. In the other four instances, the aortic or lower extremity thrombosis was entirely missed by the osteopath, internist, emergency room physician, or general surgeon involved in each of those cases.

The large number of cases of litigation following popliteal artery injury indicates a particular legal vulnerability with this type of trauma. It must be kept in mind that traumatic knee instability calls for attention to the popliteal vessels. Arteriography in all such cases might be a wise policy to pursue.

The Ben Taub Hospital group has pointed out that, in patients requiring amputation following repair of popliteal vascular injuries, the common factors leading to failure of the procedure are extensive time delay (> 36 hours), associated bone and soft tissue injuries leading to postoperative wound infection, and early occlusion of the popliteal artery repair or delay in performance of fasciotomy.[16] These factors were all represented in the amputations seen in the current group of litigation cases. It was clear that attorneys concerned with these cases were aware of the report of Lim et al at the University of Illinois, in which 31 consecutive popliteal artery injuries were treated without amputation.[17] In that series, penetrating trauma was the most frequent cause of injury, but attorneys did not distinguish between blunt injury and penetrating trauma in discussing these cases in which dislocation of the knee or blunt trauma was the most frequent form of injury. In Flint and Richardson's review of the University of Louisville experience, popliteal artery injuries associated with fracture were also consistently repaired with excellent results and no amputations.[18]

The problem of failure to perform fasciotomy or a late fasciotomy was noted in nearly all of these cases. Compartment pressure measurements were taken in one case, but were not used effectively in the decision to perform fasciotomy. It should be recognized that the injured extremity inevitably has tissue edema. This is often the reason for expanding compartment pressure. If need for revascularization is present and this is done, tissue edema and muscle ischemia secondary to the lack of blood flow prior to revascularization both contribute to elevated compartmental pressure. In patients with trauma, compartment pressures below 10 cm saline are considered to be normal, and concern about compartment syndrome occurs whenever such pressures exceed 30 cm saline.[19] Compartment pressures in the conscious or, especially, in the unconscious patient should be estimated clinically or by measurement in all cases of severe extremity trauma.

A plan of management of knee injuries should include a physical examination to evaluate stability of the joint. Many dislocations spontaneously reduce, even at the scene of the accident. The only clue may be instability of the knee or a popliteal space hematoma seen in the emergency room. If knee dislocation is confirmed, the foot should be examined for the classical signs of ischemia. In the absence of these, orders must be written for the observation of distal tissue perfusion and the performance of Doppler ankle pressures on a serial basis. If peripheral neuropathy develops and manifests as burning pain or numbness, arterial injury should be assumed and arteriography performed immediately.

The aneurysm-related emergencies are not surprising to vascular surgeons. Often, the emergency room physician or internist seeing an acute abdominal condition in an elderly patient minimizes the possibility of aneurysm expansion and rupture in favor of another diagnosis. In one of the present cases, an emergency room physician missed the diagnosis of abdominal aortic aneurysm rupture in a patient with a history of renal stones. A CT scan or B-mode scan of the abdomen would very easily have made the diagnosis of contained rupture of an aortic aneurysm. In another instance, an internist missed the diagnosis of ruptured abdominal aortic aneurysm when both a plain film of the abdomen and a B-mode scan showed the presence of an aneurysm in the patient who, by this time, had been admitted to the hospital. In another instance, an emergency room physician felt that a 17-year-old girl was hysterical, when in fact, she developed clear-cut myelopathy as a result of thoracic aortic dissection.

In the two instances of missed ischemic colitis following aortic surgery in this series of cases, one instance did not lead to litigation while the other did. In both instances, postoperative diarrhea was noted by the nurses, leukocytosis was present in the record, and in both instances the condition was treated quite late. The one successful treatment did not eventuate in graft infection while in the other, sepsis and its associated multisystem failure did lead to death.

CONCLUSIONS

This case review shows that litigation in emergency vascular surgery is linked to a bad outcome. Amputation and/or death are recognized as a hazard in most vascular emergencies. Yet, when such an undesired outcome occurs, litigation results if the patient and family are not informed before treatment is initiated or if delay in treatment precludes success of the procedure. Also, it should be recognized that even successful vascular repairs may result in neuropathy sufficient to cause disability or discomfort. When these occur, litigation may follow.

As a general rule, much litigation in emergency vascular surgery can be avoided simply by early recognition of arterial occlusion. The occlusion may be produced by iatrogenic injury, trauma, embolus, or atherosclerotic thrombosis. Twenty-nine of the 47 cases reviewed in this series were concerned with acute arterial occlusion. Within this group were the five cases of white clot syndrome of heparin-associated thrombocytopenia, as noted above. In addition, the eight popliteal artery injuries in seven patients comprised an important subgroup of patients. Knee dislocation, joint instability, or popliteal space hematoma was obvious in each of these cases and should have led to early diagnosis of popliteal artery occlusion.

Since recognition of arterial occlusion may escape the casual examiner, routine use of objective measurements, such as Doppler-derived segmental limb pressure, may alert the treating physician to the presence of diminished distal perfusion. In many of the cases reviewed, Doppler pulses were noted, but pressures were not taken. Uniform use of pressure rather than pulse-taking when the Doppler instrument is available would avoid this calamity.

Missed diagnosis of aneurysm, as expected, is another source of litigation. Avoidance of litigation in this situation is simply one of recognition that a patient with an aneurysm is likely to experience rupture of the aneurysm. This is true whether the aneurysm is atherosclerotic or traumatic, true or false. They all eventually proceed to rupture or to thrombosis.

REFERENCES

1. Smith RF, Szilagyi DE, Pfeifer JR: Arterial trauma. Arch Surg 86:825, 1963
2. Orcutt MB, Levine BA, Gaskill III HV, et al: Iatrogenic vascular injury. A reducible problem. Arch Surg 120:384, 1985
3. Youkey JR, Clagett GP, Rich NM, et al: Vascular trauma secondary to diagnostic and therapeutic procedures: 1974 through 1982. A comparative review. Amer J Surg 146:788, 1983
4. Adar R, Bass A, Walden R: Iatrogenic complications in surgery. Five years' experience in general and vascular surgery in a university hospital. Ann Surg 196:725, 1982
5. Robbs JV, Naidoo KS: Nerve compression injuries due to traumatic false aneurysm. Ann Surg 200:80, 1984
6. Rhodes GR, Dixon RH, Silver D: Heparin induced thrombocytopenia with thrombotic and hemorrhagic manifestations. Surg Gynecol Obstet 136:409, 1973
7. Rhodes GR, Dixon RH, Silver D: Heparin induced thrombocytopenia: Eight cases with thrombotic-hemorrhagic complications. Ann Surg 186:752, 1977
8. Stead RB, Schafer AI, Rosenberg RD, et al: Heterogenicity of heparin lots associated with thrombocytopenia and thromboembolism. Amer J Med 77:185, 1984
9. Salzman EW, Rosenberg RD, Smith MH, et al: Effect of heparin and heparin fractions on platelet aggregation. J Clin Invest 65:64, 1980
10. Lynch DM, Howe SE: Heparin-associated thrombocytopenia: Antibody binding specificity to platelet antigens. Blood 66:1176, 1985
11. Böttiger LE: Editorial: Heparin-induced thrombocytopenia. Acta Med Scand 218:257, 1985
12. Blaisdell FW, Steele M, Allen RE: Management of acute lower extremity arterial ischemia due to embolism and thrombosis. Surgery 84:822, 1978
13. Tawes Jr RL, Harris EJ, Brown WH, et al: Arterial thromboembolism. A 20-year experience. Arch Surg 120:595, 1985
14. Balas P, Bonatsos G, Xeromeritis N, et al: Early surgical results in acute arterial occlusion of the extremities. J Cardiovasc Surg 26:262, 1985

15. Satiani B, Gross WS, Evans WE: Improved limb salvage after arterial embolectomy. Ann Surg 188:153, 1978

16. Jaggers RC, Feliciano DV, Mattox KL, et al: Injury to popliteal vessels. Arch Surg 117:657, 1982

17. Lim LT, Michuda MS, Flanigan DP, et al: Popliteal artery trauma. 31 consecutive cases without amputation. Arch Surg 115:1307, 1980

18. Flint LM, Richardson JD: Arterial injuries with lower extremity fracture. Surgery 93:5, 1983

19. Christenson JT, Qvarfordt P: Intramuscular pressure changes during and after revascularization of the femoral arteries in humans. World J Surg 7:646, 1983

PART II

Diagnostic Aids

Hermann W. Kaebnick
Elliot O. Lipchik
Jonathan B. Towne

The Role of Angiography in Emergency Vascular Surgery

Major advances in emergency vascular surgery have been realized and developed as a result of treating vascular injuries sustained during military encounters,[1-3] and are also responsible for the improved survival in our "urban battlefields." During wartime, routine exploration of penetrating wounds was necessary because of the high velocity missile injuries with associated massive tissue destruction and unavailability of radiologic vascular imaging techniques. Most large series of civilian arterial trauma[4-6] involve penetrating trauma from low velocity missiles and sharp edged instruments, which has allowed for the development of a selective operative approach in the management of penetrating trauma. Nonpenetrating arterial trauma frequently poses a problem of recognizing that an arterial injury may be present and in the triaging of multiple complex wounds. Angiography and the vascular radiologist have become integral members of the team that assists in managing diagnostic and therapeutic problems of trauma victims.

Angiography has three major roles in the management of arterial injury: (1) to determine the precise location and extent of an arterial injury with potential multiple site or multivessel involvement; (2) to diagnose an arterial injury when the clinical presentation is equivocal; and (3) to provide access for the transcatheter control and manipulation of damaged blood vessels.

Angiograms are of particular value in patients with injuries to the base of the neck that may involve several vessels and when intrathoracic proximal control may be required. Likewise, in patients who have obvious arterial injury, but in whom the path of the bullet parallels the course of the artery or in whom multiple pellet wounds make the determination of the exact site of arterial injury difficult, arteriography enables a precise surgical approach and avoids extensive dissection of the vessels. As a diagnostic modality, arteriography should answer specific questions posed by the clinical examination and does not replace a careful history and physical examination. Diagnostic angiography is of value to avoid unnecessary surgical exploration in patients with injuries in proximity to major vascular structures without other signs or symptoms of vessel damage. It is helpful in evaluating arteries not easily assessible by clinical examination such as the internal carotid, vertebral, or profunda femoris artery. In a patient with multiple injuries and shock, the evaluation of peripheral circulation and tissue perfusion in the injured extremity may be difficult.

The goal of vascular trauma surgery is to avoid the complications and sequelae of missed arterial injury, such as gangrene, delayed hemorrhage, pseudoaneurysm formation, and arteriovenous fistula. Technical advances in vascular imaging have kept pace with the ability of the vascular radiologist to "intervene" in difficult arterial injuries. Disrupted arteries and arteriovenous fistulas that are located in difficult areas to explore and control surgically are frequently accessible to catheter embolization or balloon catheter occlusion.

Angiography requires an allotment of time unique for each institution and the capabilities of each vascular radiologist. This quotient must be considered in the diagnostic and therapeutic value of the procedure. Time lost in diagnostic studies accounts for 15 percent of the early preventable trauma deaths, two thirds of which occur on the x-ray table.[7] Loss of time is the major risk factor in the trauma victim, which in general involves a youthful population free of atherosclerotic cardiac and peripheral vascular disease. This group usually tolerates large contrast loads and percutaneous arterial catheterization well.[6,8,9] The only absolute contraindication to angiography is an anaphylactic reaction to contrast media, while low cardiac output, anuria, local infection, bleeding diatheses, allergy to contrast, and diabetes with poor renal function are relative contraindications.[10] Large series of consecutive arteriograms have been performed with no mortalities and less than 0.4 percent morbidity.[6,9,11]

The angiography suite is the appropriate area for safe and efficient vascular imaging and possible therapeutic intervention.[12] A study that is to be performed in lieu of an operation should be conducted with sterile technique and the best possible conditions to identify an arterial injury. All acutely ill patients undergoing angiographic evaluation must be accompanied by a surgeon with the resources for patient monitoring, control of airway, and with the authority to terminate the diagnostic study if the patient requires urgent surgery. A "stable" patient should not be allowed to become "unstable" while waiting for a "complete" evaluation in the arteriography suite. Intraoperative[13] or "Emergency Room"[14] arteriograms are fast, simple techniques to obtain a static single view of a selected peripheral artery. Intraoperative studies allow for the assessment of technical errors and evaluation of distal flow or injury.[15,16] Single film arteriograms performed in the emergency room may effectively reduce operative exploration and time in the angiography suite, but the validity of such a procedure awaits comparison with operative exploration and close long-term follow up to determine the rate of false negative studies and morbidity of missed injuries. Static arteriograms cannot provide the high film detail of a multiple view fluoroscopically directed catheter arteriogram. Interventional angiography requires an appropriately equipped suite and should be considered as a treatment or therapy with its own attendant risks and benefits.

TECHNIQUE

Examinations are performed utilizing a percutaneously placed intraarterial catheter to inject contrast material in the artery near the site of the injury. The transfemoral approach is preferred because of the size of the femoral artery, its constant stable location and ease

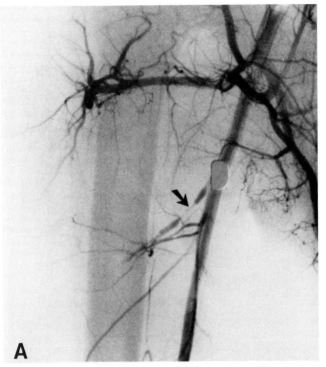

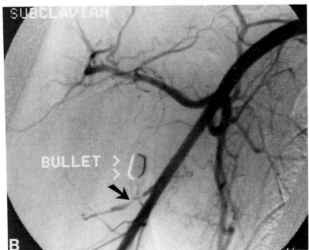

Fig. 1. (A) A subtraction view of a conventional-film arteriogram with a selective right axillary contrast injection. The track of the bullet has distorted the contour of the posterior humeral circumflex artery. (B) For comparison, an intraarterial digital subtraction angiographic study of the same patient as (A), demonstrating the same feature.

of access.[12] The right brachial/axillary approach is the second choice and may be necessary because of localized injury or inability to advance a catheter across an arterial defect. Newer imaging techniques of digital subtraction angiography[17,18] have been compared to film-based angiography (Fig. 1 A,B). Conventional angiography is preferred in uncooperative patients or when a large field is to be visualized with multiple overlying foreign bodies. Digital subtraction angiography (DSA) can be performed rapidly with the results immediately available for viewing. The image of an intraarterial DSA is comparable to conventional angiography, while allowing for a savings in film and storage costs.[19] Intraarterial DSA injection allows for a smaller amount of dilute contrast to be used than with film screen imaging. The procedure time should be shorter compared to film screen acquisition.[20,21] Intravenous DSA is recommended in certain areas, but we feel the technique is inferior as to image detail, outline, and contrast material load.

Vascular injury is identified by an arrest of contrast media, an irregularity of the contour of the vessel, internal filling defects, premature venous filling (Fig. 2 A, B),

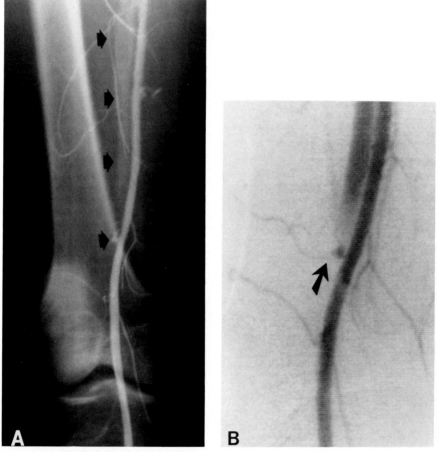

Fig. 2. (A) A conventional-film arteriogram demonstrates an arteriovenous fistula from a laceration at the distal superficial femoral artery. (B) Intravenous digital subtraction angiogram of the same patient as (A) demonstrates the enhancement of the venous phase although contours are not as sharp as conventional-film studies.

extravasation of contrast, or opacification of a false aneurysm. When the arterial media and intima are disrupted an intact adventitia may bulge outward under arterial pressure causing an increased lumen size. A torn intima can be seen as a radiolucent defect in the column of contrast media (Fig. 3). Evaluation of larger vessels requires precise adjustment of contrast flow rates and volume. Multiple views may be necessary to adequately survey the circumference of a vessel or to displace overlying osseous structures or foreign bodies. Angiography can underestimate the degree of arterial injury, especially in the larger vessels at the base of the neck. Longitudinal and tangential lacerations in an experimental canine model have demonstrated little or no angiographic defects in a significant number of animals.[22,23] This has not been the experience in the clinical setting[24] but it reiterates the need for quality angiography with close review by the vascular radiologist and vascular surgeon cognizant of the mechanisms of injury.

Angiography is ideally suited to exclude an arterial injury that may be clinically subtle.[25] A penetrating wound in proximity to a major vascular structure may have a high rate of negative exploration if a policy of routine surgical explorations[6,9,24,26] was in

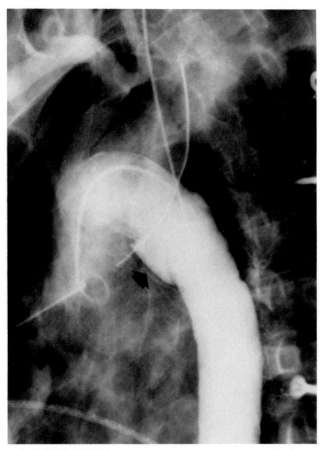

Fig. 3.   A conventional-film arteriogram of a transected thoracic aorta demonstrates the intimal defect with the bulging out of the intact adventitia.

Table 1

Algorithm for Selective Management of Transmediastinal Penetrating Wounds

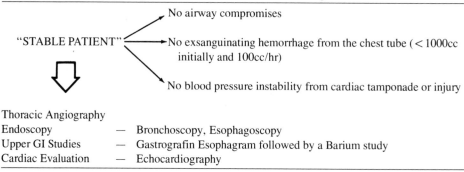

No airway compromises

"STABLE PATIENT" → No exsanguinating hemorrhage from the chest tube (< 1000cc initially and 100cc/hr)

No blood pressure instability from cardiac tamponade or injury

Thoracic Angiography	
Endoscopy	— Bronchoscopy, Esophagoscopy
Upper GI Studies	— Gastrografin Esophagram followed by a Barium study
Cardiac Evaluation	— Echocardiography

effect. Angiography allows for a higher degree of accuracy and safety in observing a clinically "stable" patient. The opposite extreme—routine angiography—should not be inferred. Obvious clinical findings do not require angiographic confirmation and unwarranted delay in treatment is unacceptable. For example, a patient with a .22 caliber bullet wound to the medial thigh with an ischemic leg and absent distal pulses does not require an angiogram to diagnose or treat the injury. Prompt surgical repair is all that is needed.

INDICATIONS FOR ANGIOGRAPHY BY SPECIFIC ANATOMIC REGIONS

Thoracic Cavity

A majority of penetrating chest injuries are managed nonoperatively with closed chest tube thoracostomy; operative indications are well established. A therapeutic dilemma arises with a transmediastinal missile injury. Selective management[27] of a stable patient includes diagnostic arch, thoracic aortic angiography, and visualization of the arch vessels (Table 1).

Parmley and his associates[28] in 1958, presented the clinical and pathologic features of a large series of patients with rupture of the thoracic aorta due to nonpenetrating chest trauma. Of the 15 percent that survived the initial event, only 5 percent survived longer than 4 months, making early diagnosis and treatment imperative. The history of a rapid deceleration injury and the x-ray findings of a widened mediastinum on an anteroposterior 100 cm supine chest radiograph constitute the major indications for obtaining a thoracic aortogram (Fig. 4) to evaluate for a transected thoracic aorta.[29] Abnormal chest radiographic findings do not show a high enough degree of specificity to make the diagnosis without a contrast study.[29-31] While an increasing number of abnormal findings on chest radiography improves specificity, clinical suspicion is adequate to warrant a thoracic angiogram. Following is a list of chest roentgenographic findings in ruptured thoracic aorta:

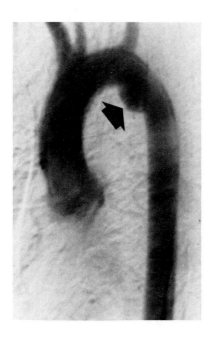

Fig. 4. Intraarterial digital subtraction angiogram of a patient involved in a motor vehicle accident with chest pain and a widened mediastinum (8.5 cm). The pseudoaneurysm formation is seen in projection.

1. Widening of superior mediastinum (≥ 8 cm).
2. Loss of sharpness or obscuring of aortic knob.
3. Deviation of nasogastric tube.
4. Deviation of trachea to the right.
5. Downward displacement of left main stem bronchus.
6. Apical pleural capping.
7. Enlarged or abnormal aortic contours.
8. Left hemothorax.
9. First and/or second rib fractures.
10. Displacement of left or right paraspinous interspace.
11. Obliteration of aortic-pulmonary window.

Thoracic Outlet/Base of Neck

The thoracic outlet and base of neck are the confines of the aortic arch vessels, brachial plexus, esophagus, and trachea. This area of the neck has been designated as zone 1, or below the cricoid cartilage as anatomically defined by Roon and Christenson.[8,32] Zone 3 is the portion of the neck above the angle of the mandible and zone 2 is the centrally defined portion of the neck (Fig. 5). Penetrating injury to the base of the neck represents a diagnostic and therapeutic challenge. Routine exploration of all wounds penetrating the platysma in this area has been advocated due to the lack of overt signs of major vascular injury in 30 percent of patients; half are venous injuries that would not be visualized by arteriography.[33] These patients are subject to rapid circulatory collapse, despite initial hemodynamic stability, due to the large size of the vessels injured. After initial evaluation, with close surveillance and monitoring by a surgeon, a stable patient with no evidence of hemorrhage or airway compromise, can undergo emergency arteriog-

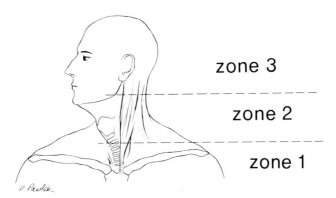

Fig. 5. Penetrating wounds to the anterior neck can be classified into injuries involving different zones. Selective management to each zone has evolved with angiography playing an important diagnostic and therapeutic role.

raphy with minimal morbidity and no mortality.[34-36] A negative arteriogram allows for nonoperative management of 30 to 80 percent of patients with base of neck penetrating injury. Appropriate incision and position can be planned in those with positive findings. Any angiographic abnormality should be operatively explored. A negative arteriogram does not constitute an absolute contraindication to exploration of a wound if the clinical examination is to the contrary.

Blunt injury to the cervicomediastinal structures is frequently associated with complex multisystem trauma. A patient with head and abdominal injuries should be under high suspicion of having sustained chest trauma as well. The presentation is not as dramatic as penetrating wounds to this area and may not present with a loss of distal pulses despite injury to innominate or subclavian vessels.[37,38] Patients with first and second rib fractures have associated aortic and brachiocephalic vascular lesions in 8 to 14 percent of injuries studies by angiography.[39] The combination of an absent distal pulse, a brachial plexus injury, and a displaced first rib fracture is very sensitive for an associated vascular injury, while isolated signs such as a widened mediastinum are not sensitive enough to accurately predict a vascular lesion.[39-41] An understanding of the mechanism of injury and clinical suspicion when structures of the mediastinum are involved should lead to angiography.

Neck

The neck represents two surgical transition areas where operative exposure is difficult and infrequently performed with a central zone of easy, rapid surgical exposure associated with minimal morbidity. The zones I and III injury as previously described (Fig. 5) are considered optimal areas to have angiographic "exclusion" of arterial injury. The major controversy surrounds the concept of routine exploration of zone II injuries—from the angle of the mandible to the cricoid cartilage. In the selective management of penetrating neck injuries, emergency four-vessel extracranial cerebrovascular angiography is an integral part of the diagnostic evaluation that can allow for safe nonoperative treatment (Table 2).[41-45] In a stable patient without exsanguinating hemorrhage, an expanding hematoma, or airway compromise, preoperative angiography can allow assessment of the carotid

Table 2
Algorithm for Selective Management for Anterior Neck Penetrating Wounds

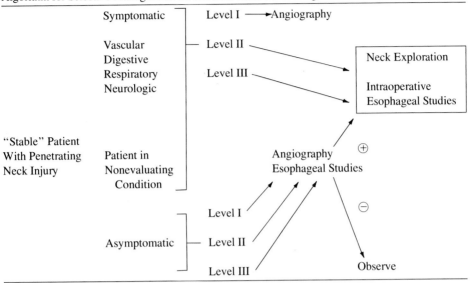

Adapted from Narrod and Moore[45]

arteries, intracerebral collateral flow, and the vertebral arteries. The vertebral arteries are not routinely explored and are difficult to expose if they are injured. In blunt or penetrating injuries to the neck that have undergone arteriographic evaluation, vertebral artery lesions have represented up to 20 percent of the vascular injuries[46] (Fig. 6).

Extremity

In most large series of extremity arterial trauma, penetrating injuries constitute 50 to 90 percent of the cases.[24,26,47,48] The distribution of injuries slightly favors the lower extremities. Arteriography is indicated to evaluate and help plan operative intervention in: (1) wounds associated with fractures and blunt trauma; (2) wounds from multiple pellets or missiles; (3) wounds in which the missile traverses a course parallel to a major artery; (4) wounds in patients with pre-existing vascular insufficiency; and (5) wounds with suspected pseudoaneurysm or arteriovenous fistula.[8,26]

Injuries with equivocal signs of ischemia, in proximity to a major vessel, and a questionable history of bleeding or hypotension constitute 50 to 75 percent of cases the vascular surgeon may be asked to evaluate.[6,9,14,24] The correlation of pulse deficit with arterial injury increases the more peripheral the injury. An injury to the subclavian or axillary artery has a 10 to 30 percent incidence of a normal distal pulse.[4,33] While distal pulses may be present despite an arterial injury, the association of a hematoma and/or neurologic deficit has been felt by some to be a more reliable finding.[22] On the other hand, an extremity pulse may be absent or diminished in 18 percent of patients with no arterial injury.[6,49] When evaluating an injured extremity with more than one of the clinical signs of arterial injury such as absent or decreased distal pulses with ischemia, pulsatile bleeding or expanding hematoma, hypotension or a corresponding neurologic deficit, an arterial injury is present in greater than 90 percent of cases.[47,50] Blunt arterial extremity

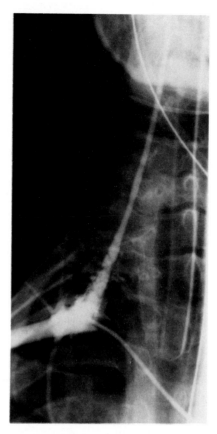

Fig. 6. Conventional-film arteriogram of a patient involved in a motor vehicle accident sustaining a right brachial plexus injury and disruption of the right vertebral artery with extravasation of contrast from the lumen of the vessel.

trauma is complicated by associated multisystem injury and shock in over 40 percent of cases.[51] Angiography is currently the accepted method of determining an arterial injury in a stable patient with equivocal clinical signs. The accuracy of this approach was 92 percent with an overall sensitivity of 97 percent and specificity of 90 percent by correlating angiograms to operative findings in a series reported by Snyder, et al.[24]

The greatest controversy surrounds the role of angiography in the evaluation of "proximity alone injuries" when there is a low incidence of arterial injury ranging from 8 to 11 percent.[24,47,48] Selective arteriography has reduced negative explorations for "proximity alone injuries" to 3 to 30 percent.[26,44] False positive angiograms represent 4 to 10 percent of cases[9,24,26] and usually are the result of cautious "over-reading" of the contrast study. A false negative arteriogram (1 to 3 percent) results from a limited angiographic study, multiple small pellet wounds, and small lacerations.[24,26,47] Proximity injuries have a low enough incidence of associated vascular injury in some series to suggest nonoperative and nonangiographic evaluation of clinically negative patients.[22,50] This policy in general is unwise because of (1) the unknown natural history of minimal arterial lesions,

(2) the noncompliant and mobile nature of the patient population involved in extremity trauma, and (3) the morbidity of delay in treating complicated vascular injuries—pseudoaneurysms, arteriovenous fistulas, and thrombosed distal vessels.

THE MCW EXPERIENCE

After reviewing our experience with extremity trauma[48] in 1978, a policy of selective preoperative arteriographic evaluation of stable patients with presumed penetrating arterial trauma was adopted. An injury in proximity to a major vessel, a nonexpanding hematoma, a history of hypotension, and equivocal physical findings were used as indications to angiographically evaluate extremity arterial trauma during the period of 1980–1986. The implementation of technical advances in vascular imaging also occurred during this period. Penetrating extremity injuries in 69 patients that underwent angiographic evaluation for upper (31 patients) and lower (38 patients) extremity trauma were reviewed. Multiple penetrating injuries were sustained in 25 percent (17/69) of the patients. Gunshot wounds accounted for the majority of the injuries (71 percent) with stab wounds (20 percent) and shotgun wounds (9 percent) comprising the remainder. The age range of the patients was 17 to 50 years old with a mean of 27.6 years. There were 60 males and 9 females. Right and left sided injury occurred with similar frequency (35/34).

Clinical indications for obtaining an extremity arteriogram were proximity to a major vessel alone in 59 percent (41/69) instances while multiple indications were present in the remainder of the cases. Other clinical indications of arterial injury were: (1) Clinically significant hematoma at the site of injury, 28 percent (19/69); (2) distal pulse deficit in 20 percent (14/69); (3) hypotension that responded to initial resuscitation, 14 percent (10/69); and (4) a corresponding neurologic deficit, 7 percent (5/69).

Abnormal angiograms were obtained in 38 percent (26/69) of the patients, half of whom proceeded to operative intervention. A distal pulse deficit was the most frequent associated finding in 9/13 (77 percent) with only 1/13 (8 percent) having a proximity injury and abnormal angiogram as the only indication for operation. Arterial repair was accomplished by primary closure or segmental resection and primary repair in 6 cases, while a vein interposition graft was used in 5 cases. One shotgun wound that was explored for having a pulse deficit, neurologic deficit, and spasm of the brachial artery noted on preoperative angiogram was negative for arterial injury. A patient who had an occluded anterior tibial artery from a shotgun blast to the popliteal fossa underwent a fasciotomy alone, only to return 2 years later with a tibioperoneal arteriovenous fistula. This represents the only false negative angiogram in the series. Negative arteriograms were followed by exploration in 2 instances. The first case was a stab wound to the groin that developed a rapidly expanding hematoma 24 hours after initial presentation secondary to a femoral vein injury, which required a lateral venorrhaphy. In one case the femoral vessels were explored despite a negative arteriogram because the bullet was overlying the vessel. The exploration was negative.

Extremity angiographic studies demonstrated minor abnormalities and resulted in nonoperative therapy in 12/13 (92 percent) of the cases. One patient with an arteriovenous fistula from a stab wound refused operation and subsequently had a normal examination on followup visits. Occlusion of side branch vessels, profunda branches of the femoral or brachial system, and isolated injuries of one of the tibial vessels were not explored in 5/13

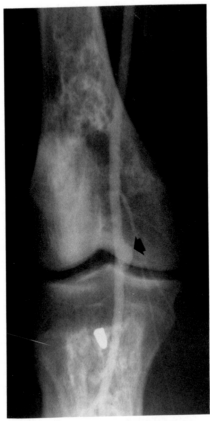

Fig. 7. A pseudoaneurysm of the left popliteal artery from a missile injury is demonstrated by conventional-film angiography.

(38 percent) patients. This included injuries to the anterior tibial, posterior tibial, profunda brachii, and lateral scapular artery. A pseudoaneurysm of the popliteal artery (Fig. 7) was demonstrated in a patient with multiple gunshot wounds and was not repaired because of coexisting life threatening multisystem injuries. He died 5 months later of uncontrolled abdominal sepsis. The injured popliteal artery remained patent with a palpable distal pulse. Two patients with extravasation from minor branch vessels of the axillary artery due to gunshot wounds were not explored and no clinical evidence of pseudoaneurysm or A/V fistula was seen at 4 and 21 months. Spasm of the brachial artery from a gunshot wound and associated humeral fracture was seen by arteriography in one patient. Six penetrating injuries had associated fractures, half of which had abnormal angiograms involving an isolated tibial artery or side branch vessels of profunda brachial system and were not explored but had external fixation of the fracture. These fractures were treated as closed fractures without developing ischemic contractures or arterial insufficiency.

Intraarterial digital subtraction angiography was instituted in the evaluation of extremity injuries in 1984. This represents 24/69 (35 percent) of the patients who were evaluated by this technique. Conventional angiography was initially used in combination with DSA in 7/24 (29 percent) and only DSA films were obtained in 17/69 (25 percent).

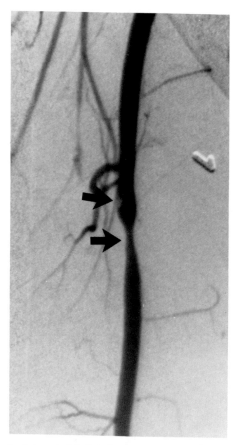

Fig. 8. An intraarterial digital subtraction angiogram of a patient with a "proximity alone injury" to the right upper arm. The intimal defect was confirmed at operation. Note spasm distal to intimal defect.

During the last 2 years intraarterial DSA was the primary study performed in a cooperative patient without multiple fragments or pellets overlying a possible arterial injury. The technique has been able to demonstrate a small intimal defect in the brachial artery from a gunshot wound (Fig. 8) as well as accurately define a transected thoracic aorta. These studies were performed with percutaneously placed 5 Fr angiographic catheters with selective placement in an artery near the site of suspected injury under fluoroscopic control. Entrance and exit wounds were marked on the skin with an opaque object and multiple views were obtained as needed.

The physical examination was sensitive in determining which patient would need operative exploration in that 92 percent (12/13) of the patients with arterial trauma had more than one clinical indication of arterial injury. The only false negative angiogram (1/69—1 percent) occurred in a patient that sustained a shotgun injury and presented later with an arteriovenous fistula that was not demonstrated on the initial arteriogram. This reiterates the need for an aggressive operative approach and longterm follow-up of the treacherous injury. A "proximity alone injury" represented the majority of the cases (59

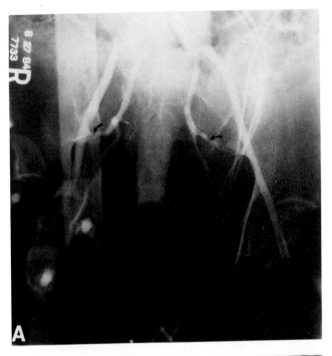

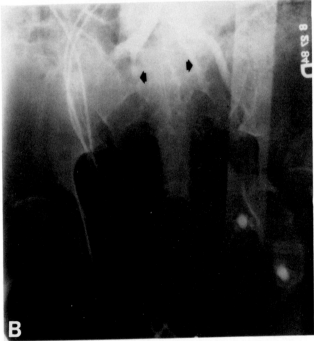

Fig. 9. (A) Conventional-film pelvic arteriogram demonstrating bilateral injuries to the superior gluteal arteries. (B) After transcatheter gelfoam embolization of both superior gluteal arteries. There is no extravasation noted.

percent) taken care of by the vascular service, yet the rate of angiographic abnormalities demonstrated was only 2 percent (1/41). This lone abnormality may have been ideally managed without operation in a reliable patient. Not all angiographic abnormalities require operation. Occluded minor side branch vessels without extravasation have not developed pseudoaneurysms or arteriovenous fistulas in follow-up examinations.

Technical advances in digital subtraction angiography are applicable to the evaluation of the trauma victim. The rapidity with which the examination can be performed along with the instant review reduces overall procedure time. The capability to subtract overlying osseous structures aids visualization of arterial structures particularly at the base of the skull, the thoracic cavity, and the pelvis.

THE ROLE OF COMBINED ANGIOGRAPHY AND INTERVENTIONAL RADIOLOGY IN VASCULAR TRAUMA

The management of severe pelvic fractures is the best example of how angiography and the advances in interventional radiology have enabled better control of exsanquinating hemorrhage in an injury with a high mortality from bleeding.[52-54] The morbidity of a retroperitoneal exploration and hypogastric arterial ligation are felt to outweigh nonoperative management with blood replacement.[55] The radiographic film of a disrupted pelvis cannot of itself predict which patient will have an associated arterial injury.[53] Exclusion of other sites of injury and ongoing resuscitation with pelvic stabilization (MAST suit, external fixation) are frequently necessary prior to or during documentation of pelvic arterial injury by angiography[52,53] (Fig. 9 A,B). The necessity for a coordinated effort between the trauma surgeon, orthopedic surgeon, vascular radiologist, and ancillary staff is vital. Pelvic arterial injury is poorly controlled by direct ligation, but it is accessible to percutaneous transcatheter embolization or balloon occlusion.[54,56,57]

Traumatic injury to the extracranial vertebral arteries can result in thrombosis, disruption, arteriovenous fistula, or pseudoaneurysm. While no treatment is needed for the thrombosed artery, nonoperative occlusion of the vessel is possible with coil embolization[58,59] or balloon catheter occlusion.[60,61] This can be done at the time of the angiogram with selective catheter placement of the embolization material to occlude the artery. Lesions of the high internal carotid artery represent rare injuries and difficult surgical exposures. The axiom of proximal and distal control with an arteriovenous fistula in this region is technically difficult. Balloon catheter occlusion of the communication or of the inflow and outflow vessels (Fig. 10 A,B) can aid the operative management of selected patients.[62,63]

CONCLUSION

Angiography is a diagnostic and therapeutic tool assuming an ever increasing role in the selective management of penetrating and nonpenetrating trauma. This expanded role should not be due solely to increasing technology but also to appropriate selection of patient groups who will benefit from these modalities. Close interaction between surgeon and vascular radiologist is important to this end.

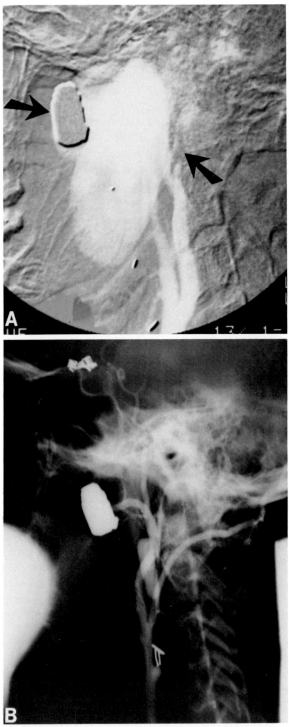

Fig. 10. (A) Intraarterial digital subtraction angiographic demonstration of a high flow arteriovenous fistula between the internal carotid artery and jugular vein at the base of the skull. (B) Transcatheter placement of occluding balloons was unsuccessful in obliterating the fistula selectively. An internal carotid artery balloon was placed proximally and distally prior to extra-cranial/intra-cranial arterial bypass.

72

REFERENCES

1. Debakey ME, Simeone FA: Battle injuries of the arteries in World War II: An analysis of 2,471 cases. Ann Surg 123:534, 1946
2. Hughes CW: Arterial repair during the Korean War. Ann Surg 147:555, 1958
3. Rich NM, Baugh JH, Hughes CW: Acute arterial injuries in Vietnam: 1000 cases. J Trauma 10:359, 1970
4. Drapanas T, Hewitt RL, Weichert RF, Smith AD: Civilian vascular injuries: A critical appraisal of three decades of management. Ann Surg 172:351, 1970
5. Perry MO, Thal ER, Shires GT: Management of arterial injuries. Ann Surg 173:403, 1971
6. Smith RF, Elliott JP, Hageman WH, et al: Acute penetrating arterial injuries of the neck and limbs. Arch Surg 109:198, 1974
7. Foley RW, Harris LS, Pilcher DB: Abdominal injuries in automobile accidents: Review of care of fatally injured patients. J Trauma 17:611, 1977
8. Freeark RJ: Role of angiography in the management of multiple injuries. Surg Gynecol Obstet 128:761, 1969
9. Geuder JW, Hobson RW, Padberg FT, et al: The role of contrast arteriography in suspected arterial injuries of the extremities. Am Surg 51:89, 1985
10. Pollard JJ, Nebesar RA: Abdominal angiography. N Engl J Med 279:1035, 1968
11. Lang EK: Prevention and treatment of complications following arteriography. Radiology 88:950, 1968
12. Ben-Menachem Y: Angiography in Trauma: A Work Atlas. Philadelphia, WB Saunders, Co, 1980
13. Lumpkin MB, Logan WD, Couves LM, Howard JM: Arteriography as an aid in the diagnosis and localization of acute arterial injuries. Ann Surg 147:353, 1958
14. O'Gorman RB, Feliciano DV, Bitondo CG, et al: Emergency center arteriography in the evaluation of suspected peripheral vascular injuries. Arch Surg 119:568, 1984
15. Pasch AR, Bishara RA, Lim LT, et al: Optimal limb salvage in penetrating civilian vascular trauma. J Vasc Surg 3:189, 1986
16. Roberts RM, String ST: Arterial injuries in extremity shotgun wounds: Requisite factors for successful management. Surgery 96:902, 1984
17. Weinstein MA, Pavlicek WA, Modic MT, et al: Intra-arterial digital subtraction angiography of the head and neck. Radiology 147:717, 1983
18. Davis PC, Hoffman JC: Work in progress. Intra-arterial digital subtraction angiography: Evaluation in 150 patients. Radiology 148:9, 1983
19. Crummy AB, Stieghorst MF, Turski PA, et al: Digital subtraction angiography: Current status and use of intra-arterial injection. Radiology 145:303, 1982
20. Goodman PC, Jeffery RB, Brant-Zawadzki M: Digital subtraction angiography in extremity trauma. Radiology 153:61, 1984
21. Gavant ML, Gold RE, Fabian TC, et al: Vascular trauma to the extremities and lower neck: Initial assessment with intravenous digital subtraction angiography. Radiology 158:755, 1986
22. Mufti MA, LaGuerre JN, Pochaczevsky R, et al: Diagnostic value of hematoma in penetrating arterial wounds of the extremities. Arch Surg 101:562, 1970
23. Lain KC, Williams GR: Arteriography in acute peripheral arterial injuries: An experimental study. Surg Forum 21:179, 1970
24. Snyder WH, Thal ER, Bridges RA, et al: The validity of normal arteriography in penetrating trauma. Arch Surg 113:424, 1978
25. Gerloch AJ, Mathis J, Goncharenko V, et al: Angiography of intimal and intramural arterial injuries. Radiology 129:357, 1978
26. Sirinek KR, Levine BA, Gaskill HV, et al: Reassessment of the role of routine operative exploration in vascular trauma. J Trauma 21:339, 1981

27. Richardson JD, Flint LM, Snow NJ, et al: Management of transmediastinal gunshot wounds. Surgery 90:671, 1981

28. Parmley LF, Mattingly TW, Manion WC, et al: Non-penetrating traumatic injury of the aorta. Circulation 17:1086, 1958

29. Fisher RG, Hadloch F, Ben-Menachem Y: Laceration of the thoracic aorta and brachiocephalic arteries by blunt trauma. Radiol Clin North Am 19:91, 1981

30. Lipchik EO, Robinson KE: Acute traumatic rupture of the thoracic aorta. Am J Roentgenol 104:408, 1968

31. Barcia TC, Livoni JP: Indications for angiography in blunt thoracic trauma. Radiology 147:15, 1983

32. Roon AJ, Christensen N: Evaluation and treatment of penetrating cervical injuries. J Trauma 19:391, 1979

33. Flint LM, Snyder WH, Perry MO, et al: Management of major vascular injuries in the base of the neck. Arch Surg 106:407, 1973

34. Hunt TK, Blaisdell FW, Okimoto J: Vascular injuries of the base of the neck. Arch Surg 98:586, 1969

35. Busuttil RW, Acker B: Management of injuries to the brachiocephalic vessels. Surg Gynecol Obstet 154:737, 1982

36. Lim LT, Saletta JD, Flanigan DP: Subclavian and innominate artery trauma. Surgery 86:890, 1979

37. Richardson JD, Flint LM: Cervicomediastinal injuries following blunt trauma. Am Surg 48:141, 1982

38. Zelenock GB, Kazmers AK, Graham LM, et al: Nonpenetrating subclavian injuries. Arch Surg 120:685, 1985

39. Livoni SP, Barcia TC: Fracture of the first and second rib: Incidence of vascular injury relative to type of fracture. Radiology 145:31, 1982

40. Phillips EH, Rogers WF, Gaspar MR: First rib fractures: Incidence of vascular injury and indication for angiography. Surgery 89:42, 1981

41. Thomas AN, Goodman PC, Roon AJ: Role of angiography in cervicothoracic trauma. J Thorac Cardiovasc Surg 76:633, 1978

42. Merion RM, Harness JK, Ramsbaugh SR, et al: Selective management of penetrating neck trauma. Arch Surg 116:691, 1981

43. Golueke PS, Goldstein AS, Sclafarri SJ, et al: Routine versus selective exploration of penetrating neck injuries: A randomized prospective study. J Trauma 24:1010, 1984

44. Hiatt JR, Busuttil RW, Wilson SE: Impact of routine arteriography on management of penetrating neck injuries. J Vasc Surg 1:860, 1984

45. Narrod JA, Moore EE: Selective management of penetrating neck injuries. Arch Surg 119:574, 1984

46. Meier PE, Brink BE, Fry WJ: Vertebral artery trauma. Arch Surg 116:236, 1981

47. Turcotte J, Towne JB, Bernhard VM: Is arteriography necessary with management of vascular trauma of the extremities. Surgery 84:557, 1978

48. Borman KR, Snyder WH, Weigelt JA: Civilian arterial trauma of the upper extremity. Am J Surg 148:796, 1984

49. McCormick TM, Burch BH: Routine angiographic evaluation of neck and extremity injuries. J Trauma 19:384, 1979

50. McDonald EJ, Goodman PC, Winestock DP: The clinical indications for arteriography in trauma to the extremity. Radiology 116:45, 1975

51. Ransom KA, Shatney CH, Soderstrom CA, et al: Management of arterial injuries in blunt trauma of the extremity. Surg Gynecol Obstet 153:241, 1981

52. Flint LM, Brown A, Richardson JD, et al: Definitive control of bleeding from severe pelvic fractures. Ann Surg 189:709, 1979

53. Kam J, Jackson H, Ben-Menachem Y: Vascular injuries in blunt pelvic trauma. Radiol Clin North Am 19:171, 1981

54. Margolies MN, Ring EJ, Waltman AC, et al: Arteriography in the management of hemorrhage from pelvic fracture. N Engl J Med 287:317, 1972

55. Ravitch MM: Hypogastric artery ligation in acute pelvic trauma. Surgery 56:601, 1964

56. Jander HP, Russinovich NA: Transcatheter gelfoam embolization in abdominal, retroperitoneal, and pelvic hemorrhage. Radiology 136:337, 1980

57. Paster SB, Van Houten FX, Adams DF: Percutaneous balloon catheterization: A technique for the control of arterial hemorrhage caused by pelvic trauma. JAMA 230:573, 1974

58. Rossi P, Passariello R, Simonetti G: Control of a traumatic vertebral arteriovenous fistula by a modified Gianturco coil embolus system. Am J Roentgenol 131:331, 1978

59. Gianturco C, Anderson JH, Wallace S: Mechanical devices for arterial occlusion. Am J Roentgenol 124:428, 1975

60. Debrun G, Negre J, Kasbarian M, et al: Endovascular occlusion of vertebral fistulae by detachable balloons with conservation of the vertebral blood flow. Radiology 130:141, 1979

61. Wiener I, Flye MW: Traumatic false aneurysm of the vertebral artery. J Trauma 24:346, 1984

62. Debrun G, Larour P, Vinuela F, et al: Treatment of 54 traumatic carotid-cavernous fistulas. J Neurosurg 55:678, 1981

63. Scialfa G, Vaghi A, Benardi L, Toron L: Neuroradiologic treatment of carotid and vertebral fistulas and intracavernous aneurysms. Neuroradiology 24:13, 1982

Robert L. Vogelzang
Madeleine R. Fisher

Computed Tomography and Magnetic Resonance Imaging in Vascular Surgical Emergencies

Computed tomography (CT) scanning is now universally accepted as an extremely useful tool in the investigation of disease throughout the body. It can be stated without exaggeration that CT has revolutionized the practice of medicine in virtually every specialty. In vascular surgery the routine use of CT in a variety of problems has changed the way diagnoses are made. It allows prompt recognition of conditions that were difficult if not impossible to diagnose using older techniques. Nowhere is this concept better epitomized than in the realm of vascular surgical emergencies. In these cases, life or limb threatening conditions such as hemorrhage, prosthetic graft infection, or vascular occlusion exist as the result of aneurysm, trauma, dissection, tumor, or previous arterial surgery. Prompt and appropriate diagnosis of the immediate problem and its cause is afforded by the use of contrast enhanced CT. This frequently obviates the need for angiography and eliminates less accurate tests such as plain films, barium studies, nuclear medicine scans, and/or ultrasound.

In the past several years magnetic resonance imaging (MRI) of the body has become a practical reality. The technique offers promise in the imaging of many disease processes. In the neural axis it has become a preferred modality due to inherently higher contrast resolution and freedom from artifacts. Progress in body imaging has been slower due to problems with motion artifact but early results in cardiovascular imaging demonstrate that MRI offers theoretical advantages over CT that may make it the imaging test of choice in vascular disease.

The purpose of this chapter is to identify those vascular surgical emergencies in which we found CT and MRI to be most useful and to clarify and illustrate the diagnostic features of the various conditions encountered.

Vascular Surgical Emergencies
ISBN 0-8089-1843-5

COMPUTED TOMOGRAPHY

Methods

In most vascular surgical emergencies the decision to use intravenous contrast material is based on the disease process that is suspected. For example, in ruptured abdominal aortic aneurysms a noncontrast scan will clearly and quickly demonstrate the high density hematoma outside the aorta as well as the aneurysm itself. However, with contrast enhancement, the abnormalities may be more vivid. In other circumstances, such as in the exclusion of aortic dissection, contrast material is mandatory in order to identify the intimal flap and clarify the relationship of the lumen to surrounding abnormalities. Patterns of flow in the two lumens can also be recognized from dynamic scan sequences. In general, we use intravenous contrast material routinely and reserve noncontrast scans for those patients in whom ruptured aortic aneurysm or hemorrhage is suspected and who may be subject to renal failure from hypovolemic shock.

Abdominal Aorta

Ruptured Aortic Aneurysm

It is widely recognized that CT compares favorably with angiography for the routine preoperative evaluation of abdominal and thoracic aneurysms.[1-10] CT demonstrates the

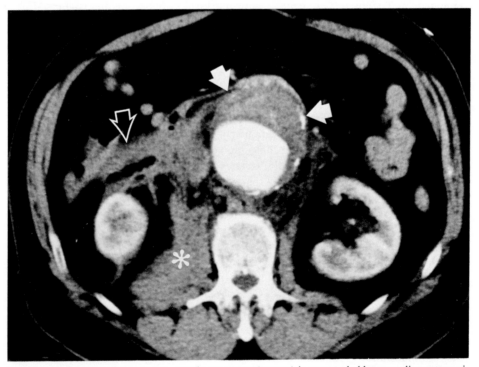

Fig. 1. Ruptured aortic aneurysm. Aortic aneurysm (arrows) is surrounded by spreading retroperitoneal collections in the anterior perirenal space (open arrow) as well as in the right psoas muscle which is enlarged (*). Also note irregularity adjacent to the aorta on the left.

relationship of the aneurysm to the renal and iliac arteries equally as well as angiography and depicts size with far greater accuracy due to its identification of mural thrombus. At Northwestern University Medical School CT has replaced aortography in the majority of these cases; angiography is reserved for situations when CT is not entirely diagnostic or the problem is complicated by occlusive disease or prior vascular reconstruction. In our hands this group of patients represents about 5 percent of the total and includes those with unusual aneurysms (thoracoabdominal, mycotic, inflammatory, or posttraumatic) or confusing CT findings, as may occur because of tangential sections through a tortuous aorta (partial volume averaging).

Rupture of an abdominal aortic aneurysm is a catastrophic event described elsewhere in this volume. The survival time of between 9 hours and 10 days if treatment is not initiated does allow prompt diagnosis.[11,12] When the classic triad of pain, a pulsatile abdominal mass, and hypotension is found, the diagnosis is made clinically and surgery is performed immediately. More commonly, however, other abdominal processes must be excluded. Up to one third of patients with ruptured abdominal aortic aneurysms may be treated for other conditions prior to establishment of a correct diagnosis.[10,13,14]

Rupture generally occurs into the retroperitoneum, which can usually be seen on CT. Graham et al report an incidence of 86 percent.[14,15] The majority of reports indicate a retroperitoneal perirenal location although a small number may involve the vena cava, psoas muscle, duodenum, or renal vein.[10,16-18] The CT findings of ruptured aneurysm are: (1) the presence of an aortic aneurysm, (2) high density (40–60 Hounsfield units [HU]) perinephric or other retroperitoneal collections. Intraperitoneal collections may also be seen, (3) An indistinct aortic margin in the vicinity of the collections (Fig. 1). Some authors also have discussed the findings associated with so called "unstable" aneurysms or those that are at risk for imminent rupture. Johnson et al define the aneurysms as those that exhibit an eccentric lumen with no thrombus between the lumen and the outer wall. A second criterion is the presence of contrast insinuating into the thrombus. In their experience these CT features accurately depicted the presence of surgically documented instability (either an aortic bubble or an elliptical shape of the aneurysm) in 4 of 5 patients.[19] Obviously this work requires corroboration but it may hold promise in surgical decision making concerning which aneurysms require surgery and which may be managed conservatively.

Perianeurysmal fibrosis or inflammatory aneurysm may occasionally be mistaken for a leaking abdominal aneurysm since these patients may have back pain that mimics the clinical appearance of a rupture. The CT findings in this condition that may involve 5–10 percent of aneurysms reflect the pathologic appearance of an aneurysm surrounded by a smooth white rind of fibrous tissue with a chronic inflammatory infiltrate within. A characteristic CT appearance consisting of a rim of periaortic soft tissue that enhances after contrast administration has been reported by a number of authors.[20-25] The sharply defined rind is distinctly different from the spreading perirenal collections seen in aneurysm rupture. In addition, trapping and medial deviation of the ureters within the mass may be seen (Fig. 2.)

Other less common nonaortic aneurysms at risk for rupture may also be identified and staged more expeditiously with CT. These include iliac aneurysms as well as isolated visceral artery aneurysms[26] (Figs. 3 and 4).

An aortic aneurysm may occasionally rupture, seal off, and form a chronic contained rupture.[27,28] We have had the opportunity to see three patients in whom the diagnosis of remote rupture could be made by the presence of a thrombosed extraaortic mass (Fig. 5).

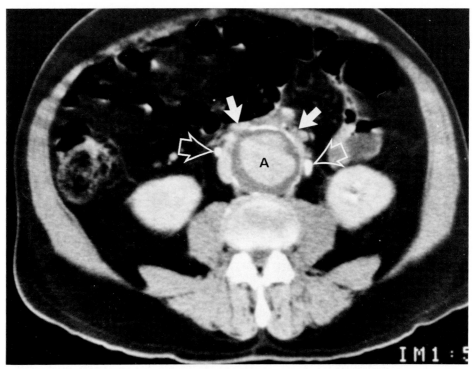

Fig. 2. Perianeurysmal fibrosis. Typical CT appearance with aortic aneurysm (A) surrounded by contrast enhancing rind (arrows). Note ureters (open arrows) deviated medially by the mass. This is in contrast to the lateral deviation usually seen with other large masses.

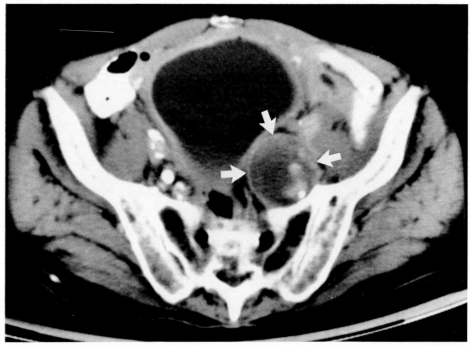

Fig. 3. Internal iliac aneurysm. Large left internal iliac aneurysm (arrows). Note small diameter lumen compared to amount of low density thrombus.

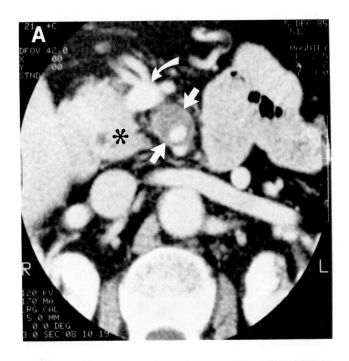

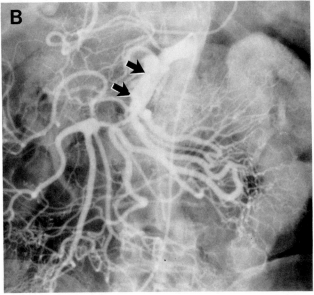

Fig. 4. CT (A) demonstrates superior mesenteric artery aneurysm (arrows). Note two opacified lumens. At surgery chronic rupture was found with formation of false lumen. Also note superior mesenteric vein (curved arrow) as well as pancreatic head (*). Superior mesenteric arteriogram (B) shows mass effect of the aneurysm with filling of the false lumen (arrows) from which proximal jejunal branches arise.

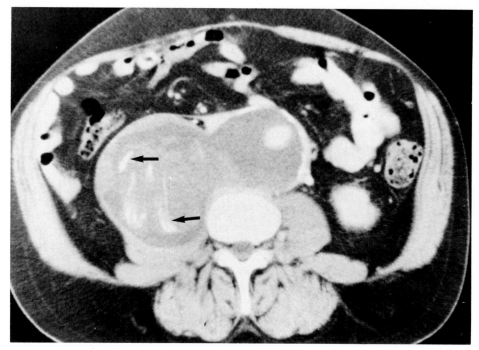

Fig. 5. Chronic contained rupture into the psoas muscle. Large right periaortic mass with laminated calcifications (arrows) arises off the infrarenal aneurysm. Calcification indicates chronicity.

Two of the patients had had a remote clinical episode that in retrospect probably was the inciting event.

Thoracic Aorta

Ruptured Thoracic Aortic Aneurysm

There are very few reports in the literature concerning the CT appearance of ruptured thoracic aneurysm since in most cases these patients are quite unstable and if any test is done angiography is usually elected. Aneurysm rupture can, however, produce periaortic thickening or fluid as well as pleural or extrapleural hematomas.[10] Rarely (about 5 percent of cases) a left-sided descending aortic aneurysm may present with right-sided extrapleural rupture.[29] We have recently reported two such cases.[30] In both patients little or no fluid was seen in the left hemithorax and a large hematoma was present on the right (Fig. 6). On the basis of this experience and the known utility of CT in the identification of both hematomas and aneurysms we believe that CT is likely to be the most diagnostic test in this situation.

Pseudoaneurysm

Thoracic aortic pseudoaneurysms may form as a result of anastomotic leak after surgery or blunt thoracic injury. These pseudoaneurysms are at substantial risk for free rupture and CT can provide a valuable method of localizing the masses and relating them to the surrounding structures. Gundry et al reported 11 such patients after motor vehicular

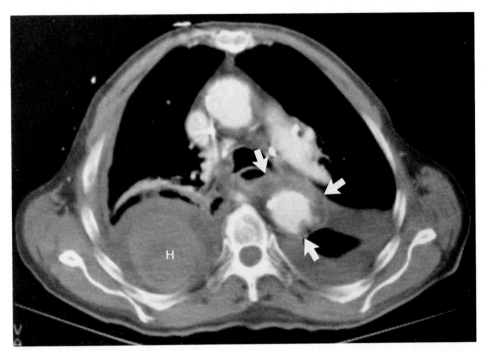

Fig. 6. Right-sided rupture of descending thoracic aneurysm. Thoracic aneurysm (arrows) has ruptured across the mediastinum and presents with a large extrapleural hematoma (H) and pleural effusion. There is pleural effusion on the left as well.

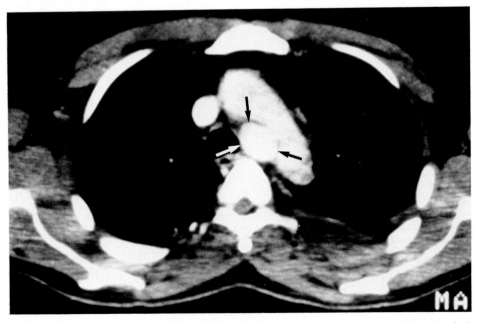

Fig. 7. Thoracic aortic pseudoaneurysm after blunt chest trauma. This 26-year-old patient had been in a motor vehicle accident. Persistent mediastinal widening prompted this CT at the level of the aortic arch. Notice small saccular pseudoaneurysm (arrows) off the medial aspect of the arch.

trauma. Two of these were detected primarily by CT, which was performed for evaluation of mediastinal widening.[31] Other single case reports also emphasize the utility of CT in these situations[32-34] (Fig. 7).

Aortic Transection and Rupture

In the acutely injured patient with blunt chest trauma angiography has traditionally been the mainstay in those patients who survive and are suspected of having aortic rupture.[35] Plain chest radiographs may provide an early diagnostic clue. CT may, however, play a role. This was demonstrated by Heiberg et al who successfully imaged four cases of aortic transection. In their cases CT findings included (1) false aneurysm, (2) linear lucency within the lumen, (3) marginal irregularity of the aorta, and (4) periaortic or intramural hematoma and dissection.[36] Aortography will probably, however, remain the dominant modality in this life threatening emergency.

Other Aneurysms

Mycotic aneurysms of the thoracic or abdominal aorta are uncommon, potentially catastrophic, and have an extremely poor prognosis. These aneurysms are usually ascending aortic in location although scattered cases of descending and abdominal aortic aneurysm can be found.[37] Angiographic diagnosis has usually been based on the finding of a saccular aneurysm in an unusual location free of atherosclerotic disease. Typical CT features in this disease are not known since only two cases with CT correlation have been described.[38,39] We have, however, seen three cases of primary mycotic aneurysm of the aorta that were primarily diagnosed by CT. One was located at the thoracoabdominal junction and the other two were in the infrarenal aorta. In two cases, changes in an adjacent structure such as vertebral body erosion, paraspinous fluid collection, and contained rupture into the psoas muscle allowed a confident diagnosis (Fig. 8). In a third case, sudden enlargement of a small abdominal aortic aneurysm in a septic patient led to the correct diagnosis. As a result of these experiences we believe that CT should be used primarily in the detection of these lethal aneurysms.

Aortic Dissection

Dissection of the thoracic aorta is one of the most common vascular surgical emergencies with 50 percent mortality in the first few weeks and 90 percent mortality within the first year if untreated.[40,41] Prompt recognition of the presence and extent of a dissection is therefore vital if appropriate medical or surgical therapy is to be initiated. In the past 6 years, it has become clear that contrast enhanced CT using rapid scans (2 seconds or less) is as accurate as angiography in the diagnosis of aortic dissection.[40,42-48] This fact is by virtue of its ability to display the aorta and surrounding structures in cross section and visualize displaced intimal flaps and calcification as well as other mural abnormalities without concern for proper radiographic positioning. Most authors have demonstrated nearly 100 percent correlation with angiography and those institutions using fast scanners generally had no false negative diagnoses and a very low false positive rate.[40,41,47,48] In one series of 21 dissections aortography did not demonstrate proximal extension in 2 patients while CT clearly showed the presence of an ascending aortic flap.[48] Another case report documented a ruptured type 3 dissection that was not diagnosed by biplane aortography and was directly detected with CT.[49]

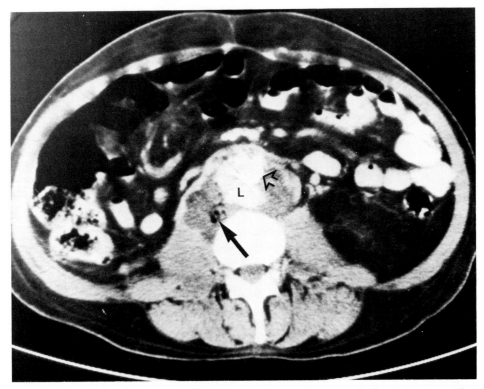

Fig. 8. Mycotic infrarenal aneurysm. Diabetic man with fever and sepsis. Contrast opacified lumen (L) is seen outside the confines of dense aortic calcification (open arrowhead). Free retroperitoneal rupture in the psoas muscles bilaterally is indicated by low density hematoma there. Infectious nature is also shown by the presence of gas (arrow) in the right psoas hematoma.

CT Findings in Aortic Dissection

The pertinent CT findings in dissection include: (1) Intimal flap with two lumens. (2) Delayed flow through the false lumen on dynamic scan. (3) Central displacement of intimal calcifications. (4) Compression or flattening of the true lumen. (5) High density blood in a thrombosed false lumen on precontrast scans. (6) Mediastinal, pericardial, or pleural hematomas.

Direct visualization of the intimal flap and two channels is pathognomonic for the disease (Fig. 9). The demonstration of slow flow in the false lumen by dynamic scanning is not essential to the diagnosis but may be helpful. If the false channel is thrombosed the diagnosis can be made on the basis of intimal calcification displacement or true luminal flattening (Fig. 10). Occasionally, a circumferential false lumen that is thrombosed may be difficult to distinguish from an aorta peripheral plaque or an aneurysm with thrombus; aortography will usually serve to facilitate the diagnosis (Fig. 11). Free rupture into the pericardial sac with high density pericardial hematoma (Fig. 12) is an ominous sign that cannot be demonstrated with angiography. Pleural blood, on the other hand, may be a reflection of either aneurysm rupture or dissection.

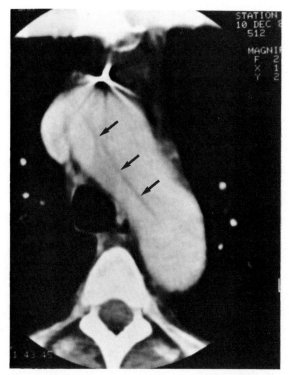

Fig. 9. Dissection of the aortic arch. Note well defined intimal flap (arrows) separating the two lumens. This dissection would be classified as proximal.

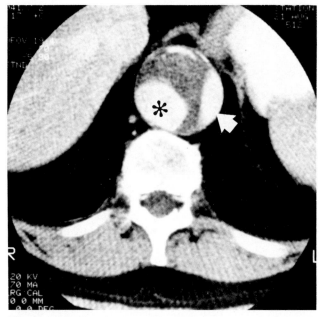

Fig. 10. Distal aortic dissection. Two opacified lumens. The true lumen (arrow) is characteristically flattened and compressed laterally while the false lumen (*) is partially thrombosed.

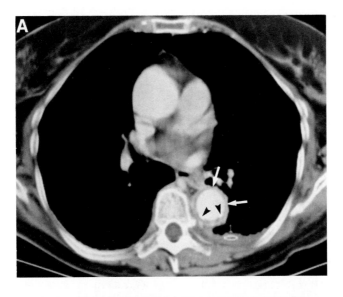

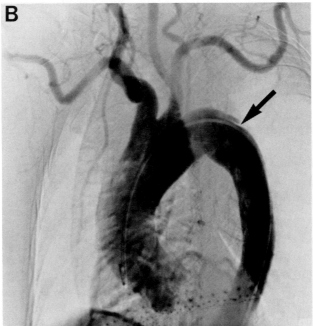

Fig. 11. Circumferential false lumen with thrombosis. CT (A) shows opacified true lumen with thin rim of surrounding thrombosed false lumen (arrows). Note central displacement of intimal calcifications (arrowheads) and small left pleural hematoma (1). Thoracic aortogram (B) shows a small intimal tear (arrow) indicating the presence of a dissection.

Limitations of CT in Dissection

Aortic branch involvement and the direction and patterns of flow in the true and false lumens cannot reliably be assessed by CT. Aortography, however, can easily document these findings. Aortic regurgitation is shown on angiography but not on CT and the site of an intimal tear is more reliably seen on angiography although this information may not be essential to the management of this condition.[50] False negative examinations can potentially occur due to streak artifacts or from partial volume averaging of adjacent calcifications in the aortic arch, which may spuriously suggest displacement into the lumen.[10,51] Neointimal calcifications on the luminal surface of old mural thrombus may also be mistaken for intimal calcification displacement.

In general, we strongly believe that CT should be ordered first in cases of suspected dissection and aortography reserved for situations in which CT is not diagnostic or incompletely diagnostic. Aortography also is indicated when surgery is contemplated and complete evaluation of branch vessels is necessary although in most cases CT can provide adequate information.

Graft Infection

One of the more common vascular surgical semiemergencies in which CT has been particularly helpful is prosthetic graft infection. This lethal and morbid complication is seen in approximately 2 percent of all operations despite appropriate preventive measures. Morbidity and mortality range between 22 and 75 percent.[52-55] Early diagnosis and appropriate therapy are thus of vital importance since exsanguinating hemorrhage can occur from graft-enteric fistulae and/or anastomotic pseudoaneurysms associated with infection. Without the use of CT the diagnosis of an infected graft or graft-enteric fistula is difficult since most conventional radiologic evaluation is less useful. The occasional exception is gallium, ultrasound, and indium labeled white blood cells. CT is clearly the only reliable diagnostic test for the presence of graft infection since it alone can detect perigraft fluid and/or gas. Open groin wounds and anastomotic pseudoaneurysms can also easily be identified.

CT Findings in Graft Infection

The majority of patients with significant graft infection demonstrate perigraft fluid or soft tissue density as well as gas in or around the graft[56] (Figs. 13 and 14). Graft thrombosis often accompanies these findings.

Proximal or distal anastomotic pseudoaneurysms may also be seen in infection although their presence is not completely diagnostic since a pseudoaneurysm may form as a result of suture line disruption without infection (Fig. 15). Open groin wounds and sinus tracts are frequent findings since graft infection often begins in the groins and spreads to involve the retroperitoneal portions of the graft.[57,58] Injection of these groin sinus tracts with dilute contrast material ("CT sinography") has been helpful in identifying the extent of graft infection and whether or not the sinus communicates with more proximal portions of the graft.[56]

In the early postoperative period perigraft hematomas and gas may give the misleading impression of infection but careful follow-up will usually demonstrate resolution of these findings within 3–6 weeks of surgery.[52,53,59] If the findings are equivocal or the collection is enlarging, CT guided aspiration can be utilized as advocated by Cunat et al.[60]

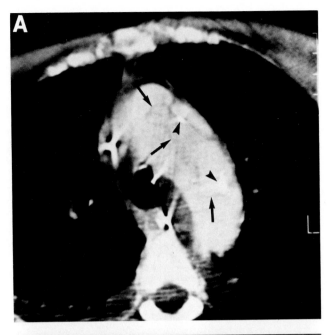

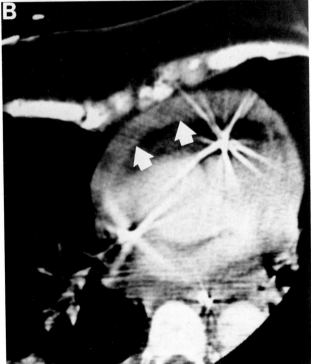

Fig. 12. Proximal aortic dissection with pericardial rupture. Scan at the level of the aortic arch (A) demonstrates dissected intima (arrows) with displaced intimal calcifications (arrowheads). At the level of the heart (B) pericardial blood (arrows) is demonstrated indicating free pericardial rupture. The patient expired shortly after performance of the CT.

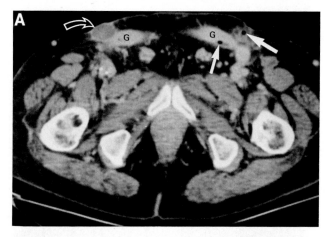

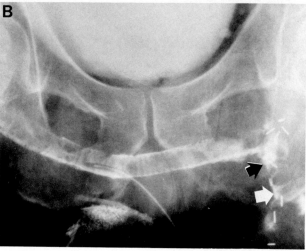

Fig. 13. Infected axillobifemoral graft. CT (A) at the level of the crossover portion of the graft demonstrates gas (arrows) and soft tissue surrounding the left sided anastomosis. Perigraft abscess (curved arrow) is seen anterior to the right sided anastomosis. Sinogram (B) through a draining sinus shows contrast surrounding the crossover portion of the graft with filling of some small perigraft abscesses (arrows) in the left groin.

Perhaps the most catastrophic of infectious complications is the development of a graft-enteric fistula (GEF). GEF probably develops as a sequela of chronic low-grade infection of the suture line and subsequent pseudoaneurysm formation or as a result of pressure between the duodenum and the suture line.[61] In the past 2 years several reports have documented the utility of CT in this heretofore difficult to diagnose disease in which up to 60 percent of patients die if gastrointestinal hemorrhage intervenes.[57,58,62] These reports, as well as our own experience at Northwestern University, indicate that virtually all patients with GEF will have some abnormality demonstrated on CT. In most cases the presence of proximal anastomotic gas, fluid, or pseudoaneurysm should be viewed with

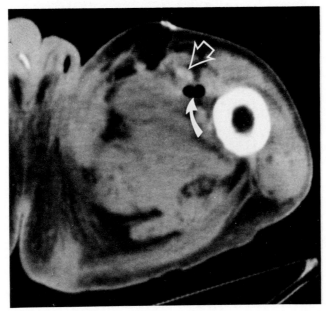

Fig. 14. Infected femoropopliteal graft. Gas (curved arrow) demonstrated adjacent to graft (open arrow).

alarm since many of these patients will have a fistula. Extravasation of orally ingested contrast material from the duodenum around the aortic graft is a rare finding, having been noted once in a report by Kukora et al.[63] Another report by Lineaweaver et al showed contrast extravasation from the aorta into the duodenum.[26] At Northwestern Memorial Hospital we have had the opportunity to evaluate three patients with surgically documented graft enteric fistula; all three had proximal anastomotic perigraft fluid and gas (Fig. 16). Finally, it should be noted that graft enteric fistula should be suspected whenever abnormalities are seen in the region of the proximal anastomosis despite an absence of clinical findings as was the case in two patients reported by Mark et al.[62]

Intraabdominal (Nongraft) Abscesses

A septic postsurgical patient may present significant problems in management since a patient with fever may not necessarily have a graft infection and may in fact have an intraabdominal or subcutaneous wound infection that does not threaten the graft. CT is superior to other modalities in the detection of these abscesses in retroperitoneal collections and has the significant advantage of identifying the relationship of the abscess to the graft. Percutaneous drainage of intraabdominal abscess guided by CT has become the standard approach to postsurgical abscesses.[56]

Hemorrhage

CT is very sensitive to the presence of extravasated blood and thus serves to accurately identify a hematoma in a patient who has bled before, during, or after surgery. When acute hemorrhage is suspected, CT without intravenous contrast will aid in appreci-

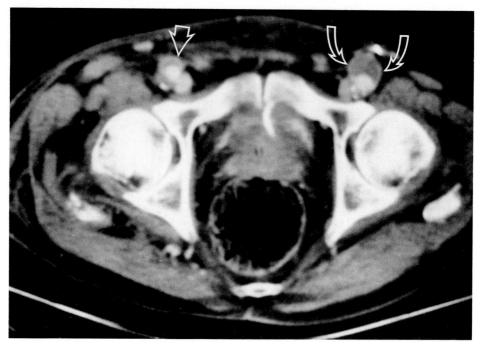

Fig. 15. Bilateral anastomotic pseudoaneurysms. Bilateral femoral-popliteal grafts have been placed. Larger left pseudoaneurysm (curved arrow) and smaller right pseudoaneurysm (open arrow) are demonstrated. Neither was evident on arteriography but the left pseudoaneurysm was clinically obvious.

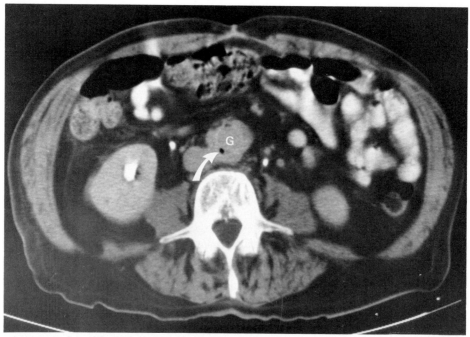

Fig. 16. Graft–enteric fistula. Aortic graft (G) is surrounded by fluid and gas (curved arrow). The findings are strongly suggestive of the presence of graft–enteric fistula.

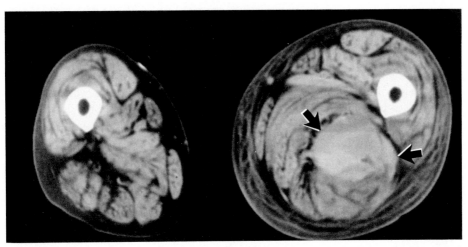

Fig. 17.   Large left thigh hematoma (arrows) is characteristic of the presence of fresh blood.

ation of the increased attenuation so characteristic of fresh blood in the abdomen, retroperitoneum, or extremities[64] (Fig. 17). Later on in their evolution hematomas decrease in attenuation and diminish in size. In general, CT can only occasionally identify the source of hemorrhage; angiography is better suited to that role.

Vascular Occlusion and Embolization

Limb threatening arterial thrombosis or ischemia is obviously treated emergently with angiography followed by thrombectomy or embolectomy and CT generally has little role acutely except in unusual cases. In those patients with repetitive episodes of arterial embolization, CT may suggest a cause such as graft enlargement and mural thrombus proximally or significant aortic atherosclerotic disease that was not fully appreciated angiographically.

Conclusions

CT plays a vital role in the evaluation of many vascular emergencies. It is the examination of choice in detection of thoracic and aortic aneurysm rupture as well as in the identification of mycotic aneurysms. In thoracic aortic dissection CT should precede angiography in virtually all cases since the superior information it provides outweighs the few small disadvantages it possesses. In graft infection with pseudoaneurysm or graft enteric fistula CT should be ordered early since it can directly image the two most important signs of graft infection: fluid and/or gas in or around the graft. Finally, CT plays a small but definite role in the identification of hematomas in the vascular surgical patient and in the identification of repetitive embolization and occlusive disease.

MAGNETIC RESONANCE

Magnetic resonance has become an increasingly used tool in a few short years for a variety of conditions. Several advantages offered by MR are similar to other imaging modalities without the associated disadvantages. Unlike ultrasound, MR provides a larger field of view and is not dependent on the patient body habitus or the operator's skill. Both CT and MR provide superb spatial resolution but MR provides better soft tissue contrast resolution.[65] Intravenous injection of contrast media is unnecessary as flowing blood results in natural contrast between the blood and cardiovascular structures.[66,67] Among the disadvantages of MR are image degradation because of patient motion, which occurs as a result of slower scanning times.[68] Patients may also become claustrophobic in most currently designed units. Also, certain patients are excluded from MR evaluation such as those with pacemakers and other internal prostheses with ferromagnetic properties, such as intracranial aneurysm clips.

Early reports indicated the potential usefulness of MR imaging for vascular abnormalities.[69,70] The multiplanar capabilities of this modality, that is, direct acquisition of sagittal, coronal, and transverse planes, are particularly useful for assessment of many vascular abnormalities. The following section will discuss the use of magnetic resonance in a variety of vascular emergencies. Evaluation of aortic dissections, aortic aneurysms, the complications of aneurysms such as rupture with hematoma and the differentiation of this from inflammatory aneurysms, and vascular graft complications will be included.

MR imaging of aortic dissections can demonstrate both type A and type B forms and show their extent.[71-74] Detection of the intimal flap, the most specific sign of dissection, has been reported as seen in 100 percent of cases[72,73] and in 58 percent of cases in another series.[74] The flap is seen by MR as a thin linear soft tissue density contrasted by the lack of signal from flowing blood within the true and false lumen (Fig. 18). Occasionally,

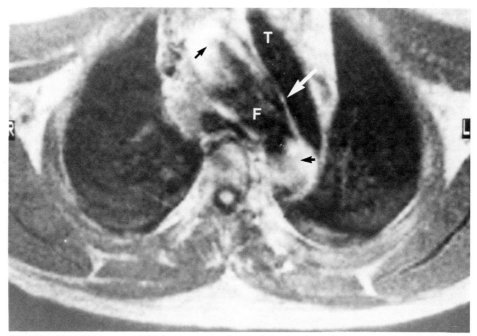

Fig. 18. Gated transverse MR image at the level of the aortic arch in a patient with Marfan's syndrome complicated by aortic dissection. Note the intimal flap (white arrow) highlighted by the lack of signal from flowing blood within the true (T) and false (F) lumen. The bright regions of intensity within the false lumen (small arrows) are secondary to slower blood flow allowing identification of this lumen.

difficulty arises in identification of the intimal flap when the false lumen is thrombosed resulting in the problem of distinguishing a thrombosed dissection from a thoracic aneurysm with mural thrombus. Other signs of dissection include: compression of the true lumen by the false lumen, the differences in flow between the true and false lumens, and the less reliable signs of disparate size of the ascending and descending thoracic aortic segments. Often there is slower blood flow within the false channel of a dissection. This is usually seen on MR as a difference in signal intensity between the true and false channels. Because of slower blood flow in the false channel the signal intensity in the false channel is greater on both the first and second echo images or on the second echo image alone. When the false channel also contains thrombus several findings have been used to differentiate slow flow from thrombus. One finding is a relative decrease in signal intensity from the first to second echo image for the organized thrombus while slow flow shows a relative increase in signal intensity from the first to second echo image. Another finding is through the use of cardiac gating where changes in blood flow between diastole and systole differentiate slow flow from thrombus where, in contrast, no changes in signal intensity occur relative to the cardiac cycle.[72] The ability to image in multiple planes allows MR, unlike CT, to determine the extent of the dissection and any involvement of the arch vessels. With CT, reformatted images in the coronal and sagittal plane are possible but provide limited spatial resolution compared to MR. MR also demonstrates the origins of the celiac, superior mesenteric, and renal arteries from either the true or false lumen. Despite the overall advantage of MR there are some disadvantages. It is only possible to evaluate the hemodynamically stable patient as limited monitoring capabilities currently exist with MR. The high magnetic field strength excludes patients with pacemakers and ventilators. Overall, MR appears to be a very promising noninvasive modality for imaging aortic dissections in the stable patient.

MR imaging of aortic aneurysms has demonstrated the dimensions, internal constituents, and involvement of the branch vessels (Fig. 19). Studies have shown there is good agreement among MR, ultrasound (US), and CT in quantifying the maximum diameter of an aneurysm.[74-77] The internal constituents such as thrombus and atherosclerotic debris within aneurysms have been identified with MR.[74,75,77] Organized thrombus identification was based on similar criteria mentioned above wherein the thrombus decreases in relative signal intensity from the first to second echo. The atheromatous debris, in contrast, was found to remain at nearly the same signal intensity on the first and second echo images.[75] Involvement of the aortic arch branches has been seen with MR.[74] Involvement of the renal arteries is well demonstrated with MR identifying them in greater than 90 percent.[75-78] Extension of the aneurysm into the iliac arteries and involvement of the visceral vessels is possible to assess with MR. Comparison of MR to US shows US less reliably demonstrates the renal arteries, iliac extension, and involvement of the visceral vessels by aortic aneurysms.[75-78] Comparison of MR to angiography has shown MR is superior for delineation of thrombus and demonstration of aortic wall thickness. Angiography is superior for visualizing renal artery stenosis and for the demonstration of multiple renal arteries.[78] MR is an accurate method for providing the information necessary for surveillance and surgical correction of aortic aneurysms. Other modalities, such as US, may be used for screening aneurysms while MR may be reserved for the cases where US fails to provide information about the renal, visceral, and iliac arterial involvement.

MR imaging has also been used for the study of posttraumatic false aneurysms.[79] It was found that the major advantage of MR over CT was the ability of MR to acquire direct sagittal and coronal images without loss of spatial resolution. This allowed imaging of the mediastinal vessels along their axes.

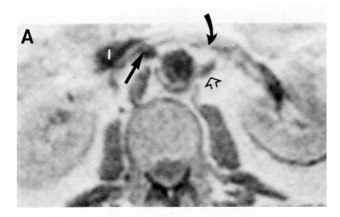

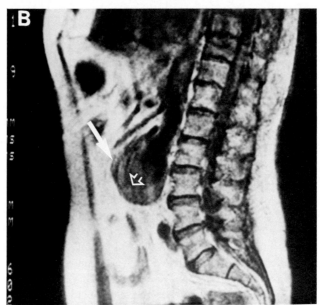

Fig. 19. (A) Transverse MR image at the level of the renal arteries in a patient with an infrarenal abdominal aortic aneurysm. Note demonstration of the left (open arrow) and right (closed arrow) renal artery without the use of contrast media and the lack of aneurysmal dilatation at this level. The left renal vein is coursing anterior to the aorta (curved arrow) into the inferior vena cava (1). (B) Sagittal MR image demonstrating the infrarenal abdominal aortic aneurysm (white arrow) filled eccentrically with organized thrombus of low intensity (open arrow).

One of the most life threatening complications of aortic aneurysms is rupture. In certain circumstances difficulty arises with CT in differentiating between hemorrhage surrounding the aorta and inflammatory fibrosis. MR imaging allows differentiation between these two entities. When acute hemorrhage occurs the MR appearance is that of tissue with greater intensity than muscle but less than that of fat on the T1 weighted sequence while on the T2 sequence the hemorrhage has similar intensity to that of fat (Fig. 20).

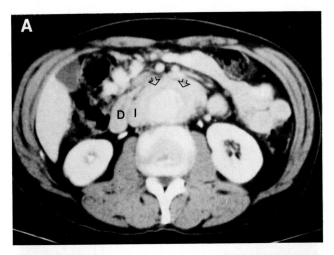

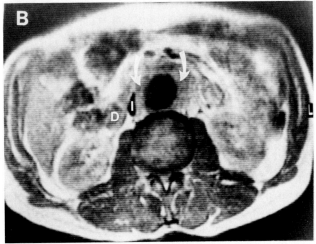

Fig. 20. (A) Transverse CT section at the level of an abdominal aortic aneurysm in a patient with persistent back pain suspected of rupture. Note the collection of material around the aorta (open arrows) involving the inferior vena cava (I). The duodenum is lateral to the inferior vena cava (D). (B and C) Transverse first echo MR image (B) demonstrates low intensity material surrounding the aortic aneurysm (curved arrows) that decreases further in relative intensity on the second echo image (C curved arrows).

Fig. 20 C continued on next page

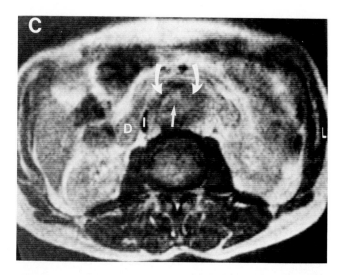

(Fig. 20. C continued from previous page)   On the second echo
image (C), the signal within the aortic lumen (small lumen) most
likely indicates slower blood flow within the aneurysm. The MR
intensity patterns demonstrated in this patient are not characteristic
of an aortic rupture with hematoma. The intensity is more typical
of a fibrous reaction such as occurs with inflammatory fibrosis
around the aorta. The inferior vena cava is adherent to the fibrous
material and distorted in shape (closed arrow). D = duodenum.

Chronic hematoma surrounding the aorta on MR has intensity similar to fat and slightly
more than muscle on both the T1 and T2 weighted sequences. MR is also useful in
differentiating this material from adenopathy.

Assessment of aortoiliofemoral grafts is often necessary to determine patency and
such complications as infection. As a consequence of the increased morbidity and mortality associated with infections of these grafts it is imperative to detect and manage this
problem as quickly as possible. The diagnosis of an infected graft by many radiologic
modalities, especially in an early stage, has been difficult.[58,80–82] Preliminary results with
MR have shown it is very sensitive in detecting graft infection without the use of contrast
material. MR was capable of demonstrating the extent of infection, the development of an
associated abscess, the patency of the graft, and the possible involvement of veins.[83]

In summary, abnormalities of the aorta that either enlarge (aneurysm) or diminish
(coarctation) the aortic lumen size, cause internal defects (dissection) or external defects
(rupture with hematoma) are demonstrable with MR. The multiplanar imaging capabilities of MR allow assessment of the relationship of these abnormalities to the arch and
visceral vessels. This information often can only be estimated on transverse CT images
and many times requires angiography. MR is particularly helpful in those patients in
whom iodinated contrast material is relatively or absolutely contraindicated by renal
insufficiency, allergy, or cardiac disease. Present problems in monitoring of critically ill
patients have restricted the use of MR to more stable patients for the present. Advances in
hardware and software for magnetic resonance should decrease the imaging time allowing
faster studies for the patient with a vascular emergency. Currently, MR of the vascular

system, particularly of the aorta, inferior vena cava, and major blood vessels shows great potential. MR allows delineation of anatomic structures and in the future it may provide more information on tissue metabolism.

REFERENCES

1. Eriksson I, Hemmingsson A, Lindgren PG: Diagnosis of abdominal aortic aneurysms by aortography, computer tomography and ultrasound. Acta Radiol Diagnos 21:209, 1980
2. Larsson EM, Albrechtsson U, Christenson JT: Computed tomography versus aortography for preoperative evaluation of abdominal aortic aneurysm. Acta Radiol Diagnos 25:95, 1981
3. Anderson PE, Lorentzen JE: Comparison of computed tomography and aortography in abdominal aortic aneurysms. J Comput Assist Tomgr 7:670, 1983
4. Sanders JH Jr, Malave S, Neiman HL, et al: Thoracic aortic imaging without angiography. Arch Surg 114:1326, 1979
5. Gomes MN, Wallace RB: Present status of abdominal aorta imaging by computed tomography. J Cardiovasc Surg 26:1, 1985
6. Pond GD, Hillman B: Evaluation of aneurysms by computed tomography. Surgery 89(2):216, 1981
7. Dixon AK, Springall RG, Kelsey Fry I, et al: Computed tomography (CT) of abdominal aortic aneurysms: determination of longitudinal extent. Br J Surg 68:47, 1981
8. Wolk LA, Pasdar H, McKeown JJ Jr, et al: Computerized tomography in the diagnosis of abdominal aortic aneurysms. Surg Gynecol Obstet 153:229, 1981
9. Gomes MN, Hufnagel CA: CT scanning: a new method for the diagnosis of abdominal aortic aneurysms. J Cardiovasc Surg 20:511, 1979
10. Godwin DJ, Korobkin M: Acute disease of the aorta: diagnosis by computed tomography and ultrasonography. Radiol Clin North Am 21(3):551, 1983
11. Christenson JT, Eklof B, Gustafson I.: Abdominal aortic aneurysms: Should they all be resected? Br J Surg 64:767, 1977
12. Cooley DA, DeBakey ME: Ruptured aneurysm of the abdominal aorta. Excision and homograft replacement. Postgrad Med 16:334, 1954
13. Lawire GM, Morris GC Jr, Crawford ES: Improved results of operation for ruptured abdominal aortic aneurysms. Surgery 85:483, 1979
14. Graham AL, Najafi H, Dye WS: Ruptured abdominal aortic aneurysm. Surgical management. Arch Surg 97:1024, 1968
15. Rosen A, Korobkin M, Silverman PM, et al: CT diagnosis of ruptured abdominal aortic aneurysm. AJR 143:265, 1984
16. Lippey ER, de Burgh M: Concurrent extraperitoneal and intracaval rupture of an abdominal aneurysm. Med J Aust 1:517, 1978
17. Sagel SS, Siegel MJ, Stanley RJ: Detection of retroperitoneal hemorrhage by computed tomography. AJR 129:403, 1977
18. Ginaldi S, Long WD: Concurrent dissection and intracaval rupture of an abdominal aortic aneurysm: CT findings. J Comput Assist Tomgr 9(2):369, 1985
19. Johnson WC, Gale ME, Gerzof SG, et al: The role of computed tomography in symptomatic aortic aneurysms. Surg Gynecol Obstet 162:49, 1986
20. Aiello MR, Cohen WN: Inflammatory aneurysm of the abdominal aorta. J Comput Assist Tomgr 4:265, 1980
21. Branch WT, Turley K, Crowell BH: Aortic aneurysm with retroperitoneal fibrosis and ureteral obstruction. Urology 9:292, 1977
22. Feldberg MAM, van Waes PFGM, ten Haken GB: CT diagnosis of perianeurysmal fibrotic reactions in aortoiliac aneurysm. J Comput Assist Tomgr 6:465, 1982

23. Pahira JJ, Wein AJ, Barker CF: Bilateral complete ureteral obstruction secondary to an abdominal aortic aneurysm with perianeurysmal fibrosis: diagnosis by computed tomography. J Urol 121:103, 1979

24. Ramirez AA, Riles TS, Imparato AM: CAT scans of inflammatory aneurysms: a new technique for preoperative diagnosis. Surgery 91:390, 1982

25. Vint VC, Usselman JA, Warmath MA: Aortic perianeurysmal fibrosis: CT density enhancement and ureteral obstruction. AJR 134:577, 1980

26. Lineaweaver WC, Clore F, Alexander RH: Computed tomographic diagnosis of acute aortoiliac catastrophes. Arch Surg 117:1095, 1982

27. Clayton MJ, Walsh JW, Brewer WH: Contained rupture of abdominal aortic aneurysms: sonographic and CT diagnosis. AJR 138:154, 1982

28. Christenson JT, Norgren L, Ribbe E, et al: A ruptured aortic aneurysm that "spontaneously healed." J Cardovasc Surg 25:571, 1984

29. Schecter LS, Held BT: Right sided extrapleural hematoma: an unusual presentation of ruptured aortic aneurysm. Chest 65:355, 1984

30. Kucich VA, Vogelzang RL, Hartz RS, et al: Ruptured thoracic aneurysm: an unusual presentation with early diagnosis by computed tomography. Radiology 160:87, 1986

31. Gundry SR, Burney RE, Mackenzie JR, et al: Traumatic pseudoaneurysms of the thoracic aorta. Arch Surg 119:1055, 1984

32. Moore EH, Farmer DW, Geller SC, et al: Computed tomography in the diagnosis of iatrogenic false aneurysms of the ascending aorta. AJR 142:1117, 1984

33. Harrington DP, Barth KH, White RI Jr, et al: Traumatic pseudoaneurysm of the thoracic aorta in close proximity to the anterior spinal artery: a therapeutic dilemma. Surgery 87:153, 1980

34. Chew FS, Panicek DM, Heitzman ER: Late discovery of a posttraumatic right aortic arch aneurysm. AJR 145:1001, 1985

35. Symbas PN, Tryas DH, Ware RE, et al: Rupture of the aorta. Ann Thorac Surg 15:405, 1973

36. Heiberg E, Wolverson MK, Sundaram M, et al: CT in aortic trauma. AJR 104:1119, 1983

37. Johansen K, Devin J: Mycotic aortic aneurysms. A reappraisal. Arch Surg 118:583, 1983

38. Pripstein S, Cavoto FV, Geritsen RW: Spontaneous mycotic aneurysm of the abdominal aorta. J Comput Assist Tomogr 3:681, 1979

39. Atlas, SW, Vogelzang RL, Bressler EL, et al: CT diagnosis of a mycotic aneurysm of the thoracoabdominal aorta. J Comput Assist Tomogr 8:1211, 1984

40. Thorsen MK, Sretto MAS, Lawson TL, et al: Dissecting aortic aneurysms: accuracy of computed tomographic diagnosis. Radiology 148:773, 1983

41. Viljanen T, Landtman M, Luosto R: Late results of the surgical treatment for aortic dissections. Thorac Cardiovasc Surgeon 33:8, 1985

42. Egan TJ, Neiman HL, Herman RJ, et al: Computed tomography in the diagnosis of aortic aneurysm dissection or traumatic injury. Radiology 136:141, 1980

43. Godwin JD, Herfkens RL, Skioldebrand CG, et al: Evaluation of dissections and aneurysms of the thoracic aorta by conventional and dynamic CT scanning. Radiology 136:125, 1980

44. Gross SC, Barr I, Eyler WR, et al: Computed tomography in dissection of the thoracic aorta. Radiology 136:135, 1980

45. Larde D, Belloir C, Vasile N, et al: Computed tomography of aortic dissection. Radiology 136:147, 1980

46. Moncada R, Churchill R, Reynes C, et al: Diagnosis of dissecting aortic aneurysm by computed tomography. Lancet 1:238, 1981

47. Parienty RA, Couffinhal JC, Wellers M, et al: Computed tomography versus aortography in diagnosis of aortic dissection. Cardiovasc Intervent Radiol 5:285, 1982

48. Oudkerk M, Overbosch E, Dee P: CT recognition of acute aortic dissection. AJR 141:671, 1983

49. Chaudhry A, Romero L, Pugatch RD, et al: Diagnosis of aortic dissection by computed tomography. Ann Thorac Surg 35:322, 1983

50. Miller DC, Stinson EB, Oyer PE: Operative treatment of aortic dissection. Experience with 125 patients over a sixteen-year period. J Thorac Cardiovasc Surg 78:365, 1979

51. Gallagher S, Dixon AK: Streak artifacts of the thoracic aorta: pseudodissection. J Comput Assist Tomogr 8:688, 1984

52. Bunt TJ: Synthetic vascular graft infections I. Graft infections. Surgery 93:733, 1983

53. Bunt TJ: Synthetic vascular graft infections II. Graft-enteric erosions and graft-enteric fistulas. Surgery 94:1, 1983

54. Jamieson CW, DeWeese JA, Rob CG: Infected arterial grafts. Ann Surg 181:850, 1975

55. Spanos PK, Gilsdorf RB, Sako Y: The management of infected abdominal aortic grafts and graft-enteric fistulas. Ann Surg 183:397, 1976

56. Vogelzang RL: The role of CT in reoperative aortic surgery, in JJ Bergan and JST Yao (eds.): Reoperative Arterial Surgery. Orlando: Grune & Stratton, 1986, pp. 33–58

57. Hilton S, Megibow AJ, Naidich DP: Computed tomography of the postoperative abdominal aorta. Radiology 145:403, 1982

58. Mark A, Moss AA, Lusby R: CT evaluation of complications of abdominal aortic surgery. Radiology 145:409, 1982

59. O'Hara PJ, Borkowski GP, Hertzer NR: Natural history of periprosthetic air on computerized axial tomographic examination of the abdomen following abdominal aortic aneurysm repair. J Vasc Surg 1:429, 1984

60. Cunat JS, Haaga R: Periaortic fluid aspiration for recognition of infected graft. AJR 139:251, 1982

61. Buchbinder D, Leather R, Shah D: Pathologic interactions between prosthetic aortic grafts and the gastrointestinal tract. Am J Surg 140:192, 1980

62. Mark AS, Moss AA, McCarthy S, et al: CT of aortoenteric fistulas. Invest Radiol 20:272, 1985

63. Kukora JS, Rushton FW, Cranston PE: New computed tomographic signs of aortoenteric fistula. Arch Surg 119:1073, 1984

64. Sagel SS, Siegel MJ, Stanley RJ: Detection of retroperitoneal hemorrhage by computed tomography. AJR 129:403, 1977

65. Pykett IL: MR imaging in medicine. Scientific American 246:78, 1982

66. Bradley WG, Waluch Y: Blood flow: Magnetic resonance imaging. Radiology 154:443, 1985

67. Axel L: Blood flow effects in magnetic resonance imaging. AJR 143:1157, 1984

68. Crooks LE, Ortendahl DA, Kaufman L, et al: Clinical efficiency of nuclear magnetic resonance imaging. Radiology 146:123, 1983

69. Higgins CB, Goldberg H, Hricak H, et al: Nuclear magnetic resonance imaging of vasculature of abdominal viscera: Normal and pathologic features. AJR 140:1217, 1983

70. Herfkens RJ, Higgins CB, Hricak H, et al: Nuclear magnetic resonance imaging of atherosclerotic disease. Radiology 148:161, 1983

71. Amparo EG, Higgins CB, Hoddick W, et al: Magnetic resonance imaging of aortic disease: Preliminary results. AJR 143:1203, 1984

72. Amparo EG, Higgins CB, Hricak H, et al: Aortic dissection: Magnetic resonance imaging. Radiology 155:399, 1985

73. Geisinger MA, Risius B, O'Donnell JA, et al: Thoracic aortic dissections: Magnetic resonance imaging. Radiology 155:407, 1985

74. Glazer HS, Gutierrez FT, Levitt RG, et al: The thoracic aorta studied by magnetic resonance. Radiology 157:149, 1985

75. Amparo EG, Hoddick WK, Hricak H, et al: Comparison of MR imaging and ultrasonography in the evaluation of abdominal aortic aneurysms. Radiology 154:451, 1985

76. Flak B, Li DK, Ho BB, et al: Magnetic resonance imaging of aneurysms of the abdominal aorta. AJR 144:991, 1985

77. Lee JKT, Ling D, Heiken JP, et al: Magnetic resonance imaging of abdominal aortic aneurysms. AJR 143:1197, 1984

78. Evancho AM, Oabkken M, Weidner W: Comparison of NMR imaging and aortography for preoperative evaluation of abdominal aortic aneurysm. Magnetic Resonance in Med. 2:41, 1985

79. Moore EH, Webb WR, Verrier ED, et al: MRI of chronic posttraumatic false aneurysms of the thoracic aorta. AJR 143:1195, 1984

80. Hedgcock MW, Eisenbert RL, Godding GAW: Complications relating to vascular prosthetic grafts. J Canad Assoc Radiol 31:137, 1980

81. Causey DA, Fajaman WA, Perdue GC, et al: Gallium-67 scintigraphy in postoperative synthetic graft infections. AJR 134:1041, 1980

82. Stevick CA, Fawcett HD: Aortoiliac-graft infection: Detection by leukocyte scan. Arch Surg 116:939, 1981

83. Justich E, Amparo EG, Hricak H, et al: Infected aortoiliofemoral grafts: Magnetic resonance imaging. Radiology 154:133, 1985

D.E. Strandness, Jr.

Noninvasive Tests in Vascular Emergencies

Noninvasive tests are not required for the evaluation of most vascular emergencies. The decision with regard to treatment must be based upon the clinical problem, the perceived time frame in which intervention must be planned, and the desired endpoint. For most vascular emergencies it is unusual for the results of most tests to change the therapy. On the other hand, the information gained may modify the therapeutic approach and permit a better evaluation of the end result. Unfortunately, there is no large body of data available to dictate the exact indications for testing, the interpretation of the results, and the ultimate place for the modality being used in vascular emergencies. For this reason, the reader is cautioned that the views expressed are largely those of the author and based upon experience rather than any controlled studies.

ACUTE ARTERIAL OCCLUSION

Patients with acute limb ischemia must be considered in the two major categories where arterial occlusion is known to occur. The first is related to trauma—blunt or penetrating where the injury to the vessel is but one part of the clinical picture. The other occurs when the arterial occlusion occurred because of a "disease endpoint," i.e. thrombosis on an atherosclerotic plaque or emboli from a site proximal to the site where the obstruction occurs.

The five "Ps"—pain, pallor, paresthesias, paralysis, and pulselessness are well known endpoints of acute ischemia and serve to emphasize those highlights of the clinical problem that are important in evaluating the location of the occlusion and the extent of the ischemia. To this list of five items should be added another "P," the physician, because it is his or her perception of the event that is the most critical to the outcome.

Before going into the clinical evaluation, it is important to ask which noninvasive tests might be used in such a setting. They must be useable within the time-frame of a well-conducted but often rapid clinical review of the patient's status. The only device that

Vascular Surgical Emergencies
ISBN 0-8089-1843-5

readily fits this category is a continuous wave Doppler with a blood pressure cuff for making measurements of ankle blood pressure.[1-3] The use of this device will not delay implementation of other diagnostic tests or therapeutic interventions.

DEGREE OF ISCHEMIA

For the patients with limb-threatening ischemia who present with pain, pallor, loss of cutaneous sensation, and early changes in motor function, the issue is clear—nothing short of some associated life-threatening complication should delay operative correction of the arterial occlusion. If a continuous wave (CW) Doppler is used in these patients, there will be no detectable flow signals from either the dorsalis pedis, posterior tibial, or peroneal arteries at the level of the ankle. One useful bit of information can be obtained by assessing the noninvolved limb by noting the velocity patterns (monophasic versus triphasic) and measuring the ankle/arm index (AAI).[4] If the velocity patterns and ankle pressures are within a normal range (AAI $\geq$ 1.0), it is reasonable to assume that the circulatory status of the involved limb was normal prior to the event that led to the occlusion and the ischemia.[2,3] If the AAI is abnormal ($<$ 1.0), it is reasonable to assume that the patient had chronic arterial disease in both limbs prior to the emergency.

One might argue that the acute event could involve both limbs—particularly when it is secondary to emboli and confuse the interpretation in the last paragraph. In my experience, acute arterial occlusions nearly always result in the development of some symptoms unless they involve a single arterial segment, such as the peroneal artery, which does not normally provide a major portion of the flow to the foot.

There are situations in which ischemia is present but not limb-threatening. How can these situations be recognized and distinguished from those in which immediate action is required? In my experience this can be recognized by the following elements: (1) pain is absent; (2) the patient describes numb toes but light touch sensation is preserved; (3) the foot is cool but not cold. In this circumstance, the Doppler assessment may provide confirming information. The findings often fall into the following categories:

1. Velocity signals are present in the tibial arteries but monophasic. Interpretation—collateral flow is usually adequate to maintain viability.
2. AAI $>$ 0.5, limb viability is not in question, collaterals are excellent and flow will improve even if nothing is done.
3. AAI $<$ 0.5. Under these circumstances, it is most important to examine the absolute values of the systolic pressure. If the pressure is greater than 50 mmHg, limb viability is not threatened. If it is below 50 mmHg, collateral function is marginal *at that time.*

Under these circumstances, there is no immediate need for operative correction (within the first four hours) and the work-up may be more systematic and include preoperative arteriography.

LEVEL AND EXTENT OF OBSTRUCTION

The lack of pulses confirms two things—that the perfusion pressure at the site of examination is low and the most proximal level of the arterial occlusion. For example, absence of pulses distal to a normal femoral pulse tells the examiner that the most proximal occlusion is the superficial femoral artery. Unfortunately, it does not tell the observer if there are other areas of occlusion. This is, of course, important information that could be obtained by a quick and suitable survey with the CW Doppler.

To do this effectively and accurately there are several cardinal rules that must be followed:

1. Always examine comparable sites for both limbs. Why? The findings from the noninvolved limb usually serve as the normal control. The exception to this is when there was preexisting arterial disease. This would have been suspected by the finding of an AAI of less than 1.0 in the unaffected limb.
2. Always examine the same sites—common femoral, midsuperficial femoral, popliteal, tibial, and peroneal arteries.
3. Remember that normal velocity signals are always triphasic in the lower limb arteries. There is forward flow, reverse flow, forward flow, all within each heart cycle.
4. Velocity signals when detectable distal to sites of acute occlusion are always monophasic.
5. Absence of a flow signal from a vessel segment close to the site of occlusion is strongly suggestive that the artery is also occluded. Example, if the superficial femoral artery is occluded, the lack of detectable flow in the popliteal artery suggests it is also blocked.
6. Absence of a flow velocity signal from the tibial and peroneal arteries at the ankle does not necessarily suggest that the artery in question is occluded unless one of the other vessels at that level has flow. If no flow is detected from both of the tibial vessels, it could be secondary to an occlusion, but could also be due to the fact that the perfusion pressure at this point in time is extremely low ($<$ 20–30 mmHg).
7. Audible flow velocity signals just proximal to an acutely occluded artery may have a "thumping" sound. This is easily recognized.
8. If the acute occlusion is associated with blood loss such as with a fracture, there will be accentuation of the reverse flow component of the triphasic waveform in the unaffected limb. This is because of the fact that as the peripheral resistance rises to maintain the central aortic perfusion pressure, the reverse flow component becomes more prominent.

THERAPEUTIC APPROACH

As stated earlier, the results of any noninvasive test in the emergency situation rarely influence the decision for operative correction when the ischemia is severe enough to threaten limb viability. There is one situation in which nonoperative management may be indicated and suggested by the results of the survey with the CW Doppler and measurements of the ankle pressure. If the occlusions are confined to the tibial arteries and the collateral circulation is adequate to maintain viability, a nonoperative approach may be used.[5] This can be suggested by the following findings: (1) the presence of normal velocity signals in the popliteal artery; (2) the presence of blood flow in one or both tibial arteries at the ankle; and (3) an ankle systolic pressure above 50 mmHg. If flow is not detectable from either the dorsalis pedis or posterior tibial artery, it is important to determine if there is a contribution to the foot by the peroneal artery as it courses around the lateral malleolus.

It has been my experience that chronic occlusions distal to the popliteal trifurcation will generally not lead to the development of severe intermittent claudication.[6] In addition, the collateral circulation is so good below the knee that following an acute occlusion, perfusion pressure will increase considerably over the ensuing days to weeks as the collaterals open and dilate to accommodate the developing increase in blood flow.[5]

The one situation that requires considerable judgment is when there is normal popliteal artery flow and no detectable flow signals at the ankle level. If the foot is clearly viable and there is no rest pain, it can be predicted that flow will improve over the ensuing days. Any time the occlusion is in or proximal to the popliteal artery, surgical correction is indicated even if the foot is clearly viable. This is due to the fact that the patient will have intermittent claudication if the obstruction is not corrected.

UPPER EXTREMITY

Most of the principles enumerated above also apply to the arm with the management dictated by the location and extent of the occlusion. The Doppler survey can quickly be done and complimented by the measurement of upper arm and wrist pressures. The issue with regard to exercise-induced ischemia when acute occlusions are treated nonoperatively is not as clear as it is with the legs, presumably because of the excellent collateral circulation and the occupational requirements for arm use. Obviously the surgeon must err on the side of restoring blood flow at the time when it is most easily accomplished. This is best done as close to the time the obstruction occurred as possible.

ACUTE VENOUS THROMBOSIS

Acute occlusion of the venous system should be considered in terms of the anatomic location, superficial or deep, and the clinical implications of the occurrence. The term thrombophlebitis is commonly used to include acute thrombosis of both the superficial and deep veins but in the author's view, this is not correct. Acute thrombosis of most superficial veins is often secondary to an inflammatory event and properly deserves the classification of thrombophlebitis.[7] On the other hand, deep venous thrombosis is not associated with significant inflammation and thus should not be included in the category of "phlebitis."

Superficial venous thrombophlebitis is usually easily recognized by the erythema, exquisite local tenderness, and the presence of a palpable cord. If there is any question about the diagnosis, the CW Doppler can easily be used to settle the issue. There will be no flow in the involved vein because it always thromboses as a part of the inflammatory event. If flow is detected from the vein in the inflamed area, it is very likely that cellulitis is the diagnosis and not thrombophlebitis.

With acute deep venous thrombosis, the diagnosis must always be confirmed or rejected by some objective direct or indirect test.[8] Given the experience with several different modalities, it is now possible to recommend a reasonable approach that is dictated by the availability of the testing methods. It is also clear that the results of the noninvasive tests are sufficiently accurate to permit the diagnosis to be rapidly made so that the proper treatment can be instituted without any unusual delay.

Those patients who are suspected of harboring deep venous thrombi during the waking hours should have the noninvasive test performed immediately. When the diagnosis is suspected during the evening or night, it may be appropriate to start heparin therapy and delay the performance of the test for the following morning. This probably adds very little risk for the patient and only postpones the testing procedure to a time when it can be more efficiently performed. However, if the noninvasive laboratory functions on a call schedule, it is certainly possible to establish the diagnosis early and decide about the proper course of therapy to be employed.

The following noninvasive tests may be used to confirm or reject the diagnosis: (1) continuous wave Doppler;[9] (2) impedance or strain gauge plethysmography;[10,11] (3) phleborheography;[12] and (4) ultrasonic duplex scanning.[13]

The CW Doppler assessment is based upon the examination of those major veins that are accessible to this form of energy. These include the external iliac, common femoral, superficial femoral, popliteal, and posterior tibial veins. In the arm, it is feasible to assess the subclavian, axillary, and brachial veins. The application is based upon the loss of flow in the occluded segment and the detection of abnormal flow patterns in veins proximal to the sites of involvement. The technique has been extensively described so it will not be covered further at this time.

The accuracy of the Doppler technique depends heavily upon the experience of the operator but can be used to detect occlusions at each of the sites listed above. The sensitivity for detecting thrombi in proximal veins (popliteal and above) should approach 90 percent with a specificity of 90 percent. For thrombi confined to the veins of the calf, the accuracy is in the range of 80 percent.[14]

The plethysmographic methods depend upon measurement of changes in venous emptying when a cuff is placed on the thigh to temporarily block venous outflow. These approaches produce very good results with proximal venous occlusions. The reported sensitivity and specificity are in the range of 90 percent for these methods. They are not useful for the detection of thrombi confined to the calf.

The latest method to be utilized is ultrasonic Duplex scanning, which is the most promising technique yet to appear. Its great virtue is that it can be used to directly visualize and assess the patency of all the major veins that are commonly the site of venous thrombosis. Thrombi are readily observed, particularly when they are quite fresh. In addition, it is possible to assess propagation, lysis, organization, and recanalization. Not enough work has yet been done to correctly assess its final role but it appears that this will be the definitive test for the future.[13]

The proper role for these noninvasive tests now appears quite clear. If the noninvasive test is unequivocally positive, then it is appropriate to treat without a confirming phlebogram. For the patient with a normal test, it is safe to withhold treatment with certain provisos. If calf vein thrombosis is suspected, it may be necessary to consider doing a phlebogram unless Duplex scanning is available, which can be used to visualize the veins below the knee. It must be emphasized that phlebography should always be used if the noninvasive tests listed above are not available.

For the patient with a venous injury secondary to blunt or penetrating trauma, it is not feasible to utilize any of the noninvasive tests that require application of cuffs or gauges to the limb. The CW Doppler can be used and is probably the technique of choice if information is desired with regard to either disruption or occlusion of a major venous segment. There is virtually no experience with Duplex scanning in this regard, so we can only speculate on its utility. Since venous injuries are so commonly associated with arterial injury, the urgency to revascularize the limb will obviously dictate the type and timing of the diagnostic tests to be utilized.

CEREBROVASCULAR EMERGENCIES

If a noninvasive test is to be used in this setting, it will have to provide useful clues that might alter the need for an arteriogram. With a suspected injury to the carotid artery, there is a need for arteriography regardless of the findings by noninvasive testing. The one situation in which this might not hold true is if the carotid artery is found to be totally occluded. Under these circumstances, arteriography might be avoided, but at present most surgeons would feel most comfortable with arteriographic confirmation. The same would appear to be true with acute dissections even though they may have been suspected by ultrasonic Duplex scanning.

If a noninvasive test is to be used, which should it be? This will be determined by the urgency of the situation, the time required to do the study and the information that is desired. These can be considered in terms of the following categories: (1) indirect tests—supraorbital Doppler and oculoplethysmography—OPG-Gee;[15,16] and (2) the direct methods—CW Doppler and Duplex scanning.[17,18]

The indirect tests will become positive if the internal carotid artery is occluded or the diameter is severely reduced ($>$60 percent). The major problem with the indirect tests is that they cannot distinguish between a high grade stenosis or total occlusion, a fact that is of considerable importance from a therapeutic standpoint.[15,16] The direct tests—particularly Duplex scanning—are very good for detecting an acute occlusion as well as grading the degree of stenosis.[18]

When an operative procedure has been performed the surgeon will require immediate confirmation of the result if ischemic complications occur in the first 24 hours.[19] It is mandatory to reexamine the carotid artery and if possible identify the basis for the event. While the presence of a fresh wound compromises the testing procedure, it is now possible to apply a sterile drape to the wound, which protects the sterility of the area and permits transmission of ultrasound. If an OPG-GEE is available, this may also be used. However, no single institution has enough experience in this setting to provide firm guidelines as to which testing procedures should be done. Obviously when time is of the essence, a rapid trip back to the operating room may be the only suitable approach since correction of a technical problem may prevent irreversible cerebral damage. In the operating room, it is often useful to apply one of the direct methods such as CW Doppler to assess the state of the internal carotid artery.[20] If it is occluded, the vessel must be opened to extract the thrombus and assess the basis for the occlusion. If the carotid artery is patent, the surgeon must do an arteriogram to determine if an intimal flap with an associated thrombus is present.

When a neurologic event occurs during the period when the patient is back on the ward, a noninvasive test may be usefully applied. The finding of a total occlusion by Duplex scanning would at least document the basis for the event. If a high grade stenosis were found, it would strongly suggest a technical error. The management at this point would depend upon the nature of the neurological event and the judgment of the surgeon.

The following guidelines are suggested but admittedly are not based upon a great deal of experience:

1. A transient ischemic event with the finding of a total occlusion by Duplex scanning. An arteriogram is optional but could be done to verify the Duplex scan.
2. A completed stroke with total occlusion. In this setting, the surgeon may be advised to accept the adverse event with the hope that improvement may occur.
3. A transient ischemic event with the finding of a patent internal carotid artery. In this setting contrast arteriography is certainly warranted even if the Duplex study is reported as normal. The reason is that documentation is essential since the finding of an intimal flap or residual stenosis may be the grounds for reexploration and correction.
4. A completed stroke with the finding of a patent internal carotid artery. Accept the adverse event because very little would probably be gained by a more aggressive approach.

MONITORING

An important adjunctive role for noninvasive tests is to assist the surgeon in the documentation of the outcome of the chosen therapeutic approach. There are a few general rules that apply and can be used both in the operating room and during the early postoperative period. These are as follows:

1. Complete correction should leave the patient normal in hemodynamic terms.
2. Partial correction will result in an increase in pressure and flow but not to the level found normally. It is in this situation that a great deal of judgment is required on the part of the surgeon.

The only equipment required is a gas sterilized continuous wave Doppler probe that can be used both in the operative field and in vessels distal to the site of the operative intervention.[20,21] The rules to be followed are simple in concept, i.e., the velocity signal and pressures at the sites furthest removed should be restored to normal.[22] As many surgeons know, however, there are combinations and permutations that require considerable judgment. My own practice has been to order an arteriogram for *any finding* that suggests the correction has been incomplete.

Some of the more difficult situations arise when the patient has sustained an acute occlusion in the setting of preexisting occlusive arterial disease. It may not be feasible in this setting to completely correct both the acute and chronic changes that exist in the arterial supply. The goal is oftentimes to simply remove the acute occlusion while at the same time protecting and preserving the collateral circulation that was functioning at the time of the acute event. While the status of the circulation may not have been known, the rules with regard to the effectiveness of the collateral circulation in chronic arterial occlusion generally apply. These have been covered earlier and will not be repeated here.

In the case of the carotid artery, all monitoring methods used in the neck are designed to document the results in the operated segment and the first few centimeters distally.[23,24] At the present time, arteriography is the obvious gold standard and the one most widely applied. It is the opinion of this author that arteriography is mandatory whenever an emergency procedure is done to correct an acute event in the carotid artery. We would still utilize the gas sterilized Doppler probe to scan the operative arterial segment but still insist upon anatomic verification of the immediate result.

Because of the widespread use of invasive diagnostic and therapeutic arteriographic approaches, it is important to document the status of the arterial circulation prior to and following each procedure. This is not commonly done even in our own institution and failure to do so occasionally leads to confusing situations. This is particularly true when there is preexisting disease and the development of a new event. It is very helpful to know what the AAI was before a catheter is placed. If this is unknown, then one can never be sure what the magnitude of the new event represents. Of course, if the patient has a normal AAI it should remain so. On the other hand, a change in the degree of abnormality and its significance depends entirely upon the status of the circulation prior to the invasive procedure. Thus, the simple measurement of ankle systolic blood pressure should be a routine procedure whenever an invasive arterial study or therapy is planned.

CONCLUSIONS

When faced with a vascular emergency, the prime consideration is preservation of life and limb. Under these circumstances, the judgment of the surgeon is critical with regard to timing of intervention and the necessary diagnostic tests to permit this to occur. Most diagnostic tests, invasive and noninvasive, will not change the proposed therapy. Yet, useful information may be obtained that may modify the therapeutic approach and certainly provide a better basis for evaluating the outcome.

REFERENCES

1. Strandness DE Jr, Schultz RD, Sumner DS, et al: Ultrasonic flow detection: A useful technique in the evaluation of peripheral vascular disease. Am J Surg 113:311, 1967
2. Yao JST, Hobbs JT, Irvine WT: Ankle systolic pressure measurements in arterial diseases affecting the lower extremities. Br J Surg 56:676, 1969
3. Carter SA, Lezack JD: Digital systolic pressures in the lower limbs in arterial disease. Circulation 43:905, 1971
4. Knox RA, Strandness DE Jr: Ultrasound techniques for evaluating lower extremity arterial occlusion. Sem Ultrasound 2(4):264, 1981
5. Strandness DE Jr: Acute arterial occlusion, in Strandness DE Jr. (ed.): Peripheral Arterial Disease: A Physiologic Approach. Boston, Little, Brown and Co. 1969, p. 217
6. Strandness DE Jr: Effect of arterial obstruction on exercise. in Strandness DE Jr (ed.): Peripheral Arterial Disease: A Physiologic Approach. Boston, Little, Brown and Co., 1969, p. 61
7. Strandness DE Jr, Thiele BC: Venous thrombosis and pulmonary embolism, in Strandness DE Jr and Thiele BC (eds.): Selected Topics in Venous Disorders: Pathophysiology, Diagnosis and Treatment. Mt. Kisco, New York, Futura Publishing Co., 1981, p. 79
8. Haeger K: Problems of acute deep venous thrombosis. 1. The interpretation of signs and symptoms. Angiology 20:219, 1969
9. Sumner DS: Doppler evaluation of the venous circulation, in Rutherford RB (ed.): Vascular Surgery, 2nd Ed. Philadelphia, WB Saunders, 1985, p. 185
10. Hull R, Van Aken WG, Hirsh J, et al: Impedance plethysmography using the occlusive cuff technique in the diagnosis of venous thrombosis. Circulation 53:696, 1976

11. Cramer MM, Langlois YE, Beach KW, et al: Standardization of venous flow measurement by strain gauge plethysmography in normal subjects. Bruit 7:33, 1983
12. Cranley JJ, Canos AJ, Mahalingham K: Diagnosis of deep venous thrombosis by phleborheography in Bergan JJ and Yao JST (eds.): Venous Problems, Chicago, Year Book Publications, 1978, p. 187
13. Strandness DE Jr: Echo-Doppler (duplex) ultrasonic scanning. J Vasc Surg 2:341, 1985
14. Barnes RW, Russell HE, WU KK, et al: Accuracy of Doppler ultrasound in clinically suspected venous thrombosis of the calf. Surg Gynecol Obstet 143:425, 1976
15. Barnes RW, Russell HE, Bone GE, et al: The Doppler cerebrovascular examination: improved results with refinements in technique. Stroke 8:468, 1977
16. Gee W: Ocular pneumoplethysmography. Ophthalmology 29:276, 1985
17. Nix ML, Barnes RW, Rittgers SE, et al: Direct carotid Doppler examination: technique and results. Bruit 3:13, 1979
18. Thiele BL, Strandness DE Jr: Ultrasound imaging in the detection of carotid disease, in Kempczinski RF and Yao JST (eds.): Practical Noninvasive Vascular Diagnosis. Chicago, Year Book Medical Publishers, 1982, p. 239
19. Baker WH: Management of stroke during and after carotid surgery. in Bergan JJ and Yao JST (eds.): Cerebrovascular Insufficiency. Orlando, FL, Grune & Stratton, 1983, pp. 481–495
20. Zierler RE: Intraoperative Doppler techniques for arterial evaluation. Semin Ultrasound 6:73, 1985
21. Mozersky DJ, Sumner DJ, Barnes RW, et al: Intraoperative use of a sterile ultrasonic flow probe. Surg Gynecol Obstet 136:279, 1973
22. Williams LR, Flanigan DP, Schuler JJ, et al: Intraoperative assessment of limb revascularization by Doppler-derived segmental blood pressure measurements. Am J Surg 144:578, 1982
23. Zierler RE, Bandyk DF, Thiele BL: Intraoperative assessment of carotid endarterectomy. J Vasc Surg 1:78, 1984
24. Anderson CA, Collins GC, Rich NM: Routine operative arteriography during carotid endarterectomy: A reassessment. Surgery 83:67, 1978
25. Flanigan DP, Sigel B, Schuler JJ: Intraoperative ultrasonic carotid artery imaging, in Bergan JJ and Yao JST (eds.): Cerebrovascular Insufficiency. Orlando, FL, Grune & Stratton, 1983, p. 343

Donald Silver
Ricardo Rao

Hematological Assessment in Acute Vascular Surgery

Hemostasis is an essential component of successful surgery; failure of hemostasis may result in uncontrollable bleeding and adversely affect the outcome of any surgical procedure. The uncontrollable bleeding usually occurs, at least initially, from interrupted major blood vessels but may occur when one or more of the naturally occurring mechanisms for maintaining hemostasis goes awry. Vascular surgeons frequently interfere with the hemostatic process with anticoagulants and/or platelet function inhibiting agents thus creating situations that may contribute to excessive bleeding. This chapter will attempt to help the vascular surgeon identify and manage those patients who are bleeding, or likely to bleed, from congenital or acquired deficiencies of the hemostatic process.

HEMOSTASIS

Surgical bleeding occurs from inadequate control of severed blood vessels much more often than it does from defects of the hemostatic process. Surgeons who are careful in their dissections and promptly control severed vessels with hemostat, cautery, clip, or ligature will be rewarded with infrequent perioperative bleeding—even in the patient with compromised hemostatic mechanisms.

The nonmechanical mechanisms responsible for controlling bleeding from small blood vessels include vasoconstriction, platelet plug formation, and the formation of a fibrin clot. The vasoconstriction and platelet plug formation occur very soon after vascular injury and have been called primary hemostasis. The incorporation of the platelet plug into a resilient fibrin clot has been called secondary hemostasis. The resultant coagulum of platelets, fibrin, and other cellular elements maintains hemostasis until vascular repair or obliteration by scarring has occurred. Vascular integrity may be restored by natural or induced thrombolysis. Thromboses that do not lyse undergo organization and varying degrees of recanalization.

Vascular Surgical Emergencies
ISBN 0-8089-1843-5

Vessel wall

The smooth muscle of small arteries and veins contracts when the vessel is injured and reduces or stops blood flow through the injured area. The stimulus for the vasoconstriction is quite complex and has humoral, neurogenic, and myogenic components. The thromboxane A_2 released from adherent platelets is a potent vasconstrictor.

A number of congenital and acquired disorders that affect vascular integrity have been recognized. These may be responsible for formable hemorrhage in the surgical or trauma patient. Bleeding from these disorders, although relatively infrequent, is difficult to recognize and manage.[1] The congenital vascular disorders include the Ehlers-Danlos syndrome, Marfan syndrome, pseudoxanthoma elasticum, and hereditary hemorrhagic telangiectasia. Bleeding in patients with these disorders is very difficult to control. We have experienced a 40 percent mortality from bleeding and a 60 percent recurrent bleed rate in 5 patients with Ehlers-Danlos syndrome. Seventy percent of the patients with type IV Ehlers-Danlos have been reported to die of hemorrhage from spontaneous arterial rupture.[2] Acquired vascular disorders are more common than the congenital ones and include: purpura, inflammatory disorders, amyloidosis, diabetes, and drug induced disorders.

Platelets

The 200,000–400,000 platelets/mm^3 in human blood are produced by megakaryocytes and have a circulating life of 9–10 days. Platelets transport and/or synthesize coagulation proteins, procoagulants (platelet factor III), anticoagulants (platelet factor IV), bioactive amines, and prostaglandins. Platelets have a very important role in initiating hemostasis; therefore an inadequate number of platelets or platelets with altered function can have deleterious effects on the hemostatic mechanism.

Platelets normally do not adhere to other platelets or to normal vascular endothelium. Prostacyclin produced by endothelial cells helps prevent this adhering. Within 10–20 seconds after vascular injury, however, platelets begin to adhere to the collagen fibrils in the exposed subendothelial layers of the injured vessel. The adhered platelets undergo a change in shape and release several bioactive substances that cause additional changes in the platelet surface that cause platelets to adhere to other platelets, i.e., platelet aggregation.

The platelet factor III and the coagulation factors released during aggregation lead to activation of the coagulation mechanism with the conversion of fibrinogen to fibrin. The fibrin network that is produced helps stabilize the platelet hemostatic plug. Contraction of platelet microfilaments, stimulated by activated coagulation factor XIII, leads to clot retraction. The platelet plug–fibrin coagulum persists until lysis, embolization, or organization occurs.

Although inherited platelet disorders are quite rare, acquired platelet disorders are among the common causes of abnormal bleeding. Bleeding disorders may be caused by too few or too many platelets or by platelets with congenital or acquired storage or release disorders. Increased vascular fragility and permeability is associated with severe, prolonged thrombocytopenia especially when the platelet count falls to 20,000/mm^3 or less. Thirty thousand to 50,000/mm^3 normal platelets are usually adequate for hemostasis in surgical patients. Bleeding may be associated with platelet counts less than 30,000/mm^3, but rarely occurs when the count is more than 100,000/mm^3 unless defects in the vasculature or coagulation mechanism are present. The transfusion of platelet rich plasma from a single unit of fresh blood will increase the platelet count in the average adult by 10,000–20,000 platelets/mm^3. The transfusion of 4–6 units of platelet concentrates will normally restore hemostasis in patients with platelet disorders. An excessive number of platelets, usually associated with thrombosis, may be associated with bleeding, which most often occurs from the mucous membranes or the gastrointestinal tract. The platelet count in a patient with thrombocytosis is usually above 1,000,000/mm^3 and may reach more than 10,000,000/mm^3.

Qualitive platelet disorders should be suspected when bleeding occurs in the presence of normal tests of coagulation and normal platelet counts. The qualitative platelet disorders contribute to spontaneous bleeding less frequently than do the quantitative disorders. Although abnormal platelet function rarely causes significant bleeding, it may exacerbate existing bleeding from trauma and surgery. While inherited platelet disorders are quite rare, the acquired platelet disorders are among the common causes of bleeding. The acquired qualitative defects are frequently caused by drugs that adversely affect platelet adhesion, release, or aggregation. Aspirin irreversibly reduces the platelet's ability to synthesize prostaglandins (including thromboxane A$_2$) by irreversible acetylation of cyclooxygenase. Other drugs, e.g., indomethacin, sulfinpyrazone, ibuprofen, and steroids, alter platelet function for shorter periods of time, e.g., 6–8 hours. Dipyridamole inhibits platelet function by reducing platelet phosphodiesterase activity. Tricyclic antidepressants and antihistamines also have poorly defined inhibiting effects upon platelet function. If platelet function cannot be improved by elimination of the offending medications for several days prior to surgery, normal platelet function can be restored by platelet transfusions.

Coagulation

The activation of factor X leads to the conversion of prothrombin to thrombin and the subsequent conversion of fibrinogen to fibrin, the final pathway of coagulation. Activation of factor X may occur through the intrinsic and/or extrinsic pathways of coagulation (Fig. 1). The extrinsic system is activated by the release of tissue thromboplastin from injured tissues. The prothrombin time is used to monitor the extrinsic system. Activation of the intrinsic system begins with the activation of factor XII when it comes in contact with foreign surfaces—especially collagen or basement membrane. The partial thromboplastin time is used to monitor function of the intrinsic system. Surgery and trauma activate both systems of coagulation.

Disorders of coagulation, coagulopathies, may be caused by congenital or acquired abnormal production of coagulation factors, consumption of coagulation factors faster than they can be replaced, or losses of coagulation factors during bleeding with inadequate replacement. Congenital deficiencies have been described for all of the clotting factors except III and IV. A congenital deficiency of a clotting factor may occur from reduced production of the factor or by the production of a factor that is antigenically similar but with reduced or absent procoagulant activity because structural changes have occurred in the factor. The patient with congenital clotting disorders usually has a single factor deficiency while the patient with acquired clotting disorders frequently has deficiencies of several factors. Patients with congenital deficiencies of clotting factors usually bleed only when stressed by surgery or trauma since only 5–10 percent of normal factor activity is needed to maintain hemostasis under normal conditions.

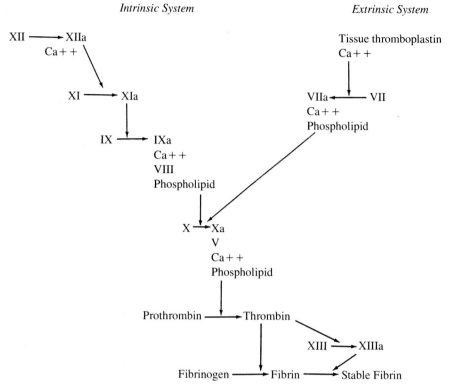

Fig. 1. Pathways of Coagulation.

Acquired disorders of coagulation are caused by deficient production, inaccurate replacement, and/or excessive consumption of coagulation factors, or by anticoagulant therapy. The liver produces all coagulation factors except factors III and VIII (the endothelial component of the liver does contribute to factor VIII production); therefore, impaired liver function may contribute to deficient production of coagulation factors. The synthesis of factors II, VII, IX, and X (and proteins C and S) depend on the liver having an adequate supply of vitamin K. In addition to the problems encountered by patients with an inadequate supply and/or absorption of vitamin K, many drugs interfere with the absorption or availability of vitamin K and the vitamin K antagonists (e.g. warfarin).[3]

Most coagulation factors, except the labile factors V and VIII, are stable in stored blood. After 2–3 weeks of storage, the labile factors may decrease to 10–20 percent of normal. In addition, platelets in banked blood are usually low in number and are nonfunctional. Therefore large numbers of blood transfusions, 5–6 units per hour, to normal patients and lesser amounts to patients with depression of their coagulation proteins, may cause bleeding through dilution of the clotting factors and platelets.

An increased number of patients are receiving heparin or coumarin pre- and intraoperatively as prophylaxis for venous thromboembolism. This drug alteration of the coagulation mechanism may contribute to perioperative bleeding.

The effect of the activated clotting factors is usually tempered by dilution and by the naturally occurring coagulation inhibitors. Therefore coagulation is a limited process and intravascular coagulation is controlled. However, occasionally the rate of intravascular coagulation is excessive, e.g., with sepsis, amniotic fluid embolism and incompatible blood transfusions, so that coagulation factors are consumed more rapidly than they can be produced. The depletion of fibrinogen, prothrombin and factors V, VIII, IX, X, XII, and XIII and platelets that occurs during a consumptive coagulopathy is frequently associated with bleeding.

Fibrinolysis

Plasminogen, the inactive precursor of plasmin, circulates bound to fibrinogen and remains bound to fibrin during coagulation. Plasminogen is converted to plasmin by a variety of activators—the plasminogen activator of the vascular endothelium has an important role in restoring vessel patency by initiating thrombolysis. Plasmin preferentially digests fibrin but also digests fibrinogen and other coagulation proteins and plasma proteins. Fibrinolysis occurs whenever the plasmin produced exceeds the available antiplasmins. Excessive activation of plasminogen occurs most often as a response to diffuse intravascular coagulation but may also occur with profound hypotension or hypoxemia, electric shock, extensive trauma,[4] or infusion of fibrinolytic activators, e.g., urokinase or streptokinase. The hyperfibrinolysis that occurs in response to diffuse intravascular coagulation is called secondary fibrinolysis and occurs much more commonly than does primary hyperfibrinolysis. During surgery, hyperfibrinolysis may cause clots to lyse and may impair clotting by digesting the coagulation proteins. Intraoperative fibrinolysis should be suspected when there is diffuse intraoperative bleeding, especially when there is bleeding from previously "dry" surfaces.

DIAGNOSIS

History

A complete history, thorough physical examination and a few laboratory tests should help the surgeon identify, preoperatively, most patients with congenital and many patients with acquired bleeding disorders. A competent hematologist and a sophisticated laboratory may be necessary to identify some coagulation disorders.

The history is invaluable for detecting hemorrhagic disorders and should help distinguish a congenital bleeding disorder from an acquired one (Table 1). The type of congenital hemostatic disorder may be suspected from the pattern of inheritance, e.g., hemophilia A and B have a X-linked recessive pattern of inheritance with the males being afflicted and the females transmitting the disease.

The age at which the bleeding disorder presents is important. When excessive bleeding occurs early, e.g., with umbilical cord separation, with circumcision, with the minor trauma of childhood, or with menses, an inherited bleeding disorder should be suspected. The acquired hemorrhagic disorders usually occur later in life, frequently associated with other disorders, e.g., hepatic or renal diseases. Patients should be questioned about bleeding after tooth extractions, tonsillectomy, minor trauma, and surgical procedures. Excessive bleeding after any of these conditions requires additional laboratory evaluation while the absence of excessive blood loss with these conditions makes it unlikely that the patient has an inherited bleeding disorder.

The type of bleeding provides insight into the etiology of the bleeding. Petechiae are

Table 1
Bleeding Disorders: History and Physical Findings

	Coagulation Disorders		Vascular and Platelet Disorders	
	Acquired	Congenital	Acquired	Congenital
Positive family history		+		+
Early bleeds		+		+
Late bleeds	+		+	
Positive drug history	+		+	
Hepatic and renal failure	+		+	
Hypersplenism			+	
Hemangiomas skin and mucous membrane				+
Malignancies	+		+	
Starvation	+			
Petachiae	rare		common	
Hematomas and hemarthroses	common		rare	
Nose bleeds	rare		common	
Bleeds from superficial wounds	rare		common	
Delayed bleeding	common		rare	

usually associated with platelet or vascular abnormalities, e.g., functional disorders of platelets, thrombocytopenia or von Willebrand's disease, while ecchymoses may occur with any of the bleeding disorders. The bleeding associated with platelet or vascular disorders is usually eventually controlled while the bleeding associated with coagulation defects is poorly controlled and may be associated with hemarthroses, hematuria, and retroperitoneal hematomas. Congenital factor defects are usually the cause of hemarthroses.

Drug induced bleeding disorders occur with such frequency that it is important to obtain a detailed history about drugs being taken at the times bleeding has occurred. Bleeding from multiple sites, needle punctures, gastrointestinal tract, and areas of trauma may be caused by excessive anticoagulation, hyperfibrinolysis, or intravascular consumptive coagulation with a secondary hyperfibrinolysis. Hemorrhagic diatheses may be caused or aggravated by liver or renal insufficiency, leukemia, and collagen or vascular disorders.

Physical Examination

The physical examination may produce evidence of previous bleeding episodes, of active bleeding, or of conditions that predispose to bleeding (Table 1). The examination should include an inspection for the presence and distribution of petechiae, purpura, ecchymoses, hemangiomas, tumors, jaundice, hematomas, and hemarthroses. Ecchymoses occurring with hematuria and gastrointestinal hemorrhage suggest an acquired coagulation defect. Hemarthroses and expanding hematomas are common sequlae of congenital coagulation factor deficiencies. Hemangiomas of the skin and mucous membranes may suggest the presence of hereditary hemorrhagic telangiectasia.

Disorders that accompany or cause coagulation problems may be detected during the physical examination. Thrombocytopenia may be caused by an enlarged large spleen.

Malignancies may be associated with reduced clotting factors and platelet synthesis and/ or accelerated consumption of coagulation factors. Several disorders are associated with "circulating anticoagulants," e.g., lupus erythematosus, malignancies and some collagen disorders.[5] Hepatic insufficiency may be associated with decreased production of coagulation factors and increased fibrinolytic activity. Bleeding may occur during times of starvation, periods of intestinal sterilization, and in patients with altered fat absorption because factors II, VII, IX, and X are frequently reduced in these patients.

Laboratory Testing

If the personal history and the family history are negative for bleeding, it is unlikely that the patient has, or will develop, a bleeding disorder. If a bleeding disorder is suspected or is present, screening tests and on occasion specific tests are indicated.[6] The commonly utilized screening tests include the prothrombin time (PT), partial thrombinplastin time (PTT), thrombin time (TT), platelet count, and template bleeding time. These tests are simple to perform, inexpensive, and widely available.

The PT, a measure of the activity of the extrinsic pathway of coagulation, is prolonged by the deficiencies of factors I, II, V, VII, and X and by inhibitors of coagulation, e.g., heparin. The PTT, a measure of the activity of the intrinsic pathway of coagulation, is prolonged by deficiencies or inhibitors to the clotting factors of the intrinsic pathways. The PTT does not detect deficiencies of factor VII or XIII. The TT, a measure of the conversion of fibrinogen to fibrin by thrombin, is prolonged in the presence of low fibrinogen and abnormal fibrinogen, heparin, and fibrin and fibrinogen degradation products. The platelet count detects quantitative deficiencies of platelets. The template bleeding time measures the formation of the hemostatic plug.[7] The bleeding time is prolonged by deficiencies of platelets, decreases of coagulation factors I and V and von Willebrand's factor, and by vessel wall abnormalities. If the screening tests are abnormal, specific factor assay and tests for circulating inhibitors, platelet function, primary platelet activity, and fibrin solubility may be required to determine specific defect(s) of hemostasis.

Bleeding from acquired disorders of hemostasis occurs much more commonly than does bleeding from congenital disorders. The bleeding from an acquired disorder usually occurs intraoperatively or postoperatively and frequently occurs in a patient with a negative history for bleeding and normal screening tests. These acquired defects of hemostasis include: the thrombocytopenia and/or factor deficiency, especially factors V and VIII, that occurs with the transfusion of large quantities of older bank blood during brisk bleeding; the interference with the coagulation process of excessive amounts of intraoperative anticoagulants—especially heparin; and/or the consumption of coagulation factors (as in disseminated intravascular coagulation) faster than they can be produced. The consumptive coagulopathy may be accompanied by a secondary hyperfibrinolysis. The acquired bleeding occurs mainly in patients who require large volumes of blood, e.g., with major surgery, ruptured aneurysms, and multiple trauma—including major vascular trauma. Many coagulationists recommend replacing the factors with a unit of fresh frozen plasma for each 5–6 units of bank blood transfused during brisk bleeding.

The intravascular coagulation that accompanies sepsis, large aneurysms, giant hemangiomas, and AV fistulae may not consume coagulation factors sufficiently preoperatively to cause bleeding preoperatively. However, the increased consumption of the coagulation factors and platelets that is induced by surgery, and the partial replacement factors by older bank blood, may cause the consumption to exceed the production of platelets and factors. If this occurs, bleeding will ensue. This type of bleeding is best controlled by eliminating the cause of the bleeding, e.g., the abscess, the aneurysm, and so forth.

The control of nonmechanical intraoperative bleeding requires thoughtful consultation between the vascular surgeon, the anesthesiologist, and the coagulation laboratory director. The amount of heparin administered should be determined; did the patient receive 7000 units or 70,000 units? The blood bags should be reviewed to insure that the patient received only properly crossed matched and labeled blood. The relation of the bleeding to hypotension, acidosis, or other systemic disorders that affect the coagulation–lytic mechanisms should be determined and these disorders should be corrected. The surgeon should note the type of bleeding: if incised surfaces bleed excessively and no clots are forming, a platelet and/or factor(s) deficiency is present; and if previously dry surfaces begin to bleed and incised surfaces continue to bleed, it is likely that hyperfibrinolysis is present in addition to platelet and factor deficiencies.

The laboratory evaluation of intraoperative bleeding includes the TT, PT, PTT, platelet count, fibrinogen assay, and an assay for fibrinolytic activity, usually the whole blood or euglobulin lysis time (Table 2). Low platelet counts are corrected (to at least 50,000/mm^3) with platelet transfusions. Prolongation of the PT and/or PTT indicate the need for factor(s) replacement. There is no time for testing for the specific factor deficiency during intraoperative bleeding. Therefore, all factors are replaced with fresh frozen plasma and/or cryoprecipitate until hemostasis is secured or the PT and PTT approach the normal values for the coagulation laboratory. If hyperfibrinolysis is a problem after the intravascular coagulation is controlled, the fibrinolytic inhibiting agent, epsilon-aminocaproic acid (EACA) may be required. The usual dose of EACA is 5 gm as a loading dose and 1 gm an hour until the fibrinolysis is controlled.

The bleeding encountered in the vascular patient postoperatively is usually mechanical, e.g., from an unsecured vessel, a suture line or graft leak, the slippage of tie or clip, and so forth. Occasionally, postoperative bleeding will occur in a patient from excessive anticoagulation. This should be readily detected by the standard laboratory tests. If the patient is bleeding from excessive heparin, the heparin can be neutralized with protamine sulfate. One milligram of protamine sulfate will neutralize 100 units of heparin. One usually gives part (usually a third to half) of the calculated dose of protamine slowly intravenously because excessive protamine can act as an anticoagulant and protamine given rapidly can cause hypotension. It has been suggested that protamine given intraarterially has less of a hypotensive effect.[8] Platelet counts and coagulation factors are usually

Table 2

Laboratory Tests and Hemostatic Function

	BT*	PT	PTT	TT	Platelets	Lysis time
Platelet deficiency	P†	N	N	N	L	N
Hemophilia "states"	N	N	P	N	N	N
Vitamin K factor deficiency	N	P	P	N	N	N
Consumptive coagulopathy	P	P	P	P	L	N
with secondary lysis	P	P	P	P	L	S
Heparin therapy	P	P	P	P	N	N
Hyperfibrinolysis (primary)	N-P	N-P	N-P	N-P	N	S

*BT = bleeding time; PT = prothrombin time; PTT = partial thromboplastin time; TT = thrombin time
†P = prolonged; N = normal; L = low; S = shortened

rapidly restored to normal postoperatively in patients with normal bone marrow and liver function and are not likely to be a cause of bleeding in the vascular patient.

Bleeding that occurs in the operative site, in the vascular patient, during the recuperative or later periods is most often related to suture line or graft problems, e.g., disruption, leak, false aneurysm, fistula, infection, and so forth and require special efforts to control the bleeding.

Nonmechanical bleeding in vascular patients

If vascular patients are carefully evaluated and managed, they are at no greater risk for postoperative hemorrhagic complications than are other surgical patients. The postoperative hemorrhagic complication rate in the vascular patient is approximately 1.6 percent.[9] A review of 152 of our recent patients having vascular surgery revealed that 33 of them required more blood replacement than expected. Twenty-one of the 33 patients required excessive, by our standards, blood replacement during the immediate perioperative period. None of these patients had an identifiable coagulopathy; the increased blood loss in each patient was directly related to the surgical procedure.

SUMMARY

Vascular surgeons through their use of anticoagulants and platelet inhibiting agents in the perioperative period may encounter slightly more operative bleeding than do other surgeons. However, patients with vascular surgical disorders do not bleed more from acquired or congenital defects of hemostasis than do other patients and are not at increased risk for postoperative hemorrhage if the surgery is done well. A careful history, physical examination, and, when appropriate, screening battery of laboratory tests will most often detect those vascular surgery patients likely to have excessive bleeding and will allow preoperative correction of their defects of hemostasis.

REFERENCES

1. Bick RL: Vascular disorders associated with thrombohemorrhagic phenomena. Semin Thrombosis Hemostasis 5:167, 1979
2. Cikrit D, Miles J, Silver D: Spontaneous arterial perforation: the Ehlers-Danlos specter, presented at Internat Soc Cardiovasc Surg, New Orleans, LA (in press), June 1986 J Vasc Surg
3. Giddings JC, Evans BK: Drugs affect blood coagulation and hemostasis, Int Anesth Clinic 23:103, 1985
4. Kapsch DN, Metzler M, Harrington M, et al: Fibrinolytic response to trauma. Surgery 95:473, 1984
5. Margolius A Jr, Jackson DP, Ratnoff OD: Circulating anticoagulants: A study of 40 cases and a review of the literature. Medicine 40:145, 1961
6. Sirridge M: Laboratory evaluation of the patient. Clin Lab Med 4:285, 1984
7. Mieke CH Jr, Kaneshiro MM, Maheb IA, et al: The standard normal Ivy bleeding time and its prolongation by aspirin. Blood 34:204, 1969
8. Wakefield TW, Whitehouse WM Jr, Stanley JC: Depressed cardiovascular function and altered platelet kinetics following protamine sulfate reversal of heparin activity. J Vas Surg 1:346, 1984
9. Bergquist D, Kallero S: Reoperation for postoperative haemorrhagic complications: Analysis of a 10 year series. Acta Chir Scand 151:17, 1985

PART III

Acute Cerebrovascular Emergencies

Steven P. Okuhn
Ronald J. Stoney

Carotid Artery Dissection

Dissection of the carotid artery is an uncommon cause of cerebrovascular insufficiency. Many cases resolve spontaneously or occur without dramatic local or neurologic symptoms. However, hemorrhage with exsanguination or airway compromise and cerebrovascular accidents have been described in association with carotid dissection making this entity a true (potential) vascular surgical emergency. This chapter will review the three general categories of carotid artery dissection: traumatic, spontaneous, and those occurring in vessels weakened by some identifiable cause. The pathology and clinical presentation of these lesions will then be reviewed. Finally, surgical methods and results of a series of spontaneous carotid artery dissections treated at the University of California, San Francisco, will be presented in hopes of placing our treatment algorithm in clinical perspective.

Etiology

Dissection of the carotid artery may be caused by inflammatory or degenerative disease, blunt or penetrating trauma, or it may be spontaneous without any apparent inciting event. Congenital malformations, local arteritis, cystic medial necrosis, fibromuscular dysplasia, Marfan's syndrome, syphilis, and pharyngeal infections have all been implicated in isolated cases of carotid dissection.[1-12] Surprisingly few patients have evidence of atherosclerotic disease or hypertension associated with dissection.[6,11,12] Penetrating trauma from knife or missile wounds or needle puncture from angiography can result in severe carotid injury including dissection.[13-16] Similarly, blunt trauma to the neck and deceleration or hyperextension injuries can all lead to carotid dissection.[13,17-20] Spontaneous dissection of the carotid artery has also been described with increasing frequency and may be more common than was previously appreciated.[1-12,21-33] It usually involves the cervical internal carotid artery and since many cases resolve without treatment or occur without dramatic local or neurologic symptoms, the prevalence of this entity is probably underestimated. Although by definition, trauma is not an etiologic factor in

Vascular Surgical Emergencies
ISBN 0-8089-1843-5

spontaneous dissection, it is likely that mild hyperextension during athletic events or minor trauma may stretch and disrupt the carotid intima.[30,32,34-35] Similarly, coughing has been described as the cause of spontaneous dissection in what was presumably an already weakened vessel.[30] Although fibromuscular dysplasia, cystic medial necrosis, and intimal disruption from hyperextension and coughing have occasionally been associated with spontaneous carotid dissection, the etiology is still unknown in the majority of cases. The sequelae of carotid dissection, false aneurysm formation and disruption, can occur following dissection from any of the above listed causes.

Pathology and Pathogenesis

Carotid dissections, whether occuring spontaneously, secondary to blunt trauma, or involving a pathologically weakened vessel, all seem to affect the internal carotid artery with an overwhelming preponderance. There have been reported cases of blunt trauma or hyperextension/deceleration injuries causing common carotid dissection but these are exceedingly rare.[17] Three patterns of disease have been noted in the cervical carotid artery. Dissections can begin: (1) approximately 2.5 cm beyond the origin of the carotid bulb (Fig. 1); (2) in the mid cervical internal carotid artery; and (3) in the distal internal carotid artery 2 to 4 cm from the bony foramen. Traumatic dissections more commonly affect the distal internal carotid artery, for here the vessel is fixed as it enters the skull and impacted energy is likely to cause the type of intramedial or intimal injury that can lead to dissection.[13] Spontaneous dissections usually begin in the two more proximal locations

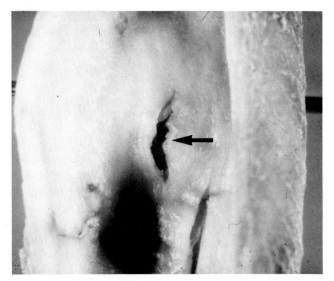

Fig. 1. Specimen showing an intimal tear at the starting point of a spontaneous dissection in the proximal internal carotid artery (arrow). (Reproduced from Krupski WC, Effeney DJ, Ehrenfeld WK: Fibromuscular dysplasia, aneurysms, and spontaneous dissection of the carotid artery, in JJ Bergan, JST Yao (eds.): *Cerebrovascular Insufficiency,* Copyright 1983, by Grune & Stratton, Inc., Orlando, FL. With permission.)

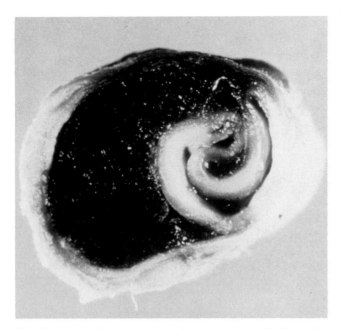

Fig. 2. Proximal cross-section of a resected carotid dissection specimen, showing the dissection within the deep layers of the arterial media with thrombus in the false lumen ("jelly-roll appearance") compressing the inner media and intima. (Reproduced from Krupski WC, Effeney DJ, Ehrenfeld WK: Fibromuscular dysplasia, aneurysms, and spontaneous dissection of the carotid artery, in JJ Bergan, JST Yao (eds.): *Cerebrovascular Insufficiency,* Copyright 1983, by Grune & Stratton, Inc., Orlando, FL. With permission.)

and typically extend to the point where the internal carotid enters the petrous canal. The dissection may rarely extend from the cervical carotid artery to involve intracerebral vessels.[6,10,30]

Whether resulting from blunt trauma or occurring spontaneously, either intramural hemorrhage or intimal disruption must be the primary pathologic event.[1,3,6] Progression of the dissecting hematoma within the media leads to acute external enlargement of the vessel wall and compression of the true lumen (Fig. 2). This may result in complete occlusion of the true lumen. Alternatively, microemboli from the thrombus in the region of intimal disruption may occlude distal intracerebral vessels. Other pathologic progressions may include reentry of the intramural bleeding back through the intima creating a false lumen (Fig. 3), or extension of the dissection into the plane between the media and adventitia with false aneurysm formation. These aneurysms are usually saccular and may result in local bleeding or the release of emboli into the distal circulation.[1-3,6,21] In the absence of complicating thrombosis or arterial disruption, recanalization of either the true or false lumen is the most likely outcome.[3,23,24]

Exploration of a carotid artery dissection reveals a sharply demarcated transition between the normal artery and the diseased vessel.[6] The dissected segment is moderately dilated with a bluish hue owing to thrombus in the characteristic second (false) lumen in

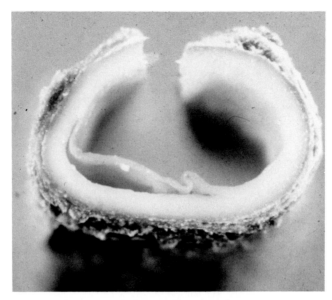

Fig. 3. Distal cross-section of the same specimen as depicted in Figure 2, displaying a more superficial dissection plane as the false lumen rejoins the true lumen.

the outer media.[1,6,10] On histologic examination of spontaneously dissected arteries, the smooth muscle cells are fragmented and decreased in number.[6] The elastic tissue is also deficient with degeneration and fragmentation of the internal elastic membrane. There is also a characteristic deposition of a mucoid substance throughout all layers of the vessel wall. While there has been no histologic evidence of cystic medial necrosis, FMD, atherosclerosis, or vasculitis in resected spontaneous dissections from this institution, these abnormal findings suggest that some underlying arterial pathology is at least partially responsible. This premise is further supported by angiographic evidence of FMD in the carotid artery contralateral to a spontaneous dissection noted in three of our patients as well as general arterial ectasia seen angiographically in five others.[6,29]

Clinical Findings

Spontaneous dissection is usually a disease of middle age although it has been reported to occur over a wide range of ages with the youngest reported case in a 4-year-old.[3] Thirty patients have presented with spontaneous dissection of the carotid artery at the University of California, San Francisco, during the past 20 years. The group consists of 12 women and 18 men ranging from 11 to 66 years of age.

The clinical presentation of these patients is summarized in Table 1. The most common presenting symptoms were either transient ischemic attacks (56 percent) or completed stroke (30 percent). Several patients had recurrent TIAs after the initial episode presumably caused by embolization of thrombus from the dissected segment. The sudden onset of ipsilateral headache, tinnitus, or neck pain were also fairly common presentations.[30,33] Unilateral periorbital facial pain seen in association with an incomplete

Table 1

Symptoms at Presentation

Symptom	No.	%
Transient ischemic attacks	17	56
Completed Stroke	9	30
Amaurosis Fugax	5	17
Headache	6	20
Neck Pain	4	13
Tinnitus	2	7
Incomplete Horner's Syndrome	1	3

Horner's syndrome is very suggestive of internal carotid artery dissection.[25] The incomplete Horner's syndrome is thought to represent local dilation of the pericarotid sympathetic plexus with preservation of the external carotid sympathetics that control sweating of the face. None of these 30 patients gave a history of cervical trauma or unusual movements preceding the onset of symptoms.

Findings associated with carotid dissection from blunt carotid trauma, hyperextension, or deceleration injury range from asymptomatic to full-blown stroke. The key to accurate diagnosis is a high index of suspicion when a history of neck trauma is combined with any evidence of cerebral ischemia, Horner's syndrome, or local evidence of injury.[13,18] In fact, it is typical for hyperextension or deceleration carotid injuries to be silent initially, with medial dissection leading to symptomatic vessel occlusion hours later.[13,18-20] An angiogram is mandatory in these patients to rule out associated injuries and to safely plan the operative repair. For hemodynamically or neurologically unstable patients, the angiogram can be performed in the operating room if necessary.

Angiographic Findings

Three arteriographic patterns of carotid dissection have been noted and these simply demonstrate the three patterns of disease mentioned earlier.[6,28-29] The most common abnormality seen with spontaneous dissection is an irregular tapered narrowing eccentrically placed in the cervical internal carotid artery. This wave-like narrowing begins approximately 2.5 cm distal to the carotid bifurcation and is referred to as the "carotid string sign" (Fig. 4). It probably represents elevation and folding of the intima in the dissected segment. The long narrow column of contrast extends to the petrous canal where the vessel regains its normal caliber. A lucent filling defect may be seen at the origin of the dissection representing an elevated intimal flap. Because of the minimal amount of flow through this region there is a significant delay of contrast filling the vessel and subtraction techniques may be required to visualize the lumen. Occasionally, despite these best efforts, a patent vessel appears thrombosed on angiography. Although the "carotid string sign" is a classic finding in spontaneous dissection, other pathology may present with a similar angiographic picture including, for instance, an atherosclerotic preocclusive lesion in the carotid bulb with an nonadherent trailing thrombus.[36]

The next general radiographic pattern of dissection includes abnormalities that involve the midsegment of the cervical carotid artery. These vessels typically regain their normal size before entering the skull. The last pattern consists of distal internal carotid

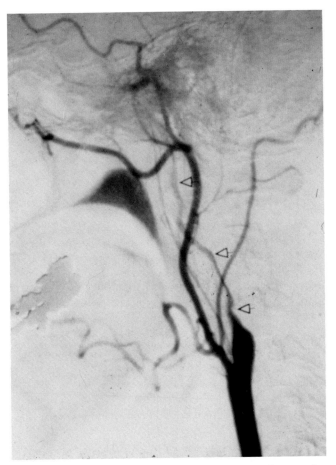

Fig. 4. "Carotid string sign" (arrows) seen on an angiogram of a
spontaneous dissection of the internal carotid artery.

artery occlusion near its entry into the petrous canal and distal to some length of tapered
narrowing (Fig. 5). Other radiographic abnormalities are often seen in association with
carotid dissection, including contralateral FMD, false aneurysms, and ipsilateral embolic
occlusions of the middle cerebral artery and its branches.

Surgical Methods and Results

Therapy of carotid dissection is governed primarily by arteriographic and clinical
findings while the mechanism of injury plays a lesser role in determining treatment.
Because isolated dissection is handled the same whether it occurs spontaneously or results
from blunt trauma, spontaneous dissection of the internal carotid artery will be used as the
primary example in the following discussion. Special considerations that arise in blunt
traumatic dissection will also be examined. Treatment of penetrating trauma will be
omitted from this chapter.

Early in our experience with managing spontaneous dissection of the internal carotid

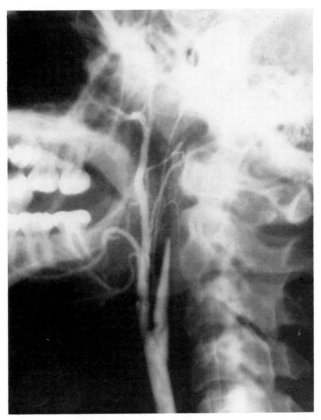

Fig. 5. Angiogram depicting tapered segment of narrowing ("dunce's cap") with occlusion of the internal carotid artery in a case of spontaneous dissection.

artery, it was felt that some form of surgical therapy was the preferred approach.[6] Of 11 patients undergoing operations, treatment consisted of segmental resection with interposition saphenous vein grafting in 3 patients, 1 of whom suffered a mild postoperative stroke from subsequent graft occlusion. Graduated intraluminal dilation was performed in another patient with a short, surgically inaccessible lesion. Removal of mural thrombus and dissected intima with balloon catheters was attempted in two others. One of these latter patients had a markedly abnormal intraoperative arteriogram with numerous persistent intimal defects. He underwent internal carotid ligation without complication after the stump pressure was measured to be over 70 mmHg. A second patient with recurrent transient ischemic attacks, mural thrombus and a stump pressure of 65 mmHg also had internal carotid ligation without neurologic sequelae. Four additional patients with stump pressures less than 70 mmHg had procedures limited to carotid exploration alone. One of these patients underwent concomitant superficial temporal to middle cerebral artery bypass for persistent TIAs despite adequate anticoagulation. Of these seven surgically manipulated vessels (excluding the four simple explorations) there were only two documented patent internal carotid arteries on follow-up.

This disappointing experience contrasted sharply with the remaining 19 patients in

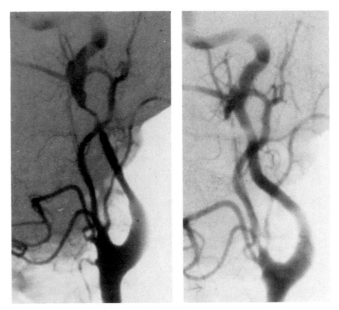

Fig. 6. Short, segmental dissection of the internal carotid artery. Left, the middle portion of the internal carotid artery shows an irregular, tapered narrowing while the proximal and distal portions appear normal. Right, repeat carotid arteriogram three months later following conservative therapy with a normal appearing internal carotid artery. (Reproduced from O'Dwyer MB, Moscow N, Trevor R, et al: Spontaneous dissection of the carotid artery. *Radiology* 137(2):379–385, 1980. With permission.)

the series who had no attempt at arterial reconstruction. These patients were anticoagulated and observed and they suffered no further ipsilateral neurologic symptoms after their initial presentation. Repeat arteriograms performed 1–16 months after the original study in 11 patients showed reexpanded carotid artery lumens in 10 patients (Figs. 6 & 7).

Therapy for Spontaneous Dissection of the Carotid Artery

Once the local neck findings or neurologic symptoms lead to an angiogram and the diagnosis of spontaneous carotid dissection is established, appropriate treatment is then initiated. In light of the excellent results obtained with expectant management of this lesion, observation and anticoagulation is now recommended for most patients.[2,6,23,24,29,30] Heparin, followed by coumadin therapy prevents further intramural and intraluminal thrombus formation and limits the possibility of distal embolization. These agents may also facilitate more rapid recanalization of the vessel. Contraindications to anticoagulation include a cerebral infarct, intracerebral hemorrhage, or associated injury to the carotid artery or surrounding tissues. This latter situation will be further discussed in the following section. The optimal duration of therapy is unknown; however, there is no evidence that long-term anticoagulation is necessary. In fact, since most conservatively managed

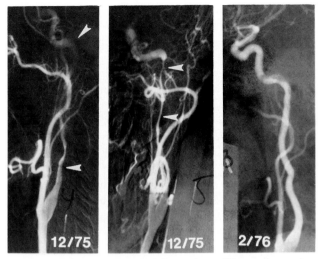

Fig. 7. Left, lateral view of left internal carotid artery in a patient who experienced one sudden episode of right arm and leg weakness associated with headache and left neck pain persisting for three hours. This arteriogram demonstrates the tapered narrowing of the cervical internal carotid artery with reexpansion intracranially (arrows). Center, anteroposterior view showing dissection limited to the cervical internal carotid artery (arrows). Right, lateral view of the left carotid artery with a normal vessel lumen after 2 months of conservative treatment. (Reproduced from Ehrenfeld WK, Wylie EJ: Spontaneous dissection of the internal carotid artery. *Arch Surg* 111:1294–1301, 1976. Copyright 1976, American Medical Association. With permission.)

dissections display a near-normal angiographic appearance by one year, with some normalizing as early as one month, a relatively limited treatment period seems indicated.[24]

These patients should be closely monitored for regression of their lesions. However, if progressive stenosis is documented, or neurologic symptoms develop despite anticoagulation, operative repair may be indicated. Along with arteriography, carotid duplex scanning and ophthalmoplethysmography (OPG-Gee) may each provide useful prognostic information in individual patients.[24]

While decisions regarding intervention must take into account the observation that with time the lumen may return to normal, surgical therapy is indicated for spontaneous carotid artery dissections under certain circumstances. The threat of distal embolization, or carotid occlusion outweighs the low risk of operation in those young asymptomatic patients whose dissected segment is totally accessible and whose original neurologic deficit was brief. Although carotid recanalization demonstrated by angiographic normalization is the likely outcome in these patients, the long-term natural history of the dissected vessels is unknown.[6,24,33,37] For this reason, resection and graft replacement is the treatment of choice under these circumstances. Asymptomatic patients with unfavorable lesions, the overwhelming majority, should be expectantly managed as outlined above.

The generally accepted contraindication to revascularizing patients with acute, completed strokes would also apply to patients who suffer such an event as a result of a spontaneous carotid dissection. However, operation *is* indicated in patients with recurrent

TIAs despite adequate anticoagulation. Embolization of thrombus is the cause of neurologic findings in some of these patients. Surgical treatment is offered in hope of preventing stroke by either removing the embolic focus through resection and grafting or excluding the focus by ligating the internal carotid artery.

The choice between excision and exclusion is determined by the anatomy of the dissection as seen on preoperative arteriography. Attempting to repair a dissection that approaches the base of the skull (a long carotid string sign) may be fraught with hazard. The possibility of retention of intraluminal blood clot or loosely attached intimal fragments after instrumental dilation or thrombectomy with balloon catheters makes these techniques unsafe. To adequately reconstruct the internal carotid artery at this level, one must expose the base of the skull by disarticulating and splitting the vertical ramus of the mandible, dividing the digastric muscle, and removing the bony styloid process. Even surmounting this technical challenge with risk of injury to cranial nerves IX–XII and associated vascular structures, there is the possibility that the dissected artery will not be reconstructable.

It is with this scenario in mind that the recommendation against routine repair of these high internal carotid dissections is made. Instead, if adequate collateral blood supply to the ipsilateral cerebral hemisphere is documented, then simple ligation of the involved proximal internal carotid artery is the preferred treatment. Arterial ligation in these and other patients with inaccessible embolizing lesions has shown that a carotid stump pressure in excess of 70 mmHg is indicative of adequate collateral blood flow.[38] The correlation of intraoperative stump pressure and postligation neurologic status is summarized in Table 2. In this series all 13 patients whose stump pressures exceeded 70 mmHg had no neurologic sequelae. In contrast, 6 of the remaining 11 patients whose stump pressures ranged from 50 to 68 mmHg developed a postligation stroke. Anticoagulation should be used to help prevent clot propagation with distal carotid embolization or thrombosis following proximal carotid ligation.

Preoperative OPG-Gee with digital occlusion of the ipsilateral common carotid artery may provide useful prognostic information. However, this technique should not be employed in place of carotid stump pressure determination performed at ward blood pressure under the controlled conditions available in the operating room. For symptomatic patients with low stump pressures, the surgical team should be prepared to do either extracranial to intracranial bypass or mandibular osteotomy as described above.

Whether ligation should be performed after EC/IC bypass would depend on the presumed etiology of the neurologic symptoms and the confidence placed in continued bypass patency. Specifically, symptoms demonstrated to be embolic by angiography would be best treated by ligation. In contrast, hemodynamic (low flow) symptoms would

Table 2

Correlation of Carotid Stump Pressure With
Neurologic Status After Internal Ligation

	Neurologic Status	
Carotid Stump Pressure (mmHg)	Stroke	No Stroke
50–68	6	5
>70	0	13

better respond to EC/IC bypass without ligation in hope of early augmentation of flow from the bypass and late normalization of the dissected carotid artery. Anticoagulated patients with persistent cerebral ischemic symptoms and angiographic evidence of distal occlusion may also benefit from EC/IC bypass once occlusion is confirmed by intraoperative examination. Unfortunately, the recent multicenter study on the efficacy of EC/IC bypass does not address these difficult clinical situations.[39]

When there is angiographic evidence of aneurysm formation in association with spontaneous dissection of the carotid artery, prompt surgical repair is indicated. Resection and anastomosis with interposition grafting if necessary is the recommended treatment for accessible lesions. This aggressive treatment is warranted whether or not the lesion is symptomatic in order to prevent the grave complications of aneurysm rupture or distal embolization of thrombus. If the aneurysm is not surgically accessible or is associated with a dissection that would otherwise be nonrepairable, then stump pressure determination and carotid ligation should be considered. Expectant management with anticoagulation as described above would be extremely dangerous in this setting and is not recommended.

Therapy For Blunt Traumatic Carotid Artery Dissection

Considerations in the care of isolated blunt traumatic dissections are similar to those in spontaneous dissection with two notable exceptions. First, anticoagulation is extremely dangerous in the trauma setting and should not be used unless a meticulous search for associated arterial and soft tissue injuries is negative. Second, angiographic evidence of carotid occlusion does not obviate the need for carotid exploration, even in patients without neurologic symptoms. Unless a severe fixed neurologic deficit is present, these patients should be taken to the operating room where open examination and stump pressure determination of the carotid artery can be performed. Patent arteries may appear occluded even on adequate biplanar angiograms. Left alone these patients run the risk of late carotid occlusion with distal propagation of clot and subsequent stroke. If occlusion is confirmed intraoperatively, revascularization should not be attempted. Successful proximal restoration of carotid blood flow would only result in further neurologic insult from embolization of inaccessible distal thrombus or transform a pale infarct into a larger, dangerous hemorrhagic infarct.

When repair of traumatic dissection appears feasible, complete resection of the affected segment should be performed. If this is impossible then decisions regarding ligation rest on intraoperative stump pressure determination as they did in the case of spontaneous dissection. If blunt traumatic carotid dissection is associated with a false aneurysm or soft tissue hematoma then prompt operative exploration is indicated to prevent the complications of arterial disruption and hemorrhage or thrombosis and distal embolization.

ACKNOWLEDGMENT

Supported in part by the Pacific Vascular Research Foundation, San Francisco, California.

REFERENCES

1. Bostrom K, Liliequist B: Primary dissecting aneurysm of the extracranial part of the internal carotid and vertebral arteries. Neurology 17:179, 1967
2. Bradac GB, Kaernbach A, Bulk-Weischedel D, et al: Spontaneous dissecting aneurysms of cervical cerebral arteries: Report of six cases and review of the literature. Neuroradiology 21:149, 1981
3. Friedman WA, Day AL, Quisling RG, et al: Cervical carotid dissecting aneurysms. Neurosurgery 7:207, 1980
4. Lloyd J, Bahnson HTL: Bilateral dissecting aneurysms of the internal carotid arteries. Am J Surg 122:549, 1971
5. Wylie EJ, Ehrenfeld WK: Extracranial Occlusive Cerebrovascular Disease: Diagnosis and Management. Philadelphia, WB Saunders, 1970
6. Ehrenfeld WK, Wylie EJ: Spontaneous dissection of the internal carotid artery. Arch Surg 111:1294, 1976
7. Anderson CA, Collins CG Jr, Rich NM, et al: Spontaneous dissection of the internal carotid artery associated with fibromuscular dysplasia. Am Surg 46:263, 1980
8. Ringel SP, Harrison SH, Norenberg MD, et al: Fibromuscular dysplasia: Multiple spontaneous dissecting aneurysms of the major cervical arteries. Ann Neurol 1:301, 1977
9. Garcia-Merino JA, Guterrez JA, Lopez-Lozano JJ, et al: Double lumen dissecting aneurysms of the internal carotid artery in fibromuscular dysplasia: Case report. Stroke 14:815, 1983
10. Brice JG, Crompton MR: Spontaneous dissecting aneurysms of the cervical internal carotid artery. Br Med J 2:207, 1964
11. Thapedi IM, Ashenhurst EM, Rozdilsky B: Spontaneous dissecting aneurysm of the internal carotid artery in the neck. Arch Neurol 23:549, 1970
12. Vanneste JAL, Davies G: Spontaneous dissection of the cervical internal carotid artery. Clin Neurol Neurosurg 86:307, 1984
13. Perry MO: The Management of Acute Vascular Injuries. Baltimore, Williams & Wilkins, 1981
14. Fleming JFR, Park AM: Dissecting aneurysms of the carotid artery following arteriography. Neurology (N.Y.) 9:1, 1959
15. Sirois J, Lapointe H, Cote PE: Unusual local complication of percutaneous cerebral angiography. J Neurosurg 11:112, 1954
16. Crawford T: The pathological effects of cerebral arteriography. J Neurol Neurosurg Psychiat 19:217, 1956
17. Aranson M, Kramer R: Traumatic disruption of the left common carotid artery following blunt trauma. Surg Rounds 12:47, 1985
18. Jernigan WR, Gardner WC: Carotid artery injuries due to closed cervical trauma. J Trauma 11:429, 1971
19. Solheim K: Common carotid artery aneurysm after blunt trauma. J Trauma 19:707, 1979
20. Yamada S, Kindt GW, Youmans JR: Carotid artery occlusion due to nonpenetrating injury. J Trauma 7:333, 1967
21. Anderson R McD, Schechter MM: A case of spontaneous dissecting aneurysm of the internal carotid artery. J Neurol Neurosurg Psychiat 22:195, 1959
22. Hodge CJ, Lee SH: Spontaneous dissecting cervical carotid artery aneurysm. Neurosurgery 10:93, 1982
23. McNeill DH, Dreisbach J, Marsden RJ: Spontaneous dissection of the internal carotid artery: Its conservative management with heparin sodium. Arch Neurol 37:54, 1980
24. Gee W, Kaupp HA, McDonald KM, et al: Spontaneous dissection of internal carotid arteries: Spontaneous resolution documented by serial ocular pneumoplethysmography and angiography. Arch Surg 115:944, 1980

25. Mokri B, Sundt TM, Houser W: Spontaneous internal carotid dissection, hemicrania and Horner's syndrome. Arch Neurol 36:677, 1979

26. Maitland CG, Black JL, Smith WA: Abducens nerve palsy due to spontaneous dissection of the internal carotid artery. Arch Neurol 40:448, 1983

27. Miyamoto S, Kikuchi H, Karasawa J, et al: Surgical treatment for spontaneous carotid dissection with impending stroke. J Neurosurg 61:382, 1984

28. O'Dwyer JA, Moscow N, Trevor R, et al: Spontaneous dissection of the carotid artery. Radiology 137:379, 1980

29. Effeney DJ, Krupski WC, Ehrenfeld WK, et al: Spontaneous dissection of the carotid artery. Aust NZ J Surg 53:533, 1983

30. Fischer CM, Opimann RG, Roberson GH: Spontaneous dissection of cervicocerebral arteries. Can J Neurol 5:9, 1978

31. Luken MG, Archerl GF Jr., Correll JW, et al: Spontaneous dissecting aneurysms of the extracranial internal carotid artery. Clin Neurosurg 26:353, 1979

32. Barker WF, in discussion Ehrenfeld WK, Wylie EJ: Spontaneous dissection of the internal carotid artery. Arch Surg 111:1294, 1976

33. Fischer CM: The headache and pain of spontaneous carotid dissection. Headache 22:60, 1982

34. Beatty RA: Dissecting hematoma of the internal carotid artery following chiropractic cervical manipulation. J Trauma 17:248, 1977

35. Boldrey E, Maass L, Miller E: The role of atlantoid compression in the etiology of internal carotid thrombosis. J Neurosurg 13:127, 1956

36. Mehigan JT, Olcott C: The carotid "string" sign: Differential diagnosis and management. Am J Surg 140:137, 1980

37. Houser OW, Mokri B, Sundt TM, et al: Spontaneous cervical cephalic arterial dissection and its residuum: Angiographic spectrum. AJNR 5:27, 1984

38. Ehrenfeld WK, Stoney RJ, Wylie EJ: Relation of carotid stump pressure to safety of carotid ligation. Surgery 93:299, 1983

39. The EC/IC Bypass Study Group: Failure of extracranial–intracranial arterial bypass to reduce the risk of ischemic stroke: Results of an international randomized trial. N Engl J Med 313:1191, 1985

Roger M. Greenhalgh, Charles N. McCollum
B.M. Bourke, Rachel Dain
G.D. Perkin, F. Clifford Rose

Emergency Carotid Endarterectomy

Performing a carotid endarterectomy in a patient with an acute neurological deficit has been controversial for more than 22 years.[1] Early reports suggested a high incidence of complications when surgery was performed in the first few days after the development of an acute deficit. These complications were believed to be associated with the restoration of flow to an area of ischaemic brain producing hemorrhage in an area of infarction.[2] The Joint Study of Extracranial Arterial Occlusion in 1969 reviewed data on 255 acute stroke patients with altered consciousness. Of these, 187 were admitted in coma, semicoma, or stupor and were treated medically. At the time of discharge 53 percent were improved, 22 percent were the same, 5 percent were worse, and 20 percent had died during during the period in hospital. Fifty patients were operated upon within the first 2 weeks of acute stroke and of these 34 percent were improved, 18 percent were unchanged, 6 percent were worse, and 42 percent died. In other words, the surgically treated group had a mortality twice as great as the medically treated group. The surgically treated group appeared to be comparable with the nonsurgical group, although a random allocation study was not performed. Concerning operation for total internal carotid artery occlusion, the joint study made no definite conclusions regarding indications for operation, but noted that "the earlier an operation is performed, the greater the chance of reestablishing patency and the higher the risk of converting an anaemic infarct into the much more lethal haemorrhagic infarct."

DEFINITIONS

We use the terms recommended in the Marseille classification.[3] The term *acute stroke* always has a rather imprecise definition. The term *transient ischaemic attack* (TIA) has universal acceptance. This implies a neurological deficit that usually lasts minutes, but by definition, is completely cleared within a 24-hour period. The Marseille classification allows for the term *transient stroke* as a stroke that persists longer than 24 hours but it is completely cleared within a 3-week period. The term *established stroke* is reserved for a

Vascular Surgical Emergencies
ISBN 0-8089-1843-5

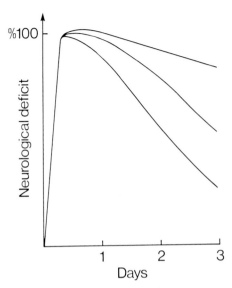

Fig. 1. Acute stroke.

stroke that persists for more than 3 weeks. An established stroke can either have a good outlook such that, for example, there can be no detectable deficit at 4 or 5 weeks or else it can have a bad outlook in which case the established stroke could be accompanied by a deficit that is present months later and may be regarded as permanent. The term *acute stroke* as can be seen in Figure 1 is very difficult to define. It is quite impossible to be certain within the first 24 hour period whether the patient will subsequently be seen to have a transient ischaemic attack, transient stroke, or an established stroke with a good or bad outcome. The term *crescendo transient ischaemic attack* (CTIA) implies a succession of transient ischaemic attacks in which succeeding TIAs are more severe or more frequent. In Figure 2 CTIA is depicted as an attack in which a number of TIAs occur within a

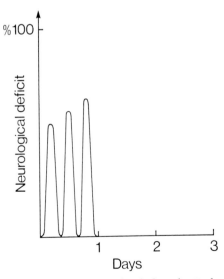

Fig. 2. Crescendo transient ischaemic attacks.

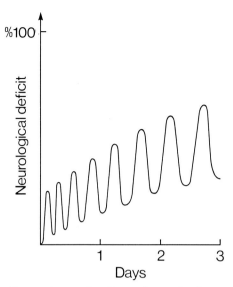

Fig. 3. Progressing stroke: fluctuating stroke (stuttering hemi-plegia).

24 hour period during which the deficit is more severe than the previous one. The term *crescendo transient ischaemic attack* is also used where attacks of similar severity occur with progressively shorter intervals between attacks.

By the term *progressing stroke* we understand that progression of a neurological deficit has occurred over at least a 24 hour period. Progressing stroke can be of one of at least two recognizable types. Fluctuating stroke has otherwise been referred to as *stuttering hemiplegia* (Fig. 3). In this form of progressing stroke there is a progressive worsening of deficit over at least a 24 hour period, but within the 24 hour period, deficit waxes and wanes and becomes more and less severe but never clears completely. Another type of progressing stroke is the stroke in evolution (SIE) (Fig. 4) in which progression occurs

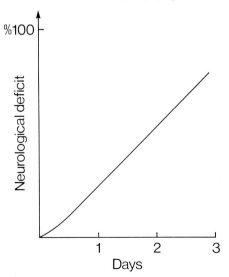

Fig. 4. Progressing stroke (stroke in evolution).

over at least a 24 hour period and there is no waxing and waning, but gradual increase in deficit.

INDICATIONS

Following the clear historical warning of the hazards of emergency carotid surgery, the indications for urgent intervention for stroke have quite properly been extremely limited. We reviewed our experience of the most recent 200 carotid procedures at Charing Cross Hospital in London. Emergency carotid intervention was performed in only 25 of these 200 procedures. By far the commonest indication was progressing stroke in 15 patients, followed by crescendo transient ischaemic attacks in 7 patients. The remaining three procedures were following an angiogram on one occasion and technical problems following carotid surgery on two occasions. These 3 patients will be described briefly here for completeness before describing the other 22 patients with progressing stroke and crescendo transient ischaemic attacks in greater detail.

One patient underwent urgent carotid surgery followed an arch angiogram. He was a 55-year-old man with a history of 2 established strokes 18 months apart after which good recovery had taken place on both occasions. The arch angiogram demonstrated a 60 percent left internal carotid stenosis and immediately after the procedure he developed signs of stroke and homonymous hemianopia. Emergency left carotid endarterectomy was performed at once. There was loose material at the level of the stenosis but total occlusion had not occurred. The patient made a good recovery. At 1 and 3 months postangiogram and surgery a very slight deficit was detectable. It is quite impossible in such circumstances to be certain whether surgery is of value and no satisfactory control trial has been performed for this problem.

The first patient for whom emergency reoperation was necessary recovered at first completely normally after the primary carotid endarterectomy. Then after some hours she developed early signs of stroke and was returned to the operating room urgently. A kink had occurred in the internal carotid after removal of the atherosclerotic stent and this vessel had thrombosed. The clot was evacuated and the back bleed was good. A Javid shunt was inserted at once. The kink was corrected and a patch inserted to minimize the risk of further kinking. The patient made a satisfactory recovery with no detectable motor or sensory deficit, but 3 months after this procedure evidence of personality changes were noted by those who knew her well. The other patient had a neurological deficit following carotid surgery performed for a number of attacks related to a carotid arteritis. After carotid surgery the whole carotid system thrombosed. The patient was returned to the operating room, clot evacuated, and a shunt instantly reinserted. The artery was patched and the patient was treated with intravenous heparin and increased doses of steroids. Three months after the procedure, despite considerable improvement there was some residual deficit. Again, the justification for such reoperation procedures is open to question, although there remains a strong impression that rapid reintervention is better than leaving the internal carotid occluded if the time interval is short.

We have not otherwise performed emergency carotid endarterectomy on patients with acute carotid occlusion. Meyer and his colleagues[4] at the Mayo Clinic reported recently 34 patients who underwent emergency carotid endarterectomy for acute internal carotid occlusion. Before operation all of their patients had profound neurologic deficits including hemiplegia and aphasia. In 9 patients, occlusion occurred within 1 hour of cerebral angiography and in 5 patients occlusion followed carotid surgery. Thirty–three of the 34 were hospitalized when the internal carotid occlusion took place. Whereas a commendable 94 percent success rate was achieved in restoring patency, at follow-up, 9 patients (26.5 percent) had a normal neurological examination and 4 (11.8 percent) had a minimal deficit. In other words, 13 (38 percent) had a good outcome. On the other hand 7 (20.6 percent) died.

NATURAL HISTORY

Before considering operative intervention for progressing stroke and CTIA, it is important to know the natural history of these conditions. There are no control studies of the efficacy of operation for CTIAs or progressing stroke, but nonoperative series have been reported. Millikan[5] reviewed the natural history of 204 consecutive patients with progressing stroke. This series served as a control for a clinical study evaluating the effects of carbon dioxide inhalation in patients with progressing stroke caused by carotid artery disease. At the end of 14 days, only 12 percent were normal, 69 percent hemiparetic, 5 percent monoparetic, and 14 percent of the patients had died. Mentzer et al[6] identified 55 patients with fluctuating neurological deficits from the records of 485 consecutive patients with cerebral ischaemia. The fluctuation deficits were either CTIAs or progressing stroke. Of the 55 patients 31 were managed nonoperatively and 24 had emergency operation. The operative and nonoperative groups had similar age and sex distribution and incidence of associated medical problems. Of the five nonoperative CTIA patients, one recovered completely, three were moderately to severely impaired at the time of discharge, and one died of complications of cerebral infarction. Seven operated CTIA patients recovered completely and were free of symptoms at the time of discharge. For progressing stroke the operative and nonoperative groups were comparable for degree of neurological deficit at the time of diagnosis. Of the 26 nonoperated progressing stroke patients, only 2 made a complete neurological recovery, 3 had a mild residual deficit, 17 a moderate to severe deficit, and 4 patients died. In the operative group, of 17 patients described as having progressing stroke, only 12 were admitted to hospital with the primary condition, while 4 developed signs after arteriography and 1 after an elective carotid endarterectomy. However, after surgery, 4 of the 17 had complete neurological recovery and 8 were left with a mild deficit, 4 with a moderate to severe deficit and 1 patient died. In other words 12 out of 17 of the operative group (70.6 percent) against 5 of 26 of the nonoperative (19.2 percent) were in the mild to normal category with respect to degree of neurological deficit at the time of hospital discharge.

THE CHARING CROSS SERIES

We have operated upon 22 patients including 7 with CTIAs and 15 with progressing stroke. All patients were fully conscious and well orientated. All of the 15 progressing stroke patients had a mild stroke with mild deficit and this deficit worsened over a period of at least 24 hours of observation. There was no return of deficit to normal at any time during the period of observation. In some patients there was fluctuation in deficit (fluctuating stroke) and in others there was a gradual deterioration without fluctuation (stroke in

Table 1
Progressing Stroke

Patient	Sex	Age	Hypertension	Presentation	CT Scan	Stenosis (%)	Stump Pressure (mmHg)	Shunt	Outcome
JG	M	66	No	CTIAs. Fluctuating stroke over 7 days	Infarction	90	100	No	No progression Improved
AN	M	58	Yes	2 months before established stroke. Good recovery. Fluctuating stroke over 9 days	Infarction	90	105	No	No progression
NR	F	63	No	No TIAs. Gradual SIE over 3 days	Infarction	50	45	Yes	No progression Then stroke Carotid screen NAD
JW	F	80	Yes	No TIAs. Gradual SIE over 2 days	Normal	80	60	No	No progression Improved
EP	F	61	No	No TIAs. Fluctuating stroke over 13 days	Infarction	50	50	Yes	No progression Improved
KD	F	70	Yes	No TIAs. Gradual SIE over 2 days	Infarction	90	50	No	No progression Improved
WE	M	64	No	Established stroke. Good recovery 14 months before. Fluctuating stroke over 3 days	Infarction	90	70	No	No progression Almost normal

144

	Sex	Age		History	CT				Outcome
TD	F	58	Yes	CTIAs. Then SIE over 2 days	Normal	90	30	Yes	No progression / Improved
BA	M	46	No	Established stroke. Good recovery 2 months before. Then SIE over 2 days	Infarction	40	80	No	No progression / Improved / Almost normal
BR	M	59	No	CTIAs for 24 hours. Then SIE over 24 hours	Not done	50	0	Yes	No progression / Normal
VM	F	74	Yes	CTIAs for 5 days. Then SIE over 24 hours	Infarction	90	45	Yes	No progression / Normal
ED	F	61	Yes	TIAs over 5 days. Then SIE over 2 days	Not done	90	70	No	No progression / Improved / Almost normal
DP	M	77	No	CTIAs. Then SIE over 24 hours	Infarction	85	60	Yes	No progression / Improved
BK	M	70	Yes	CTIAs for 12 days. Then SIE over 2 days	Infarction	Aneurysmal disease	60	No	No progression / Normal
RW	F	79	No	CTIAs for 2 weeks. Established stroke, mild deficit. Progression over 3 days	Infarction	70	Low	Yes	No progression / Improved

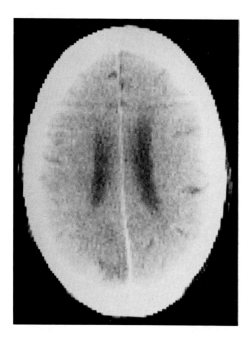

Fig. 5. CT scan of patient JG, showing diminished density in the left occipital region.

evolution). The finding of an occluded internal carotid artery was regarded as a contraindication for surgery.

The Progressing Stroke Patients

The series of 15 patients is summarized in Table 1. Seven were men and eight women. Ages ranged from 46 to 80 with a mean of 65.7 years. Seven out of 15 were hypertensive. Seven of the patients had crescendo transient ischaemic attacks preceding progressing stroke and three had had an established stroke and made a good recovery and then developed progressing stroke in the same carotid territory. The remaining five patients had no evidence of previous transient ischaemic attacks or strokes and four of the five developed a gradual stroke in evolution over a period of days. The last patient had no previous history of stroke or transient ischaemic attack and developed a fluctuating type of progressing stroke.

Cerebral CT scan was performed on 13 of the 15 patients and infarction was demonstrated in 11 of these. In patient JG, a 66-year-old male, CTIAs were followed by fluctuating stroke over a period of about 7 days. The angiogram showed stenosis of about 90 percent in the left internal carotid artery. The intracranial angiogram showed that the left posterior cerebral artery arose from the left internal carotid. The first CT scan (Fig. 5) showed a diminished density in the left occipital area, which was thought to be an infarct related to the left carotid disease because of the abnormal intracranial anatomy. His neurologic deficit increased over 24 hours and his stroke progressed. The CT scan 24 hours later (Fig. 6) showed some extension in the left occipital region. Twenty four hours after this, further neurological deterioration had occurred and the CT scan (Fig. 7) was performed. This is the only patient in whom serial CT scans have been performed on successive days in association with clinical evidence of progression of neurologic deficit.

Urgent arch angiography with carotid and intracranial views was performed for all of

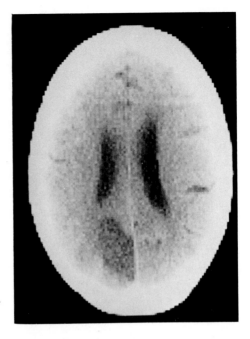

Fig. 6. CT scan of patient JG 24 hours after
the first CT scan.

the patients and in each, demonstrable arterial disease was noted. One patient had aneurysmal disease and in another a stenosis of 40 percent was found. However, in the
remainder, stenoses of 50 percent or more were demonstrated and in 7 the stenoses were
greater than 90 percent. Figure 8 is the angiogram of patient WE. Above the tight stenosis
in the internal carotid artery there is an obvious filling defect.

When the neurological deficit had worsened over a 24 hour period, progressing stroke

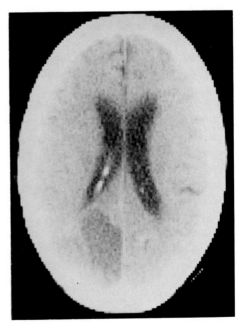

Fig. 7. CT scan of patient JG 48 hours after
the first CT scan.

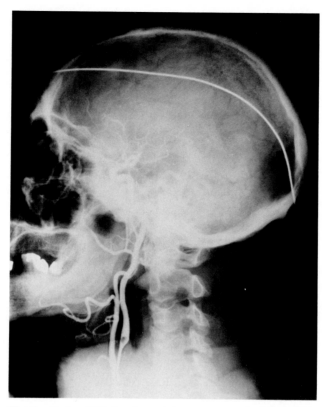

Fig. 8. Patient WE showing a tight stenosis of the region of the internal carotid artery with a filling deficit beyond the stenosis.

was diagnosed and emergency carotid endarterectomy under general anaesthesia was performed. The stump or back pressure was recorded at the time of surgery and there was a great variation (Table 1). It was our policy to use a Javid shunt for cerebral protection on occasions where the stump pressure was 50 mmHg or less. This resulted in the shunt being used on 7 occasions.

Progression of stroke was arrested after surgery in all 15 patients and 6 patients became and remained either completely neurologically normal or almost normal. After arrest of progression, eight patients began to have an improving neurological deficit after the operation, but the deficit did not return completely to normal. Good results were therefore considered to have been achieved for 14 out of 15 patients (93 percent). In the remaining patient, the progression of stroke was halted for a week after surgery and then a stroke in the relevant territory occurred. Carotid imaging was performed for this patient, but no abnormality was detected. Patient NR was a 63-year-old woman who was not hypertensive and who had developed a gradual stroke in evolution without previous TIA or stroke. At operation the stump pressure was 45 mmHg and a shunt had been used. It is very difficult to explain why this patient suddenly had an established stroke 1 week after surgery and this patient is considered to be the only one of the 15 patients who had an unfortunate outcome.

Table 2
Crescendo Transient Ischaemic Attacks

Patient	Sex	Age	Hypertension	Presentation	CT Scan	Stenosis (%)	Stump Pressure (mmHg)	Shunt	Outcome
NG	M	64	No	CTIAs	Infarction	95	0	Yes	Normal
WW	M	61	Yes	Crescendo amaurosis fugax	Infarction	90	50	Yes	Normal
MA	F	60	No	Established stroke. Good recovery. Crescendo TIAs	Normal	Kinked irregular carotid	25	Yes	No TIAs Good recovery Improved
KE	M	55	No	CTIAs and amaurosis fugax	Infarction	90	50	Yes	Normal
RO	M	72	No	CTIAs	Not done	90	40	Yes	Normal
RB	M	56	No	CTIAs	Not done	99	40	Yes	Normal
IP	F	69	No	CTIAs	Infarction	99 →100	0	Yes	Died

Crescendo Transient Ischaemic Attacks

Of the 7 patients, 5 were male and 2 female, age range was 55–72 years with a mean age of 62.4 years. Only one of the patients was hypertensive. As can be seen from Table 2, 1 patient (MA) was a 60-year-old woman who had previously had an established stroke and made a good recovery. She then developed CTIAs in the same distribution. Oddly enough, her CT scan was normal at that stage and she was subsequently shown to have kinked carotid vessels on angiography.

For all patients arch angiography with carotid and intracranial views was performed and other than the patient with a kinked irregular carotid artery all had a stenosis of greater than 90 percent (Table 2), one had an internal carotid stenosis of 95 percent, and 2 of approximately 99 percent. Emergency carotid endarterectomy was performed for all patients and once again the stump or back pressure was recorded. Again, this was variable but in every instance the stump pressure was 50 mmHg or less and a Javid intraluminal shunt was used for cerebral protection on every occasion. Five patients were completely normal after emergency carotid surgery and patient MA, the 60-year-old woman who had previously had an established stroke with good recovery and with a kinked carotid artery was greatly improved after carotid surgery but did have some very mild deficit. It was considered that good results were achieved therefore in 6 out of 7 in this series (87 percent). One patient died after the procedure—she was not hypertensive and presented with CTIAs without any previous stroke or symptoms. The CT scan had demonstrated infarction and angiography showed 99 percent stenosis. A period of 6 hours elapsed before surgery was performed and at operation the internal carotid artery was found to be occluded with a recent clot in the lumen beyond the atherosclerotic stenosis. This clot was flushed out and a Javid shunt inserted. This patient did not recover and the error that occurred here was clearly related to the thrombosis that occurred after arteriography with an excessive time lapse before surgery. Since this experience we have performed noninvasive assessment of the carotid vessels immediately before surgery on every occasion in case "silent" internal carotid occulsion has occurred.

It is quite unjustified to compare by implication nonoperated results of, for example, Millikan with the operated results that we have achieved for progressing stroke or any other such comparison. The surgical results certainly appear to be much better than nonsurgical, but one has to remember that the series took place in different parts of the world and at different times and there is no guarantee that such series are comparable. However, others have achieved encouraging results with emergency carotid procedures for progressing and transient ischaemic attacks. Goldstone and Moore[7] reported a series of 26 patients in whom emergency carotid endarterectomy was performed. Eight of the 26 patients in the series had CTIAs and 18 had progressing stroke of whom 10 exhibited slowly progressing stroke in evolution and 8 had fluctuating stroke of the waxing and waning type. All of their patients had critical arterial lesions of the carotid bifurcation appropriate to the symptoms. All of their 26 patients had a "dramatic complete and so far permanent neurological recovery following operation. There was no morbidity from either the angiographic or surgical procedures." These results do appear to be very good indeed and are comparable with ours, but in our case, particularly for the progressing stroke patients, we acknowledge that some patients had a neurologic deficit in the postoperative period and could not be regarded as completely normal. Nevertheless, of ours only one patient had a stroke after surgical intervention and surgery always arrested progression of stroke. This is the critical issue. That surgical intervention stopped the progression of the stroke is important rather than the neurological status after several weeks. The degree of irreversible ischaemic damage is to some extent determined before the operation begins.

It certainly looks as if there is the possibility that surgical intervention for progressing stroke and CTIAs is justified compared with the expected natural history for nonintervention. No satisfactory control trial has been performed either for CTIAs or progressing stroke and this certainly should be performed in an attempt to justify carotid surgery for these indications. It will be argued by some that it is not ethical to withhold carotid surgery in view of the expected 88 percent poor outcome for nonintervention as reported by Millikan[5] and the good results reported here and by Goldstone and Moore.[7] This would certainly be a dangerous view point as indications for carotid surgery are under great scrutiny at the present time. It could well be that we can prove scientifically the value of carotid surgery for these indications at a time when some neurologists believe that there is no proof or cast iron indication for carotid endarterectomy on any occasion. If the results of surgery compared with nonintervention are so favorable it would require only about 15 patients in each group to produce an answer. Most centers are likely to see two or three progressing strokes per year and so a multicenter trial is necessary. In such a trial it will be prudent to choose those centers with a good record in performing carotid endarterectomy with low morbidity and mortality over the last 200 cases. The vascular surgeons would need to work with neurological colleagues who would need to assess the patients independently both before surgery and after surgery at fixed periods. CT scan and angiography would be necessary on all patients and where possible the surgical procedure would need to be standardized. The neurologic assessment would need to be quantitative to some extent in order that it could be seen whether surgical intervention had arrested the deterioration in neurological deficit as the stroke was progressing.

In conclusion, good results have been achieved for emergency carotid endarterectomy, for CTIAs, and progressing strokes. While emergency carotid surgery for acute stroke or for an occluded internal carotid artery is still controversial, the results for CTIA and progressing stroke are so good compared with the natural history that a multicenter trial to compare operated and nonoperated groups is recommended.

REFERENCES

1. Wylie EJ, Hein MF, Adams JE: Intracranial hamorrhage strokes. J Neurosurg 21:212, 1964
2. Blaisdell WF, Clauss RH, Galbraith JG, et al: Joint Study of Extracranial Arterial Occlusions. JAMA 209:1889, 1969
3. Courbier R (Ed): Basis for a Classification of Cerebral Arterial Disease. Amsterdam, Excerpta Medica, 1985
4. Meyer FB, Piepgras DG, Sandok BA, et al: Emergency carotid endarterectomy for patients with acute carotid occlusion and profound neurological deficits. Arch Surg 203(1):82, 1986
5. Millikan CH: Clinical management of cerebral ischaemia, in MacDonnell FL, Brennan RW (eds.): Cerebral Vascular Disease—Eighth Conference, New York. New York, Grune & Stratton, 1973, p. 209
6. Mentzer RM, Finkelmeier BA, Crosby IK, et al: Emergency carotid endarterectomy for fluctuating neurological deficits. Surgery 89(1):60, 1981
7. Goldstone J, Moore WS: A new look at emergency carotid artery operations for the treatment of cerebrovascular insufficiency. Stroke 9:599, 1978

William J. Fry
Richard E. Fry

Management of Carotid Artery Injury

Through the earliest years of recorded surgical history, the surgeon's preoccupation was with the staunching of hemorrhage from cervical wounds. But it was not until 1803 that successful ligation of the common carotid artery was carried out. This was done by David Fleming.[1] Ligation as a form of therapy for carotid artery trauma persisted until the middle of the 20th century. Reports of the ability to suture arteries and the well devised techniques of Alexis Carrel did not seem to influence the care of the lacerated carotid artery. Ligature remained the primary treatment throughout both World War I and World War II, and this resulted in a 44 percent mortality rate and a 30 percent incidence of major neurologic deficit. Following World War I many authors favored Makin's[2] advocacy of the nonoperative approach to penetrating neck wounds. Even with this conservative approach, the mortality rate remained at 35 percent.

It was not until the Korean Conflict that it was seen as possible, indeed routinely so, to repair traumatic lesions of the carotid artery. This significant advance derived from recognition and dissemination of peripheral vascular surgical principles, most of which began with Carrel. Several controversies arose from the ability to repair arteries and restore circulation to the brain. The most important was the question of conversion of an ischemic infarct to an hemorrhagic infarction after reinstitution of blood flow. Little controversy developed regarding management of the patient with carotid artery disruption and no neurologic deficit. However, differences of opinion still exist regarding revascularization of patients with neurologic deficits.

INCIDENCE

Carotid injuries represent somewhat over 5 percent of all arterial injuries. The majority of these are secondary to penetrating trauma with only 2–3 percent being caused by blunt trauma. With the use of routine arteriography,[3] vertebral artery injury has been demonstrated much more frequently than had previously been thought. For example, in our clinic, we have found the vertebral artery injured in association with penetrating neck wounds in 10 percent of cases.

Vascular Surgical Emergencies
ISBN 0-8089-1843-5

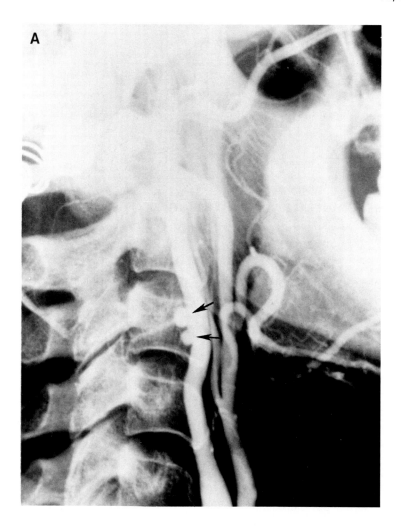

TYPES OF INJURY

Carotid injuries may be classified according to layers of the artery that are involved.

1. Intimal tear—defect seen on arteriogram showing discontinuity of the smooth intimal surface. There may or may not be thrombus adherent to the defect. In older patients atherosclerotic plaque formation may be confusing on arteriography. Comparison with the contralateral carotid artery is helpful to rule out injury.
2. Partial disruption—these lesions may form a false aneurysm, minor defects of the arterial wall, complete thrombosis of the vessel or an arteriovenous fistula if an adjacent vein is also injured.
3. Complete disruption—these lesions may have almost normal flow on arteriogram, partial flow, or complete thrombosis. The thrombus surrounding the severed artery may extend into the lumen and cause distal embolization either spontaneously or by rough handling at the time of operative repair.
4. Dissection—intimal disruption may progress to subintimal dissection. In our experience this is most common in the internal carotid artery. It most often extends to the

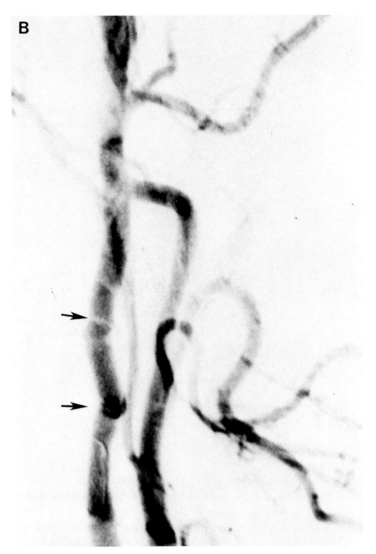

Fig. 1. (A) Arteriogram demonstrating stretch injury to internal carotid artery. Arrows point to two aneurysms caused by acute stretching of the neck and partial disruption of the internal carotid artery. (B) Postoperative arteriogram showing vein interposition graft replacing segment of internal carotid artery involved in partial disruption.

base of the skull. Minor dissections secondary to blunt trauma usually will heal spontaneously. Extensive dissections, usually secondary to extensive blast effect do not heal readily and may pose a therapeutic dilemma.

Blunt injury to the carotid artery in the neck is secondary to a direct blow or a combination of stretching and compression of the artery (Fig. 1). Intraoral injury or fracture of the base of the skull may cause internal carotid injury. Intraoral injury is most common in children.

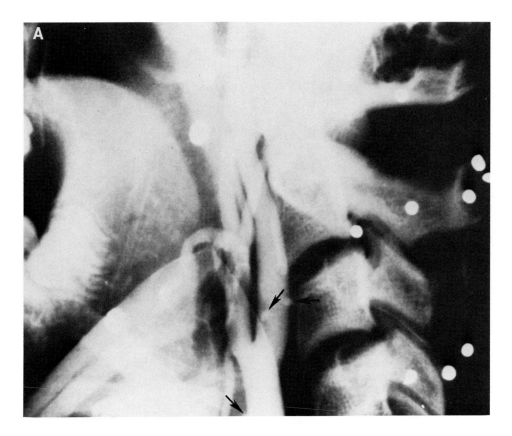

PENETRATING CERVICAL INJURY

Considerable controversy exists throughout trauma centers in the United States about the proper management of penetrating neck wounds.[4] Policies vary from routine exploration of all patients with penetrating trauma with wide dissection of the carotid arterial system on the involved side, to selective operations in the patient with penetrating neck trauma who undergoes routine arteriography. There are strong proponents of both systems; however, we believe that the routine use of arteriography and the selective use of operation is best.

While arteriography in all patients with penetrating trauma of the neck is desirable, this is sometimes impossible because of the unstable condition of the patient as observed in the emergency room. Patients who have active arterial bleeding from the wound and/or patients with rapidly expanding hematomas and secondary airway difficulties should be taken immediately to the operating room. Delay may cause death from exsanguination or airway obstruction.

ROLE OF ARTERIOGRAPHY

The majority of penetrating neck wounds do not appear as the true emergency described above. Therefore, routine arch aortography and selective arteriograms on the affected side can be obtained. This serves as a guide to the surgeon in planning a repair of

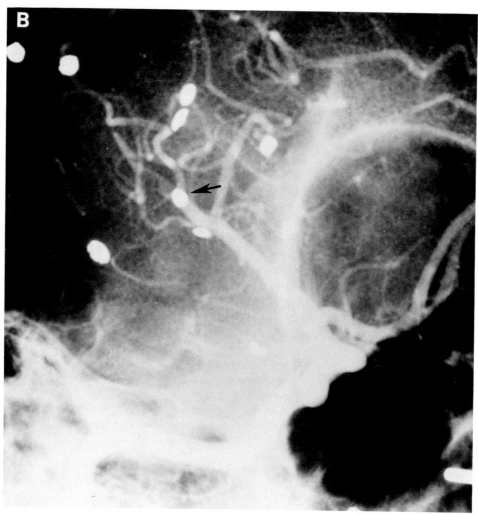

Fig. 2. (A) Arteriogram showing subtle changes of multiple false aneurysms secondary to penetration by shotgun pellets. Multiple views and high quality films are required for accurate assessment of these injuries. (B) Intracranial arteriogram demonstrating shotgun pellet embolus to the middle cerebral artery. The wound of entrance is demonstrated in Figure 2A. This was successfully removed by craniotomy and microvascular technique and reestablishment of normal blood flow. The patient recovered with minimal neurologic defect.

a lesion of the carotid artery and helps him or her to determine whether the patient should be operated upon or not. We believe that a normal well done arteriogram of the extracranial vessels with multiple views rules out injury of the arterial system.[5] The only exception to this is seen in shotgun wounds (Fig. 2). In such wounds, if there is any question, these patients should be operatively explored to rule out the chance for arterial injury. Those who argue that routine exploration may be done safely with minimum morbidity and mortality seem to be eluding the goal of all surgeons. That is to eliminate unnecessary operative procedures. One must remember that operative morbidity includes more than simple postoperative complications. Cost and unnecessary time spent in the hospital must also be considered. This is particularly true with the relative rare carotid and vertebral arterial disruptions. While extracranial arteriography may be time consuming, it still requires less time than an operative procedure, is more economical, and has potentially less side effects than general anesthesia and a formal neck exploration.

There are additional benefits to arteriography. Missiles and knives do not have predictable trajectories. Penetration in the mid neck may injure a vessel in the mediastinum or in the high internal carotid artery. In addition, the detection of thrombus in an area of disruption or partial disruption helps to plan exposure so that this is not dislodged to form a distal embolus. Armed with an accurate and well done arteriogram, the surgeon is able to plan the operative procedure from proper exposure to the type of repair needed. The surgeon can thus, spend less time in the operating room and can perform a thoughtful and expeditious repair of the involved vessel.

One third of all carotid injuries observed in this clinic over the past 10 years involved the internal carotid artery. Many of these were in the mid to distal portion of the internal carotid artery and posed problems with exposure. The knowledge of the location of such an injury allows the surgeon to plan preoperatively. We have utilized nasotracheal intubation in these patients with subsequent subluxation of the mandible in order to allow exposure of the internal carotid artery to the base of the skull.[6,7] We currently place one wire around the mandible taking care to avoid major nervous and vascular structures. A second wire is placed through the nasal spine. The jaw is subluxed anteriorly and held in place by connecting the two wires with a third wire (Fig. 3). This technique has proven to be very useful in extending the exposure of the internal carotid artery easily to the base of the skull. We have seen no morbidity or functional impairment from the use of this technique.

Because of the relatively common associated injuries to the vertebral artery, the surgeon should be familiar with the easy exposure of the vertebral artery. Refinement of the techniques described by Henry has been useful when this injury is encountered.[8,9] This has completely avoided the seemingly unmanageable problem of an uncontrollable hemorrhage from the depths of a neck wound along the tract of a bullet or a knife.

TECHNIQUE

The routine incision to expose the cervical vessels is a long vertical incision made at the anterior border of the sternocleidomastoid muscle. This incision may be used for either exposure of the entire cervical carotid artery or the first through the third portions of the vertebral artery. The incision is carried through the platysma muscle and the anterior layer of the deep cervical fascia as it overlies the anterior border of the sternocleidomastoid muscle. By then reflecting the sternocleidomastoid muscle laterally, the carotid sheath is exposed. If there is a major disruption of the carotid artery, attempt to gain proximal and distal control prior to directly approaching the lesion. This is not always possible, particularly if the bleeding from the artery has not tamponaded within the carotid sheath. Great care must be taken not to push around a partial disruption with great vigor as this may dislodge thrombus that will be carried distal to the brain.

Most stab wounds of the common carotid artery may be repaired by direct suture. Since there is no blast effect with the stab wound, there is little necessity to debride the area of injury except where it may be fragmented due to multiple wounds. With isolated neck trauma we routinely heparinize the patient at the time that proximal and distal control has been achieved. In patients with multiple trauma it may not be prudent to heparinize the

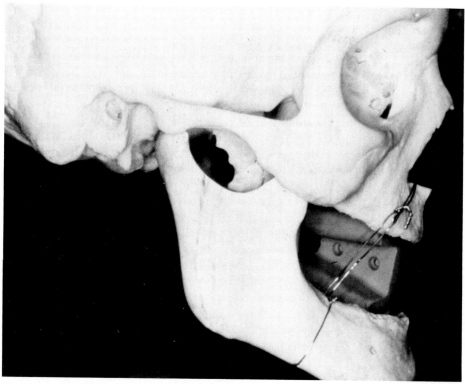

Fig. 3. Photograph showing the method of wiring the jaw in the unilateral anterior and subluxated position. After nasotracheal intubation, the wires are placed and the jaw held in the anterior position. Upon completion of the operation, the wires are removed and the mandible returned to the normal position.

patient. Under these conditions we carefully flush the vessel prior to completing the repair and copiously irrigate the vessel locally with heparinized saline.

In patients with gunshot wounds of the common carotid artery, it is important to debride the artery adequately in order to excise all devitalized tissue. This may automatically require an interposition graft. We prefer to use the saphenous vein as it more nearly resembles the size of the carotid artery. The jugular vein is a second choice, however it is much larger than the carotid artery and the flow characteristics are not as good as with the saphenous vein. In patients with injuries of the common carotid artery, a shunt is not routinely used while the vessel is debrided and the repair is being done. It would seem prudent to use the shunt if there are multiple arterial injuries in the neck or in the atherosclerotic patient with an occluded contralateral carotid artery. Many gunshot wounds of the carotid artery may be repaired with a patch graft rather than an interposition graft. The saphenous vein is preferred; however, the jugular vein is adequate for the patch. Great care must be taken in fashioning a patch so that one does not inadvertently fashion an aneurysm of the carotid artery. We have seen patch grafts that are too large, forming an aneurysm or diverticulum of the vessel that then accumulates laminated clot. This may give rise to intermittent transient ischemic attacks caused by embolization of thrombus.

Isolated injuries of the external carotid artery seldom require more than simple ligation of either the main trunk of the vessel or the branches that are divided. These are particularly common in gunshot wounds to the face, which may involve several branches. Simple ligation of the main external carotid artery when more distal branches are interrupted is not sufficient to prevent continued bleeding, false aneurysm formation, or arterial venous fistulae. The rich anastomotic plexus between the contralateral external carotid artery requires individual ligation of interrupted branches of the external carotid artery in order to prevent late complications.

Injuries of the internal carotid artery present a much greater challenge to the surgeon than either the common carotid or external carotid artery. The ability to plan the operative procedure is important and therefore mandates whenever possible a preoperative arteriogram. Lesions in the mid and upper portions of the internal carotid artery require special exposure principles as outlined earlier. The use of nasotracheal intubation with forward subluxation of the jaw is mandatory to enable the surgeon to have adequate exposure. In most instances the anterior belly of the digastric muscle must be divided in order to expose the entire internal carotid artery. Great care must be taken to avoid injury to the IX, X, XI, and XII cranial nerves. High injuries of the internal carotid artery are usually above the point where the XII nerve crosses the internal carotid artery and one may direct all attention to the area above the XII nerve. At times the XII nerve will lie in the immediate vicinity of the lesion and require that the ansa hypoglossi nerve be cut as it emerges from the XII nerve. This enables one to free the XII nerve and reflect it medially, exposing the entire carotid artery. The X nerve runs immediately posterior to the internal carotid artery at its mid portion and in an area of trauma with hemorrhage great care must be taken to avoid injuring it. The IX nerve will only be encountered when dissecting the distal half of the internal carotid artery. In this area, it lies posterior medial to the internal carotid artery and will generally not be seen if one stays immediately in the adventitia of the internal carotid artery. Wide dissections for false aneurysms may involve the IX nerve and great care should be taken to avoid injuring it. The postoperative morbidity from injury to the IX nerve is significant and dictates great care in dissection.

The principles of repair of the internal carotid artery are the same as in any major vascular injury. There is generally enough room to excise a centimeter of the internal carotid artery and effect an end-to-end anastomosis without tension. This can be accomplished by completely freeing the entire internal carotid artery. We prefer the use of a saphenous interposition graft rather than prosthetic graft when replacement of a portion of the internal carotid artery is necessary. In interruptions of the internal carotid artery we use an indwelling shunt. The vein graft is placed over the shunt allowing the distal anastomosis and a portion of the proximal anastomosis to be completed before the shunt is removed. In some lesions that are very high, it has been impossible or very difficult to utilize a shunt. In these instances, we have finished the distal anastomosis and then placed an indwelling shunt to allow a more leisurely proximal anastomosis. The use of the Pruitt-Inahara shunt may obviate the necessity of shunt clamps or tourniquets to hold the shunt in place.

Some authors have recommended the use of the external carotid artery as a replacement for the internal carotid artery. Whenever possible we have preferred to use an interposition saphenous vein graft rather than sacrificing the external carotid artery to replace a defect in the internal carotid artery. The saphenous vein has worked very well in our experience. This has maintained a normal collateral system to the brain by preserving the external carotid artery.

Extensive dissections of the internal carotid artery caused by gunshot wounds pose a problem that has required the use of the ECIC bypass in order to maintain circulation to that side of the brain. These large lesions do not avail themselves to direct arterial repair as the dissection is so extensive and the tissues so damaged that they do not hold a stitch. We have resorted to extracranial–intracranial bypass with subsequent ligation of the internal carotid artery in order to avoid rupture of these lesions, and at the same time maintain cerebral circulation.

Extensive dissections from direct injury are quite different from those seen with dissections from either stretching of the neck or from an external blow. The dissections caused by these two mechanisms present as a small tubular enlargement of the internal carotid artery, which should be treated conservatively. We have followed these lesions with serial arteriographs and have found them to heal spontaneously in 6 weeks to 3 months.[10] The large lesions caused by direct blow from a missile do not heal and become larger; ultimately, they will rupture if left unattended.

The controversy continues as to when revascularization should be carried out in the face of neurologic deficit. We feel that any patient with a profound neurologic deficit should not have carotid artery flow reestablished. Those patients with minor neurologic deficits and particularly those that wax and wane should have carotid artery flow reestablished. We currently believe that extracranial–intracranial bypass is an important adjunct in the therapy of some patients with carotid artery disruption.[6,11,12] This is particularly true in those patients that have extensive dissections of the internal carotid artery or lesions at or in the base of the skull. These are best treated by ECIC rather than attempts at finding the distal end of the internal carotid artery in the bony canal.

The general principle of reestablishing blood flow in the neurologically normal patient is important, because only 20 percent of patients have a complete Circle of Willis.[13] The sequence of a period of normal neurologic function followed by neurologic dysfunction that continues to a profound hemiplegia is due to thrombus extending up the carotid stump and occluding the anterior and posterior communicating arteries. This usually occurs 36–48 hours following the injury. It is important to recognize this sequence of events. One should not be lulled into complacency by the patient with a disrupted carotid artery and no initial neurologic deficit. Since it is very difficult to assess the Circle of Willis and collateral circulation on an emergency basis, we believe that an aggressive attempt should be made to revascularize these lesions.

The mortality rate seen in our clinic with carotid artery injuries has been in association with gunshot wounds. They have been multiple in nature. The great majority of patients who have died, entered the hospital with profound neurologic deficit. The mortality rate for all carotid injuries has remained just 10 percent. The neurologic deficit for all carotid injuries has remained at 5 percent. These have all been secondary to gunshot wounds. All have been relatively minor defects, none of which have been made worse by revascularization. The mortality in isolated carotid artery injury is 4 percent in our clinic.

The care of carotid artery injuries remains as one of the great challenges to the vascular and trauma surgeon. This is because of the inadequacy of intracranial collateral circulation in 80 percent of all patients.

REFERENCES

1. Watson WL, Silverstone SM: Ligature of the common carotid artery in cancer of the head and neck. Ann Surg 109:1, 1939

2. Rich N, Spencer FC: Carotid and vertebral artery injuries, in Rich N, Spencer FC (eds.): Vascular Trauma. Philadelphia, W.B. Saunders, 1978, pp 260–286

3. Meier DE, Brink BE, Fry WJ: Vertebral artery trauma. Arch Surg 116:236, 1981

4. Sankaran S, Walt AJ: Penetrating wounds of the neck: Principles and some controversies. Surg Clin North Am 57:139, 1977

5. McCormack TM, Burch BH: Routine angiographic evaluation of neck and extremity injuries. J Trauma 19:384, 1979

6. Fry RE, Fry WJ: Extracranial carotid artery injuries. Surgery 88(4):581, 1980

7. Fisher DF, Clagett GP, Parker JI, et al: Mandibular subluxation for high carotid exposure. J Vas Surg 1(6):727, 1984

8. Meier DE, Brink BE, Fry WJ: Vertebral artery trauma. Arch Surg 116:236, 1981

9. Henry AK: Extensile Exposure. Baltimore, Williams and Wilkins, 1970, pp 53–58

10. Ehrenfield WK, Wylie EJ: Spontaneous dissection of the internal carotid artery. Arch Surg 111:1294, 1976

11. Gewertz B, Samson D, Ditmore QM, et al: Management of penetrating injuries of the internal carotid artery at the base of the skull utilizing extracranial-intracranial bypass. J Trauma 20(5):365, 1980

12. Samson D, Boone S: Extracranial-intracranial (EC-IC) arterial bypass: past performance and current concepts. Neurosurgery 3:79, 1978

13. Bradley EL: Management of penetrating carotid injuries: an alternative approach. J Trauma 13:248, 1973

PART IV

Arterial Injuries

Malcolm O. Perry

Penetrating Trauma to the Extremities

Vascular wounds are the sole cause or major contributing event in causation of many deaths related to trauma. Even those patients who survive may experience severe disability from vascular injuries that lead to amputation or those that produce impaired function.[1] For example, 20 percent of arterial injuries involve the femoral vessels (Table 1). Acute ligation of the common femoral artery results in an amputation rate of approximately 50 percent, only slightly less than that following acute occlusion of the popliteal artery. Those limbs not amputated are physiologically impaired. Moreover, large veins and important nerves are found within the femoral triangle and injury to them also produces disability. In vascular wounds of the upper extremity the brachial plexus is often involved,[2] and its damage can produce profound disability.

In most situations there is little difficulty in ascertaining that the patient has a serious injury when he or she has experienced penetrating trauma, but patients who have multiple wounds present a severe test of the judgment, discipline, and training of every surgeon. A careful assessment of all injuries and the establishment of priorities in treatment are essential to a successful outcome.

ETIOLOGY

Because aggressive acts of violence are the usual causes of penetrating wounds of the extremities, the greatest incidence of such wounds is seen in urban areas. Most of the wounds are caused by knives and bullets, but accidental wounds may result from injuries inflicted by shards of glass or metal projections during motor vehicle accidents or industrial mishaps. In a smaller number of patients, blunt trauma is at fault (Table 2).

Stab wounds are much more common than gunshot wounds of the extremities, but since such injuries are not as deep they are less likely to produce vascular wounds, and often can be treated with relatively minor corrective procedures. Gunshot wounds, on the other hand, penetrate deeply and often involve the trunk or thorax as well as the extremities, and therefore are likely to produce widespread damage. The vessels of the extremi-

Table 1

Arterial Injuries: Distribution

Extremity	501
Aorta	31
Visceral	37
Cervical	96
Total	665

Table 2

Vascular Trauma Etiology—
665 cases

Trauma	%
Gunshot	55
Edged instruments	36
Blunt trauma	9

ties are most often involved because they are longer and located superficially. In some cases the victims may attempt to defend themselves with their arms or legs, and thus invite injuries to the extremities.

MECHANISMS OF INJURY

In penetrating wounds caused by stabbing or bullets traveling at a low velocity the damage is mainly confined to the wound tract. Knife wounds usually cause lacerations or punctures of the artery; bullets not only inflict direct damage to the neurovascular structures in their path, but the concussive effects caused by high velocity missiles may produce widespread damage. The cavitation effect of the high velocity bullet (2000–3000 feet per second) can damage a vessel remote from the wound tract, and when the blast cavity collapses a suction effect is generated that can draw surface structures such as dirt and clothing into the wound, thus contributing to the possibility of infection.

A high velocity bullet or metal fragment is capable of producing a great deal of tissue damage if it strikes bone and all of the energy is dissipated in the target. Such destructive effects may not be suspected from an initial examination of the skin surface where there may be only a small entrance and exit wound, yet the interior damage can be extensive. In such wounds wide debridement is required if invasive sepsis is to be avoided.

The muzzle velocity of a shotgun pellet is similar to that produced by a 22 caliber rifle bullet (approximately 1200 feet per second), but the damage inflicted by multiple pellets is often widespread, and the shotshell wadding and bits of clothing carried into the wound enhance the possibility of infection. As is the case with wounds inflicted by high velocity missiles, close-range shotgun blasts often cause a great deal more damage to the interior structures than is apparent from inspection of the entry site (Fig. 1).

Vascular injuries in the extremities usually can be readily identified because of the penetrating wound, and the presence of severe hemorrhage or hematoma, but deeper wounds may not be quite so evident.[3] Diminished or absent pulse, major hemorrhage with hypotension, large or expanding hematoma, bruit at or distal to injury, anatomically-related neurological defect, and ischemia are the findings that suggest the presence of a

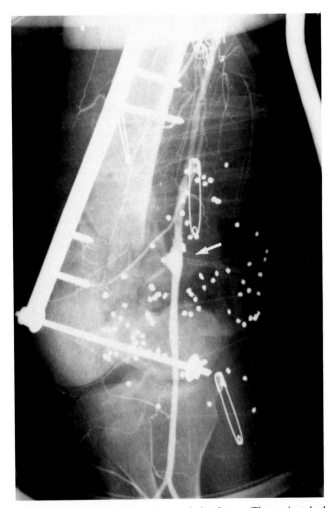

Fig. 1. The shotgun blast fractured the femur. The patient had normal distal pulses, and only when postoperative bleeding occurred was an arteriogram obtained. This revealed the vascular wound of the superficial femoral artery (arrow).

vascular wound—often a combination of these clinical features is present. The most common findings include hemorrhage, hematoma, and deficits in the distal pulses. These findings in the presence of a penetrating wound of the extremity are sufficient to establish the diagnosis. When present, ischemia is an important finding but its absence does not preclude a significant vascular injury. The pulse wave is a pressure wave. It attains velocities up to 10 meters per second, and can pass beyond intimal flaps, through soft clot and collateral vessels. Blood flow has a velocity of 40–50 cm per second and is distinct from the pulse wave; the physical examination must take this discrepancy into account. Moreover, wounds of arteries crossing the shoulder or the pelvis, areas with rich collateral circulation, are likely to be associated with intact although diminished distal pulses. In addition, injuries of the profunda femoris or the deep brachial arteries usually do not cause

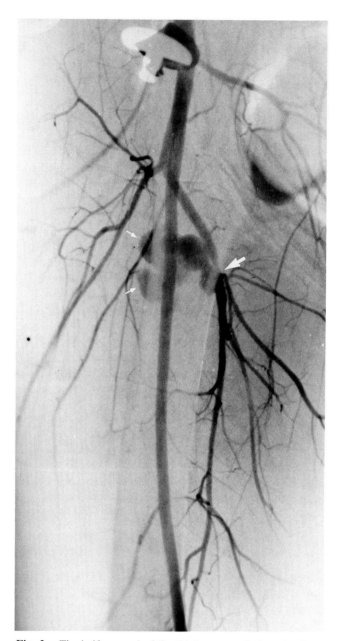

Fig. 2. The knife wound of the thigh was not believed to have caused a serious injury, but the arteriogram showed a wound of the profunda femoris (large arrow) and extravasation of contrast medium into an acute false aneurysm (small arrows).

detectable changes in the distal pulses (Fig. 2). Major venous wounds, of course, may occur without any alteration in the pulses or blood flow. The only finding in such patients may be hematomas, a history of or persistent bleeding.

Doppler techniques for the detection of blood flow and the measurement of limb blood pressures are useful adjuncts. These methods are limited by the same hemodynamic forces that govern blood flow and pulse wave generation. They can be misleading and are best used in concert with a careful physical examination.

ARTERIOGRAPHY

In a stable patient who has sustained penetrating trauma to the upper or lower extremity preoperative biplane arteriography may be of great value, not only in identifying an arterial injury, but in assessing the extent of the injury and in detecting distal thromboembolism. The indications for preoperative arteriography that appear to be useful are (1) blunt trauma, fractures; (2) penetrating injuries, chest; (3) cervical injuries, base of skull; (4) assessment of multiple pellet wounds; and (5) injuries to forearm, leg. These are of value especially in patients who have multiple injuries. In a prospective study of 143 patients with penetrating trauma to the extremities, the validity and usefulness of arteriography was established (Fig. 3). All of the patients had arteriograms and were operated upon for the listed indications regardless of the arteriographic findings. On subsequent evaluation one patient was noted to have a false negative examination, and there were 28 false positive examinations. There were 32 true positive studies. It was concluded from this study that biplane arteriography offers reliable, but not infallible evidence as to the presence or absence of arterial injuries.[4] Particular difficulty is encountered in the assessment of the great vessels near the arch of the aorta because in this area it is difficult to obtain good biplane films without overlapping images.

In a study by O'Gorman and his associates single view arteriograms were obtained by simple arterial puncture of the common femoral artery. These were used to assess the possibility of vascular injury in patients who had penetrating trauma to the extremity.[5] In over 500 patients the assessment proved to be valuable in detecting such injuries. The studies were quite safe; no patient died or had morbidity as a result of the single arterial puncture performed with an 18-gauge Cournand needle. Although follow-up was not obtained in all the patients, late complications were not encountered in the study. Those patients who had firm indications for operative exploration were operated upon. The arteriographic study was used mainly to exclude the presence of vascular injury in patients who had no other indications for surgery.

It is clear that if firm indications for operation are present, arteriograms may be unnecessary. Any untoward delay is undesirable and in some situations can be dangerous. If the patient is unstable the evaluation is best performed in the operating room. This may include an arteriogram performed either at the beginning of the operation or during the operation, as required to assess the distal circulation and to evaluate the patient for other injuries or incidental thromboembolism. In unstable patients if sudden cardiovascular collapse does occur immediate operation can be undertaken and control of bleeding can be achieved rapidly. Such patients should not be sent to the radiology department for study, nor should they be admitted to an intensive care unit if they are unstable since an emergency operation can be required at any time.

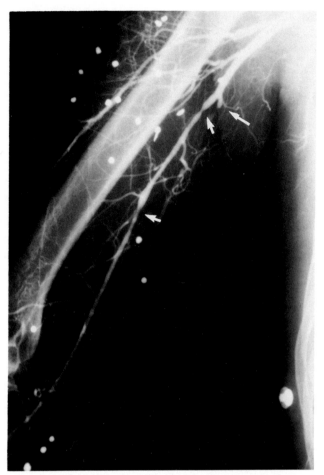

Fig. 3. The pellets from the shotgun resulted in occlusion of the profunda brachial artery (large arrow) and spasm of the brachial artery (small arrows).

PREPARATION FOR SURGERY

Many of these patients will have associated injuries and certain priorities must be set if a successful conclusion is to be gained. Initial attention to the airway and control of bleeding must always be the first priority, but it is usually obvious what is required. A more dangerous situation can exist when the patient has achieved some degree of cardio-pulmonary stability via compensatory mechanisms, and then suddenly the internal adjust-ments required to maintain this state deteriorate; the collapse is sudden, and irreversible shock may occur.

Multiple access lines to the circulation are needed. One large intravenous line is committed only for fluid replacement; it is not used for drug administration nor for anesthetic manipulations. Venous autografts may be needed for repair of injured arteries in the extremities, and it is often prudent to preserve the saphenous or cephalic vein in an uninjured extremity, but the treatment of shock takes precedence. The saphenous vein at the ankle is almost always available, and easily cannulated. Fluid requirements in patients with multiple injuries are often impressive. Shires and his associates showed that there are internal shifts of extracellular fluid caused by trauma and surgery.[6] For resuscitation of these people, a combination of blood and a balanced salt solution (Ringer's lactate) is recommended. It is wise not to overtransfuse trauma patients, especially if chest trauma or cardiac disease is present. A whole blood hematocrit of approximately 30 percent is optimum; further increases in hemoglobin during this stage are unnecessary and may increase the possibility of cardiac overload. If such patients are hemodynamically unstable arterial lines or Swan Ganz catheters are extremely helpful. Difficult subclavian vein punctures can produce an additional vascular injury, and it is best to insert these lines with a great deal of care. The central line can be inserted from a peripheral vein and advanced into the heart and pulmonary circulation rather than from a direct subclavian puncture.

WOUND PROTECTION

During the initial treatment of patients with penetrating injuries there may be a tendency to overlook the problem of wound care. The incidence of infection and subsequent complications can be directly related to contamination of the wounds at the time of resuscitation. Undamaged tissue should be conserved so it may be utilized in covering repaired vessels. When multiple wounds are present several exploratory incisions may be required, especially if there are fractures and other injuries. If these incisions are poorly placed intervening tissue may be devitalized, important collateral vessels may be divided unnecessarily, and final cover of the vessels may be difficult to arrange.[1] Wound protection is an important part of the initial measures in the care of these patients, and especially if there is extensive soft tissue damage such as may be seen with close-range shotgun wounds and high velocity missile wounds. Remote bypass grafts to restore blood flow may be required because of heavy contamination of the primary wound, and therefore exploratory incisions should be placed so as to preserve areas for the use of these subcutaneous grafts.

Although distal clot propagation can occur in such patients, especially if they are hypotensive, and thrombosis can convert an initially reasonable situation to one with increased risk of tissue loss, such problems are unusual. If there is to be a long delay between admission to the operating room and conclusion of the repairs, it may be useful in such situations to temporarily insert shunts into the arteries and veins in order to restore distal flow to an ischemic extremity. Such maneuvers are especially helpful in the popliteal circulation where the collateral pathways are relatively sparse. Once the temporary inlying shunts are in place the ischemia will be relieved. The shunts also offer access for arteriographic visualization of the distal arterial tree to assess the possibility of other injuries, or to detect distal clots.

OPERATIVE MANAGEMENT

The selection of the anesthetic agent is important, especially in patients who are already hypotensive.[3] The cardiodepressant action of anesthetics should be kept in mind as the operation begins. In the patient with multiple injuries certain precautions should be observed as well. Careful positioning of the neck during introduction of anesthesia is necessary in order to avoid dislodging clots in patients who have associated cervical injuries, and of course some of the patients may have cervical spine or cranial injuries that deserve attention. Patients usually are placed supine in the anatomic position, thus affording access to the chest, the abdomen and all four extremities. In some patients with penetrating trauma to the extremities it may be necessary to extend an incision into the chest or the abdomen to obtain proximal control of bleeding.

In most situations vertical exploratory incisions are recommended—they can be extended easily in either direction to permit proximal and distal control of the arteries, or entry into the trunk or thorax as needed. Vertical incisions parallel the neurovascular structures and thus reduce the chance of injuring superficial veins that may be needed for autografts.

Control of Bleeding

Usually external bleeding from penetrating trauma of the extremities can be controlled with direct digital pressure. In most patients brisk hemorrhage has stopped by the time they are admitted, but large hematomas are often present, and in some patients bleeding may persist. If the wound is not bleeding it is best not to disturb it during the resuscitation; penetrating objects that are still in the wound must be protected during transportation, but they should not be removed until the patient is in the operating room and it is possible to gain proximal and distal control. No attempt should be made to blindly clamp vessels deep in the wound prior to taking the patient to the operating room. In cases in which fatal hemorrhage appears imminent, the wound can be extended and vascular clamps applied precisely under direct vision.

Preoperative preparations are performed prior to the administration of anesthesia if the patient is cooperative and especially if the patient is hemodynamically unstable, since the administration of anesthesia may precipitate severe hypotension. It is often wise to prepare wounds prior to administering the anesthetic, and to insert and secure the access lines to allow the surgical team to intervene quickly if the patient suddenly undergoes cardiovascular collapse.

Once the wounds have been identified and the surgical plan established, the injuries are approached directly through vertical incisions. If the hematoma is large or there is continued bleeding, it is often best to expose the vessels proximally and gain control in an area where the artery and vein can be clearly visualized. In extremities with multiple distal wounds and large hematomas, exposure of the vessels can be difficult, and it is helpful to place an orthopedic tourniquet around the extremity proximal to the injury. If severe bleeding is encountered prior to direct exposure and control of the artery, the orthopedic tourniquet can be quickly inflated, thus arresting the hemorrhage while precise identification is made and control is obtained.

In most situations proximal control of the artery may be obtained utilizing soft vascular tapes, latex tubing, or vascular clamps. These measures when combined with adequate suction and direct pressure with fingers or sponge sticks are usually adequate to obtain control of hemorrhage while the injuries are identified and vascular clamps are properly put into place.

Once the injury has been identified, the clots should be evacuated carefully and the extent of the wound examined. Every effort is made to avoid fragmenting and dislodging clots or extending the damage to the vessel, a problem especially in patients who have atherosclerosis and fragile arteries. In some patients it may be necessary to insert a Foley catheter or a Fogarty catheter with an attached 3-way stopcock to control hemorrhage. (There are available special Pruitt-Inahara balloon occlusion and irrigation catheters with attached stopcocks.) The catheter is inserted directly into the arterial wound, inflated, and gently retracted until bleeding is stopped, and then left in place while more precise proximal and distal control is obtained. Repairs are not begun until all the hemorrhage is arrested and the entire extent of associated injuries assessed. It is often wise to pause at this point in the resuscitation and be certain that there is no persistent bleeding and that the patient has received adequate blood and fluid replacement.

Basic Techniques

Selection of suture materials for repair of vascular injuries is largely the choice of the operating surgeon, but over recent years there has been a tendency to select the less reactive plastic monofilament sutures rather than the braided cardiovascular sutures popular in the past.[3] In direct vascular repairs healing can be anticipated and permanent sutures are not necessarily required in every instance, but since the monofilament sutures are less reactive and may perhaps have less of a tendency to harbor bacteria than the braided sutures, they are chosen more often than not. Small sutures should be employed in most of these cases since healing of autogenous tissue is expected and long-term suture line integrity does not depend on the suture material.

Vessels are repaired by the usual vascular technique: continuous over and over sutures are quite effective and can be used in almost all vessels. It is often prudent in small vessels (less than 4 mm in diameter) to use interrupted sutures in order to insure intimal coaptation, although with magnification it has been demonstrated that continuous sutures even in small arteries are effective if properly inserted. The vessels frequently are in spasm, and this is especially true in young people, and if a constricting continuous suture is used there will be a moderate amount of stenosis produced when in the postoperative period the spasm relents and the vessels resume a more normal size. In all children and in young adults interrupted sutures are recommended. The repair may be facilitated by transecting the artery obliquely, or perhaps constructing a spatulated lumen to obtain a larger suture line. Although tangential lacerations of larger vessels such as the vena cava often can be repaired by simple direct repair, this is unusual in the extremities since femoral and brachial vessels generally are too small to permit such a repair.

Debridement is as important in the management of vascular injuries as in other wounds, and it is best not to make a firm decision as to the type of repair until the vessel is satisfactorily debrided. Since most civilian vascular wounds are inflicted by knives or missiles traveling at a low velocity wide debridement is generally not required. In the presence of the usual gunshot wound it is often necessary to debride only that amount of vessel that can be seen to be injured. In wounds caused by high velocity missiles the injury often extends beyond that which is immediately visible to the naked eye, and it is advisable to remove approximately 5 mm of vessel beyond the apparent damage.[1]

Resection and end-to-end anastomosis is usually chosen for the restoration of vascular continuity in vessels of the upper and lower extremity. The most commonly injured vessels (femoral and brachial) can be mobilized to permit resection of 1 cm or so of the artery and still permit a satisfactory end-to-end anastomosis without tension. If the extent of the injury is so wide that end-to-end anastomosis cannot be accomplished without tension, it is best to interpose a suitable vein autograft rather than to accept an improper repair. The saphenous vein is usually chosen for such autografts, but the hypogastric artery, external iliac, or other arterial autografts may be employed in certain circumstances.

When grafting procedures are needed autografts are favored, although recent studies suggest that disruption caused by subsequent infection is not increased by the presence of plastic prostheses such as polytetrafluorethylene.[7] It has been suggested that these plastic substances may be used even when heavy bacterial contamination is present, but this opinion is not shared by all vascular surgeons and most prefer that an autogenous graft be used if available in appropriate sizes.[8]

In those situations in which adequate autografts are not available, plastic grafts have been used, and usually have performed satisfactorily. If bacterial contamination is heavy, it is probably best not to perform an in-line repair, but to bypass the wound with autogenous tissue through clean tissue planes, thus rerouting the vessel to a remote position. Various remote subcutaneous routes have been chosen, but axillofemoral and femoral-femoral, iliofemoral and obturator canal grafts have been used in these circumstances. In patients who have infected popliteal lesions or heavily contaminated areas of the distal femoral and popliteal, iliopopliteal or femoral-popliteal grafts placed in the lateral position have been satisfactorily employed.[9] Once repair is completed the graft should be covered with clean tissue. This may require transposition of various muscle groups, such as the use of a sartorius muscle flap, to provide adequate cover for vascular repairs in the femoral triangle areas.

TIBIAL ARTERY INJURIES

Injuries to the tibial arteries present a special problem because in most cases they do not result in severe ischemia unless two of the three arteries are interrupted. In patients who have penetrating trauma to the lower leg, but who otherwise would not require operative exploration (one tibial artery occluded and no bleeding), such an injury can be accepted without repair. Arteriographic survey of these patients is essential in order to determine if indeed there is a significant problem. This is especially true in a patient who has multiple wounds as the result of a shotgun blast. In the absence of other indications for surgery, surgical exploration of a tibial artery customarily would be performed only if it were bleeding or if an AV fistula or false aneurysm were seen on the arteriogram. If a person has interruption of a single tibial artery (with the other two patent and with adequate flow to the foot), that patient would probably be observed with serial studies rather than direct operation. In contrast, those patients who have wounds of two tibial arteries should have these vessels repaired in order to insure adequate function of the extremity.

ASSESSMENT OF REPAIR

In most cases vascular repair is followed by the immediate return of distal pulses. In patients who are incompletely resuscitated and who remain hypotensive and cold, it can be difficult to determine if the repair is satisfactory, and other measures may be required. A sterile Doppler probe is useful in documenting distal patency in such circumstances. It may be possible to position a sterile Doppler probe over the distal vessels (or the ulnar or radial artery) and with a syringe gently produce miniature waves in a heparin saline irrigating solution. These flow waves can be detected by the Doppler probe. If there is any question about the patency or the adequacy of repair, or if distal clots are suspected, an operative arteriogram is required (Fig. 4). In many situations, this should be a routine, although it is not possible in all operating rooms to obtain high quality films. In the postoperative period and in the recovery room if there is any question as to the adequacy of flow an arteriogram is needed. The sine qua non of viability of the extremity is continued perception of light touch and adequate intrinsic motor function. Any deterioration in these modalities is a compelling reason to perform an arteriogram, regardless of skin color, temperature, presence or absence of pulses, or limb blood pressures.

ADJUNCTIVE METHODS

Management of Spasm

Arterial spasm often is seen in patients with vascular trauma, especially young patients, and in rare cases may be responsible for stasis and thrombosis. When spasm is thought to be the cause of poor distal flow following a vascular repair, arteriography almost invariably reveals distal clots. If there is some question as to patency an operative arteriogram will usually reveal the vessel to be open, and although there may be irregular

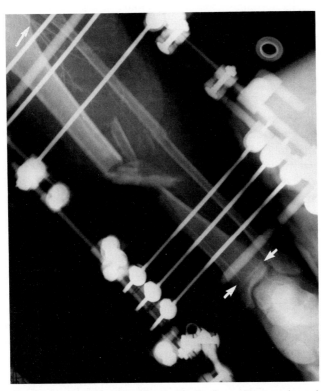

Fig. 4. An operative arteriogram via the femoral artery showed an open popliteal artery (large arrow) and open tibial arteries (small arrows).

areas of narrowing from spasm, a smooth intimal surface is seen. In these situations the spasm will resolve over the following hours, Doppler signals will become stronger, the blood pressure will rise and subsequently distal pulses will become palpable.

In rare cases, such as those reported by Kinmonth, spasm can be relentless and it may be necessary to employ other methods of treatment.[10] Mechanical or hydraulic dilation may be helpful in these situations and a variety of vasodilators have been recommended, but the results are indifferent. Tolazoline, nitroglycerin, papavarine, and nifedipine have been used in certain circumstances, but there are conflicting reports as to their effectiveness.[11] In most situations if an arteriogram reveals the vessels to be open the spasm will resolve on its own and does not require specific treatment. The important point is to determine that there is no distal occluding clot.

Fasciotomy

Patman and his associates recommended that fasciotomy be considered for the following conditions: (1) combined arterial and venous injury, (2) massive soft tissue damage, (3) delay between wounding and definitive repair, (4) prolonged hypotension, and (5) swelling of extremity.[12] Matsen has stated that when the compartmental pressures exceed 45 mmHg, cell damage is likely to occur unless decompression is performed.[13] If fasciotomy is performed on the basis of these pressure measurements, or because of hypesthesia in the distribution of the deep peroneal nerve, and before obvious swelling has occurred, the results are quite good. If fasciotomy is delayed until the extremities are swollen and until there has been prolonged disturbance in neuromuscular function, it is less likely to be of benefit. In such patients muscle debridement is often necessary, and long-term disability can be severe.

Studies by the author suggest that evaluation of flow in the tibial veins using Doppler techniques may assist in establishing the diagnosis of increased compartmental pressures. When tissue pressures exceed resting tibial venous pressures, flow should be restricted, and when the pressure exceeds 50 torr venous flow should cease. If spontaneous and augmented tibial vein Doppler signals are absent in a patient with the clinical findings suggesting a compartmental syndrome, measurements of tissue pressure are usually elevated above 50 torr, and fasciotomy is indicated. Measurements of tissue pressure and Doppler evaluation of tibial venous flow were performed in ten limbs in six patients, and good correlation was found in all six patients. This method may subsequently prove to be useful in evaluating compartment syndromes during their early stages.

When swelling is minimal or absent adequate fasciotomy can be performed through limited skin incisions and the skin can be closed primarily. If limb swelling is already present, or if there is significant edema of the skin, and subcutaneous tissues, wide dermotomy may be required, and long incisions are necessary in such limbs to decompress all the muscle compartments. In most instances the compartments can be decompressed through two incisions, one over the fibula that permits entry to the anterior and posterior compartment on either side of the fibula, and a supplementary medial calf incision. In the author's experience fibulectomy has not been necessary to insure adequate decompression of the deep muscle compartments. Such incisions should be carefully protected from contamination since infection is a possibility in all such wounds. Early repair is recommended, and if the wounds are not closed primarily they should be covered with split thickness skin grafts in 2–3 days.

Table 3
Results of Treatment—665 cases

Result	%
Failure of repair	5.2
Bleeding	2.0
Infection	3.1
Amputation	1.8
Mortality	10.4

RESULTS

As listed in Table 3 the results of operative repair of penetrating injuries of vessels of the extremities are quite good if the patients are operated upon before ischemic damage has supervened. In most situations this is possible because isolated wounds of the brachial and superficial femoral arteries, two of the more commonly injured arteries, usually do not produce sufficient ischemia to cause distal problems. In contrast, occlusive injuries of the common femoral artery or popliteal artery are likely to be followed by severe ischemia, and in such patients early repair is necessary to restore function and insure a pain-free extremity.

Amputation rates have been significantly reduced during the past 2 decades by an aggressive approach to the identification and repair of all vascular injuries.[14] Injuries of the popliteal artery, especially as a result of blunt trauma, are still likely to incur a significant risk of amputation or prolonged limb disability.

Injuries to two tibial arteries and injuries of radial and ulnar artery also are likely to produce significant distal extremity problems, and such wounds should be primarily repaired whenever possible. Repair of these small arteries requires meticulous surgical technique, using magnification and completion arteriography to insure good results. With such methods one can anticipate that most people with penetrating trauma to the extremities will do well, and they can be expected to have a normal extremity following convalescence.

REFERENCES

1. Perry MO: The Management of Acute Vascular Injuries. Baltimore, Williams and Wilkins, 1981
2. Flint LM, Snyder WH, Perry MO, et al: Management of major vascular injuries in the base of the neck. Arch Surg 106:407, 1973
3. Snyder WH, Thal ER, Perry MO: Peripheral and abdominal vascular injuries, in Rutherford RR (ed.): Vascular Surgery. Philadelphia, W.B. Saunders, 1984, pp 460–500
4. Snyder WH, Thal ER, Bridges RA, et al: The validity of normal arteriography in penetrating trauma. Arch Surg 113:424, 1978
5. O'Gorman RB, Feliciano DV, Bitundo GG, et al: Emergency center arteriography in the evaluation of suspected peripheral vascular injuries. Arch Surg 119:568, 1984
6. Shires GT, Canizaro PE, Carrico CJ: Shock, in Schwartz SI (ed.): Principles of Surgery, Chapter 4. New York, McGraw-Hill, 1979, pp 115–164

7. Lau JM, Mattox KL, Beall AC, et al: Use of substitute conduits in traumatic vascular injury. J Trauma 17:541, 1977
8. Rich N, Spencer F: Venous injuries, in Vascular Trauma. Philadelphia, W.B. Saunders, 1978, pp 156–190
9. Perry MO: Remote bypass grafts for managing infected popliteal artery lesions. Arch Surg 114:605, 1979
10. Kinmonth JB: Physiology and relief of traumatic arterial spasm. Br Med J 1:59, 1952
11. Dickerman RM, Gewertz BL, Foley DW, et al: Selective intraarterial tolazoline infusion in peripheral arterial trauma. Surgery 81:605, 1977
12. Patman RD: Fasciotomy: indications and techniques, in Rutherford RB (ed.): Vascular Surgery, Chapter 50. Philadelphia, W.B. Saunders, 1979
13. Matsen F: Compartmental syndromes. Hosp Prac 15:113, 1980
14. Pasch AR, Bishara RA, Lim LT, et al: Optimal limb salvage in penetrating civilian vascular trauma. J Vasc Surg 3:189, 1986

Robert A. McCready
Gordon L. Hyde

Autogenous Tissue in the Revascularization of Traumatic Vascular Injuries—its Value and Limitations

In the treatment of traumatic vascular injuries, primary repair of the damaged vessels is the preferred method of management. Primary repair can be accomplished by resection of the damaged segment with end-to-end anastomosis or by lateral arteriography. However, extensive damage to a long segment of the vessel precludes primary repair and necessitates using some type of vascular conduit. Some surgeons have advocated using only autogenous tissue to repair traumatic vascular injuries to avoid the risk of a prosthetic graft subsequently becoming infected in a contaminated wound.[1] Other surgeons, however, have used prosthetic grafts almost exclusively for the repair of traumatic vascular injuries including those that are potentially contaminated.[2-7] These authors feel that prosthetic grafts have distinct advantages over autogenous grafts should a perigraft infection develop. In addition their reported short-term patency rates are very good.

Most series dealing with vascular trauma have a paucity of long-term follow-up as the majority of patients sustaining traumatic vascular injuries have acquired their injuries secondary to acts of violence and long-term follow-up is difficult to obtain. Only 18 percent of the patients in one series came for postoperative evaluation in spite of being offered a financial reward.[6] Our preference has been to use autogenous veins to reconstruct traumatic vascular injuries and to use prosthetic grafts only in the repair of large arteries such as the thoracic or abdominal aorta. We recently reviewed our experience with autogenous tissues in the reconstruction of traumatic vascular injuries with particular reference to long-term follow-up.

METHODS AND MATERIALS

From 1963 to 1985 we treated 99 patients at the University of Kentucky in whom autogenous tissue (vein) was used in the reconstruction of traumatic arterial injuries. In 22 patients autogenous veins were also used for repair of associated venous injuries. Six injuries involved the carotid artery and all were repaired by resection of the damaged segment and interposition vein grafting. Saphenous vein was used in four patients and jugular vein in two patients. One patient had a postoperative stroke but no postoperative arteriogram was performed to evaluate patency. The other five patients did well but the majority did not have postoperative arteriograms to ascertain graft patency.

Saphenous vein interposition grafts were used in two patients with intraabdominal vascular injuries. Excellent results were obtained in one patient with a gunshot wound to the external iliac artery. The other patient sustained bilateral renal artery thromboses secondary to blunt trauma. One renal artery was repaired by resection of the damaged segment with primary anastomosis, and an aortorenal saphenous vein graft was used to bypass the other renal artery lesion. A postoperative arteriogram demonstrated occlusion of the saphenous vein graft. The other renal artery repair was patent. The type of autogenous tissue used and the results of arterial repair are listed in Table 1.

EXTREMITY VASCULAR INJURIES

Among the remaining 91 patients with extremity vascular injuries, the subclavian or axillary arteries were involved in 14 patients, the brachial artery in 28 patients, and the common femoral, superficial femoral, or popliteal arteries in 29 patients. Two of the extremity arterial repairs were vein-patch angioplasties whereas the remainder were interposition vein grafts.

AXILLARY-SUBCLAVIAN ARTERIAL INJURIES

Among the 14 patients with axillary or subclavian artery injuries, there was 1 late graft failure in a patient who developed an infected pseudoaneurysm (Staphylococcus aureus) 8 months postoperatively, which was treated by ligation. Because of excellent collateral circulation, he has a nearly normal extremity. Excellent results were obtained in the remainder. Of the venous injuries, four were repaired with interposition saphenous vein grafts, and one with a saphenous vein patch. The subclavian vein was ligated in three patients, and no edema developed in these patients. The venous repairs appeared to be patent although no postoperative venograms were performed.

Table 1
Nonextremity Arterial Injuries

Location of Arterial Injury (No. Pts.)	Type of Autogenous Graft		Results of Arterial Repair		
	SV	JV	Excellent	Early Failure	Late Failure
Renal (1)	1			1	
External Iliac (1)	1		1		
Carotid (6)	4	2	5	1	

SV-Saphenous Vein, JV-Jugular Vein

BRACHIAL ARTERY INJURIES

Among the 28 patients with brachial artery injuries, there were 4 early failures, 2 of which appeared to be caused by technical errors resulting in graft thrombosis with both patients having viable but ischemic extremities.

The other 2 graft failures developed in patients who had large soft-tissue defects that had precluded adequate soft-tissue coverage of their vein grafts at the time of revascularization. Their wounds subsequently became infected with multiple gram-positive and gram-negative organisms being cultured from their wounds. Both patients bled massively several days postoperatively, with one patient nearly exsanguinating. At reexploration the bleeding sites were in the midportions of the vein grafts well away from the anastomoses, and it appeared that a portion of the vein wall had necrosed. In one patient, a second saphenous vein graft was placed, but it also became infected with recurrent massive hemorrhage. The brachial arteries were subsequently ligated in each patient with both having viable but ischemic extremities. The venous injuries among the patients with brachial artery injuries were treated by ligation and no patient had postoperative edema.

Four patients with brachial artery injuries required amputation of their upper extremities because of extensive muscle necrosis. Three patients had severely ischemic extremities on admission and there had been a several hour delay between injury and restoration of circulation in all. Two of the three arterial repairs were patent at the time of amputation. In the other patient an above-elbow amputation was performed 10 months postinjury for a painful and functionless arm secondary to the initial nerve injury. The arterial repair was patent at the time of amputation.

LOWER EXTREMITY ARTERIAL INJURIES

Among the 49 patients with lower extremity arterial injuries, there were 2 patients with common femoral artery injuries, 18 patients with superficial femoral artery injuries, and 29 patients with popliteal artery injuries.

Among the 29 popliteal artery injuries, there were 4 early graft failures, all of which resulted in amputation. Technical error appeared to be the cause of graft failure in one patient in whom the distal pulses were lost after the orthopedic injuries were repaired. Although the distal anastomosis was redone, there were no palpable distal pulses at the completion of the procedure. Outflow occlusion appeared to be the cause of the graft failure in one patient who had been explored initially at another institution at which time the popliteal artery and vein were ligated for control of hemorrhage. At reexploration at our institution it was not possible to restore patency of the popliteal vein. In addition, the saphenous vein used to repair the popliteal artery had been harvested from the injured extremity and undoubtedly increased the venous hypertension. The third graft failure occurred in an elderly patient in whom all three tibial vessels were severely atherosclerotic and the cause of the graft failure in this patient appeared to be inadequate outflow compounded by a several hour delay between the injury and subsequent revascularization.

The fourth graft failure occurred in a patient with a large soft-tissue defect that had precluded adequate soft-tissue coverage of the graft. The wound subsequently became infected with multiple organisms. Several days postoperatively profuse hemorrhage developed from the vein graft. At reexploration, a hole in the midportion of the vein graft was repaired, but massive bleeding recurred a day later and a new saphenous vein graft

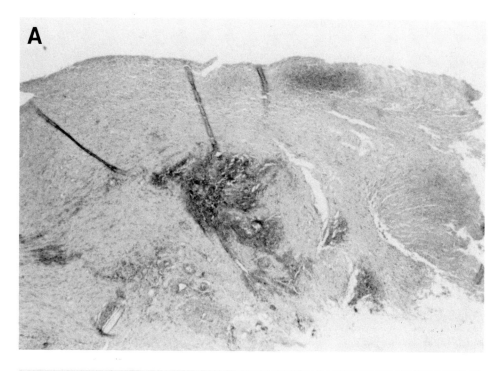

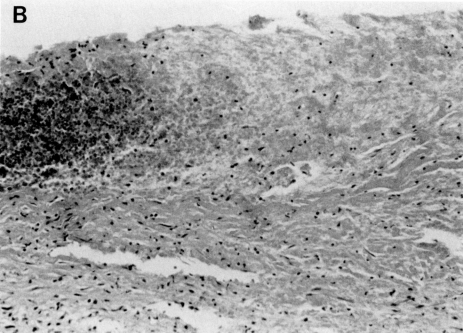

Fig. 1. (A) Low-power photomicrograph of the saphenous vein graft demonstrating acute inflammation and necrosis. (H & E stain, original magnification ×18). (B) Higher power view demonstrating focal necrosis with numerous inflammatory cells (H & E stain, original magnification ×200).

182

was placed. It also became infected and rebled with a third interposition graft being placed. Several weeks later, however, a large infected pseudoaneurysm of the vein graft developed and the patient underwent an above-knee amputation. Pathologic examination of the saphenous vein graft demonstrated aneurysmal dilatation and necrosis of the vein wall (Fig. 1).

A total of six amputations were performed in the early postoperative period. All four early graft failures resulted in amputation. In the two other patients, the extremities were severely ischemic at the time of revascularization and in retrospect the patients probably should have undergone primary amputation. Their grafts were patent at the time of amputation. Five of the six patients requiring amputations had associated venous injuries, three of which were repaired. The popliteal veins were ligated in the other two patients. All six patients requiring amputation had fasciotomies performed at the time of the vascular repair. Eighteen of the 29 patients with popliteal injuries had fasciotomies either at the initial operation or in the early postoperative period.

Among the 29 patients with superficial femoral or popliteal vein injuries, interposition saphenous vein grafts were used in 14 patients and saphenous vein patch repairs were used in two patients. Eleven patients underwent primary repair of the venous injuries. Two of the patients with popliteal vein injuries had ligation of their popliteal veins. Both of these patients eventually required amputation.

Of the 14 interposition vein grafts used to repair venous injuries, there were 2 failures documented by venography. Three patients required support stockings to control milk edema but no venographic studies were done in these patients to determine the patency of the venous repairs. The remainder of the patients undergoing venous repairs are asymptomatic.

FOLLOW-UP

Of the 99 patients in our series, there were 5 deaths and 10 patients were lost to follow-up. The five deaths were the result of multiple associated injuries. Follow-up among the remaining 84 patients ranged from 1 to 207 months with an average of 33.5 months.

Because several patients were lost to long-term follow-up, it is certainly possible that our incidence of late graft failure might have been considerably higher had we been able to obtain long-term follow-up on all patients. Some of the grafts could have thrombosed with the patients remaining asymptomatic because of the development of collateral circulation. In the military experience in Vietnam, Rich et al noted that 24 of 34 patients with thrombosed arterial repairs did not require operative intervention, attesting both to the ability of collateral circulation to prevent ischemia as well as to the fact that these patients are often limited in their activities by their associated neurologic deficits.[19] However, in those patients in whom we have long term follow-up, the results have been very encouraging as demonstrated by the patient with normal vascular laboratory studies 112 months following the repair of a popliteal artery injury (Fig. 2). Figure 3 demonstrates patent interposition saphenous vein grafts in both the popliteal artery and vein 39 months following the vascular repair. Even though our incidence of late graft failure may be higher than we are aware of, we believe that our low incidence of graft infection with autogenous grafts is accurate as these patients would have most likely returned to us for treatment of any subsequent graft infection.

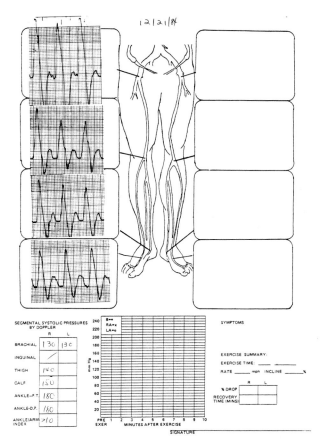

Fig. 2. Vascular laboratory study demonstrating normal segmental pressures and waveforms 112 months following saphenous vein interposition grafting of a popliteal artery transection.

There are conflicting results reported with prosthetic grafts in the repair of traumatic vascular injuries. In their report on prosthetic grafts that had been used to repair contaminated vascular wounds in Vietnam, Rich and Hughes noted that 20 of 26 patients (77 percent) in whom prosthetic grafts were used had subsequent graft failures with infection developing in 9 patients and thrombosis occurring in 9 patients.[1] Massive hemorrhage accompanied the infection in the majority of patients due to disruption at the prosthetic graft-host artery anastomosis. Thirty-one percent of the patients with graft failures required amputations. Prosthetic grafts were used to replace damaged iliac veins in two patients but both became infected and had to be removed. In a previous report from Vietnam these authors described a patient who died as a result of an infected prosthetic graft in the iliac artery.[8] Because of their high failure rate with prosthetic grafts among patients with wartime vascular injuries, they strongly advised against using prosthetic grafts whenever there is potential contamination of the wound.

Contrary to the military experience, there are a number of reports from large urban trauma centers describing satisfactory results with prosthetic grafts in the repair of vascular injuries both in the arterial and venous systems.[2–7] In their series of 20 patients with

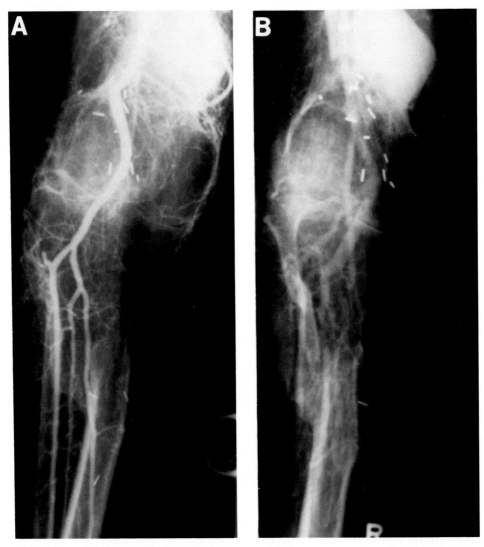

Fig. 3. (A) Postoperative arteriogram (39 months following injury) demonstrating a patent saphenous vein graft which had been used to repair a popliteal artery injury. (B) The late venous phase demonstrates patency of the popliteal vein that had also been repaired with a saphenous vein interposition graft.

traumatic vascular injuries (20 arterial and 5 venous injuries) all of which were repaired with polytetrafluorethylene (PTFE), Shah et al reported occlusion of only 1 arterial and 1 venous graft 3 months postoperatively secondary to infection and thrombosis.[7] The patency rate was 91 percent, but only 10 patients had 2 years follow-up. Jaggers et al reported an excellent patency rate with PTFE grafts in the repair of popliteal artery injuries, but the follow-up was very short and many patients were lost to follow-up.[4]

In a more recent report from the same Baylor group describing their results with 236 PTFE grafts used to repair traumatic vascular injuries, both the early and late failure rates were high.[6] Only 38 patients (18.4 percent) of the entire series were available for late study, and the mean follow-up was 25 months. Among these 38 patients, graft occlusion had occurred in 11 or 29 percent. Of the eight PTFE grafts that had been used to repair venous injuries and that were studied by venography or isotope studies postoperatively, all were significantly narrowed or occluded. Even though few patients were available for follow-up, the 29 percent occlusion rate is disturbingly high especially when one considers the young age (average age 29 years) of their patients and the fact that the average duration of follow-up was only 25 months. With a longer duration of follow-up, it is reasonable to assume the patency rate would have decreased even further. Seven grafts in their series became infected with four of the infections resulting in dehiscence at the host artery-graft anastomosis. One of these patients died from dehiscence of a PTFE graft that had been used to replace the superior mesenteric artery.

Intuitively, one would expect a high incidence of infection among prosthetic grafts that are placed in contaminated wounds. However, except for the report from Rich and Hughes from Vietnam, other studies suggest that prosthetic grafts may be superior to autogenous grafts in contaminated wounds.[2,5,7,9] In a series of 122 patients from Baylor who received interposition grafts for vascular injuries, Dacron grafts were used in 57 patients and saphenous vein grafts in 65.[2] Of the 12 perigraft infections 5 occurred in patients with Dacron grafts and 7 occurred in patients with saphenous vein grafts. Gram-negative organisms were cultured in all seven patients with infected vein grafts. Five of the seven patients with infected vein grafts had profuse hemorrhage from the wound, and in these five patients the entire vein graft had disrupted. By contrast, among the five patients with infected Dacron grafts, three patients had intermittent anastomotic bleeding with pseudoaneurysm formation but there were no episodes of gross hemorrhage. Importantly in the patients with infected Dacron prostheses, there were "sentinel" bleeding episodes that heralded the anastomotic breakdown with pseudoaneurysm formation but there were no episodes of profuse hemorrhage. These sentinel bleeding episodes allowed time to take the patient to the operating room for graft removal and either ligation of the native artery or the construction of an extraanatomic bypass.

If the prosthetic graft is placed in a major body cavity such as the abdomen or chest, however, a prosthetic graft-host artery dehiscence may lead to exsanguination as occurred in one of the four graft-artery dehiscences in Feliciano et al's series.[6] In the patient who died from the dehiscence, a PTFE graft had been inserted in the superior mesenteric artery, but it became infected from a pancreatic leak with subsequent dehiscence of the graft. Although there is clinical and experimental evidence to support the use of prosthetic grafts in contaminated vascular wounds, prosthetic grafts are certainly not immune to infection with all of its attendant hazards.

Clinically there are a number of anecdotal reports of patients exsanguinating as a result of dissolution of an infected saphenous vein graft after repair of traumatic vascular injuries.[10-12] One of our patients nearly exsanguinated as a result of this complication. In the patients in whom this complication has been reported, there has been massive soft-tissue loss with subsequent wound infections. Dissolution of the vein grafts usually occurred several days postoperatively at a time when the patients were out of the intensive care units and not under constant observation. Once a vein graft becomes infected and bleeds, the native artery should be ligated both proximally and distally at a point where the native artery is healthy and not surrounded by infection or inflammation. In two of our three patients with infected vein grafts that bled, multiple attempts at revascularization with fresh autogenous tissue were made, but profuse, recurrent hemorrhage recurred in both. Similar disastrous results with multiple attempts at revascularization in the presence of gross infection were reported by Rich et al from Vietnam.[13]

Experimentally, prosthetic grafts appear to tolerate infection better than autogenous grafts.[5,14–17] In one experimental study comparing infected PTFE and infected vein grafts in the femoral arteries of dogs, transmural necrosis leading to exsanguinating hemorrhage occurred in six of seven infected vein grafts whereas only two of seven PTFE grafts bled.[14] Bleeding in the animals with PTFE grafts was due to necrosis of the host artery at the anastomotic site. Other experimental studies have confirmed the tendency of autogenous vein grafts to undergo transmural necrosis when they become infected.[5,15–17] In contrast, the bleeding seen with infected prosthetic grafts is due to the host artery necrosis at the anastomotic site, which rarely leads to exsanguinating hemorrhage. As pointed out by Lau, this usually allows time for definitive treatment such as removal of the infected graft and ligation of the infected artery.[2]

The critical factor that seems to predispose to autogenous graft infection appears to be the lack of adequate soft-tissue coverage.[2] An autogenous graft depends upon its nutrition from both the intraluminal diffusion of nutrients as well as from its contact with the surrounding soft tissues. It has been postulated that the bacterial infection prevents contact between the vein graft and host tissue by its inflammatory action. The infection may also introduce an element of collagenase activity that can lead to transmural necrosis and disruption of the vein graft. Massive soft-tissue injury that precluded adequate viable soft-tissue coverage of the graft was present in our three patients with vein graft dissolution, and this seems to be a common factor among other patients who developed vein graft infections reported in the literature.[10–12] Gram-negative enteric organisms seem especially virulent in this setting.[2] Gram-negative organisms were present in our 3 patients with vein graft necrosis as they were in all 7 patients in Lau et al's series who experienced massive hemorrhage.[2]

Ledgerwood and Lucas have described good results using porcine skin grafts to cover exposed vascular repairs until adequate soft-tissue coverage can be provided.[18] However, Feliciano et al did not have much success with this technique in their patients with exposed PTFE grafts.[6] Rotation of a muscle flap or a "free flap" is another option that could be used to provide soft-tissue coverage of an exposed graft at the time of the initial vascular repair or in the early postoperative period. A latissimus dorsi flap was used in one of our patients to cover a brachial artery repair, but it was thought to compress the vein graft with subsequent thrombosis of the graft. Ledgerwood and Lucas have also reported poor results with rotating major muscle flaps over vascular anastomoses at the time of the initial vascular repair.[18] Based on our experience and theirs, it does not appear that major soft-tissue reconstruction should be undertaken in the acute situation. Because of the extreme importance of early coverage of any type of vascular conduit with viable tissue, we certainly would concur with Feliciano et al's recommendation that early consultation with a plastic surgeon in the care of such patients is highly desirable.[6]

When there is massive soft-tissue loss precluding adequate soft-tissue coverage of a vascular graft, prosthetic grafts may be superior to autogenous grafts in a contaminated wound if an extraanatomic bypass with an autogenous or prosthetic graft through undamaged tissue planes cannot be performed. Placing an autogenous graft in a potentially contaminated wound without adequate, viable soft-tissue coverage risks subsequent infection and transmural necrosis of the graft with the potential for life-threatening hemorrhage.

Prosthetic grafts seem to tolerate infection better than autogenous grafts in that anastomotic hemorrhage may develop in infected prosthetic grafts whereas infected vein grafts may undergo transmural necrosis with the potential for exsanguinating hemorrhage. In addition the short-term patency rates are acceptable.[2-7] Although we have not had experience with prosthetic grafts in traumatic vascular injuries, our experience with autogenous grafts in wounds with massive soft-tissue loss in which the vein grafts became infected and dissolved resulting in massive hemorrhage suggests that there is a definite role for prosthetic grafts in patients with large, open wounds in which contamination is likely. Our preference would be to use a PTFE graft as a temporizing measure until the wound is clean and is ready for soft-tissue coverage. At that time definitive soft-tissue coverage could be provided by rotating a major muscle flap or by utilizing a free flap. At the time of the soft-tissue reconstruction, strong consideration should be given to replacing the prosthetic graft with an autogenous graft because of the superior patency rates with autogenous tissue in lower extremity revascularization.

In the few patients in whom we had long-term follow-up, the patency rates with autogenous tissue were excellent as illustrated by a patient who has normal pedal pulses more than 17 years following repair of a popliteal artery injury. Figures 2 and 3 illustrate normal vascular laboratory and arteriographic studies several years following the vascular repairs. The excellent long-term patency rates seem especially important with traumatic injuries. Most patients with such injuries are very young with long life expectancies.

Our satisfactory long-term results with autogenous tissue have encouraged us to use autogenous tissue for the reconstruction of traumatic vascular injuries whenever primary repair is not feasible. There are, however, situations in which prosthetic grafts may be preferable, if not mandatory, such as in the repair of large intrathoracic or abdominal arteries when the large size of the arteries dictates using a large prosthetic graft. Patients with life-threatening injuries in whom an expedient operation must be performed may also be better served with a prosthetic graft to save the time required to harvest and prepare a vein graft. As Leather has pointed out, the fact that prosthetic grafts have an inferior patency rate for small-vessel revascularization compared to saphenous vein does not mean that there is no role for prosthetic grafts in vascular trauma.[20] Using a prosthetic graft in the acute vascular repair preserves the saphenous vein for elective revascularization, under optimal conditions, in the few patients who require further revascularization.

REFERENCES

1. Rich NM, Hughes CW: The fate of prosthetic material used to repair vascular injuries in contaminated wounds. J Trauma 12:459, 1972
2. Lau JM, Mattox KL, Beall AC, et al: The use of substitute conduits in vascular trauma. J Trauma 17:541, 1977
3. Vaughan GD, Mattox KL, Feliciano DV, et al: Surgical experience with expand polytetrafluoroethylene (PTFE) as a graft replacement for traumatized vessels. J Trauma 19:403, 1979
4. Jaggers RC, Feliciano DV, Mattox KL, et al: Injury to popliteal vessels. Arch Surg 117:657, 1982
5. Shah RM, Ito K, Clauss RH, et al: Polytetrafluoroethylene (PTFE) graft in contaminated wounds. J Trauma 23:1030, 1983
6. Feliciano DV, Mattox KL, Graham JM, et al: Five-year experience with PTFE grafts in vascular wounds. J Trauma 25:71, 1985

7. Shah DM, Leather RP, Corson JD, et al: Polytetrafluoroethylene grafts in the rapid reconstruction of acute contaminated peripheral vascular injuries. Am J Surg 148:229, 1984

8. Rich NM, Hughes CW: Vietnam Vascular Registry: A preliminary report. Surgery 65:218, 1969

9. Cheek RC, Pope JC, Smith HF, et al: Diagnosis and management of major vascular injuries: A review of 200 operative cases. Ann Surg 41:755, 1975

10. Lucas CE: (Discussion following Rich NM, Hughes CW) The fate of prosthetic material used to repair vascular injuries in contaminated wounds. J Trauma 12:467, 1972

11. Mattox KL: (Discussion following Vaughan GD, Mattox KL, Feliciano DV, et al) Surgical experience with expanded polytetrafluoroethylene (PTFE) as a graft replacement for traumatized vessels. J Trauma 19:408, 1979

12. Ledgerwood AM: (Discussion following Lau JM, Mattox KL, Beall AC, et al) Use of substitute conduits in traumatic vascular injury. J Trauma 17:545, 1977

13. Rich NM, Baugh JH, Hughes CW: Acute arterial injuries in Vietnam: 1,000 cases. J Trauma 10:359, 1970

14. Stone KS, Walshaw R, Sugiyama GT, et al: Polytetrafluoroethylene versus autogenous vein grafts for vascular reconstruction in contaminated wounds. Am J Surg 147:692, 1984

15. Cheek RC, Cole FH, Smith HF: Comparison of Dacron and aortic autografts in wounds contaminated with fecal matter. Ann Surg 40:439, 1974

16. Bricker DL, Beall AC, DeBakey ME: The differential response to infection of autogenous vein versus Dacron arterial prosthesis. Chest 58:566, 1970

17. Knott LH, Crawford FA, Grogan JB: Comparison of autogenous vein, Dacron, and Gore-Tex in infected wounds. J Surg Res 24:288, 1978

18. Ledgerwood AM, Lucas CE: Split thickness porcine graft in the treatment of close-range shotgun wounds to extremities with vascular injury. Am J Surg 125:690, 1973

19. Rich NM, Baugh JH, Hughes CW: Significance of complications associated with vascular repairs performed in Vietnam. Arch Surg 100:646, 1970

20. Leather RP: (Discussion following Feliciano DV, Mattox KL, Graham JM, et al) Five-year experience with PTFE grafts in vascular wounds. J Trauma 25:71, 1985

David V. Feliciano

Use of Prosthetic Grafts in Extensive Arterial Injuries

With the increased magnitude of civilian vascular injuries in recent years, segmental replacement of injured arteries has been frequently required in trauma centers.[1] While autogenous saphenous vein has long been favored as the substitute vascular conduit for segmental replacement,[2] it is clear to experienced vascular trauma surgeons that this conduit cannot be used in all instances. The major practical and theoretical reasons for this have been discussed elsewhere,[3] but will be reviewed again as follows:

1. Inadequate luminal size—When a saphenous vein will not dilate to a diameter greater than 3–4 mm, experience in elective vascular surgery with long bypasses suggests that long-term patency will not be ideal.[4–6]
2. Poor quality vein—Diseased saphenous veins with intimal thickening, fibrotic stenoses, or aneurysmal dilatations such as varicosities also do not have satisfactory long-term patency when inserted into the arterial tree.[4,5]
3. Size discrepancy between vein graft and vessel to be grafted—When the subclavian, axillary, or common femoral arteries are injured, conduits with a diameter of 8–10 mm are generally required for ease of reconstruction and to maintain smooth arterial flow. If the saphenous vein in a young trauma patient does not dilate over a diameter of 4–5 mm, it simply will not fit into these larger vessels in a satisfactory fashion. Panel vein grafts have been proposed as a solution, but are rarely justified when one is dealing with an ischemic extremity in a young trauma patient.
4. Severely injured extremity—When a patient presents with combined extensive arterial and venous injuries in one extremity, early restoration of blood flow is critical. This is particularly true when a delay in definitive treatment has occurred because of difficulty in extrication, a long prehospital transit time, or an interhospital transfer. In order to properly harvest enough length of saphenous vein for both repairs from the uninjured extremity, a delay of 30 minutes or more may occur. The dangers of this delay can only be avoided by using two operating teams, inserting temporary intraluminal shunts, or by inserting a synthetic conduit.[1,7]
5. Saphenous vein may become the only venous outflow from an injured lower extremity—In the patient with bilateral lower extremity vascular injuries, excision of

the saphenous vein from either lower extremity may be hazardous, as occlusion of a repair in the deep femoral venous system will leave the patient without a conduit for venous return.

6. Multiply injured patient—In the patient with multiple truncal injuries and extremity vascular injuries requiring operation in various areas of the body, rapid repair is mandatory to avoid the hypothermia, acidosis, and coagulopathies that occur with shock and massive transfusion. When loss of life is the major threat to the patient, a synthetic conduit may be justified in the interest of shortening operating time without sacrificing an ischemic extremity.

For these reasons, a variety of laboratory and clinical studies have been performed in the last 20 years to evaluate the performance of prosthetic grafts in traumatic vascular injuries.

LABORATORY RESEARCH

Much of the research comparing prostheses with "natural" tissues has focused on the risk of infection in heavily contaminated wounds as well as the response of each conduit to infection.[8] In 1958, Harrison compared freeze-dried aortic homografts with woven Teflon grafts inserted into mongrel dogs that also had fecal contamination of retroperitoneal tissue around the grafts.[9] In the animals with aortic homografts, 50 percent died, primarily as a result of exsanguination from rupture of the grafts. Deaths related to the graft in the woven Teflon graft group occurred in only 19 percent of animals. Harrison concluded that "Teflon grafts are superior to homografts . . . the complications are more amenable to therapy and less likely to cause death."

In a remarkably similar study published in 1959, J.H. Foster et al compared the response of freeze-dried homograft aortas to woven nylon grafts inserted in the canine abdominal aorta and once again contaminated with feces.[10] With a survival of 73 percent in the nylon graft group and 19 percent in the homograft group, Foster felt that "the synthetic prosthesis proved superior both in terms of survival and maintenance of aortic continuity." He also noted "that persistent residual infection may be found in the long-term survivor with a synthetic prosthesis."

Brown's similar canine study in 1961 showed that formalin-preserved rather than freeze-dried aortic homografts had an early complication rate equivalent to that of crimped Teflon prostheses in the presence of fecal infection.[11] He also documented the late degenerative changes that would eventually eliminate the homograft from clinical usage.

In the oft-quoted study by W.S. Moore et al in 1962, arterial bypass or segmental replacement of canine carotid arteries with external jugular veins was performed in wounds contaminated with coliform organisms.[12] Excluding the six vein grafts that occluded, there was only one suture line disruption in the remaining nine grafts. The authors concluded that "autogenous vein grafts will survive and remain patent in the presence of standard coliform infection."

Bricker's study in 1970 compared the response to coagulase negative Staphylococcus aureus of 6-mm Dacron grafts and external jugular veins or femoral veins (in two dogs) inserted into the common iliac arteries in one group and the common femoral arteries in another group.[13] One infected vein graft ruptured in both the iliac and femoral groups;

however, the occlusion rates of the Dacron grafts, 7/10 in the iliac group and 5/10 in the femoral group, clearly compromised the results of the study. The authors concluded that "if this report merely disrupts the complacency associated with the tacit acceptance of the vein graft as a universally superior prosthesis in contaminated wounds, its purpose will be served."

In 1974, Cheek et al compared canine aortic autografts with 6-mm Dacron grafts soaked in 1 percent cephalothin for 60 minutes before implantation under conditions of retroperitoneal fecal contamination.[14] As none of the Dacron grafts suffered an anastomotic disruption while three of the aortic autografts did, it was concluded that "in fields contaminated by fecal matter, antibiotic-soaked Dacron graft is superior to arterial autograft for arterial replacement."

Moore, in 1975, compared canine femoral artery autografts, allografts, and 4-mm knitted Dacron grafts used as bypasses around ligated femoral arteries contaminated with coagulase positive, Staphylococcus aureus.[15] Anastomotic disruption occurred with 3/8 Dacron grafts, but in only 1/12 autografts and 2/12 allografts. Also, the patency rate of the Dacron grafts (2/8) was poor as compared to that of the autografts (7/12) and allografts (9/12). The conclusion reached was that "fresh live arterial autograft and allograft arteries are suitable materials for arterial reconstruction in infected fields."

In one of the early studies on the response of polytetrafluoroethylene (PTFE) prostheses to infection, Weiss et al compared 8-mm Dacron grafts and 8-mm Gore-Tex grafts inserted into the canine aorta and then subjected to intravenous injections of Staphylococcus aureus.[16] There were no significant differences between histologically infected or uninfected Dacron and Gore-Tex grafts in terms of negative initial blood cultures, early prolonged bacteremia, or percentage of positive blood cultures. The authors concluded that their "observations do not support the use of Gore-Tex in an infected environment." They did question, however, whether the extensive tissue ingrowth and complete neointimal development noted with implanted Gore-Tex grafts would "provide a greater resistance to late bacterial challenge or increase the response of a graft infection to antibiotic therapy."

The responses of 4-mm Gore-Tex, autogenous vein, and 4-mm Dacron grafts inserted in canine common femoral arteries were compared after wound exposure to Staphylococcus aureus by Knott et al in 1978.[17] All animals received perioperative cefazolin for a period of 24 hours. Anastomotic disruptions occurred in 4/5 animals with Gore-Tex grafts and in 3/5 animals with Dacron grafts. In 2/4 of the vein disruptions, there was gross dissolution of portions of the graft. It was noted that "wound hemorrhage was similar whether synthetic or autogenous materials were used."

A similar study was performed by Ward et al in 1982.[18] Canine common femoral artery autografts were compared to 4-mm PTFE bypass grafts and autogenous vein bypass grafts in the femoral area under conditions of fecal contamination on one side. As 3/10 animals with autografts, 5/10 animals with autogenous vein grafts, and 9/10 animals with PTFE grafts died from anastomotic disruption or graft autolysis, the authors concluded that "PTFE seems to be the least favorable of the three substitute conduits studied."

In 1983, Shah et al compared the response of 6-mm PTFE grafts and autogenous (jugular) vein grafts inserted in opposite common femoral arteries and subjected to contamination with Staphylococcus aureus and Escherichia coli.[19] Intravenous cefoxitin was administered to one group of five dogs, while another group of five dogs received no antibiotics. Three vein grafts and one thrombosed PTFE graft disrupted in the nonantibiotic group. In the antibiotic group, cultures from 5/5 PTFE sites and from 4/5 vein graft sites were positive for the infecting organisms. The authors concluded that "dissolution of vein wall can occur in the presence of active infection" and that the implications of positive bacterial cultures at 3 weeks (after inoculation) in antibiotic-treated dogs were unclear.

Stone et al, in 1984, compared the response of 6-mm PTFE grafts and autogenous (external jugular) vein grafts inserted as opposite end-to-side femoral arteriovenous shunts and contaminated with an inoculum of 10^3 coagulase-positive Staphylococcus aureus.[20] All 6 dogs receiving antibiotics for 5 days had normal healing and patency of all grafts at the time of sacrifice 6 weeks after operation. In the group of seven dogs that did not receive antibiotics, vein graft disruption occurred in 6/7 instances, while only 2/7 PTFE anastomoses disrupted (p < 0.05). The authors noted that PTFE "has been shown to maintain its structural integrity in the presence of well-entrenched infection" and advocated its use "for controlled clinical trials in patients with contaminated vascular injuries."

As PTFE prostheses have been the most frequently utilized in clinical trials in recent years,[3,19,21] it is interesting to review the results of the previously described five laboratory trials involving this graft.[16–21] In Weiss's[16] and Ward's[18] studies in which no antibiotics were used in the presence of intravenous or topical bacterial contamination of the newly inserted graft, PTFE was felt to perform the same as a porous prosthesis[16] or much worse than autogenous vein.[18] When perioperative antibiotics were utilized[17,19,20] under conditions of topical bacterial contamination (primarily Staphylococcus aureus) of the newly inserted graft, PTFE performed as well as autogenous vein[17] or better.[19,20]

CLINICAL STUDIES

As synthetic prostheses were not used during the Korean War,[22] the earliest reports on their use in traumatic vascular injuries were from civilian trauma centers.[23–27]

In 1959, Schramel and Creech reported on the use of a crimped nylon tube inserted into the superficial femoral artery of a patient sustaining a close range shotgun wound.[23] In the postoperative period, the graft became exposed following debridement of necrotic muscle in the thigh. While the exposed graft remained patent, the presence of persistent wound infection with Staphylococcus aureus led to removal of the graft on the 122nd postoperative day. The authors noted that "synthetic arterial prostheses retain their function . . . even in the presence of infection or when covered by soft tissue." They also commented that exposed prostheses "act as foreign bodies, hindering control of the infection and resisting attempts to cover them."

In 1960, Morris et al reported on the use of 9 knitted Dacron grafts and 14 homografts in a series of 220 patients with arterial injuries.[24] Results with these 2 conduits were not separated in the paper, but appear to be satisfactory in that only 3 amputations and 1 death occurred in the group of 23 patients.

In 1970, Fromm et al described two patients who required Dacron aortoiliac bifurcation graft insertion and one patient who required a Dacron tube graft from the aorta to the right common iliac artery after sustaining penetrating wounds of the abdomen.[25] All three patients had concomitant injuries to the small bowel, but did well in the postoperative period. The authors noted that this was the first report of successful replacement of the injured aorta by a prosthetic aortoiliac graft. They stated that their success "refutes the concept that these grafts will necessarily become infected" and emphasized the importance of careful reperitonealization of the graft, "followed by thorough irrigation of the peritoneal cavity with warm saline prior to closure."

Drapanas et al used prostheses in 14 of 188 (7.6 percent) arterial repairs reported from Charity Hospital in 1970.[26] Prostheses were used when vein grafts were too small to serve as a conduit; however, the results after repair with prosthetic grafts were not specified. In the 181 patients with injuries to arteries of the limbs, the amputation rate was 7.1 percent and mortality was 5.5 percent. Therefore, it must be presumed that the prostheses functioned satisfactorily in some patients.

In the large Parkland Memorial Hospital series of 1971, prosthetic grafts were used in seven of 207 (3.4 percent) arterial repairs.[27] The authors commented that prostheses were used only in the aortoiliac system, but the results with these grafts were not specified.

The fate of prosthetic grafts used for arterial repair in Vietnam (two patients actually sustained trauma in Germany) was reported by Rich and Hughes in 1972.[28] In 26 surviving patients, there were 20 failures (77 percent) including 9 infections, 9 thromboses, 1 stenosis, and 1 false aneurysm. Also, there was a 100 percent failure rate when wounds to the axillary, external iliac, superficial femoral, and popliteal arteries were considered. The amputation rate was 31 percent (8/26). The authors noted that the 77 percent failure rate was 2½ times the overall complication rate for vascular repairs in Vietnam and was "not acceptable in managing these arterial injuries." Exact details of delay in operative therapy, extent of soft tissue injury and contamination, indication for use of a prosthetic graft, operative technique, extent of debridement, type of wound coverage and closure, and perioperative use of antibiotics were not specified in the review.

Mattox et al, in 1974, reported the use of Dacron prosthetic replacement in four patients with injuries to the suprarenal aorta and two patients with injuries to the suprarenal vena cava.[29] The exact outcome of the grafted patients is not clear in this report, but postoperative graft infection is not mentioned as a complication.

Cheek et al from Memphis later reported on the use of 20 Dacron grafts in 136 (14.7 percent) arterial repairs performed from 1969–1974.[30] It is of interest to note that 9 Dacron grafts that had been soaked in 1 percent cephalosporin solution were then placed in the aortoiliac position in the presence of "heavy" contamination. None of these patients had suture line complications, while 5/9 primary repairs (55.6 percent) disrupted in the postoperative period. The authors, citing their own previous laboratory work,[31] recommended that

"an antibiotic soaked Dacron graft covered by healthy tissue such as peritoneum or omentum is the procedure of choice for restoring vascular continuity in gunshot wounds of the aorta and iliac arteries, even with associated fecal contamination."

In 1977, Lau et al described a 5 year experience with 57 Dacron grafts and 65 autogenous vein grafts used as substitute conduits in patients with traumatic vascular wounds.[32] "Potential" contamination was present in 40 patients with Dacron grafts and 62 patients with autogenous vein grafts, while documented contamination was present in another 17 patients with Dacron grafts and 3 patients with saphenous vein grafts. Twelve perigraft infections were seen postoperatively, five in patients with Dacron grafts and seven in patients with vein grafts. Three of the patients with Dacron infections had intermittent anastomotic leaking, but no evidence of thrombosis or hemorrhage. Two others suffered late deaths, both related to the perigraft infection. In the saphenous vein graft group, two patients had graft thrombosis resulting in amputation and five patients had graft dissolution with profuse hemorrhage. The authors concluded that "we, too, believe that the ideal substitute conduit in potentially contaminated traumatic vascular injuries is a Dacron prosthesis."

Two years later, the same group reported on a preliminary experience with Gore-Tex prostheses in traumatic vascular wounds.[33] A total of 49 Gore-Tex conduits were inserted, primarily in the brachial (12 grafts), femoral (9 grafts), axillary/subclavian (8 grafts), popliteal (6 grafts), and renal/visceral vessels (6 grafts). Four patients died from shock and organ failure within 4 days of injury, while 1 patient died 25 days after injury, also with multiple organ failure. Another patient required amputation of the arm at 4 days because of vascular compromise and extent of the original injury. One patient with late presentation of a bilateral renal artery thrombosis treated with splenic artery bypass on the left and Gore-Tex interposition on the right required maintenance hemodialysis, although a postoperative renogram revealed blood flow to both kidneys. Based on this preliminary experience, the authors recommended that 4–6mm Gore-Tex prostheses continue to be evaluated as substitute vascular conduits in medium and small arteries and veins.

RECENT REPORTS

Based on the clinical series noted above, several trauma groups have continued to evaluate prosthetic grafts in traumatic vascular wounds. P.M. Shah et al, whose animal experiments have previously been described,[19] reported in the same paper on a 2 year experience with 25 PTFE grafts inserted into arterial wounds in 22 patients. In two patients, lower extremity amputations related to the original magnitude of the injury were required. The remaining 20 patients did well after surgery, and all grafts were patent at the time of discharge. Long-term follow-up in 16 patients at an average of 9 months following injury revealed that all wounds were well healed and all distal pulses were present. The authors concluded that "reinforced expanded PTFE (is) an acceptable graft to use in potentially contaminated wounds of trauma victims, provided surgical principles are rigorously followed."

In 1984, D.M. Shah et al described a 3.5 year experience with 25 vascular reconstructions in 20 patients using Gore-Tex grafts.[21] Twenty arterial grafts (popliteal=6, iliofemoral=6) and five venous grafts were inserted during this period. One patient with multiple abdominal vascular injuries died from shock, while another patient with a large open thigh wound had postoperative occlusion of grafts placed in both the femoral artery and vein. One patient developed a wound abscess after an extensive iliofemoral wound, but this healed without further complication. A below knee amputation not related to a proximal Gore-Tex insertion was required in one patient, as well. All other patients did well and had patent grafts, though follow-up beyond 24 months was available for only 8 grafts. The authors felt that in patients with peripheral vascular injuries "PTFE was an acceptable choice for primary reconstruction."

The largest American report on the use of Gore-Tex grafts in potentially and truly contaminated traumatic vascular wounds by Feliciano et al was published in 1985.[3] For a 5 year period, Gore-Tex prostheses were used whenever interposition grafting was required in injured vessels of appropriate graft size in adult patients in a busy urban trauma center. A total of 206 arterial and 30 venous prostheses were inserted in 206 patients during the period of the study. Prostheses were most commonly inserted into the femoral (64 grafts), brachial (54 grafts), popliteal (29 grafts), and axillary (21 grafts) arteries.

Venous prostheses were placed in the femoropopliteal system in 25 instances. A complete description of outcomes in the study is beyond the scope of this report, but the major conclusions are summarized as follows:

1. PTFE was found to be an acceptable prosthesis for interposition grafting in arterial wounds, but long-term patency was clearly inferior to that generally found when autogenous vein grafts are used as substitute vascular conduits. Early arterial graft occlusions were mainly related to technical problems or delayed presentation of injury. And, as the greatest number of early and late graft occlusions in the study occurred with 4-mm PTFE grafts inserted in the brachial arteries, this size graft is not recommended for interposition in the brachial artery.
2. Graft infection occurred only when grafts were left exposed or when osteomyelitis developed in adjacent fractured bone.
3. Delay in graft coverage always leads to occlusion, infection, or delayed dehiscence of the prosthetic graft–artery suture line.
4. PTFE grafts inserted in proximal extremity veins functioned as excellent temporary conduits that decreased hemorrhage in blast cavities and fasciotomy sites; however, venograms, palpation of exposed grafts, or reoperation revealed occlusion in all 11 grafts in which these modalities were performed in the postoperative period.

Other reports on the occasional use of Gore-Tex in traumatic vascular wounds have appeared, as well.[34] Also, improved results with elective use of PTFE with or without external support as an interposition graft in large veins have been noted recently.[35,36]

PRESENT APPROACH

The saphenous vein remains the conduit of choice for peripheral vascular injuries requiring segmental replacement based on its ready availability, low infection rate, and excellent long-term patency. When a satisfactory saphenous vein is not available or other critical patient factors as previously described are present, PTFE prosthetic grafts are an acceptable alternative.

Limited debridement of the wound and injured artery should be performed prior to inserting the prosthesis. The appropriate size of the prosthesis to be used may be difficult to assess as intense spasm of the transected arterial ends is usually present. It is frequently helpful to trim the adventitia off the last 2–3-mm of the end of the artery, and then pass Garrett calibrated dilators before deciding on the appropriate size of the prosthesis. Based on previous experience, the following graft sizes should be used in the arterial tree:

Subclavian	8-mm	Iliac	6–8-mm
Axillary	6-mm	Common femoral	6–8-mm
Brachial	5–6-mm	Superficial femoral	6–8-mm
	Popliteal	6–8-mm	

The appropriate length of graft is then cut using a #11 scalpel blade rather than a scissors. It should be remembered that PTFE in the older thicker conformation or when externally supported is a rigid prosthesis. If the inserted prosthesis is too long, this may lead to kinking of one of the anastomoses and subsequent thrombosis of the graft.[37]

In awkward locations beneath the clavicle or inguinal ligament or behind the knee joint, it may be preferable to perform the distal, smaller anastomosis first to allow for better thrombectomy and flushing through the larger proximal vessel. The open PTFE prosthesis will usually allow for a rapid anastomosis to the native artery without fixation sutures. When exposure is not ideal, the posterior 1/3 of the anastomosis should be performed in an open fashion (no posterior knot is tied) and only then should the two ends of the suture be pulled tight to approximate the end of the graft with the end of the artery. A 5-0 or 6-0 polypropylene suture is used for this running suture line or for an interrupted anastomosis if one chooses to use this technique on small vessels. Once the first anastomosis is complete, it is usually helpful to pass a Fogarty catheter through the two ends (one artery, one graft) in order to clear any thrombotic or embolic material from the arterial tree before completing the second anastomosis. Also, passing embolectomy catheters at this point means that the surgeon will only have to "grab" one end of the artery, and this should minimize intimal damage. When both ends of the artery are clean, 7–10 ml of heparin solution (50 units/ml) are injected into either end and small vascular clamps are reapplied. The second anastomosis is then performed in a manner similar to the first; however, the last few loops of the running suture are left loose. Proximal and distal flushing is completed through this opening. The proximal clamp is then reapplied, while the distal clamp is left off to flush air out of the interval between the clamps as the suture ends are pulled up tight and tied. Large leaks are repaired using interrupted sutures of 6-0 polypropylene, before the proximal clamp is released. The proximal clamp is then released, and the distal extremity pulses and skin color change are checked by viewing the hand or foot through a plastic bag that was placed at the time of draping.

In the upper extremity, completion arteriography is not commonly performed if pulses at the wrist immediately return upon release of the vascular clamps (Fig. 1). Distal thrombosis or embolism in the upper extremity is quite rare unless a tight arterial tourniquet has been in place for several hours prior to repair. In the lower extremity, completion arteriography is always performed by injecting 35 ml of diatrizoate meglumine dye through a 20-gauge Teflon-over-metal catheter inserted proximal to the prosthesis. Prior to injection it is helpful to place a small, metal tissue clip near each of the anastomoses so that they may be precisely localized on the arteriogram. It is also helpful to have the first toe pointing directly at the ceiling during the injection as abduction of the lower extremity may cause overlying bone to obscure a vascular repair near the knee joint or in the leg. Any anastomotic narrowing or distal clot formation noted on the arteriogram should be immediately corrected, and a repeat arteriogram performed.

Once arterial inflow has been restored, vigorous debridement of nonviable tissue is appropriate. The wound is then copiously irrigated with saline, the last liter of which includes 50,000 units of bacitracin and 1 gm of kanamycin in my institution.

If extensive blast cavities are present underneath a prosthesis inserted into the femoral artery, an attempt should be made to approximate some muscle under the graft and insert open and/or suction drains through the posterior thigh to allow for dependent drainage. An exposed graft is covered at the first operation if at all possible. When the patient is unstable, the graft is covered with a porcine xenograft and antibiotic-soaked gauze for 24 hours. The patient is then returned to the operating room for skin or myocutaneous flap coverage.

Based on extensive laboratory and civilian clinical experience, the combination of antibiotic irrigation of the graft and wound prior to closure and perioperative intravenous

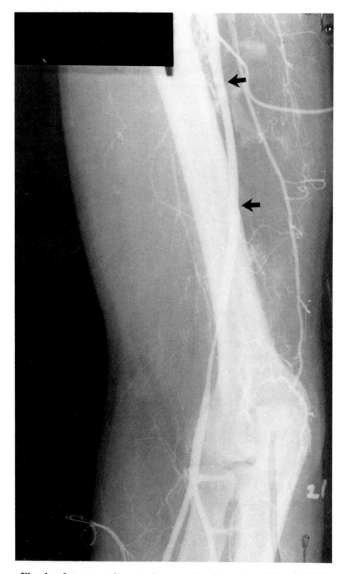

Fig. 1. Intraoperative arteriogram after insertion of 6-mm PTFE prosthesis (black arrows) in brachial artery. Diminished pulses at the wrist were due to distal spasm.

antibiotics for a 3 day period makes the risk of infection in peripheral arterial PTFE grafts exceedingly small.[3,19,21,33,38-43] Also, patients are instructed on the need for lifetime supplemental antibiotics whenever other invasive maneuvers, serious illnesses, or operative procedures occur.[37]

As there is laboratory evidence demonstrating that neointimal hyperplasia may occur at PTFE-artery suture lines, it has been my policy to place all patients on daily aspirin and dipyridamole for a 3 month period after discharge.[44-46]

CONCLUSION

Prosthetic grafts, especially those made of PTFE, are acceptable alternatives for segmental arterial replacement in selected patients after trauma. By following the principles described, excellent short-term results should be obtained. Long-term data on the use of these prostheses is not available at this time.

ACKNOWLEDGMENT

I acknowledge the technical assistance of Mary LeJeune.

REFERENCES

1. Feliciano DV, Bitondo CG, Mattox KL, et al: Civilian trauma in the 1980s. A 1-year experience with 456 vascular and cardiac injuries. Ann Surg 199:717, 1984
2. Rich NM, Baugh JH, Hughes CW: Acute arterial injuries in Vietnam: 1000 cases. J Trauma 10:359, 1970
3. Feliciano DV, Mattox KL, Graham JM, Bitondo CG: Five-year experience with PTFE grafts in vascular wounds. J Trauma 25:71, 1985
4. Szilagyi DE, Elliott JP, Hageman JH, et al: Biologic fate of autogenous vein implants as arterial substitutes: Clinical, angiographic and histopathologic observations in femoro-popliteal operations for atherosclerosis. Ann Surg 178:232, 1973
5. Szilagyi DE, Hageman JH, Smith RF, et al: Autogenous vein grafting in femoropopliteal atherosclerosis: The limits of its effectiveness. Surgery 86:836, 1979
6. Fuchs JCA, Mitchener JS III, Hagen P-O: Postoperative changes in autologous vein grafts. Ann Surg 188:1, 1978
7. Johansen K, Bandyk D, Thiele B, Hansen ST Jr: Temporary intraluminal shunts: Resolution of a management dilemma in complex vascular injuries. J Trauma 22:395, 1982
8. Martin TD, Mattox KL, Feliciano DV: Prosthetic grafts in vascular trauma: A controversy. Comp Ther 11:41, 1985
9. Harrison JH: Influence of infection on homografts and synthetic (Teflon) grafts. Arch Surg 76:67, 1958
10. Foster JH, Berzins T, Scott HW Jr: An experimental study of arterial replacement in the presence of bacterial infection. Surg Gynecol Obstet 108:141, 1959
11. Brown RB, Hoofer WD, Greenberg JJ, Edmunds LH Jr: Vascular replacement in grossly contaminated wounds: An experimental study comparing formalin preserved homografts and plastic prosthesis. J Trauma 1:322, 1961
12. Moore WS, Blaisdell FW, Gardner M, Hall AD: Effect of infection on autogenous vein arterial substitutes. Surg Forum 13:235, 1962
13. Bricker DL, Beall AC Jr, DeBakey ME: The differential response to infection of autogenous vein versus Dacron arterial prosthesis. Chest 58:566, 1970
14. Cheek RC, Cole FH, Smith HF: Comparison of Dacron and aortic autografts in wounds contaminated with fecal matter. Amer Surgeon 40:439, 1974
15. Moore WS, Swanson RJ, Campagna G, Bean B: The use of fresh tissue arterial substitutes in infected fields. J Surg Research 18:229, 1975
16. Weiss JP, Lorenzo FV, Campbell CD, et al: The behavior of infected arterial prostheses of expanded polytetrafluoroethylene (Gore-Tex). J Thorac Cardiovasc Surg 73:630, 1977
17. Knott LH, Crawford FA Jr, Grogan JB: Comparison of autogenous vein, Dacron and Gore-Tex in infected wounds. J Surg Research 24:288, 1978

18. Ward RE, Hudson ML, Flynn TC: Gram-negative infections of arterial substitutes. J Surg Research 33:510, 1982

19. Shah PM, Ito K, Clauss RH, et al: Expanded microporous polytetrafluoroethylene (PTFE) grafts in contaminated wounds: Experimental and clinical study. J Trauma 23:1030, 1983

20. Stone KS, Walshaw R, Sugiyama GT, et al: Polytetrafluoroethylene versus autogenous vein grafts for vascular reconstruction in contaminated wounds. Am J Surg 147:692, 1984

21. Shah DM, Leather RP, Corson JD, Karmody AM: Polytetrafluoroethylene grafts in the rapid reconstruction of acute contaminated peripheral vascular injuries. Am J Surg 148:229, 1984

22. Hughes CW: Arterial repair during the Korean War. Ann Surg 147:555, 1958

23. Schramel RJ, Creech O Jr: Effects of infection and exposure on synthetic arterial prostheses. Arch Surg 78:271, 1959

24. Morris GC Jr, Beall AC Jr, Roof WR, DeBakey ME: Surgical experience with 220 acute arterial injuries in civilian practice. Am J Surg 99:775, 1960

25. Fromm SH, Carrasquilla C, Lucas C: The management of gunshot wounds of the aorta. Arch Surg 101:388, 1970

26. Drapanas T, Hewitt RL, Weichert RF III, Smith AD: Civilian vascular injuries: A critical appraisal of three decades of management. Ann Surg 172:351, 1970

27. Perry MO, Thal ER, Shires GT: Management of arterial injuries. Ann Surg 173:403, 1971

28. Rich NM, Hughes CW: The fate of prosthetic material used to repair vascular injuries in contaminated wounds. J Trauma 12:459, 1972

29. Mattox KL, McCollum WB, Jordan GI Jr, et al: Management of upper abdominal vascular trauma. Am J Surg 128:823, 1974

30. Cheek RC, Pope JC, Smith HF, et al: Diagnosis and management of major vascular injuries: A review of 200 operative cases. Amer Surgeon 41:755, 1975

31. Richardson RL Jr, Pate JW, Wolf RY, et al: The outcome of antibiotic-soaked arterial grafts in guinea pig wounds contaminated with E. coli or S. aureus. J Thorac Cardiovasc Surg 59:635, 1970

32. Lau JM, Mattox KL, Beall AC Jr, DeBakey ME: Use of substitute conduits in traumatic vascular injury. J Trauma 17:541, 1977

33. Vaughan GD, Mattox KL, Feliciano DV, et al: Surgical experience with expanded polytetrafluoroethylene (PTFE) as a replacement graft for traumatized vessels. J Trauma 19:403, 1979

34. Menzoian JO, Doyle JE, Cantelmo NL, et al: A comprehensive approach to extremity vascular trauma. Arch Surg 120:801, 1985

35. Dale WA, Harris J, Terry RB: Polytetrafluoroethylene reconstruction of the inferior vena cava. Surgery 95:625, 1984

36. Katz NM, Spence IJ, Wallace RB: Reconstruction of the inferior vena cava with a polytetrafluoroethylene graft after resection for hypernephroma of the right kidney. J Thorac Cardiovasc Surg 87:791, 1984

37. Feliciano DV: Pitfalls in the management of peripheral vascular injuries. Prob Clin Surg 3:101, 1986

38. Moore WS, Rosson CT, Hall AD, Thomas AN: Transient bacteremia. A cause of infection in prosthetic vascular grafts. Am J Surg 117:341, 1969

39. DiGiglia JWD, Leonard GL, Ochsner JL: Local irrigation with an antibiotic solution in the prevention of infection in vascular prostheses. Surgery 67:806, 1970

40. Moore WS, Rosson CT, Hall AD: Effect of prophylactic antibiotics in preventing bacteremic infection of vascular prostheses. Surgery 69:825, 1971

41. Malone JM, Moore WS, Campagna G, Bean B: Bacteremic infectability of vascular grafts: The influence of pseudointimal integrity and duration of graft function. Surgery 78:211, 1975

42. Kaiser AB, Clayson KR, Mulherin JL Jr, et al: Antibiotic prophylaxis in vascular surgery. Ann Surg 188:283, 1978

43. May ARL, Darling RC, Brewster DC, Darling CS: A comparison of the use of cephalothin and oxacillin in vascular surgery. Arch Surg 115:56, 1980

44. Oblath RW, Buckley FO Jr, Green RM, et al: Prevention of platelet aggregation and adherence to prosthetic vascular grafts by aspirin and dipyridamole. Surgery 84:37, 1978
45. Hagen P-O, Wang Z-G, Mikat EM, Hackel DB: Antiplatelet therapy reduces aortic intimal hyperplasia distal to small diameter vascular prostheses (PTFE) in nonhuman primates. Ann Surg 195:328, 1982
46. Richter RC: Antiplatelet therapy in surgery. Infect Surg 3:137, 1984

William L. Russell
R. Phillip Burns

Acute Upper and Lower Extremity Compartment Syndromes

The description of paralysis and contracture resulting from compression of the involved upper extremity was described by Von Volkmann in 1881.[1] It was initially suggested that such paralysis and contracture resulted from an interruption of arterial blood supply due to splinting and immobilization of the extremity. Other theories have been considered over the years but it is now known that Volkmann's contracture is most often due to an untreated compartment syndrome caused by a variety of factors. In most instances hemorrhage and/or edema within the involved compartment produces increased pressure and ischemia. Therefore, early decompression of the limb prevents the sequelae of paralysis and possible subsequent contracture described by Volkmann. Clear definition of anatomical compartments, understanding of the pathophysiology and reliable pressure monitoring have all allowed effective surgical decompression to be carried out. Better understanding of the pathophysiology alone has led to early and successful medical management of a compartment syndrome without subsequent fasciotomy.[2-7] These are addressed in this chapter.

ETIOLOGY

Simply stated, compartment syndromes can result from any condition that diminishes the compartment size or causes increased compartment contents. Over the years, many factors have been implicated (Table 1). The occurrence of a compartment syndrome is dependent upon the duration of the increased pressure and the absolute intracompartment pressure. Unrecognized compartment syndrome can proceed to the ischemia and necrosis of the contents of the compartment described above. In addition to contracture, renal failure, amputation or death may be the result of neglected compartment syndrome.

Vascular Surgical Emergencies
ISBN 0-8089-1843-5

Table 1

Classification of Acute Compartment Syndromes

Decreased compartment size
  Constrictive dressings and casts
  Closure of fascial defects
  Thermal injuries and frostbite
Increased compartment contents
  Primary edema accumulation
    Postischemic swelling
      Arterial injuries
      Arterial thrombosis or embolism
      Reconstructive vascular and bypass surgery
      Replantation
      Prolonged tourniquet time
      Arterial spasm
      Cardiac catheterization and angiography
      Ergotamine ingestion
    Prolonged immobilization with limb compression
      Drug overdose with limb compression
      General anesthesia with knee–chest position
    Thermal injuries and frostbite
    Exertion
    Venous disease
    Venomous snakebite
  Primarily hemorrhage accumulation
    Hereditary bleeding disorders, e.g., hemophilia
    Anticoagulant therapy
    Vessel laceration
  Combination of edema and hemorrhage accumulation
    Fractures
      Tibia
      Forearm
      Elbow, e.g., supracondylar
      Femur
    Soft tissue injury
    Osteotomies, e.g., tibia
  Miscellaneous
    Intravenous infiltration, e.g., blood, saline
    Popliteal cyst
    Long leg brace

From Mubarak SJ, Hargens AR: Compartment Syndromes and Volkmann's Contracture. Philadelphia, W. B. Saunders Co., 1981. With permission

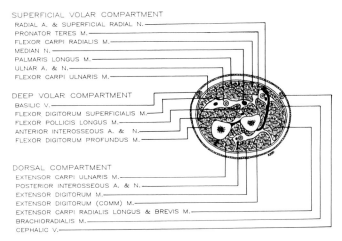

SUPERFICIAL VOLAR COMPARTMENT
RADIAL A. & SUPERFICIAL RADIAL N.
PRONATOR TERES M.
FLEXOR CARPI RADIALIS M.
MEDIAN N.
PALMARIS LONGUS M.
ULNAR A. & N.
FLEXOR CARPI ULNARIS M.

DEEP VOLAR COMPARTMENT
BASILIC V.
FLEXOR DIGITORUM SUPERFICIALIS M.
FLEXOR POLLICIS LONGUS M.
ANTERIOR INTEROSSEOUS A. & N.
FLEXOR DIGITORUM PROFUNDUS M.

DORSAL COMPARTMENT
EXTENSOR CARPI ULNARIS M.
POSTERIOR INTEROSSEOUS A. & N.
EXTENSOR DIGITORUM M.
EXTENSOR DIGITORUM (COMM) M.
EXTENSOR CARPI RADIALIS LONGUS & BREVIS M.
BRACHIORADIALIS M.
CEPHALIC V.

Fig. 1. Compartments of the lower arm.

ANATOMY

Forearm

The forearm consists of two basic compartments: the volar and dorsal compartment. On crossectional view as shown in Figure 1, the flexor carpi ulnaris, palmaris longus, flexor carpi radialis, and pronator teres are the superficial volar compartment and arise from the area of the medial epicondyle of the humerus. Deeper in the volar compartment are found flexor digitorum profundus and superficialis, flexor pollicis longus, and the pronator quadratis. The median nerve is found in the volar compartment between the more superficial and deep layers as is the ulnar nerve, artery and vein, as well as radial nerve, artery and vein.

Muscles of the dorsal compartment include extensor digitorum communis, extensor carpi ulnaris, abductor pollicis longus, and extensor pollicis longus and brevis. Nerve supply is the posterior interosseous nerve, a branch of the radial nerve. The compartment is divided by the interosseous membrane and surrounded by the intrabrachial fascia with strong septal bands.[8]

Leg

There are four compartments of the leg (Fig. 2). The anterior and lateral compartments are found anterior to the interosseous membrane with the superficial and deep posterior compartments posterior to the interosseous membrane. They are also bound by the posterior intramuscular septum between the lateral and superficial posterior compartment. Attention should be particularly drawn to the nerves present in the four compartments of the lower leg (Fig. 2); principally the deep peroneal nerve in the anterior compartment, the superficial peroneal nerve in the lateral compartment, the tibial nerve in the deep posterior compartment, and the sural nerve in the superficial posterior compartment. Sensory changes along the paths of these nerves give reliable data and diagnosis of specific compartments involved. A knowledge of the anatomy facilitates greatly the approach to appropriate fasciotomy if needed.

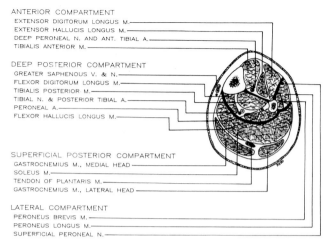

ANTERIOR COMPARTMENT
EXTENSOR DIGITORUM LONGUS M.
EXTENSOR HALLUCIS LONGUS M.
DEEP PERONEAL N. AND ANT. TIBIAL A.
TIBIALIS ANTERIOR M.

DEEP POSTERIOR COMPARTMENT
GREATER SAPHENOUS V. & N.
FLEXOR DIGITORUM LONGUS M.
TIBIALIS POSTERIOR M.
TIBIAL N. & POSTERIOR TIBIAL A.
PERONEAL A.
FLEXOR HALLUCIS LONGUS M.

SUPERFICIAL POSTERIOR COMPARTMENT
GASTROCNEMIUS M., MEDIAL HEAD
SOLEUS M.
TENDON OF PLANTARIS M.
GASTROCNEMIUS M., LATERAL HEAD

LATERAL COMPARTMENT
PERONEUS BREVIS M.
PERONEUS LONGUS M.
SUPERFICIAL PERONEAL N.

Fig. 2.   Compartments of the lower leg.

PATHOPHYSIOLOGY

Matsen[9] has defined compartment syndrome as "a condition in which increased pressure within a limited space compromises the circulation and function of the tissues within that space." This definition is comprehensive and outlines the basic changes that lead to compartment syndromes. From the anatomy review of the upper and lower extremity, the muscles, vessels, and nerves are enclosed with relatively nonexpandable boundaries made of bone, fascia, and interosseous membranes; therefore, very effectively comprising a closed space by the intrinsic rigidity.

Holden[10] classified the traumatic event into two broad types; type one consisting of direct arterial injury at a level proximal to the subsequent ischemia and type two representing direct injury to the distal part of the limb with ischemia developing at the site of the injury. It is obvious that there is more than one mechanism involved in formation of compartment syndrome; however, the final common pathway as suggested by Sarokhan and Eaton[11] is interstitial edema and ultimate disruption of the microcirculation. Tissue perfusion may then be compromised to a degree sufficient to produce muscle ischemia and possible infarction. Regardless of the inciting cause for ischemia, trauma capable of inducing an initial rise in intramuscular and intracompartmental pressure may ultimately produce a significant compromise in tissue perfusion that will persist until interrupted either by reduction of intracompartmental pressure or progressive necrosis of the involved muscles.[11] Intact macrocirculation distal to the area of interest is notoriously inaccurate as a guide to the status of local muscle perfusion.

Cellular response is based on several factors; the specific effect of increased tissue pressure on local blood flow in the tissue under consideration, metabolic demands of the tissue and the duration of increased tissue pressure. Studies in animal and human subjects, have yielded results demonstrating variations in response to pressures among individual subjects as well as tissue involved.[8,9,12,13] Nerve and muscle do have a significant potential for recovery and reconstruction following ischemic injury; however, the duration of the ischemic insult and the presence of other factors including hypotension, hemorrhagic shock, limb elevation, and local tissue injury are all modifiers of the resistance to ischemia.[14]

Table 2

Decline in Membrane PD in the Ischemic Limb*

	Group No.	Baseline	Ischemia	Reperfusion
Muscle membrane PD	I	-91.8 ± 1.1	-79.1 ± 1.1	-71.4 ± 1.3
(mV)	II	-92.0 ± 0.8	-82.7 ± 1.9	-74.2 ± 1.4
Creatine phosphate	I	17.0 ± 2.0	3.4 ± 1.8	17.5 ± 1.6
(μM/gm of wet tissue)	II	17.6 ± 0.9	15.9 ± 1.6	17.3 ± 2.6
Adenosine triphosphate	I	5.8 ± 0.6	5.9 ± 0.3	5.6 ± 0.8
(μM/gm of wet tissue)	II	6.2 ± 0.5	6.3 ± 0.4	6.2 ± 0.8

From Perry MO, Shires GT, Albert SA: Cellular changes with graded limb ischemia and reperfusion. J Vasc Surg 1 (4):539, 1984. With permission.

*Persists 3 hours following restoration of normal perfusion.

$p < 0.01$.

Perry[6] has reported cellular changes with graded ischemia and reperfusion as shown in Table 2. The continual fall in muscle membrane potential difference following restoration of normal flow strongly suggests serious membrane damage with persistent and perpetuating edema across the basement membrane. The reduction of membrane potential reflects severe metabolic derangements and apparently demonstrates failure of the sodium pump. Eklof[15] showed serious membrane damage following aortic surgical procedures in humans as much as 16 hours postoperatively from the temporary aortic occlusion. Administration of low molecular weight Dextran in these patients seemed to prevent delayed changes in high energy phosphate energetics. Very promising studies have suggested oxygen-free radicals may contribute to this serious damage in the reperfusion period.[16] Superoxide radical scavengers such as mannitol, superoxide dismutase, and allopurinol can protect ischemic muscle from reperfusion injuries.[6] The actual effect is unknown but it appears certain that diuresis is only one of the actions of these compounds.

Etiologies of Compartment Syndrome

A wide variety of injuries may place the patient at risk for compartment syndrome. Our study of 100 consecutive patients at risk for compartment syndrome is listed in Table 3. Of those, 39 percent involved fracture, 32 percent arterial occlusions, 20 percent soft tissue injury, and 9 percent other etiologic factors such as burns and wringer injuries. Thirty-three exhibited significantly elevated compartment pressures. Arterial occlusion

Table 3

Summary of 100 Patients at Risk Comparing Mechanism of Injury and Compartment Pressure Response

Mechanisms	0–10 mmHg	10–30 mmHg	>30 mmHg	Total
Soft tissue	4	11	5	20
Arterial occlusion	6	7	19	32
Fracture	8	25	6	39
Burn	1	1	—	2
Other	2	2	3	7
Total	21	46	33	100

was the most common event leading to compartment syndrome. Mubarak and Hargens[17] studied 80 prospective cases with a 45 percent incidence of fracture and 13 percent arterial injury using the wick catheter. Perhaps this represents the respective admixture of patients of vascular and orthopedic surgeons.

As noted in Table 1, compartment syndrome may result from decreased compartment size or increased compartment contents. Compartment syndrome caused by constrictive dressings and casts may involve decreased compartment size as well as increased compartment contents due to the nature of the injury for which they are utilized. Elevation of the extremity leads to decreased perfusion of compartment contents and can increase the potential for ischemic change. Burn patients should also be monitored for potential development of compartmental syndrome due to constrictive eschar and tissue changes.

The utilization of pneumatic anti-shock garments (PASG) is often seen in and around trauma centers. Chisholm[18] studied 8 healthy volunteers using a wick catheter and PASG applied to the legs and abdomen. As seen in Table 4, the intramuscular pressure with PASG inflation reached levels approximately equal to the resting intramuscular pressure plus the externally applied pressure.

Although relatively uncommon, recent case reports by Bass,[19] Godbout,[20] and Maull[21] outline the potential severity of long term high pressure PASG and establish guidelines in utilization of such garments. They stress careful monitoring of the PASG pressures and maintaining the lowest pressure possible to achieve adequate systolic pressure response. Utilization of blood and crystalloid replacement is the mainstay in establishment and maintenance of an adequate blood pressure in the trauma patient. A combination of increased intracompartmental pressure and decreased arterial perfusion pressure contribute more to muscular ischemia than either separately. Both situations exist in the hypotensive trauma patient with PASG. Continuous monitoring of intracompartmental pressure should be a companion procedure in those patients requiring PASG.[18]

INCREASED COMPARTMENT CONTENTS

Primary Edema Accumulation

Arterial occlusion, complete or partial with resultant tissue ischemia, is the most common factor in our clinical series of compartment syndrome. In these patients at risk for compartment syndrome, pre-revascularization compartment pressures were uniformly less than 30 mmHg. Following revascularization often prompt elevation of pressure to 30 mmHg and greater occurred. The predictability with which significantly increased pressure occurred was in those patients with ischemic lag phase of 6–8 hours and greater. As pointed out by Perry[7] the skin and subcutaneous tissues survive hypoxemia not otherwise tolerated by skeletal muscle and peripheral nerves. Skin, however, is the tissue easiest evaluated for signs of hypoxemia and therefore may well be misleading. This occasionally causes undue delay in the urgent need for surgical revascularization.

Once revascularization occurs, metabolites such as serum lactate increase markedly with alteration of acid base balance. The significant changes in muscle membrane potential difference also occur with resultant edema and increased vascular resistance leading to lower perfusion pressures, ischemia, and additional edema. It is, therefore, important that compartment pressure measurements be obtained pre- and post-revascularization with immediate fasciotomy undertaken, if indicated.

Table 4

Correlation Between Compartment Pressure and Pneumatic
Antishock Garment Inflation Pressure

Intramuscular Pressure (mmHg)	PASG Inflation Pressure (mmHg)				
	0	30*	60†	30‡	0
Subject 1	12.0	48.5	82.0	44.0	9.0
2	13.0	44.0	76.0	42.5	16.0
3	8.0	37.5	68.7	40.0	10.0
4	7.5	28.8	58.8	27.5	10.0
5	10.0	28.8	53.8	27.5	11.0
6	8.0	35.3	60.0	35.0	11.0
7	13.0	44.5	70.5	40.0	12.0
8	4.0	33.0	57.5	27.5	2.0

From Chisholm CD, Clark DE: Effect of the pneumatic antishock garment on
intramuscular pressure. Ann Emerg Med 13 (8):582, 1984. With permission.
*Compartment pressure mean with deviation ± 4.8 mmHg.
†Compartment pressure mean with deviation ± 4.0 mmHg.
‡Compartment pressure mean with deviation ± 4.3 mmHg.

Unique clinical situations such as free flap transfers and other complex reconstructive procedures have likewise been subject to reperfusion-type injuries.[22] While not a true compartment syndrome, the edema and increased vascular resistance in the myocutaneous flap, unless recognized, can spell disaster in the reconstructive procedure.

Compartment complications of prolonged immobilization has been reported by Lydon[23] and Reddy.[24] Patients undergoing gynecologic and urologic procedures requiring prolonged, unusual positioning should be carefully positioned and extremity pressure points well padded. A case of deep posterior compartment syndrome as reported by Reddy[24] very closely mimicked deep venous thrombis. The development of plantar hypesthesia and paresis suggested the diagnosis of deep posterior compartment syndrome and decompression was accomplished. The patient, however, was left with a residual foot drop requiring a brace.

Direct causes of edema such as thermal injuries, frostbite, and venomous snakebite most often involve the subcutaneous space. Two patients reported by Roberts,[25] however, developed compartment syndrome in the upper arm secondary to snakebite, requiring fasciotomy and carpal tunnel release. The mechanism of primary edema accumulation is that of direct cytotoxicity. Roberts[25] outlines the approach to envenomation therapy including antivenin, corticosteroids, local wound suction, and fasciotomy with debridement. Intracompartmental pressure monitoring can be utilized as an important adjunct in the monitoring and care of snakebite victims and prompt fasciotomy undertaken, if necessary.

Accumulation of Hemorrhage

Wide utilization of anti-coagulants and the advent of more invasive monitoring techniques such as arterial puncture for blood gases and utilization of indwelling arterial lines for continuous pressure monitoring, have combined to place a patient at risk for potential intracompartmental hemorrhage. Trauma to a vascular hamartoma in the forearm of a young woman as reported by Joseph[26] resulted in progressive development of a compartment syndrome with severe flexion deformities of all fingers from contractures of the deep muscles. This diagnosis was missed and 6 weeks post injury the patient underwent exploration of the forearm. The radial pulse was present throughout. This case does stress the potential for reconstruction even as late as 6 weeks to several months in the absence of necrosis and gangrenous changes in the muscles.

Combinations of Edema and Hemorrhage Accumulation

In our series of patients at risk for fasciotomy, 39 fractures were monitored for potential development of compartment syndrome. Six of these patients underwent fasciotomy. The lower extremity was the most common site of compartment syndrome with fracture of the tibia most commonly noted.[25] Other factors involved include multiple injuries, prolonged traction, and elevation of the extremity involved. Elevation reduces perfusion pressure of the compartment musculature, complicating the physical effect of hemorrhage, and casting when applied.

Upper extremity compartment syndromes with resultant Volkmann's contracture are most commonly a result of supracondylar humeral fracture. As demonstrated by Sarokhan[11] and Mubarak[8] the mechanism of injury may include direct compression of the median nerve and potential laceration of the brachial artery at its entrance to the flexor compartment. This potential combination of injuries requires careful knowledge of anatomy and pathophysiology. Resultant Volkmann's contracture is well documented and severe deformity as well as litigation may occur.

Clinical Diagnosis

Functional and sensory losses precede nerve and muscle necrosis often by a matter of hours as suggested by Matsen and Krugmire.[9] Key signs of developing compartment syndrome include pain of greater intensity than the primary factors such as fractures, ischemia, or contusion. The pain is described as a deep, throbbing, and unrelenting pressure-type sensation. In the absence of more proximal nerve injury, pain is the first and most important symptom of an impending compartment syndrome.

Paresthesias manifest as a sensory deficit. As seen in crosssectional views (Figs. 1 and 2) each compartment of the forearm and leg has at least one nerve coursing through it. Careful sensory examination of the hand or foot, therefore, is helpful in determining the compartments involved. The first sensory losses are those of soft touch and proprioception preceding hypesthesia and subsequent anesthesia.

Pain with stretching of involved muscles is commonly noted. This is subjective, however, and depends very much on the patient's threshold of pain. Following soft tissue, vascular, or orthopedic trauma this finding is often present and may be difficult to interpret. Late in the compartment syndrome anesthesia in the distribution of the involved nerve renders this test unreliable. Paresis or weakness of the involved muscle compartment is likewise difficult to interpret. It may be due to compartment syndrome, guarding secondary to pain or direct nerve involvement by the trauma involved.

The only objective finding is a swollen and tense compartment as a direct manifestation of increased intracompartmental pressure. This may be directly measured as will be discussed later in this chapter. Subcutaneous edema and hematoma, which frequently accompanies soft tissue and bony tissue injury, complicates and can mask the underlying compartment syndrome.

It must be restated that pulses distal to the involved compartment may be routinely present in the absence of proximal arterial occlusion. One must be aware of this fact and realize palpation of pulses may leave one with a false sense of security. Compartment syndrome, arterial occlusion, and neuropraxia may all coexist; therefore, careful pressure assessment, possible arteriography, and nerve conduction studies may be indicated as an aid in proper diagnosis.

An uncommonly encountered clinical situation was reported by Bohn[27] of a case of streptococcal gangrene mimicking compartment syndrome. Clostridial and microaerophilic streptococcal organisms through the release of locally destructive hyaluronidase, streptokinase, proteinase, and streptolysins cause myonecrosis. The case presented by Bohn and Coleman very closely mimicked a compartment syndrome, and only through immediate cultures and gram stains was the diagnosis of streptococcal gangrene established.

Laboratory Diagnosis

Wide use of intracompartmental pressure monitoring devices is now routinely employed in determination of tissue pressure. The infusion technique by Matsen,[9] wick catheter by Mubarak[8] and others,[28] and new solid state transducer catheter by McDermott[29] have all been recently reported. In our experience,[28] the wick catheter (Myocath®, Sorensen) was utilized in consecutive patients at risk for development of compartment syndrome who were categorized according to maximum intracompartmental pressure (Table 3). The technique of placement and monitoring is reported elsewhere.[30]

Continuous intracompartmental pressure monitoring in the critical care setting or operating theater allows continual observation by trained personnel for the possible development of compartment syndrome in those patients in skeletal traction, with neurological deficits, and intra- and post-operative patients. Most compartment syndromes can be diagnosed clinically, but the above mentioned patients as well as uncooperative or poorly responsive patients require more objective means of evaluation.

Mubarak and Hargens[8] advocate 30 mmHg as a critical measurement in consideration for fasciotomy. Other researchers including Gelberman[12] and others,[9] have advocated somewhat higher pressures of 40 mmHg or greater as indications for fasciotomy. Our experience in the alert patient would coincide with a slightly higher threshold pressure than 30 mmHg and in fact, 4 patients with pressures up to 39 mmHg who were followed clinically slowly resolved the intracompartmental hypertension and did not develop a compartment syndrome (Table 5). The trend of the continually monitored intracompartmental pressure and the cooperation and reliability of the patient should be taken into consideration in establishment of individual threshold for fasciotomy. Once the diagnosis of compartment syndrome or impending compartment syndrome is established, all efforts to relieve intracompartment pressure should be undertaken. This includes the splitting and possible removal of all casts or restrictive dressing, including pneumatic anti-shock garments if at all possible. Skeletal traction should be carefully evaluated for possibility of stretching of the compartment by overweighting. Weights should be adjusted accordingly.

Elevation of the extremity is contraindicated in the patient with established or impending compartment syndrome. The elevation only serves to diminish the arteriolar perfusion pressure, thereby increasing the perfusion deficit and resultant ischemia of the muscle. This is often overlooked as a potential inciting factor due to the usual amount of edema accompanying trauma to an extremity for which elevation is often prescribed.

Table 5
Summary of 33 Patients with Compartment Hypertension

Patient No.	Age	Lag Phase (Hours)	Pressure, Millimeters of Mercury		Mechanism
			Pre-operatively	Post-operatively	
1	81	6	28	5	Fracture
2	68	24	30	4	Arterial occlusion
3	72	24	32	7	Arterial occlusion
4	48	3	32	0	Crush
5	65	—	34	38	Arterial occlusion
6	52	4	37	—	Fracture
7	2	8	37	4	Arterial occlusion
8	23	3	37	6	Blunt trauma
9	30	24	37	9	Fracture
10	33	2	37/3	—	Fracture
11	62	24	37	5	Arterial occlusion
12	52	72	39	5	Arterial occlusion
13	32	10	39	3	Blunt trauma
14	31	7	39	—	Arterial occlusion
15	35	—	41	7	Fracture
16	62	24	41/35	9/5	Arterial occlusion
17	39	4	45	10	Arterial occlusion
18	35	3	45	6	Arterial occlusion
19	27	3	45/55	8/7	Other
20	35	2	45	11	Other
21	56	36	48	4	Arterial occlusion
22	28	3	49	9	Blunt trauma
23	60	40	50	6	Arterial occlusion
24	39	12	50/88/90	7/18/10	Arterial occlusion
25	45	—	53	6	Arterial occlusion
26	51	4	55	9	Fracture
27	22	9	57	4	Arterial occlusion
28	67	—	57	8	Arterial occlusion
29	18	6	60	5	Arterial occlusion
30	55	48	64	6	Other
31	54	>60	67	1	Arterial occlusion
32	28	4	76	3	Crush
33	66	48	90/74	9/9	Arterial occlusion
34	33	2	37/3	—	Fracture

Modified from Russell WL, Apyan PM, Burns RP: Utilization and wide clinical implementation using the wick catheter for compartment pressure measurement. Surg Gynecol Obstet 160:209, 1985.

Medical Management

The use of osmotic diuretics such as mannitol, has been advocated by many.[2,3-7] As stated by Buchbinder,[2] the reperfusion syndrome observed primarily in the myocardium and brain, characterized by hyperemia, edema, increased vascular resistance, and decreased blood flow, has been shown to be prevented by the administration by hypertonic mannitol. In his clinical series, hypertonic mannitol administered prior to revascularization seemed to prevent the symptoms of reperfusion syndrome. The mechanism of action was felt to be an osmotic effect, extracting water from the cell and clearing it via the kidney. Shah et al,[5] likewise noticed increased vascular resistance in reperfused limbs and administered hypertonic mannitol that appeared to prevent the decrease in oxygen consumption following reperfusion in the canine model. He was also able to demonstrate the prevention of cell and mytochondrial swelling in the mannitol treated model versus the untreated. Hutton and associates[4] created an experimental compartment pressure in the canine anterior compartment, measured 12 hours after a period of prolonged ischemia. The animals were then infused intravenously with normal saline and given a bolus of 25 grams of mannitol, followed by 20 percent mannitol at 15 grams per hour for 2 hours. All treated animals demonstrated a decreased compartment pressure within 5 minutes and diminished their pressure to normal levels within 2 hours after infusion. Although mannitol caused an osmotic diruresis, simple dehydration was most likely not the sole factor of lowered compartment pressures and mobilization of extravascular fluid to the intravascular space may play a role. More recent studies by Perry and associates,[6] have been mentioned previously in this chapter. The significant depression of the potential difference across the muscle membrane following a period of ischemia continues following reperfusion. A marked decrease in high energy phosphate pool, mobilization of glucose and accumulation of lactate in skeletal muscle during tourniquet ischemia is rapidly resynthesized with an immediate improvement in tissue metabolism following revascularization. This has been shown with a temporary ischemia of aortic clamping.[15] Perry suggests that the presence of oxygen free radicals may well cause serious membrane damage in the post-perfusion period.[6]

Mannitol, which was formerly thought to improve ischemic muscle by osmotic activity, is now known to be a superoxide radical scavenger and may reduce muscle damage by a reduction of these radicals. Therefore, prevention of permeability changes may be the important action of this compound. Peck and associates[31] utilized mannitol in their series of 15 patients, of whom 14 required fasciotomy. Tolazoline hydrochloride (Priscoline), a peripheral alpha-adrenergic blocking agent, was also utilized for its direct relaxant effect on smooth muscles and blockage of vasoconstrictive receptors in the arterial wall. This enhanced limb salvage in this group of trauma patients.[31]

Experimental work with hyaluronidase by Gershuni[3] demonstrated a potential for rapidly alleviating increased intracompartmental pressures. The removal of hyaluronic acid molecules was felt to allow reduced resistance to flow in the interstitial space and speed reabsorption of edema fluid and thereby perform a chemical fasciotomy.

Certainly much needs to be done to more clearly define the mechanism of action of these agents; however, the importance of recognition of the patient at risk for compartment syndrome is even more critical as the early utilization of mannitol and other agents may well avoid the surgical fasciotomy.

FASCIOTOMY

Upper Extremity Decompression

The volar forearm is decompressed by a single long incision from the area just proximal to the antecubital fossa to the mid-palm. It is recommended that carpal tunnel release be incorporated as a standard part of the forearm decompression.[8,32] As seen in Figure 1, the median, ulnar, and radial nerves are found in the volar compartment, and are therefore at risk from a volar compartment syndrome. The dorsal compartment is usually opened through a long longitudinal incision over the compartment with incision of the dorsal fascia.

Continued monitoring of the intracompartmental pressure is encouraged during and after fasciotomy to assess the adequacy of the procedure. Additional debridement of the epimysium of specific muscle groups may be indicated if inappropriate response is obtained.

The incisions are packed open with bulky, nonobstructing dressings, which are changed frequently. Attempts at approximation of skin edges may be undertaken several days following fasciotomy after nonviable tissue is removed in an effort to reduce the need for later skin grafting. This is best done with steri-strips; however, it has been our experience that skin grafting is usually required. Active and passive range of motion should be initiated shortly after fasciotomy, provided all necrotic muscle and soft tissue has been debrided. Only frankly necrotic muscles, soft tissue, and nerve should be debrided. A potential for regeneration exists, provided the involved tissue is intact.

Lower Extremity Decompression

As shown in Figure 2, the lower extremity is composed of four compartments. The anterior and lateral compartments are best exposed through a lateral incision, taking care to avoid damage to the superficial peroneal nerve. The long incision is begun just distal to the head of the fibula and taken to approximately 5–8 cm above the lateral malleolus. The anterior intramuscular septum can be identified. The lateral compartment is opened the length of the incision, and attention is turned slightly anteriorly to the anterior compartment, which will require separate decompression the length of its compartment. By monitoring the intracompartmental pressure in the anterior compartment, prompt response in intracompartmental pressure will be noted, provided adequate fasciotomy is accomplished.

The superficial and deep posterior compartments are decompressed via a medial longitudinal incision, slightly posterior to the greater saphenous vein and nerve and just posterior to the border of the tibia. The fascia of the soleus is incised, thereby exposing the deep posterior compartment, which is likewise incised the length of the skin incision. The wounds are packed open as suggested for the upper extremity patient.

Closed fasciotomy technique appears primarily of benefit in chronic or exertional compartmental syndromes, and is not felt, in our experience, to provide an adequate acute fasciotomy. This view is similarly held by Clancey,[33] Hyde,[34] and others. Four quadrant fasciotomy, unless the patient has very confined symptoms, is the suggested technique.

Fibulectomy has not been utilized effectively in our experience. As pointed out by Hyde,[34] the extensive dissection and stripping of muscle origins may well cause injury to the closely approximated peroneal artery and nerve, with possible compromise of the distal foot. It is also difficult to achieve decompression of all four lower extremity compartments using this route. With the ease and adequacy of medial and lateral incisions, fibulectomy does not appear an indicated procedure.

Prophylactic Fasciotomy

Prior to adequate compartment pressure measuring devices, prophylactic fasciotomy had been widely utilized in vascular reconstructions as well in significant lower extremity orthopedic injuries. However, with the advent of adequate pressure monitoring devices and the possibility of utilization of pharmacologic preparations such as mannitol and allopurinol, the need for prophylactic fasciotomy appears to be the exception rather than the rule.

As suggested by orthopedists such as Mubarak,[8] in patients undergoing tibial osteotomies and leg lengthening procedures, as well as debridement of tibial fractures, fasciotomy may be accomplished prophylactically as a portion of the operative procedure. In arterial revascularization, however, pre-treatment with pharmacologic agents may well avoid many compartmental syndromes previously requiring a prophylactic fasciotomy.

Complications

Complications of compartment syndrome have been alluded to throughout this chapter. Primary among the complications are those of ischemic muscle and nerve changes with resultant contracture and dysfunction; myonecrosis with resultant myoglobinuria and renal failure; amputation; and death. It is obvious, from our experience, that the lag time between the inciting traumatic event and evaluation of possible involved compartments, often exceeds the 6–8 hours felt optimum for decompression. A heightened suspicion for the potential development of compartmental syndrome and rapid decompression by pharmacologic or operative techniques is imperative. The patient should be carefully monitored for myoglobinuria and aggressive hydration and diuresis undertaken.

Careful evaluation of the involved compartment, post-fasciotomy, is imperative. Debridement of necrotic muscle and soft tissue should be judiciously undertaken. The potential for post-fasciotomy infection is real and care should be taken to avoid potential infection with subsequent closure of the wound utilizing skin sutures, steri-strips, or split thickness skin grafts as soon as possible.

Rapid rehabilitation of the involved extremity, unless contraindicated due to orthopedic injury, minimizes post-compartmental syndrome contractures and dysfunction.

Summary

Compartment syndromes have been known and investigated for generations, but still remain a persistent source of morbidity in those patients at risk. The purpose of this chapter has not been to outline the multiple experimental models, early attempts at pressure monitoring, or to dwell upon basic factors of tissue perfusion. Emphasis is placed on the importance of understanding microvascular, muscular, and cellular pathophysiology that deserves fuller attention and investigation and the expectant monitoring of patients at risk.

Suspicion of potential development of compartment syndrome, and appropriate monitoring of intracompartmental pressure cannot be overstated. Our use of the wick catheter is outlined. Widely available and easily utilized techniques are well known and should be available to any vascular or trauma surgeon.

The attention to the risks of external appliances, such as casts, constrictive dressings, and pneumatic antishock garments, is stressed. Basic physiology and response of tissue to external compression must not be overlooked in the care of the trauma patient.

Fasciotomy is a procedure with significant morbidity. Our experience has shown the almost invariable requirement for prolonged hospitalization. Skin grafting accounts for a portion of this morbidity. Exciting advances in the utilization of pharmacologic agents such as mannitol and allopurinol, with constant intracompartment monitoring allowing direct treatment on a subcellular level, may well delegate fasciotomy to a less common procedure in the treatment of compartment syndrome. Nonetheless, knowledge of the anatomy and appropriate open fasciotomy techniques should be a prerequisite for those following patients at risk for compartment syndrome.

ACKNOWLEDGMENTS

Special thanks to Nancy Tucker, David Redd, and E. Y. Chapin for invaluable assistance in preparation of this manuscript.

References

1. Von Volkmann R: Die ischaemischen muskellahmugen and kontrakturen. Zentralbl Chir 8:8091, 1881
2. Buchbinder D, Karmody AM, Leather RP, Shah DM: Hypertonic mannitol. Arch Surg 116:414, 1981
3. Gershuni DH, Hargens AR, Lieber RL, et al: Decompression of an experimental compartment syndrome in dogs with hyaluronidase. Clin Orthop (197):295, 1985
4. Hutton M, Rhodes RS, Chapman G: The lowering of postischemic compartment pressures with mannitol. J Surg Res 32(3):239, 1982
5. Shah DM, Powers SR Jr, Stratton HH, Newell JC: Effects of hypertonic mannitol on oxygen utilization in canine hind limbs following shock. J Surg Res 30(6):593, 1981
6. Perry MO, Shires GT, Albert SA: Cellular changes with graded limb ischemia and reperfusion. J Vasc Surg 1(4):536, 1984
7. Perry MO: Acute arterial insufficiency of the extremities, in Rutherford RB(ed): Vascular Surgery. Philadelphia, W. B. Saunders Co., 1984, pp 440–448
8. Mubarak SJ, Hargens AR: Acute compartment syndromes. Surg Clin North Am 63(3):539, 1983
9. Matsen FA, Krugmire RB Jr: Compartmental syndromes. Surg Gynecol Obstet 147:943, 1978
10. Holden CEA: The pathology and presentation of Volkmann's ischemic contracture. J Bone Joint Surg (Br) 61:296, 1979
11. Sarokhan AJ, Eaton RG: Volkmann's ischemia. J Hand Surg (Am) 8:806, 1983
12. Gelberman RH, Szabo RM, Williamson RV, et al: Tissue pressure threshold for peripheral nerve viability. Clin Orthop (178):285, 1983
13. Mortensen WW, Hargens AR, Gershuni DH, et al: Long-term myoneural function after induced compartment syndrome in the canine hindlimb. Clin Orthop (195):289, 1985
14. Matsen FA: Tolerance of tissue for increased pressure, in Compartmental Syndromes. New York, Grune & Stratton, 1980, pp 45–64
15. Eklof B, Neglan P, Thompson D: Temporary incomplete ischemia of the legs induced by aortic clamping in man. Ann Surg 193:89, 1980
16. Gardner TJ, Stewart JR, Casale AS, et al: Reduction of myocardial ischemic injury with oxygen derived free radical scavengers. Surgery 94:423, 1983
17. Mubarak SJ, Hargens AR: Compartment Syndromes and Volkmann's Contractures. Philadelphia, W. B. Saunders Co., 1981, pp 73–75
18. Chisholm CD, Clark DE: Effect of the pneumatic antishock garment on intramuscular pressure. Ann Emerg Med 13(8):581, 1984

19. Bass RR, Allison EJ Jr, Reines HD, et al: Thigh compartment syndrome without lower extremity trauma following application of pneumatic antishock trousers. Ann Emerg Med 12(6):382, 1983

20. Godbout B, Burchard KW, Slotman GJ, Gann DS: Crush syndrome with death following pneumatic antishock garment application. J Trauma 24(12):1052, 1984

21. Maull KI, Capehart JE, Cardea JA, et al: Limb loss following military antishock trousers (MAST) application. J Trauma 21:60, 1981

22. Franklin JD: Personal Communication, February 1986

23. Lydon JC, Spielman FJ: Bilateral compartment syndrome following prolonged surgery in the lithotomy position. Anesthesiology 60(3):236, 1984

24. Reddy PK, Kaye KW: Deep posterior compartmental syndrome: A serious complication of the lithotomy position. J Urol 132(1):144, 1984

25. Roberts RS, Csencsitz TA, Heard CH Jr: Upper extremity compartment syndromes following pit viper envenomation. Clin Orthop 193:184, 1985

26. Joseph FR, Posner MA, Terzakis JA: Compartment syndrome caused by a traumatized vascular hamartoma. J Hand Surg (Am) 9(6):904, 1984

27. Bohn WW, Coleman CR: Streptococcal gangrene mimicking a compartment syndrome. A case report. J Bone Joint Surg (Am) 67(7):1125, 1985

28. Russell WL, Apyan PM, Burns RP: Utilization and wide clinical implementation using the wick catheter for compartment pressure measurement. Surg Gynecol Obstet 160(3):207, 1985

29. McDermott AGP, Marble AE, Yabsley RH: Monitoring acute compartment pressures with the S.T.I.C. catheter. Clin Orthop (190):192, 1984

30. Russell WL, Apyan PM, Burns RP: An electronic technique for compartment pressure measurement using the wick catheter. Surg Gynecol Obstet 161:173, 1985

31. Peck JJ, Fitzgibbons TJ, Gaspar MR: Devastating distal arterial trauma and continuous intraarterial infusion of tolazoline. Am J Surg 145(5):526, 1983

32. Geary N: Late surgical decompression for compartment syndrome of the forearm. J Bone Joint Surg (Br) 66(5):745, 1984

33. Clancey GJ: Acute posterior compartment syndrome in the thigh. J Bone Joint Surg (Am) 67(8):1278, 1985

34. Hyde GL, Peck D, Powell DC: Compartment syndromes. Early diagnosis and a bedside operation. Am Surg 49(10):563, 1983

James J. Schuler
D. Preston Flanigan

Vascular Repair in Orthopedic Surgery of the Spine and Joints

In view of the fact that major vascular structures are located in close proximity to the spine, major joints, and long bones it is not surprising that vessels can be injured during the course of elective orthopedic surgical procedures on the spine or major joints or in conjunction with fracture-dislocation of major long bones and joints. However, vascular injuries occurring in conjunction with orthopedic procedures are in general very uncommon and in certain anatomic locations, such as the cervical spine, shoulder, and elbow, exceedingly rare. The majority of vascular injuries incurred during orthopedic procedures occur during the course of lumbosacral disc surgery; during hip arthroplasty or various internal fixation procedures performed for hip fracture; or during knee arthroplasty or internal fixation procedures in the area of the distal femur or tibial plateau. Other vascular injuries occur in conjunction with blunt or penetrating trauma causing fractures or dislocations or are incurred during the fixation and stabilization of these injuries.

As the average age of our population increases and as the number and success of orthopedic procedures performed for the correction of degenerative spine and joint disease increases it is likely that more vascular injuries will occur during elective orthopedic procedures. Additionally, since the incidence of both accidental as well as violent trauma shows no sign of decreasing, it is likely that vascular injuries associated with fractures and dislocations will also increase.

As in many other surgical problems the success of treatment of vascular injuries incurred during orthopedic procedures is in large part dependent upon early diagnosis and early diagnosis is in turn dependent upon a high index of suspicion and a constant awareness of those circumstances in which vascular injury is most likely to occur. This chapter will therefore review vascular injuries that occur during the course of spine, hip,

Vascular Surgical Emergencies
ISBN 0-8089-1843-5

and knee surgery; or in conjunction with fracture-dislocations with an emphasis on etiology and early detection.

VASCULAR INJURIES ASSOCIATED WITH SPINE SURGERY

In spite of the wide variety of orthopedic and/or neurosurgical procedures performed on the spine, vascular injuries occur almost exclusively in conjunction with intervertebral disc surgery in the lumbosacral region. Mixter and Barr[1] introduced surgical correction for herniated nucleus pulposus or "ruptured intervertebral disc" at the Massachusetts General Hospital in 1934 and Linton and White[2] reported the first successful repair of a vascular injury incurred during lumbar disc surgery from the same institution 11 years later. The injury consisted of an arteriovenous fistula between the right common iliac artery and inferior vena cava that presented as intractable high output congestive heart failure occurring 8 months after lumbar disc surgery, which was treated successfully by right lumbar sympathectomy followed by multiple ligations of the right common iliac artery. Since the initial report by Linton and White, there have been numerous case reports usually consisting of one or two cases[3-15] as well as a smaller number of review articles.[16-22] Many of these review articles do not present all of the pertinent data on all of the patients sustaining a vascular injury during disc surgery because some of the reviews contain many cases based on "hearsay" or responses to questionnaires sent to orthopedic and neurosurgeons;[16-18] and in others, based on literature searches, much important detail is lacking. Because of this a comprehensive analysis of the incidence, etiology, and results of treatment may not be possible and is certainly outside the scope of this chapter. However, these reviews do provide the basis for identifying the major causative factors of vessel injury and provide useful general guidelines for treatment.

Incidence

The true incidence of vascular injury during lumbar disc surgery is unknown and will probably remain so since it is quite likely that many vascular injuries are not reported and others such as arteriovenous fistulae may not become clinically manifest until many years after the disc surgery. In spite of this, it is safe to say that vascular injury as a result of disc surgery is rare. In a questionnaire review by DeSaussure[17] of the experience of 3000 orthopedic and neurosurgeons in which a "high proportion" responded there were only 106 vascular injuries reported. In a similar questionnaire survey of 100 surgeons conducted by Harbison[16] only 25 vascular injuries were reported. Hohf[23] conducted a similar questionnaire survey approximately 10 years after the above review and recorded only 59 vascular injuries associated with disc surgery among 3500 respondents. Additionally, Harbison[16] reported that some respondents to his questionnaire reported no vascular injuries in over 2400 disc excisions. From the above it can be seen that the incidence of vascular injuries during disc surgery is indeed small, and probably occurs in less than 1 percent of the procedures. It is quite likely, however, that this very low incidence of occurrence is one of the reasons why these injuries have led to mortality rates in excess of 50 percent[16,18,21] in previous series, in that if a major vascular injury is unsuspected because it is so rare, then diagnosis and treatment are necessarily delayed; often beyond the point where treatment is successful.

Anatomy

In approximately 75 to 80 percent of patients the aorta bifurcates in the retroperitoneum just to the left of the midline at the level of the body of L4. The common iliac arteries pass distally and laterally and both cross the L4–L5 interspace, the left common iliac artery passing across the left lateral margin of the L4–L5 interspace and the right common iliac artery crossing the interspace almost directly in the midline. The iliac veins pass proximally to join slightly to the right of the midline and just above the L4–L5 interspace to form the inferior vena cava. The left common iliac vein passes proximally across the body of L5 and crosses the L4-L5 disc space obliquely just posterior to the right common iliac artery. This confluence of major arteries and veins forms what has been termed by Jarstfer and Rich[19] a "broad vascular belt" that is "stretched" across the entire expanse of the L4–L5 interspace. It is also at this point that the major vessels begin to become "stretched" as they cross the sacral promontory and, therefore, lie in their closest proximity to the anterior longitudinal ligament of the spine. It is because of this close anatomic relationship that approximately 75 percent of all vascular injuries incurred during disc surgery involve the distal aorta or proximal common iliac arteries or the distal inferior vena cava and proximal common iliac veins.[16,18-22] Again, because of this same close anatomic relationship, even though vascular injuries have been reported to occur during disc surgery from L2–L3 to L5–S1[16] well over 50 percent of all vascular injuries occur during surgery on the L4–L5 interspace.[16,18,19] Knowledge of the anatomic relationship as well as the disc space being operated upon at the time of the injury may be of definite aid to the vascular surgeon who undertakes emergency exploration for intraabdominal bleeding and is confronted with a massive retroperitoneal hematoma and no obvious source of the vascular injury. By gaining proximal control of the aorta and vena cava at the level of the mid infrarenal aorta and distal control of the distal common iliac arteries and veins the vast majority of injured vessels can be controlled and hemorrhage stopped while the exact site of injury is defined.

Etiology

At first glance it might be assumed that vascular injuries occurring during disc surgery are the result of inexperience or technical carelessness. However, numerous authors have stressed that the majority of these injuries occur at the hands of skilled and experienced surgeons[16-19] who were well aware of the possibility of such an injury. Since almost all disc surgery is performed from a posterior approach with the patient prone and in somewhat of a "jackknife" position to increase the size of the intervertebral disc space it would seem that the vessels are well out of harm's way.

This is not the case for the following reasons: (1) Many patients undergoing disc surgery have chronic degenerative joint disease that has caused defects in the annulus fibrosus and anterior longitudinal spinal ligament that would ordinarily shield the vessels from injury posteriorly but which, because they are diseased, allow the sharp pituitary rongeur or bone curet to pass between their fibers and thus come in contact with the vessel wall[16,17,19,20,22,24]; (2) Since the patient is prone and in a jackknife position the intraabdominal vessels are compressed against the spinal column and may actually be pushed tightly up against the anterior spinal ligament and annulus fibrosus so that their walls are in close juxtaposition thus making injury more likely.[16,19,20] It is probable that proper positioning and avoidance of excessive arching of the back would minimize the extent to which this occurs; (3) Since most patients requiring disc surgery will have some degree of degenerative joint disease of the spine with associated inflammation and scarring it is postulated that in certain patients the vessels are actually "fixed" to the anterior longitudinal ligament and annulus fibrosus and are torn as parts of the annulus fibrosus are removed with the ruptured disc[19,20]; (4) Although not all authors agree that there is an increased risk of vascular injury in patients undergoing reoperation on a previously operated disc space there are more reports of vascular injury occurring during the course of "redo surgery" than one would expect on the basis of chance alone.[16] It is postulated that previous disc surgery causes more defects in the annulus fibrosus thus leading to a higher probability of the pituitary rongeur or curet coming in contact with the vessel walls.[12,16,22] Although a knowledge of etiology is usually most useful in planning effective preventive measures all of the above etiologic factors are obviously beyond the control of the vascular surgeon. A knowledge of these etiologic factors, however, may prove useful in those patients in whom the orthopedic or neurosurgeon recognizes that the rongeur or curet has pierced the anterior longitudinal ligament and, therefore, seeks consultation from the vascular surgeon for the purpose of observation and exploration should it be deemed necessary.

Manifestations of Vascular Injury During Disc Surgery

Unlike most vascular injuries that usually present as easily recognized excessive or alarming bleeding, less than 50 percent of vascular injuries occurring during disc surgery present as abnormal bleeding through the disc space.[16,17,19,20] In those patients who do manifest indications of vascular injury the signs and symptoms can be divided into those that are usually noted with isolated arterial or venous injury and those peculiar to a traumatic arteriovenous fistula.

The most common manifestion of a laceration or partial transection of an artery or a vein, but not both, is hypotension, usually associated with tachycardia and in most cases noted by the anesthetist or recovery room personnel.[16,17,22] The presence of a palpable abdominal mass or abdominal distention immediately following disc surgery is strongly suggestive of an isolated arterial or venous injury[16,17,22] leading to a retroperitoneal hematoma or false aneurysm and warrants immediate surgical exploration. Isolated arterial injury during disc surgery almost never causes complete transection of the injured artery and, therefore, decreased distal pulses are rarely seen;[16] however, a systolic bruit is usually audible over the lower quadrant(s) of the abdomen.[16,17,21,22] Those patients with isolated arterial or venous injuries in whom injury is not suspected intraoperatively will frequently, upon recovering from the anesthetic, present with abdominal and/or flank pain, nausea, and vomiting; all secondary to the reflex paralytic ileus, which accompanies a large retroperitoneal hematoma.[19,21]

The signs and symptoms of a traumatic arterial-venous fistula secondary to lumbar disc surgery are the same regardless of whether they occur immediately after disc surgery or as much as 8 or 9 years later.[7,12,19] These consist of high output congestive heart failure with dyspnea, orthopnea, tachycardia, rales, leg swelling secondary to regional venous hypertension, and especially a loud continuous bruit over or near the region of the fistula. This characteristic bruit is usually heard best over the abdomen or flanks but can radiate to the buttocks, groins, or upper thigh.[16,18-22] The presence of leg swelling in patients with an aortocaval or ilioiliac arteriovenous fistula is secondary to regional venous hypertension distal to the fistula. Since this is usually associated with dyspnea and pulmonary rales, however, it is frequently mistaken for edema secondary to low output congestive heart failure or deep venous thrombosis and pulmonary embolism thus causing a delay in diagnosis. A history of previous lumbar disc surgery in conjunction with the characteristic abdominal bruit establishes the correct diagnosis.

Management of Suspected Vascular Injury During Lumbar Disc Surgery

As previously mentioned, less than half of all vascular injuries associated with disc surgery present as alarming or massive bleeding through the disc space at the time of disc excision. In these patients management is straightforward and consists of blood and volume replacement, abdominal exploration, and vascular repair.[16,18,19,22] In those patients in whom excessive bleeding through the disc space stops easily with pressure or in those in whom no excessive bleeding was noted but unexplained hypotension has occurred, or the operating surgeon suspects that the rongeur or curet has entered the retroperitoneal space, close observation and expectant management are warranted. In those circumstances in which a vascular injury is suspected the following guidelines should prevail: (1) Type and cross match blood and plasma immediately; (2) Arrange to have an autotransfusion apparatus available; (3) Turn the patient supine on the operating table and perform a careful physical examination of the abdomen and flanks. Since turning the patient supine will release the tamponade caused by the prone position this period of intraoperative observation and repeated abdominal examination should continue until it is clear that no retroperitoneal hematoma or false aneurysm is forming; (4) In view of the high mortality of late diagnosis and treatment of these injuries (greater than 50 percent)[16-18,21] abdominal exploration with the foreknowledge and expectation of a certain number of negative explorations is justified in those situations where a vascular injury is strongly suspected but cannot be demonstrated with certainty by intraoperative observation and examination; (5) In those situations in which the suspicion of an injury persists but is not so strong as to warrant exploration the recovery room and intensive care unit personnel should be made aware that the possibility of a vascular injury exists and subsequent monitoring and examination should be conducted with this in mind; and (6) Although not mentioned in any of the review articles dealing with the subject it seems logical, that in the stable patient in whom no physical signs are apparent, an infusion CT scan of the abdomen and pelvis would be very helpful in either establishing or ruling out the diagnosis.

Repair of Vascular Injuries Incurred During Lumbar Disc Surgery

Since the first reported successful treatment of a vascular injury secondary to disc surgery by Linton and White in 1945[2] the repair of such injuries has in general paralleled the evolution of vascular surgical technique and grafting. Reports prior to the mid 1950s when arterial homografts and the first synthetic grafts became available indicate that vascular repair was accomplished by either lateral repair or resection and end-to-end anastomosis of lacerated or partially transected arteries and veins if possible, and by ligation if this was impossible. Arteriovenous fistulae during this time period were likewise treated with multiple ligations.[2,4,15,16] However, with advances in the technique of repair of vascular injuries and the easy availability of prosthetic grafts, ligation of major vessel injuries is no longer acceptable.[20]

Since no major vascular injury has been reported above the level of the L2–L3 interspace and injuries below the common iliac bifurcation are exceedingly rare, adequate vascular control can, in almost all instances, be obtained by gaining control of the infrarenal aorta and vena cava just below the left renal vein and of the iliac vessels just proximal to their bifurcation. The vast majority of vascular injuries will be found in the "broad vascular belt"[19] overlying the L4–L5 interspace, i.e., the area of the distal aorta and vena cava and the proximal common iliac vessels. Following vascular control the type and extent of injury will dictate the method of repair. Small arterial and venous lacerations can usually be primarily repaired with lateral suture technique or patch angioplasty.[16,18] Larger lacerations and partial transections are best treated with resection and primary end-to-end anastomosis if possible or prosthetic interposition grafting if they are very large.[16,18,22] Arteriovenous fistulae are best treated by four vessel control, resection of the fistula and lateral repair if the fistula is large.[19,20,22]

A variety of technical points that may aid in repair include: (1) Since most of the lacerations, partial transections, and arteriovenous fistulae are located posteriorly and since they occur just at or above the sacral promontory and are essentially "covered" by the right common iliac artery, it can be quite difficult to expose and accurately identify the extent of the injury. In this circumstance transection of the right common iliac artery allows the aorta and intact left common iliac artery to be mobilized so that the iliac vein confluence as well as the posterior wall of the aorta and left common iliac artery become accessible[20,22]; (2) In long standing arteriovenous fistulae both the feeding artery as well as the draining vein can become massively dilated and the surrounding tissue densely scarred thus making exact localization of the fistulae difficult. Under these circumstances, Hildreth and Turcke[20] suggest that palpation through the venous wall for the maximal thrill produced by the "arterial jet" immediately opposite the fistula can aid in exact localization; and (3) In view of the massive blood loss frequently encountered during these repairs[16,18–20,22] the use of autotransfusion during exploration and repair as advocated by Brewster and coworkers[22] appears advisable.

Vascular injuries are not the only injuries that have been reported in conjunction with lumbar disc surgery. Other injured structures include bowel, ureter, bladder and appendix.[18,25,26] In light of this it is advisable to perform a very careful search for associated bowel or urinary tract injuries during exploration and repair of vascular injuries. Although ligation of the vascular injury with extraanatomic bypass to restore distal circulation has to our knowledge not been reported in the treatment of these vascular injuries it would seem advisable in those cases where gastrointestinal or urinary tract contamination of the retroperitoneum has occurred to consider this as a treatment option. This seems especially advisable if there has been a delay in diagnosis and there is established peritonitis since there is a report of death secondary to arterial-enteric fistula following primary repair of an iliac artery injury in conjunction with an ileocecal injury.

Mortality of Vascular Injury During Disc Surgery

The mortality from vascular injuries incurred during disc surgery has ranged from a high of 78 percent for arterial injuries and 89 percent for venous injuries as reported by Birkeland and Taylor[21] to zero as reported by Brewster and coworkers.[22] As would be expected, the older series report the highest overall mortalities of approximately 50 percent.[17,18,21] In addition to the improvement in survival reported in more recent series[19,20,22] there has been noted since the first report of such an injury[2] that there seems to be a much higher mortality in those patients who sustain an isolated arterial or venous injury[21] in which exsanguinating hemorrhage is the rule as compared to the much lower mortality of approximately 10 percent[19-21] in those patients who develop an arteriovenous fistula thus minimizing external blood loss.

Most authors are in agreement that the single most important factor determining the mortality of these injuries is early diagnosis and early treatment.[16-22] Thus, the vascular surgeon called upon to evaluate and treat a patient with a suspected vascular injury must maintain a high index of suspicion, be aware of the signs and symptoms of these particular vascular injuries, be prepared to closely observe and repeatedly evaluate the patients with a suspected injury but no clinical signs, and be willing to explore uncertain cases and accept a certain percentage of negative explorations.

Summary

1. Vascular injuries secondary to spinal surgery are very rare.
2. The majority of injuries are unsuspected at the time they occur.
3. Most injuries occur in the "vascular belt" area overlying the L4–L5 interspace.
4. Following the basic vascular trauma principles of control of hemorrhage and restoration of vascular continuity leads to a high rate of life and limb salvage.
5. Late diagnosis and treatment leads to a high mortality.
6. A high index of suspicion and a constant awareness of the possibility of these injuries following spinal surgery is the vascular surgeon's most valuable asset.

VASCULAR INJURIES ASSOCIATED WITH HIP SURGERY

Arterial injuries occurring in conjunction with total hip arthroplasty or operative fixation of hip fractures are exceedingly rare. It has been estimated that there are approximately 350,000 hip arthroplasties performed per year world wide.[27] However, there exist in the English language literature to date fewer than 50 case reports of arterial injury and even fewer venous injuries incurred in conjunction with hip surgery. This information does not help in defining the true incidence of such injuries since the occurrence of such limb threatening complications usually does not evoke the urge to publish and thus many such injuries probably go unreported. In those large series where sufficient information is provided to define the incidence of such injuries this has varied from 0.025 to 0.04 percent of patients undergoing hip surgery.[28-30] The majority of the reported injuries exist in the form of isolated case reports;[31-46] however, most of the useful information regarding management of these injuries comes from three excellent recent review articles.[30,47,48]

Anatomically, only the thin distal portion of the psoas muscle and its tendon, the pectineus muscle, and the capsule of the hip joint itself separate the distal external iliac vessels from the posterior medial aspects of the acetabulum. As pointed out by Ratliff[27] an extensive search of the anatomic literature by Small[27] indicates that the precise distance of these vessels from the acetabulum and anterior aspect of the hip joint is unknown. Our own observations based on a large number of suprainguinal retroperitoneal approaches to the iliac vessels indicate that the distance between the posterior wall of the external iliac vessels and the posterior medial wall of the acetabulum is approximately 1 to 2 centimeters in most patients.

This close anatomic relationship is important in understanding the etiology of these injuries. The most common mode of injury to the distal external iliac or proximal common femoral vessels is caused by the tip of the pointed Hohmann retractor used to maintain the femur in a position of anterior dislocation during hip arthroplasty lacerating or very forcibly compressing the vessels.[30,33,41] These retractors can also cause partial transection of the medial or lateral circumflex femoral arteries leading to either extensive bleeding at the time of hip surgery or to the later development of false aneurysm formation.[30,33] The second recorded mechanism of injury is extreme traction on the external iliac or common femoral vessels. During hip arthroplasty the head of the femur is dislocated anteriorly, adducted, and externally rotated. This puts an undue amount of tension on the posterior wall of the external iliac and common femoral arteries that has been postulated to cause either intimal disruption or fracture of calcified atherosclerotic plaques leading to either immediate or early perioperative thrombosis of these vessels.[29,30,32,33] The third most common mechanism of injury is direct laceration of the external iliac-common femoral artery or branches during revision of hip arthroplasty. This results either from the more extensive retraction and dissection required during revision procedures or by avulsion or laceration of the vessels by the sharp edges and spicules of methylmethacrylate used to secure the acetabular component of the hip prosthesis in place.[30] It is postulated that when the hip prosthesis becomes "loose" or partially displaced, dense scar tissue forms around the hip capsule and postero-medial aspect of the acetabulum. The nearby vessels become encased in the scar tissue thus leading to laceration during dissection or avulsion-laceration as the old acetabular component with its attached methylmethacrylate is removed.[30] This mechanism of injury leads either to hemorrhage and/or ischemia immediately, or to the later development of false aneurysm formation.[30,33,34,37,38,41,47,48] The fourth mechanism of injury is thermal damage to the adjacent vessels from methylmethacrylate leading to immediate or early postoperative thrombosis.[30] The polymerization of methylmethacrylate is an extremely exothermic reaction which produces temperatures in excess of $110°C$ in the surrounding tissues thus leading to thermocoagulation of adjacent arteries with immediate thrombosis or severe intimal damage leading to delayed thrombosis in the early postoperative period.[30,39,40] The last mechanism of injury to the iliofemoral vessels is late laceration of the vessel walls caused by screws, threaded pins, wires, or other sharp metallic objects used for stabilization and internal fixation of hip fractures. These devices can cause immediate laceration of adjacent vessels intraoperatively but more commonly lead to late false aneurysm formation or arteriovenous fistula formation when they loosen and migrate.[30,35,36,42,44,45]

The early manifestations of iliofemoral vascular injury during hip surgery consist of intraoperative bleeding or the very early postoperative development of hypotension and pelvic or wound hematoma in the case of vessel laceration[30,33,43,47,48] or varying degrees of distal ischemia in the case of thrombosis. Late manifestations of such injuries usually consist of a painful pulsatile mass in the case of false aneurysm formation or less frequently the characteristic signs of a traumatic arteriovenous fistula.

Regardless of the mechanism of vascular injury or the way in which the injury manifests itself during or after hip surgery, the standard, well established principles of vascular surgery should prevail. These include the arrest of hemorrhage by ligation of nonessential vessels, repair or bypass of major vessels, resection or ligation of false aneurysms and arteriovenous fistulae of nonessential vessels and resection with restoration of continuity for false aneurysms or arteriovenous fistulae of major vessels. In addition to these basic principles certain guidelines may be useful in this type of vascular injury: (1) Since most patients undergoing hip surgery are elderly, in the "atherosclerotic age group" it seems advisable to obtain preoperative segmental lower extremity Doppler pressures in any patient scheduled for hip surgery who has absent or diminished femoral or distal pulses. Preoperative segmental Doppler pressures will serve to establish a baseline to which postoperative pressures can be compared in those patients with a suspected increase in their degree of ischemia postoperatively.[29,31,33] Should vascular reconstruction become necessary subsequent Doppler pressures will serve to document the success of the reconstruction. Such objective documentation of preexisting ischemia may also be beneficial should medico-legal proceedings ensue; (2) In those patients who develop iliofemoral arterial occlusion secondary to either a traction injury with intimal or plaque disruption or a thermal injury from methylmethacrylate the exact extent of the injury may be difficult to determine at the time of exploration. In such patients bypass to the distal common femoral artery well beyond the area at risk would seem preferable to local repair since some patients treated with local repair experienced rethrombosis[29,33]; and (3) Those patients who require vascular reconstruction in whom there has been drainage or bleeding from a sinus tract or the wound or in whom the possibility of an infected false aneurysm exists should be reconstructed by extraanatomic bypass since direct reconstruction in such circumstances has led to graft infection[34] and subsequent major amputation.[38]

Because of the variety of vessels injured and the different types of vascular injury incurred during hip surgery the types of vascular repair or reconstructions reported have been correspondingly diverse. These repairs have varied from simple suture or lateral repair[30] to aortofemoral bypass[29] and axillofemoral bypass.[29] The results of repairing or reconstructing these injuries have likewise been quite variable.

Of the approximately 50 arterial injuries associated with hip surgery reported, at least 6 have led to major amputations[30,32,33,38,47,48] including 1 hip disarticulation.[38] In the remainder limb salvage appears to have been achieved. In at least three of these cases[30,32,33] delay in diagnosis appears to have contributed to the failure of limb salvage. In summary, vascular injuries incurred during hip surgery are exceedingly rare, have been produced by a wide variety of causes, and have been reported to affect all vessels in the region of the hip. Prompt diagnosis and early repair has led to a high rate of limb salvage whereas late diagnosis and repair has led to a high rate of amputation.

VASCULAR INJURIES ASSOCIATED WITH KNEE SURGERY

Vascular injuries associated with knee surgery are exceedingly rare. There have been only six reported vascular injuries in the English language literature following various types of knee arthroplasty,[49-52] which is performed approximately 45,000 times per year in the United States alone.[49] The mechanism of injury in these cases[50,51] is postulated to occur as follows. Many total knee replacements are performed on knee joints having fixed flexion contracture. Following arthroplasty the knee is placed in full extension and this creates compression of the "shortened" popliteal artery thus causing luminal obstruction. In this instance surgical release of the musculofascial attachments and branches of the above knee popliteal artery has restored flow in one case[50] and removing the cast and replacing the knee in a position of flexion has restored distal pulses,[51] which remained normal as the knee was gradually put into full extension over the ensuing days. Two additional injuries were caused by (1) either a pneumatic tourniquet or excessive traction on the vessel during knee dislocation and manipulation fracturing an atherosclerotic plaque in the above knee popliteal artery leading to thrombosis and eventual above knee amputation[49]; and (2) "constricting bands" secondary to scar tissue near the prosthesis causing chronic external compression of the above knee popliteal artery leading to thrombosis and requiring femoral-tibial bypass to achieve limb salvage.[49] The last case was a false aneurysm arising from the descending geniculate artery presenting two months following knee arthroplasty[52] and successfully treated by resection. Frequent examination of the extremity for signs of ischemia in the immediate postoperative period with pre- and postoperative measurement of Doppler segmental pressures and prompt intervention with relief of external compression seem to have yielded good results in the few cases reported.

False aneurysms of the popliteal artery and its branches have been infrequently reported following excision of a meniscus of the knee.[53-58] These injuries usually appear late after knee surgery, present as a painful pulsatile mass, and are treated by ligation and/or resection of nonessential branches of the popliteal artery or by resection and bypass or primary repair if they involve the popliteal artery itself. The remaining vascular injuries that occur in the region of the knee or other joints occur so infrequently that they represent surgical curiosities and will not be discussed.

VASCULAR INJURIES ASSOCIATED WITH FRACTURES AND DISLOCATIONS

Vascular injuries associated with fractures and dislocations of the extremities have a high morbidity with amputation rates ranging from 10 to 40 percent reported following such injuries in civilian practice.[59-61] Proposed reasons for this relatively high rate of amputation include delay in diagnosis of the vascular injury,[59,62] the frequency of combined venous and arterial injuries,[60,63] and frequently associated extensive soft tissue damage.[63]

In an attempt to reduce the reported unacceptably high amputation rates[59-61] we instituted in 1979 a treatment protocol for such injuries encountered at Cook County Hospital and the University of Illinois Hospital.[64] This protocol consists of: (1) the routine use of arteriography in penetrating injuries causing fractures and the selective use of arteriography in blunt injuries causing fractures or dislocations; (2) the liberal application of fasciotomy prior to both orthopedic and vascular repair in any patient with symptoms suggestive of compartmental hypertension; (3) orthopedic fixation and stabilization of fractures and dislocations prior to vascular repair in all except the most severe cases of ischemia; (4) the liberal use of autogenous saphenous vein interposition grafts for vascular reconstructions; (5) routine repair rather than ligation of venous injuries; and (6) completion arteriography as well as sterile "on the table" segmental Doppler pressures to detect technical flaws in the reconstructed vascular segment and allow for their immediate correction.

In the 6 year period between 1979 and 1984, 38 patients with 51 vascular injuries associated with fractures and/or dislocations of the extremities were managed via the above principles. Penetrating trauma caused 57 percent of injuries and blunt trauma accounted for 43 percent. The type and anatomic region of the various vascular injuries is shown in Table 1 and the associated fractures-dislocations in Table 2. Fasciotomy was

Table 1

Overall Distribution of Vascular Injuries

Location	Number of Arterial Injuries	Number of Venous Injuries
Tibial and peroneal	19	5
Popliteal	10	3
Superficial femoral	4	2
Brachial	4	0
Axillary	2	1
Subclavian	1	0
Total	40	11

Table 2

Distribution of Othopedic Injuries

Orthopedic Injury	Number of Extremities
Fracture tibia and/or fibula	20
Ligamentous knee disruption	1
Posterior knee dislocation	2
Anterior knee dislocation	2
Fracture femoral shaft	6
Fracture proximal radius	1
Posterior elbow dislocation	1
Fracture humerus	2
Fracture scapula	1
Fracture first rib	1
Fracture clavicle	1
Total	38

required in 45 percent of patients. Sixty-one percent of the orthopedic injuries required operative stabilization and fixation. This was accomplished by external fixation in 12 patients and internal fixation in 11. Vascular repair was accomplished by autogenous vein grafting (78 percent), primary end-to-end anastomosis (5 percent), vein patch angioplasty (5 percent), and prosthetic interposition grafting (3 percent). Six isolated tibial or peroneal artery injuries were treated by ligation after arteriographic and Doppler documentation of patency of the remaining tibial vessels.

Limb salvage was achieved in 97.4 percent of these injuries.[64] There was 1 death (2.6 percent) secondary to intraabdominal sepsis from multiple colon injuries and the one amputation (2.6 percent) was secondary to an extensive crush injury. There was one instance each of fracture nonunion, delayed union, and joint instability, none of which could be attributed to ischemia or failure of vascular repair. We feel that adherence to the previously mentioned principles of management and repair can provide for a high rate of limb salvage in these complex and challenging injuries.

REFERENCES

1. Mixter WJ, Barr JS: Rupture of the intervertebral disc with involvement of the spinal canal. N Engl J Med 211:210, 1934

2. Linton RR, White PD: Arteriovenous fistula between the right common iliac artery and the inferior vena cava: Report of a case of its occurrence following an operation for a ruptured intervertebral disc with cure by operation. Arch Surg 50:6, 1945

3. Stokes JM: Vascular complications of disc surgery. J Bone Joint Surg 50(A):394, 1968

4. Seeley SF, Hughes CW, Jahnke EJ: Major vessel damage in lumbar disc operation. Surgery 35:421, 1954

5. Taylor H, Williams E: Disc surgery and arteriovenous fistula. Brit J Surg 50:47, 1962

6. DeBakey ME, Cooley DA, Morris GC, Collins H: Arteriovenous fistula involving the abdominal aorta: Report of four cases with successful repair. Ann Surg 147:646, 1958

7. Staple TW, Friedenberg MJ: Ilio-iliac arteriovenous fistula following intervertebral disc surgery. Clin Radiol 16:248, 1965

8. Horton RE: Arteriovenous fistula following operation for prolapsed intervertebral disc. Brit J Surg 49:77, 1961

9. Hufnagel CA, Walsh BJ, Conrad PW: Iliac-caval arteriovenous fistula following operation for herniated disc. Angiology 12:579, 1961

10. Shumacker HB, King H, Campbell R: Vascular complications from disc operations. J Trauma 1:177, 1961

11. Moore CA, Cohen A: Combined arterial, venous, and ureteral injury complicating lumbar disc surgery. Am J Surg 115:574, 1968

12. Boyd DP, Farha GJ: Arteriovenous fistula and isolated vascular injuries secondary to intervertebral disc surgery: Report of four cases and review of the literature. Ann Surg 161:524, 1965

13. Spittell JA, Palumbo PJ, Love JG, Ellis FH: Arteriovenous fistula complicating lumbar-disc surgery. N Eng J Med 268:1162, 1963

14. Nilsonne U, Hakelius A: On vascular injury in lumbar disc surgery. Acta Orthop Scandinav 35:329, 1965

15. Holscher EC: Vascular complication of disc surgery. J Bone Joint Surg 30(A):968, 1948

16. Harbison SP: Major vascular complications of intervertebral disc surgery. Ann Surg 140:342, 1954

17. DeSaussure RL: Vascular injury coincident to disc surgery. J Neurosurg 16:222, 1959

18. Holscher EC: Vascular and visceral injuries during lumbar-disc surgery. J Bone Joint Surg 50(A):383, 1968

19. Jarstfer BS, Rich NM: The challenge of arteriovenous fistula formation following disc surgery: A collective review. J Trauma 16:726, 1976

20. Hildreth DH, Turcke DA: Postlaminectomy arteriovenous fistula. Surgery 81:512, 1977

21. Birkeland IW, Taylor TKF: Major vascular injuries in lumbar disc surgery. J Bone Joint Surg 51(A):4, 1969

22. Brewster DC, May ARL, Darling RC, et al: Variable manifestations of vascular injury during lumbar disc surgery. Arch Surg 114:1026, 1979

23. Hohf, RP: Arterial injuries occurring during orthopaedic operations. Clin Orthop 28:21, 1963

24. Leavens ME, Bradford FK: Ruptured intervertebral disc: Report of a case with a defect in the anterior annulus fibrosus. J Neurosurg 10:544, 1953

25. Birkeland IW, Taylor TKF: Bowel injuries coincident to lumbar disc surgery: A report of four cases and a review of the literature. J Trauma 10:163, 1970

26. Kern HB, Barnes W, Malament M: Lumbar laminectomy and associated ureteral injury. J Urology 102:675, 1969

27. Ratcliff AHC: Arterial injuries after total hip replacement. J Bone Joint Surg BR 67:517, 1985

28. Schlosser W, Spillner G, Breymann TH, Urbanyi B: Vascular injuries in orthopaedic surgery. J Cardiovasc Surg 23:323, 1982

29. Matos MH, Amstutz HC, Machleder HI: Ischemia of the lower extremity after total hip replacement: Report of four cases. J Bone Joint Surg 61(A):24, 1979

30. Nachbur B, Meyer RP, Verkkala K, Zurcher R: The mechanisms of severe arterial injury in surgery of the hip joint. Clin Orthop 141:122, 1979

31. Stubbs DH, Corner DB, Johnston RC: Thrombosis of the iliofemoral artery during revision of a total hip replacement: A case report. J Bone Joint Surg 68(A):454, 1986

32. Heyes FLP, Aukland A: Occlusion of the common femoral artery complicating total hip arthroplasty. J Bone Joint Surg 67(BR):533, 1985

33. Aust JC, Bredenberg CE, Murray DG: Mechanisms of arterial injuries associated with total hip replacement. Arch Surg 116:345, 1981

34. Hopkins NFG, Vanhegan JAD, Jamieson CW: Iliac aneurysm after total hip arthroplasty: Surgical management. J Bone Joint Surg 65(BR):359, 1983

35. Dameron TB: False aneurysm of femoral profundus artery resulting from internal-fixation device (screw). J Bone Joint Surg 46(A):577, 1964

36. Possman CL, Morawa LG: Vascular injury from intrapelvic migration of a threaded pin. J Bone Joint Surg 67(A):804, 1985

37. Scullin JP, Nelson CL, Beven EG: False aneurysm of the left external iliac artery following total hip arthroplasty: Report of a case. Clin Orthop 113:145, 1975

38. Dorr LD, Conaty JP, Kohl R, Harvey JP: False aneurysm of the femoral artery following total hip surgery. J Bone Joint Surg 56(A):1059, 1959

39. Green DL: Complications of total hip replacement. South Med J 69:1559, 1976

40. Hirsch SA, Robertson H, Gorniowsky M: Arterial occlusion secondary to methylmethacrylate use. Arch Surg 111:204, 1976

41. Kroese A, Mollerud A: Traumatic aneurysm of the common femoral artery after hip endoprosthesis. Acta Orthop Scand 46:119, 1975

42. Bergqvist D, Erikson U, Grevsten S: False aneurysm in the deep femoral artery as a complication of osteosynthesis of intertrochanteric femoral fracture: Report of a case. Acta Chir Scand 138:630, 1972

43. Lozman H, Robbins H: Injury to the superior gluteal artery as a complication of total hip-replacement arthroplasty: A case report. J Bone Joint Surg 65(A):268, 1983

44. Bassett FH, Houck WS: False aneurysm of the profunda femoris artery after subtrochanteric osteotomy and nail-plate fixation. J Bone Joint Surg 46(A):583, 1964

45. Meyer TL, Slager RF: False aneurysm following subtrochanteric osteotomy. J Bone Joint Surg 46(A):581, 1964

46. Mallory TH: Rupture of the common iliac vein from reaming the acetabulum during total hip replacement: A case report. J Bone Joint Surg 54(A):276, 1972

47. Reiley MA, Bond D, Branick RI, Wilson EH: Vascular complications following total hip arthroplasty: A review of the literature and report of two cases. Clin Orthop 186:23, 1984

48. Bergqvist D, Carlsson AS, Ericsson BF: Vascular complications after total hip arthroplasty. Acta Orthop Scand 54:157, 1983

49. McAuley CE, Steed DL, Webster MW: Arterial complications of total knee replacement. Arch Surg 119:960, 1984

50. Robson LJ, Walls CE, Swanson AB: Popliteal artery obstruction following Shiers total knee replacement: A case report. Clin Orthop 109:130, 1975

51. Arden GP: Complications of total knee replacement and their treatment in Ingwerson OS, Van Linge B, Van Rens TJG, et al (eds): The Knee Joint. International Congress Series #324, Amsterdam, Excerpta Medica 1974, pp 221–227

52. Coventry MB, Upshaw JE, Riley LH, et al: Geometric total knee arthroplasty: Patient data and complications. Clin Orthop 94:177, 1973

53. Elkin DC: Aneurysm following surgical procedures: Report of five cases, in Transactions of the Southern Association. Meetings held at Hollywood Beach, FL, December 9–11, 1947. Ann Surg 121:769, 1948

54. Fairbank TH, Jamieson ES: A complication of lateral menisectomy. J Bone Joint Surg 33B:567, 1951

55. Edmunds LH, Darling RC, Linton RR: Surgical management of popliteal aneurysms. Circulation 32:517, 1965

56. Baird RJ, Sivaskankar R, Hayward R, Wilson DR: Popliteal aneurysms: A review and analysis of 61 cases. Surgery 59:911, 1966
57. Julian OC, Dye WS, Javid H, Grove WJ: The use of vessel grafts in the treatment of popliteal aneurysms. Surgery 38:970, 1955
58. Lord JW: Clinical behavior and operative management of popliteal aneurysms. J Am Med Assn 163:1102, 1957
59. Makin GS, Howard JM, Green RL: Arterial injuries complicating fractures or dislocations: The necessity for a more aggressive approach. Surgery 59:203, 1966
60. Alberty RE, Goodried G, Boyden AM: Popliteal artery injury with fractural dislocation of the knee. Am J Surg 142:36, 1981
61. Sher MH: Principles in the management of arterial injuries associated with fractures/dislocations. Ann Surg 182:630, 1975
62. Flint LM, Richardson JD: Arterial injuries with lower extremity fractures. Surgery 93:5, 1983
63. McNamara JJ, Brief DK, Stremple JF, Wright JK: Management of fractures with associated arterial injury in combat casualties. J Trauma 13:17, 1973
64. Bishara RA, Pasch AR, Lim LT, et al: Improved results in the treatment of civilian vascular injuries associated with fractures and dislocations. J Vasc Surg 3:707, 1986

D. Preston Flanigan
James J. Schuler

Pediatric Vascular Emergencies

Pediatric vascular emergencies are rather rare events; as a result few individual surgeons have accumulated significant experience in this area of vascular surgery. As a result most vascular surgeons feel somewhat uneasy caring for the pediatric patient with a vascular emergency. Further adding to the problem is the small size of the patients and hence the vessels to be operated upon. The principles of management of adult vascular emergencies are well established whereas the principles in pediatric patients are not well established and are, in part, controversial. In adults the primary consideration in clinical decision making is the viability of the part. In the pediatric group limb loss is unusual as a result of the ability of these young patients to rapidly develop collateral circulation. This behavior may lead the surgeon to believe that all is well yet the risk of growth retardation and subsequent claudication is real. These and other considerations set pediatric vascular emergencies apart from other vascular emergencies.

ETIOLOGY

The etiology of pediatric vascular emergencies can be broken down into three basic types. These types are spontaneous vascular occlusions,[1-10] violent trauma,[11,12] and iatrogenic trauma[13-22] in reverse order of frequency. Spontaneous vascular occlusions are indeed rare while both violent and iatrogenic pediatric vascular trauma are increasing.[12] Although the ratio between violent and iatrogenic etiologies depends to a great extent on the institution involved, centers having both a trauma center and a large experience with pediatric vascular cannulation procedures report a ratio of iatrogenic to violent trauma of about 6:4.[23]

Spontaneous Acute Vascular Occlusions

Spontaneous vascular occlusions have been reported in almost every artery in the body in the neonatal period and early infancy.[8] Although specific causes are difficult to identify polycythemia, dehydration, and hyperviscosity are commonly present. Spontaneous thrombosis is the most common occurrence in this group but embolization from proximal sources has also been reported.[5-9] Some children may be suffering from actual hypercoagulation states such as congenital antithrombin III deficiency.[3]

Violent Trauma

Violent pediatric trauma is clearly on the rise. A disturbing trend is that of an increasing number of injuries from gunshot wounds.[12] Stab wounds and blunt trauma make up the majority of other injuries. With the exception of birth trauma, these children have an average age that is greater than most children sustaining iatrogenic injuries.[23] This is particularly important since these violent injuries often require more extensive surgical reconstruction, often requiring bypass procedures that are not often required or possible to perform in the younger age groups.

Brachial and superficial femoral arteries are the most common vessels injured by violent trauma; however, as in spontaneous vascular occlusion, injury to nearly every vessel has been reported.[12]

Iatrogenic Trauma

Iatrogenic pediatric vascular injuries are the most common type of vascular injury seen in children. The majority of these injuries are secondary to invasive diagnostic procedures or surgery.[24]

Umbilical Artery Catheterization

Umbilical artery catheterization is far from a benign procedure. Angiographic studies performed following umbilical artery catheterization have demonstrated that 95 percent of patients have some degree of thrombosis, although the incidence of clinical thrombosis is exceedingly less common averaging about 5 percent.[25] Thrombotic complications from these catheters endanger not only the lower extremities but also the visceral organs as a result of partial or complete aortic thrombosis.[25]

Certain procedures have been found to decrease the complication rate of umbilical artery catheterization when employed. These include the use of thromboresistant catheter materials, end hole versus side hole catheters, heparin drips, and the use of the high aortic position.[22,26]

Arteriography and Cardiac Catheterization

Overall transfemoral cardiac catheterization is the most common cause of iatrogenic pediatric vascular injury.[27,28] Two major studies reported complication rates for this procedure of 40 percent and 26 percent using followup arteriography to establish the diagnosis of arterial injury. The age of the patient was particularly important as regards the risk of injury with children less than 10 years of age having nearly all the injuries reported in some series.[27] Heparinization was shown in 1 series to reduce the rate of thromboembolic complications from 40 percent to 8 percent.[2] Additionally, the use of percutaneous catheterization has been shown to reduce the incidence of injury when compared to the arteriotomy technique.[18] Recently the authors performed a prospective study of pediatric patients undergoing cardiac catheterization in which most patients were less than 10 years of age but percutaneous catheterization, and heparinization were used routinely.[24] Forty-two children were studied prospectively before and after cardiac catheterization with lower extremity segmental Doppler pressure measurement and waveform analysis to assess the incidence of arterial injury. Twenty-four percent of these children sustained vascular injuries. In many of these children there was no clinical sign or symptom to indicate the injury. Age did not correlate with the incidence of injury in our study; however, most patients were less than 10 years old.

Operative Trauma

There has been no special common denominator as regards operative trauma. The most common causes reported include injury during tumor resection and from cardio-pulmonary bypass during correction of congenital heart defects.[24,29]

DIAGNOSIS

In cases of violent trauma the diagnosis of vascular injury may be quite obvious as evidenced by hemorrhage, pulsating hematoma, absent pulses, and bruits over the area of injury.[12] However, the diagnosis of vascular occlusion or injury secondary to other etiologies may be complicated in the pediatric age group. The young age of the patients often precludes verbal communication. Also, as noted above regarding our prospective study, some patients with significant injuries have only subtle clinical signs as a result of collateral circulation. Some patients with significant injuries will have obvious clinical signs. In these patients the classic signs of coldness, pallor, pulselessness, and pain may be present. Physical examination may indeed be difficult in these little patients and confirmatory noninvasive studies are useful.[24] A standard segmental Doppler examination is possible in most children (Fig. 1). Common digit and penile pressure cuffs are the appropriate size for extremity measurements in pediatric patients. Although it has been applied successfully by some authors, arteriography for diagnostic purposes should probably be avoided to prevent the possibility of additional injury. In most cases noninvasive diagnostic techniques obviate the need for invasive procedures. Doppler segmental studies combined with history and physical examination can usually localize the site of occlusion. When a more precise localization is needed, real-time B-mode imaging ultrasound has been quite useful (Fig. 2).[24]

TYPES OF INJURIES

It is worthwhile to elucidate the types of injuries and occlusions that occur since it is pertinent to proper therapy.

Spontaneous occlusions are either thromboses or emboli. No special consideration is needed with these lesions. Violent trauma produces injuries that are the most severe. Although these injuries can be minimal as seen with mild forms of injury they are more often of a more extensive nature and are often associated with major vascular disruption, fractures, and soft tissue trauma.[24] Because of their more severe nature these injuries often require more extensive revascularization procedures consisting of grafting and bypass. Fortunately these children are, on the average, older than those sustaining iatrogenic injuries.

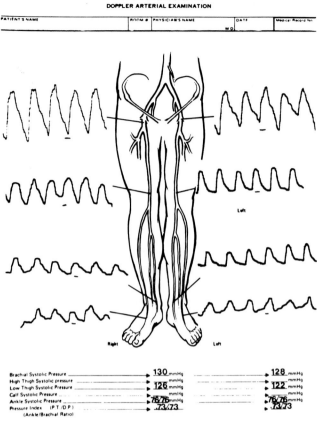

UNIVERSITY OF ILLINOIS HOSPITAL
DOPPLER ARTERIAL EXAMINATION

PATIENT'S NAME	ROOM #	PHYSICIAN'S NAME	DATE	Medical Record No.
		M D		

Brachial Systolic Pressure	130 mmHg	128 mmHg
High Thigh Systolic pressure	mmHg	mmHg
Low Thigh Systolic Pressure	126 mmHg	122 mmHg
Calf Systolic Pressure	mmHg	mmHg
Ankle Systolic Pressure	76/76 mmHg	76/76 mmHg
Pressure Index (P.T./D.P.) (Ankle/Brachial Ratio)	.73/.73	.73/.73

Fig. 1. Doppler study in a neonate following aortic thrombectomy. (From Flanigan DP, Stolar CJH, Pringle KC, et al: Aortic
thrombosis after umbilical artery catheterization. Successful surgical management. Arch Surg 117:371, 1982. Copyright 1982,
American Medical Association. With Permission.)

Iatrogenic injuries tend to produce less injury to the vessels even though the resultant
ischemia can be just as severe as that seen with more extensive trauma. The most common
site for this type of injury is the common femoral artery. The most common type of injury
is intimal disruption with resultant intimal flap formation and thrombosis. Children sustaining this type of injury are younger on the average and, thus, are often able to undergo
successful vascular repair since a limited procedure is often all that is required.

TREATMENT AND RESULTS

Although the principles of management of pediatric vascular emergencies are controversial, the principles of operative technique are standard and not dissimilar to those
applied in the adult population.

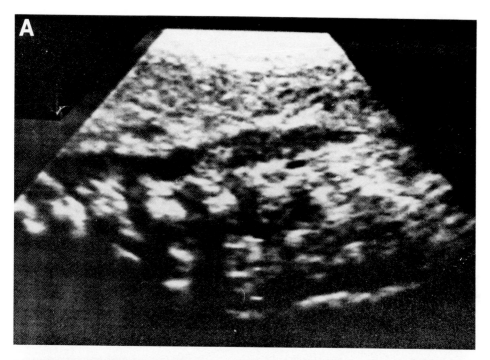

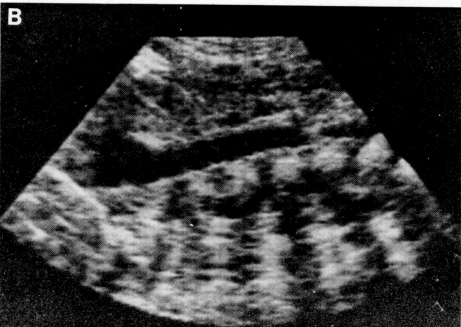

Fig. 2. Preoperative and postoperative real-time ultrasound. (A) Thrombus in the infrarenal aorta. (B) Normal study following thrombectomy. (From Flanigan DP, Stolar CJH, Pringle KC, et al: Aortic thrombosis after umbilical artery catheterization. Successful surgical management. Arch Surg 117:371, 1982. Copyright 1982, American Medical Association. With permission.)

Operations for Violent Trauma

Operations for violent trauma require the application of the same principles as are applied to adults with violent vascular trauma. These children often require initial resuscitation with fluids and blood and may need attention to associated injuries. Diagnosis is usually straightforward in these children and arteriography generally is not recommended. Prompt surgical treatment is necessary if good results are to be obtained.[12] In children with severe lower extremity ischemia and compartment syndrome fasciotomy is required.

Intraabdominal Procedures

Intraabdominal vascular injuries account for nearly all the fatalities in pediatric vascular trauma.[12] Fortunately these injuries are quite rare. Most intraabdominal injuries can be treated with primary repair. Grafting procedures are reserved for the most serious and extensive of injuries. Saphenous vein is seldom useful in these types of injuries.[12] Aortic injuries have been treated by lateral repair or primary end to end anastomosis. Vena cava injuries can usually be repaired using lateral repair and yield a much better survival than is seen in patients with aortic injuries. Occasionally ligation of intraabdominal vessels can be life saving but should be reserved for just that indication. Survival statistics for these injuries are sparse but would indicate that survival for aortic injury is unusual while patients with vena cava injuries have approximately an 88 percent survival.[12] Anecdotally injuries to aortic branch vessels have been successfully repaired.

Extremity and Cervical Procedures

Operations on the extremity and cervical vessels for violent trauma have generally been successful. Although these vessels are smaller, these injuries are less often life threatening and can usually be repaired using primary rather than grafting techniques. However, many cases using short saphenous vein interposition grafts have been successfully performed. The use of long bypasses has only rarely been required and is rarely successful unless the patient is in an older age group. Venous as well as arterial repairs have been successfully performed but long-term results are lacking for the most part. Amputation or stroke following vascular trauma in these areas is indeed uncommon. The application of microsurgical techniques has been limited but would be expected to improve current results.

Spontaneous Occlusions and Iatrogenic Trauma

It is reasonable to combine these two etiologies together for a discussion of treatment as the principles of treatment are quite similiar. Although both can produce significant ischemia and risk to life, the actual injury to the vessel is generally less than that produced by violent trauma or in the case of spontaneous occlusion, no injury may be present.

Intraabdominal Procedures

Intraabdominal arterial occlusions are usually secondary to spontaneous causes or umbilical artery catheters. With the former, any predisposing causes such as dehydration etc. should be corrected as soon as possible. In the latter, the catheter should be removed immediately. In most cases immediate administration of heparin (100mg/kg) should be performed unless otherwise contraindicated. Branch vessel occlusions may be suspected in the presence of symptoms relative to the end organ. Diagnosis of aortic occlusion is suspected in patients with bilaterally absent femoral pulses and hypertension. Most of the patients with intraabdominal arterial occlusions are either neonates or at a very young age. This fact is important in the selection of the operative approach. The size of the common femoral artery in the neonate is insufficient for the passage of a 3 Fr Fogarty catheter. A 2 Fr catheter will usually pass but is inadequate for aortic thrombectomy. Even a 2 Fr catheter will not pass distal to the common femoral artery in the neonate. Thus, thrombectomy of unilateral iliac occlusions may be attempted via the common femoral artery in these small patients but the surgeon should be experienced in microvascular techniques if a successful arterial closure is to be accomplished. Aortic occlusions should be approached transabdominally. Survival following aortic occlusion is rare. The authors have successfully treated two such patients with this condition through the use of a transverse aortotomy just proximal to the aortic bifurcation. Balloon thrombectomy was accomplished both proximally and distally. In one patient an immediate return of normal lower extremity circulation was accomplished while in the second patient a delayed return was seen even though femoral pulses returned immediately following the procedure. Delayed treatment of neonatal aortic thrombosis is uniformly fatal.[21,24]

Extremity Procedures

Iatrogenic trauma to the extremities usually involves the common femoral artery and its bifurcation in current practice, catheterization of the brachial artery being rarely used today. These procedures are performed at all ages in the pediatric age group but because of the indication of congenital heart disease most patients are less than 10 years of age. The usual injury is intimal disruption and thrombosis. In most cases this type of injury only requires simple thrombectomy and repair. We have successfully performed this procedure in children less than 2 years of age but the literature would indicate that below age 2 results have been poor. Use of magnification and other microsurgical techniques no doubt improves results. The procedure is performed via a vertical groin incision and the use of 2 Fr or 3 Fr Fogarty catheters depending on the size of the vessel. We have not attempted this procedure in neonates because of the small size of the vessels.

Ischemia can also be caused by embolization of thrombus on the catheter to distal extremity vessels. In this situation operative therapy is probably not indicated in the infant or neonate. Heparin therapy is usually the treatment of choice. We have had no success with the use of thrombolytic agents in these patients.

General Principles of Treatment

The general principles of management are the same as those applied in the adult population with a few exceptions. These exceptions take into consideration the fact that pediatric patients will grow. Thus, the use of interrupted suture techniques and the use of autogenous tissue is very important. The other consideration regarding growth is the effect that ischemia might have on the growing extremity. Numerous reports have now documented limb length discrepancies as a result of unsuccessful treatment or no treatment of pediatric arterial occlusions.[22-32] This factor assumes great importance in the overall management scheme of these patients.

Table 1

Arteries Occluded

Arteries Occluded	Number
Aorta	2
Iliac	3
Common femoral	30
Distal to common femoral*	10
Total	45

*Exact locations undetermined. Presumably thromboembolic.

THE UNIVERSITY OF ILLINOIS EXPERIENCE

Over a 32 month period 45 iatrogenic arterial injuries were seen.[24] During this period no pediatric patient with violent trauma or spontaneous arterial occlusion was seen. Of the 45 injuries 30 were secondary to cardiac catheterization procedures, 10 were due to umbilical artery catheters and 5 were a result of surgical procedures. The vessels injured are shown in Table 1. The age distribution of these children is shown in Figure 3. It can be seen that most of these patients were 4 years of age or less. Twelve surgical procedures were performed in 11 patients (Table 2). In general no patient with a palpable femoral pulse underwent surgery. Heparinization was employed in nonoperative cases when not contraindicated. The results of this approach are shown in Figure 4. Not included in this

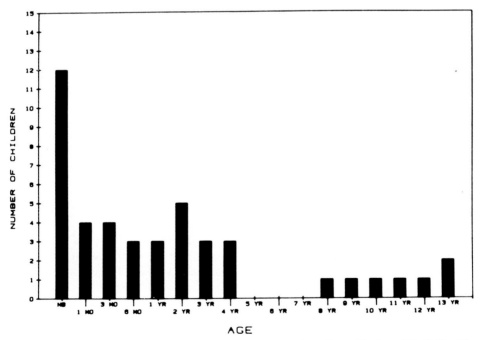

Fig. 3. Age distribution in children sustaining arterial injuries. (From Flanigan DP, Keifer TJ, Schuler JJ, et al: Experience with iatrogenic pediatric vascular injuries: Incidence, etiology, management, and results. Ann Surg 198:430, 1983. With permission.)

Table 2
Vascular Procedures Performed

Operations	Number	Ages
Aortic thrombectomy*	2	NB‡, NB
Femorofemoral bypass	2†	12 YR
Femoral patch angioplasty	1	18 MO
Femoral thrombectomy and repair	7	9 MO, 2 YR, 2.5 YR, 2.5 YR, 4 YR, 4 YR, 13 YR
Total	12	

*Transabdominal
†One patient
‡New born

analysis are several children with ischemia following catheterization procedures who had return of normal circulation within 6 hours of injury while on heparin therapy. It can be seen that, using this approach, the results of surgical treatment were excellent. Figure 5 indicates that there was a similiar age distribution between the operated and nonoperated patients. In the entire experience there was no mortality or limb loss but followup did show impairment of limb growth in some patients who had ischemia lasting more than 30 days (Table 3). Limb length discrepancies were seen in 9 percent of the surgical patients and 23 percent of the nonsurgical patients. Overall, 91 percent of children in our experience had eventual return of normal circulation.

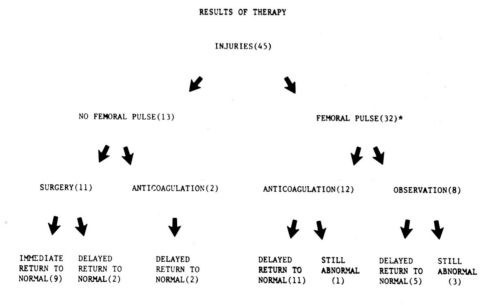

RESULTS OF THERAPY

INJURIES(45)

NO FEMORAL PULSE(13)   FEMORAL PULSE(32)*

SURGERY(11)   ANTICOAGULATION(2)   ANTICOAGULATION(12)   OBSERVATION(8)

IMMEDIATE RETURN TO NORMAL(9)   DELAYED RETURN TO NORMAL(2)   DELAYED RETURN TO NORMAL(2)   DELAYED RETURN TO NORMAL(11)   STILL ABNORMAL(1)   DELAYED RETURN TO NORMAL(5)   STILL ABNORMAL(3)

*12 DIED OR LOST TO FOLLOW-UP

Fig. 4. Types and results of therapy. (From Flanigan DP, Keifer TJ, Schuler JJ, et al: Experience with iatrogenic pediatric vascular injuries: Incidence, etiology, management, and results. Ann Surg 198:430, 1983. With permission.)

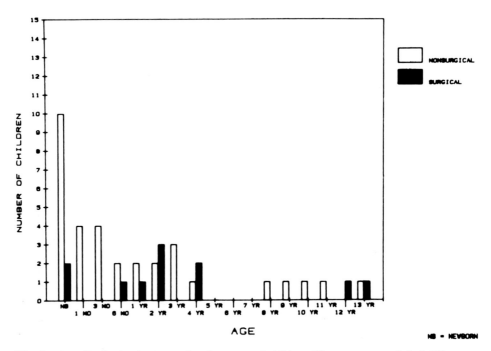

Fig. 5. Age distribution in operated and unoperated children. There was no statistical difference between groups. (From Flanigan DP, Keifer TJ, Schuler JJ, et al: Experience with iatrogenic pediatric vascular injuries: Incidence, etiology, management, and results. Ann Surg 198:430, 1983. With permission.)

RATIONALE FOR MANAGEMENT

In general the risk of death or limb loss must be compared to the risk of subsequent symptoms and growth retardation in deciding which of these lesions to treat operatively. Additionally, the expected success of the operative procedure needs to be considered. In some situations this decision is not difficult. Patients sustaining violent trauma with obvious vascular disruption and hemorrhage, pseudoaneurysm, arteriovenous fistula, or

Table 3
Children Developing Leg Length Discrepancies

Patient	Age (Mo)*	Length of Ischemia (Mo)	ABI†	Leg Length Discrepancy (cm)
1	1	5	0	0.50
2	2	2	.6	0.75
3	48	7	.78	2.25
4	3	14	.58	3.00
5	NB‡	20	0	1.00
6	13	13	.2	0.50

*At time of injury
†Immediately following injury
‡New born

severe ischemia clearly require operative intervention. The same is true for infants with aortic thrombosis, which is nearly uniformly fatal if treated nonoperatively. However, most pediatric patients with vascular occlusion (especially the iatrogenic group) do not demonstrate such obvious threat to life or limb. In fact severe ischemia is usually brief if present at all because of rapid development of collateral circulation. In this situation the risk of nonoperative treatment is limb growth impairment or later symptoms of claudication.

Several considerations are important in the decision to employ operative intervention. Of course the general condition of the patient is important. Attempts at limb salvage should not be undertaken in patients with associated life-threatening conditions. The simplicity of thrombectomy done urgently is important as subsequent bypass procedures may not be possible until a much later age and limb length discrepancies may occur during this waiting period. Infrainguinal bypass in this age group has been generally unsuccessful. Reported initial successes have resulted in severe vein graft dilatation over time.[11] Even thrombectomy, however, when performed in children less than 2 years of age has not had excellent results, although application of modern microsurgical techniques should improve upon this situation.

Our current approach is to operate on all patients with aortic thrombosis and all patients with violent trauma who have major arterial injury. In patients with isolated extremity vascular occlusions from whatever cause an operative approach is used in all patients with absent femoral pulses to palpation. In patients younger than 2 years microvascular techniques are applied to the repair of common femoral injuries. At this time patients older than 2 years with palpable femoral pulses are treated on an individual basis depending upon age. In catheter induced injury a waiting period of 6 hours on heparin is usually indicated as spasm may be the underlying problem.

REFERENCES

1. Salerno F, Collins RD, Redmond DC: External iliac artery occlusion in a newborn infant. Surgery 67:863, 1970
2. Henry W, Johnson BB, Peterson AL: Left common iliac arterial embolectomy in the newborn. West J Surg Obstet & Gynecol 68:352, 1960
3. Bjarke B, Herin P, Blomback M: Neonatal aortic thrombosis: A possible clinical manifestation of congenital antithrombin III deficiency. Acta Paediatr Scand 63:297, 1974
4. Moberg A, Reinand T: Aortic thrombosis in infancy: Two cases of different etiology. Acta Pathol Microbiol Scand 39:161, 1956
5. Braly BD: Neonatal arterial thrombosis and embolism. Pediatr Surg 58:869, 1965
6. Alstrup P, Anderson HJ, Schmidt KG: Neonatal aortic thromboembolism: Surgical treatment and coagulation studies. Dan Med J 25:261, 1978
7. Rothstein JL: Progress in pediatrics: Embolism and thrombosis of the abdominal aorta in infancy and childhood. Am J Dis Child 49:1578, 1935
8. Gross RE: Arterial embolism and thrombosis in infancy. Am J Dis Child 70:61, 1945
9. Stout C, Koehl G: Aortic embolism in a newborn infant. Am J Dis Child 120:74, 1970
10. Raffensperger JG, D'Cruz IA, Hastreiter AR: Thrombotic occlusion of the bifurcation of the aorta in infancy: A case with successful surgical therapy. Pediatrics 34:550, 1964
11. Richardson JD, Fallat M, Nagaraj HS, et al: Arterial injuries in children. Arch Surg 116:685, 1980
12. Meagher DP Jr, DeFore WW, Mattox KL, et al: Vascular trauma in infants and children. J Trauma 19:532, 1979

13. Smith C, Green RM: Pediatric vascular injuries. Surgery 90:20, 1981

14. White JJ, Talbert JL, Haller JA: Peripheral arterial injuries in infants and children. Ann Surg 167:757, 1968

15. Jacobsson B, Carlgren LE, Hedvall G, et al: A review of children after arterial catheterization of the leg. Pediatr Radiol 1:96, 1973

16. Klein MD, Coran AG, Whitehouse WM Jr, et al: Management of iatrogenic arterial injuries in infants and children. J Pediatr Surg 17:933, 1982

17. Mansfield PB, Gazzania AB, Litwin SB: Management of arterial injuries related to cardiac catheterization in children and young adults. Circulation 42:501, 1970

18. Rubenson A, Jacobsson B, Sorenson SE: Treatment and sequelae of angiographic complications in children. J Pediatr Surg 14:154, 1979

19. Wigger HJ, Bransilver BR, Blane WA: Thromboses due to catheterization in infants and children. J Pediatr 76:1, 1970

20. Goetzman BW, Stadalnik RC, Bogren HG, et al: Thrombotic complications of umbilical artery catheters: A clinical and radiographic study. Pediatrics 56:374, 1975

21. Marsh JL, King W, Barrett C, et al: Thrombotic complications of umbilical artery catheterization for neonatal monitoring. Arch Surg 110: 1203, 1975

22. O'Neill JA Jr, Neblett WW III, Born ML: Management of major thromboembolic complications of umbilical artery catheters. J Pediatr Surg 16:972, 1981

23. Shaker IJ, White JJ, Signer RD, et al: Special problems of vascular injuries in children. J Trauma 16:863, 1976

24. Flanigan DP, Keifer TJ, Schuler JJ, Ryan TJ, Castronuovo JJ: Experience with iatrogenic pediatric vascular injuries: Incidence, etiology, management, and results. Ann Surg 198:430, 1983

25. Neal WA, Reynolds JW, Jarvis CW, et al: Umbilical artery catheterization: Demonstration of arterial thrombosis by aortography. Pediatrics 50:6, 1972

26. Wesstrom G, Finnstrom O, Stenport G: Umbilical artery catheterization in newborns: Thrombosis in relation to catheter type and position. Acta Paediatr Scand 68:575, 1979

27. Freed MD, Keane JF, Rosenthal A: The use of heparinization to prevent arterial thrombosis after percutaneous cardiac catheterization in children. Circulation XLII:501, 1974

28. Mortensson W: Angiography of the femoral artery following percutaneous catheterization in infants and children. Acta Radiol Diagnos 17:581, 1976

29. Whitehouse WM Jr, Coran AG, Stanley JC, et al: Pediatric vascular trauma: Manifestations, management, and sequelae of extremity arterial injury in patients undergoing surgical treatment. Arch Surg 111:1269, 1976

30. Currarino G, Engle MA: The effects of ligation of the subclavian artery on the bones and soft tissues of the arms. J Pediatr 67:808, 1965

31. Bassett FH III, Lincoln CR, King TD, et al: Inequality in the size of the lower extremity following cardiac catheterization. South Med J 61:1013, 1968

32. Bloom JD, Mozersky DJ, Buckley CJ, et al: Defective limb growth as a complication of catheterization of the femoral artery. Surg Gynecol Obstet 138:524, 1974

Peter Carl Maurer, Johannes Heiss
Joachim Doerrler, Wilfried Burmeister

Replantation of Limbs

Reattaching or replacing severed limbs has been a dream in medicine since the earliest days of recorded history. The well known legend attributing Saints Cosmas and Damian with success in transplanting the leg of a Moor to a white-skinned patient exemplifies this dream.[1-3] However, that legend must remain a fiction even today. The unsolved immunologic questions attending limb transplantation preclude such operations. Replantation of a severed arm or leg approaches the goals of transplantation, however. This, like so many other principles of vascular surgery, lies rooted in experimental work developed even before World War I,[4-6] and includes the fruitful work of Carrel and Guthrie in Chicago in 1906.[7] Technical difficulties, such as the lack of development of blood transfusions, antibiotics, and anesthetic techniques for long operations prevented spread of this knowledge until recent time.

It is now 25 years since Malt and McKhann in Boston[8] and Chen, Chien, and Pao in Shanghai[9] simultaneously successfully replanted a severed arm. Neither knew of the others' work. Professor Churchill at the Massachusetts General Hospital retold the legend of Cosmas and Damian in commenting on Malt and McKhann's success. Nevertheless, the technique was regarded as sensational surgery of doubtful value to patients.

The Western World became aware of successes in Chinese replantation after the 1973 report entitled "American Replantation Mission to China."[10] Conversely, it was Owen's report from Australia[11] that contributed to the development of replantation surgery in a few centers in central Europe. By that time, modern techniques of anesthesia enabled the state of shock to be controlled and made long operations feasible. Improved synthetic materials and sutures, as well as optical aids and intense illumination, permitted the subtle techniques necessary for successful replantation to be carried forward.[12-22] Also, modern techniques of rescue service and transportation allowed patients and their severed limbs to be transported even hundreds of kilometers quickly enough that postischemic damage to the limbs was minimized.

Vascular Surgical Emergencies
ISBN 0-8089-1843-5

245

MICROREPLANTATION AND MACROREPLANTATION

Amputation of entire limbs happens rarely as compared to amputations of fingers, metacarpi, or hands. In the case material of the Rechts der Isar Medical Center of the Technical University of Munich, 1840 amputations of peripheral limb parts[23] and 87 amputations of entire limbs were encountered in the period from November 1975 to November 1985.

Distal limb parts consist largely of collagen, such as tendons, bone, and skin, which has a low metabolic rate. On the other hand, muscle masses of the arm and leg become more seriously threatened by autolysis and bacterial growth because of higher metabolic activity. Despite hypothermia, the time for which a whole limb tolerates ischemia is quite short when compared to the 24 hours and longer that a finger will tolerate under ideal conditions. The precise tolerable time limit for whole limbs has not been determined, nor have the possibilities of prolongation of this time limit by hypothermia, perfusion, or use of hyperbaric oxygen.[24-28] For practical considerations, limb replantations appear to have little prospect of success beyond 6 hours of ischemia.

Whole limb replantation can produce a hazardous condition for the injured patient because of postischemic damage to the limb by muscle necrosis and edema and because perfusion of myoglobin metabolites may cause toxic renal failure or septicemia.[29-31] Additionally, the long distance that neurons must traverse causes an extended period of postreplantation disability.

OBJECTIVES OF REPLANTATION

In brief, the objective of any replantation is restoration of function of the severed member. In view of this, replantation of an arm appears to be much more important than that of a leg. A leg merely serves for locomotion, but an arm must perform diverse activities. Its most important function derives from the innumerable possibilities of hand function. The function of a leg amputated below or even above the knee can be adequately replaced by a modern prosthesis. In contrast, no single prosthesis can even approximately replace a functional hand. The disadvantage of the upper extremity prosthesis is lack of sensitivity to touch. Restoration of feeling with adequate gripping function is therefore one of the important features of successful replantation.

NOMENCLATURE OF AMPUTATION INJURIES

Classification of amputation injuries follows the definition established by the People's Republic of China.[10,32-34] Accordingly, complete severance from the body is required for the definition of total amputation. Subtotal amputation implies interruption of the circulation of the main vessels, with not more than one quarter of the soft tissue covering layer preserved.

INDICATIONS FOR REPLANTATION

The most important consideration before replantation is planned is the general condition of the injured person. If he is in a critical state or if there are important concomitant injuries, replantation should not be carried out, even if the state of the amputated limb is ideal. If the injured person is in good general condition, replantation may be considered. The surgeon should under all circumstances inform the patient about the risks of the operation and about the long duration of the recovery period. He must explain that the final degree of function is not predictable. In our experience, no patient has refused a replantation trial, even after being informed of the risks. In fact, we have observed that after replantation, even in the face of poor function of the limb, the patient feels that he is one of an elite group.

The condition of the amputated member has great impact on the success of the operation. The length of the ischemic period is the most important criterion. In successful replantations, the ischemic period usually has been less than 4 hours, and the limb was treated according to the rules listed below:

1. Look for and bring severed parts with patient.
2. Do not clean or treat them in any way.
3. Stop bleeding only by compression bandage.
4. Put severed parts into clean cloth and into plastic bag. Close bag firmly and cover with ice to cool amputated part. Avoid congelation of tissue and direct contact with melting water.
5. Phone replantation center immediately. Transport patient and limb as fast as possible.

Although these principles have been published in the past,[20,21,35] they are included here for completeness.

The most favorable conditions for replantation of limbs are clean-cut injuries located as peripherally as possible. These include amputations proximal to the wrist or proximal to the ankle. More distal amputations are classified in the field of microsurgery and are not discussed here. The higher the level of amputation, the larger the amputated part, the larger the muscular portion, and the greater the special dangers of ischemia. The period of tolerable ischemia becomes shorter, and more serious complications are more likely in proximal severance of limbs. In particular, perfusion of myoglobin metabolites into the circulation leads to toxic kidney damage or anuria. Anerobic infections, including gas gangrene, and septicemia may also follow.

Amputation injuries accompanied by extensive bruising or detachment have a poorer prognosis for successful replantation and for later regeneration of the nerves. Nevertheless, replantation should not be ruled out on principle if the general condition of the patient is good and there has been a short period of ischemia, without additional peripheral damage.

The degree of contamination of the amputated part is also important. Injuries occurring in industry are frequently contaminated by oil or foreign bodies. Generous debridement of contaminated and bruised muscle and skin cannot be emphasized strongly enough. The danger of infection is great in every case and is increased if contaminated foreign material is left behind. In three of our cases, rapidly spreading infection was such a threat to the patient that reamputation had to be carried out despite patent arterial and venous anastomoses.

REPLANTATION PLAN

The single basic condition for carrying out successful replantation surgery is an organized and enthusiastic surgical team, which must be available 24 hours a day. The surgeons must be familiar with the techniques of vascular surgery and be trained in traumatology as well as in management of peripheral nerve injuries. The operating theater must be available 24 hours a day, as must good anesthetic service. Such conditions are met virtually only in a medical center that provides total service under one roof. In our own center, we have an on-call service, integrating the Department of Vascular Surgery, the Department of Plastic and Reconstructive Surgery, and the Institute of Anesthesiology. These are indispensable and inseparable, one from the other.

After the casualty arrives at the hospital, a precise examination is carried out while the patient is being treated for shock. The essential question is whether or not the patient can tolerate a replantation operation lasting 5 to 9 hours. If replantation can be considered, the amputated part is reperfused with Collins solution. Most recently, we have been using a stroma-free hemoglobin solution.[27] By massaging the severed limb, peripheral thrombi and clots can be removed. The perfusion is ended when clear fluid without clots runs from the veins.

Two surgical teams begin the operation, so that time loss can be minimized. Large-scale excision of bruised and contaminated tissue is performed on both the amputation stump and the amputated part. All tissue without adequate blood supply is removed. The vessels and nerve stumps are located, identified, and marked with atraumatic 6-0 suture. Arterial and venous stumps may be shortened until perfect wall quality is discerned. This is done irrespective of whether end-to-end anastomoses can then be performed.

Loose and devitalized bone fragments are removed, and the bone is shortened until tension-free nerve anastomoses and adequate soft tissue covering can be attained. Shortening a limb by 10 or even 15 cm can be accepted, and compensation in the upper limb with good functional result is to be expected. The particular problems of leg replantation are emphasized here, since major shortening will appreciably impair functional capacity of the leg. After adaptation of the bone ends, the osteotomy is splinted with an AO plate (Swiss Association for Osteosynthesis) and temporarily stabilized by two Lambotte pincers. Arterial spasm is relieved by gentle dilation with a No. 2 or 3 Fogarty catheter.

The arterial anastomoses are carried out as the first step in the reconstruction. Various authors have suggested that the bone be fixed prior to repair of the vascular injuries. These authors advise the use of an intraluminal arterial shunt, which is connected during the osteosynthetic reconstruction. In our opinion, priority should be given to the most rapid possible elimination of ischemia, and this is best done by immediate arterial and venous repair.

A saphenous vein graft may be used to bridge any gap created by debridement of the stump and amputated part. After reopening the artery and restoring blood flow to the limb, toxic metabolites are flushed out by allowing bleeding from small and medium-sized veins. Thus, the first pass of blood flow through the limb is not returned to the patient. Substantial loss of blood may be controlled during this time by brief clamping of the artery. Following this, ligation of small and medium-sized muscular vessels is done with absorbable sutures. Short test bleeding from the main veins is carried out, and an end-to-end anastomosis is performed using fine atraumatic sutures. The two largest vein stumps are repaired, and if it is necessary, a venous graft may be inserted.

After the venous blood flow has been reestablished, pressure plate osteosynthesis is carried out according to the principles of the Swiss Association for Osteosynthesis. Attention is paid to atraumatic handling of the limb so that the reconstructed artery and vein are not separated. If possible, yet another venous anastomosis may be carried out subsequent to the bone fixation. The anastomoses are once again checked and bleeding controlled before muscles and tendons are coapted and sutured.

With regard to the decision about primary or secondary repair of nerves, it is important to refer to Ronald Malt's statement on this subject. Malt was the first surgeon to replant successfully the right arm of a 12-year-old boy. This was done in Boston on May 23, 1962.[8,36] Malt's comment is as follows:

Thus, when the condition of the nerve, patient or surgeon is not optimal, delayed repair is chosen . . . but the surgeon cannot allow insouciance or indisposition to deprive the patient of the benefits of primary repair, if possible. At the first operation, anatomic identification is likely to be simple because scar tissue does not exist. If the site of division and the extent of damage can be identified beyond doubt, as in a clean nonlacerating injury, primary suture permits prompt regeneration and early return of function.[12]

Thus, our aim is to reconstruct the nerves immediately if the condition of the patient and the injury allow this. In most cases, direct nerve suture is possible because of the shortening of the amputated limb and of the stump. Microsurgical technique is indispensable to obtaining good functional results. If direct anastomosis is not possible, we attempt to bridge the defect with a sural nerve graft. Secondary nerve reconstructions at 3 to 8 weeks after primary replantation may be necessary in selected instances.[37]

Before reconstruction of soft tissue and closing of the skin, all devitalized tissue is removed. Finally, large-scale fasciotomies and insertion of suction drains are utilized during wound closure.

ANCILLARY MEDICATION

After adequate treatment of shock and as early as possible after the patient's admission to the emergency room, cephalosporine, 4 gm is given by injection. In badly contaminated cases, 80 mg of gentamycin twice a day is added. During the replantation procedure, another dose or two of 4 gm cephalosporine is given. This antibiotic therapy is continued over a period of 5 to 7 days. Should infection supervene in the postoperative period, organism-specific antibiotics are added. Crystalloid and colloid volume replacement is given according to established general surgical principles. In addition, low molecular weight Dextran, dipyridamole, and aspirin are used. Postoperative heparin administration is not only unnecessary but dangerous. Postoperative bleeding may cause hematoma formation, which may occlude venous reconstructions.

POSTOPERATIVE SURVEILLANCE

Patients surviving limb replantation are monitored in the intensive care unit. This allows meticulous monitoring of circulatory function, urine output, and body temperature. Special attention is paid to producing a state of diuresis so that toxic myoglobin metabolites can be flushed out. Administration of 4000 to 5000 ml of crystalloid per day is not unusual. Distal pulse monitoring is carried out hourly. If toxic renal insufficiency or general infection occurs, reamputation must be considered.

Despite exercise-stable bone fixation, the replanted arm is immobilized in a dorsal, cushioned plaster cast to decrease swelling and protect nerve anastomoses. The limb is raised above the level of the body by suspension of the splint on an extension frame. The plaster splint is changed on the third postoperative day to a lighter, moisture-resistant cast.

After upper-arm replantation, the phalangeal, metacarpophalangeal, and shoulder joints are moved passively by the physiotherapist, starting on the first postoperative day. If active therapy can be done, it is encouraged. This program can also be carried out with forearm replantations, but in distal forearm replantation, only a careful exercise program involving finger joints is carried out, since the nerve anastomoses must be preserved (Fig. 1). After final removal of the supporting bandages, all joints of the affected limb are exercised.

Occupational therapy begins at an early stage in order to familiarize the patient with the principles of treatment and to give him a positive mental attitude. Exercise of the contralateral upper extremity is especially important for the patient to regain a feeling of independence. After discharge from the hospital, the managing physician must routinely check the patient, and physiotherapy must be carried out consistently. A great deal of patience and effort are expected from the patient, who collaborates with the treating surgeon, the family doctor, the physiotherapist, and the occupational therapist to achieve successful rehabilitation. Such rehabilitation may take months to years, and supplementary rehabilitation measures may be considered. The final result of the operation can be evaluated at the earliest 1 to 1½ years after the accident. If reinnervation does not occur at expected times and with expected intensity during the follow-up period, there may be indications for nerve revision. Of course, this must be carried out in consultation with the neurologists and neurosurgeons on the team.

RESULTS OF REPLANTATION

Between November 1975 and November 1985, 87 amputation injuries of large limbs were encountered in our center. Most patients who suffered amputation injuries were referred from smaller hospitals after examination and initial treatment of shock. A few

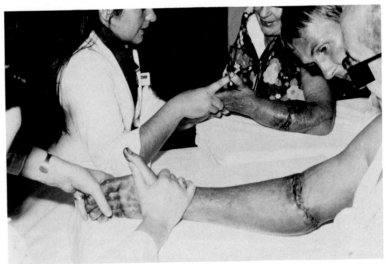

Fig. 1. Following limb replantation, a careful exercise program involving the finger joints is carried out.

LIMB – REPLANTATIONS

n = 62   (NOVEMBER 1975 – NOVEMBER 1985)

	n	REAMPUTATIONS	HEALING	REINNERVATION	FUNCTION
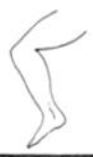	9	9*	1*	—	—
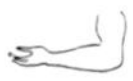	53	12	41	5	36

DEPARTMENT OF VASCULAR SURGERY,
RECHTS DER ISAR MEDICAL CENTER TECHNICAL UNIVERSITY MUNICH

Fig. 2.   Limb replantations. (*Same patient, reamputated because of poor limb functions following primary healing.)

patients came directly from the accident site, transported mostly by helicopter with a doctor on board. The site of the accident ranged up to 300 miles from the hospital, and the interval between accident and admission was from 1 to 4 hours.

In 71 cases, limb replantation was considered possible. Nine of these extremities proved not to be replantable during operative exploration because of thrombosis of peripheral vascular segments and proximal nerve lesions. Of the 62 replantations carried out (53 arms, 9 legs), success was obtained only in the upper extremity. All nine lower limbs had to be reamputated; four because of dangerous infection, three because of infection and incipient renal failure, and two because of vascular thrombosis. One lower extremity replantation healed initially, but function was insufficient and the patient was handicapped by the replanted limb. Therefore, a calf amputation was carried out 6 months after the injury.

With regard to the 53 replanted arms, 41 healed without appreciable complications (Fig. 2). Thirty of these patients have been followed more than 3 years and provided the following objective findings: Joint mobility was satisfactory to very good in passive testing of the replanted limbs. A certain degree of atrophy was nearly always observed. A loss in length between 4 and 11 cm resulted from the shortening of bone during replantation. Venous stasis was not observed, despite occlusion of anastomosed veins in 50 percent of the limbs.[38] Lymphedema was temporary in nature. In one instance of forearm replantation, ulnar and radial artery pulses were absent, but in all other cases, the pulses were palpable with Doppler-derived systemic pressures.

Evaluation of the functional results of limb replantation was carried out by checking sensitivity and muscular strength, as is usual in assessing nerve injuries.[22] The subjective feeling of the patient was appraised. In addition, it was important to determine whether the patient had been reintegrated into his work environment. We have followed the classification of Chen, and have distinguished four groups of patients,[13,22,34] as illustrated in Table 1. Thus, 25 of 30 patients belong in groups I to III, that is, those patients have attained a certain degree of function; 18 can be classified in groups I and II, with very good and good results. If we express these data in percentages, then the rate of healing is about 77 percent, the rate of functioning is about 80 percent, and good to very good functional results were obtained in about 60 percent of patients with successful replantations. Forty percent of the patients are working in the profession for which they had been trained or similar occupations.

Table 1

Functional Results after Limb Replantation

Classification According to Chen

Grade I:	Patient resumes original work. Muscular power nearly normal. Complete or nearly complete recovery of sensation. Joint motion 60% or more.
Grade II:	Patient resumes some suitable work. Muscular power overcomes strong resistance. Nearly complete recovery of sensation. Joint motion 40% or more.
Grade III:	Patient carries on daily life. Muscular power overcomes minor resistance. Partial recovery of sensation. Joint motion 30% or more.
Grade IV:	Almost no functional recovery although the replanted limb survived.

The accompanying groups of Figures (Figs. 3A–D, 4A–D, 5A–F) demonstrate three examples of limb replantation achieving the functional results of groups I and II according to Chen's classification.

DISCUSSION

In dealing with an upper extremity, even a little function is better than no function. Therefore, the results achieved in limb replantation demonstrate a major success of this treatment as compared to amputation. Even patients who are classified in group III possess an upper limb with an appreciable reduction in function but that is useful as a second hand. Such a result cannot be attained even with the most modern myoelectric prostheses. Such prostheses make specific demands upon the amputation stump that it cannot always fulfill. There is also an economic factor. The high cost of treatment and follow-up are often mentioned as an argument against limb replantation. However, objective calculations for 38 of our patients, 8 of whom were reamputated and 30 of whom healed, revealed a cost saving of 3.75 million DM for amputee pensions, which of course were not necessary after replantation. After subtracting all treatment and follow-up costs, there was still a saving of 1.2 million DM.

Favorable surgical results can only be attained by using subtle techniques and strict establishment of indications for such surgery. Success can only be achieved in large hospitals. Replantation surgery at any price may bring discredit to the procedure. For example, it is irresponsible to carry out replantation of limbs in patients with multiple injuries. It is senseless and wrong to replant limbs with large muscle masses after 6 to 8 hours of ischemia. By 10 hours, the musculature is irreversibly damaged, even though cooling has been accomplished.

Severely damaged and ischemic limbs can be a lethal danger to the entire body because of the well-known tourniquet syndrome. Limb replantation should not be sensational surgery, performed merely because it is feasible. Instead, the goal of such operations must be restoration of limb function. When this point of view is taken, it seems especially worthwhile to carry out upper limb replantations because they are the most successful and attain imminent success when the amputation is clean and distal. In the upper extremity, upwards of 10 cm of limb shortening is tolerated, and the patient can be provided with a functionally satisfactory upper limb. Unfortunately, the situation is not the same in the lower limb, since major limb shortening is not accepted by the patient, and

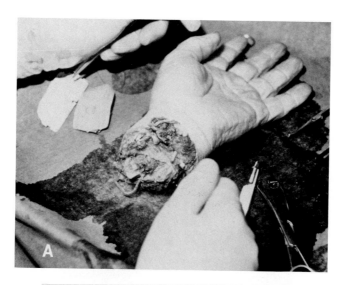

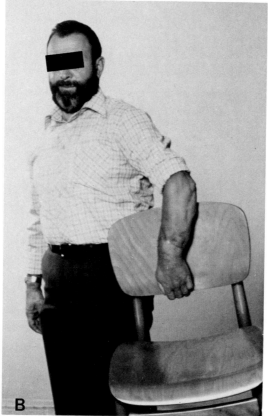

Fig. 3. (A) Complete amputation of the left forearm by a buzz saw. (B) Two months after replantation, motor function is very good, but sensitivity has not yet returned.

(continues)

253

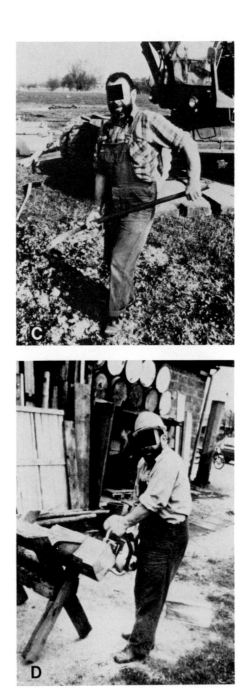

Fig. 3. (C) Ten months after the accident, the patient tries to work again at his own wish and succeeds. (D) At the end of the second year, he has regained complete motor and sensory function and does not feel limited in any way.

254

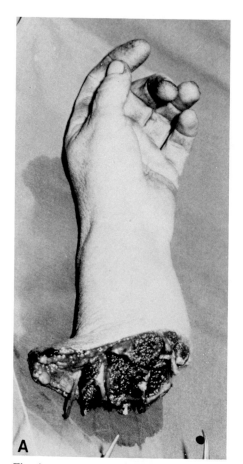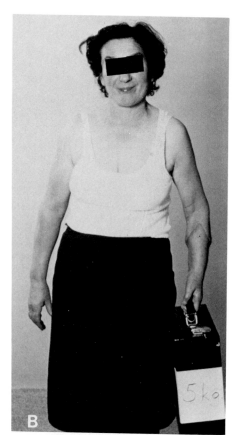

Fig. 4. (A) Total amputation of the left forearm of a farmer's wife by a harvester. (B) Functional result 5 months after replantation.

(continues)

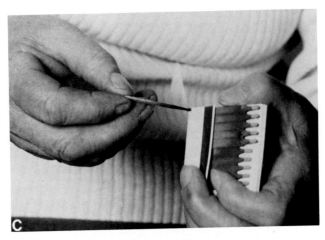

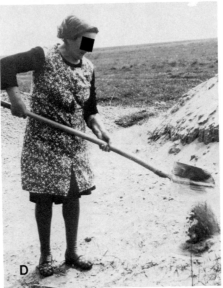

Fig. 4. (C) After 8 months, the patient can perform even meticulous work sufficiently. (D) After 21 months, the patient has resumed her previous activities completely. Here, she is preparing some construction work.

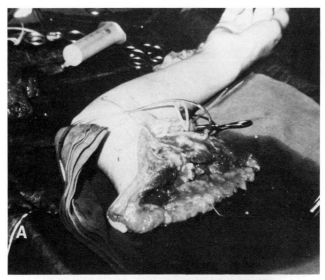

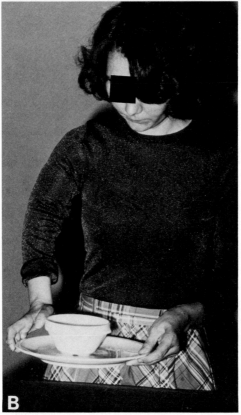

Fig. 5. (A) Complete severance of the right arm at the shoulder joint of a 26-year-old female occurred during a car accident. The patient arrived at the hospital together with the cooled arm 70 minutes after the accident. A humerus fragment 12 cm in length was completely lacerated from the muscles and devitalized. A large part of the triceps and biceps tissue had to be removed (mass left of the elbow). (B) At 15 months after replantation, the patient has regained sufficient motor function for light work. Sensitivity is still considerably diminished.

(continues)

257

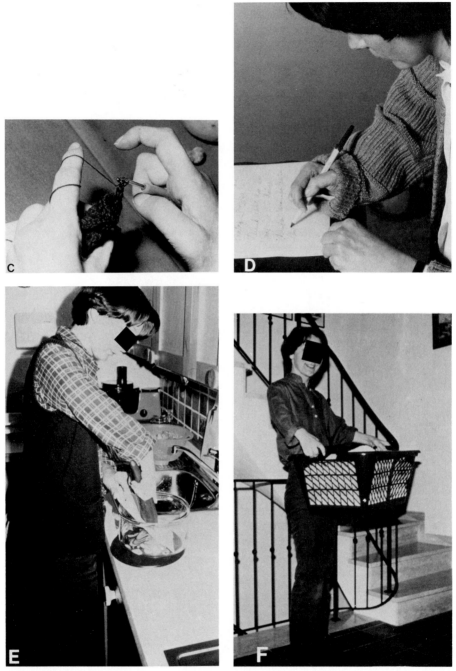

Fig. 5. (C) After 21 months, both sensitivity and motor function have considerably improved. She now can do even meticulous jobs like crochet work. (D) Thirty months after replantation, she has learned to write again with her right hand. (E) and (F) Three years after the accident, she demonstrates convincingly that she is able to manage her housekeeping all by herself.

258

it is difficult to follow the principle of attaching only healthy structures to one another without such shortening. At present, we have very markedly restricted the indications for replantation of lower limbs. The lower leg prosthesis provides a functional limb competitive with the replanted lower extremity. At present, we only consider replantation in very clean or bilateral leg amputations.

CONCLUSION

Limb replantation, especially of the upper limb, has definitely passed beyond the stage of experimental exploration. Technical problems, in general, have been solved. In the hands of experienced surgeons functioning as a team, adequate upper extremity function can be obtained today. This was an unrealistic expectation 10 years ago. A rate of healing of nearly 80 percent is now achieved, and a good functional result is obtained in 60 percent of the patients. These surprisingly good results justify the use of this reconstructive technique as the primary treatment in traumatic limb amputations.

REFERENCES

1. Fichtner G: Das verpflanzte Mohrenbein. Zur Interpretation der Kosmas und Damian Legende. Med Hist J 3:87, 1968
2. Kahan BD: Cosmas and Damian in the 20th Century. N Engl J Med 305:280, 1981
3. Black KS, Hewitt CW, Fraser LA, et al: Cosmas and Damian in the laboratory. N Engl J Med 306:368, 1982
4. Höpfner E: Über Gefässnaht, Gefässtransplantationen und Replantationen von amputierten Extremitäten. Arch Klin Chir 70:417, 1903
5. Lexer E: Verpflanzung ganzer Gliedmassen und Gewebsabschnitte. In Lexer E: Die freien Transplantationen, Band 2. Stuttgart, Enke, 1924, pp 641–648
6. Jeger E: Die Chirurgie der Blutgefässe und des Herzens. Stuttgart–New York, Springer Verlag, 1913 (Reprint 1973)
7. Carrel A, Guthrie C: Complete amputation of the thigh with replantation. Amer J Med Sci 131:297, 1906
8. Malt RA, McKhann CF: Replantation of severed arms. JAMA 189:716, 1964
9. Chen CW, Chien YC, Pao YS: Salvage of the forearm following complete traumatic amputation: Report of a case. Chin Med J 82:632, 1963
10. American Replantation Mission to China: Replantation surgery in China. Plast Reconstr Surg 52:476, 1973
11. Owen ER: Replantation of amputated extremities. Langenbecks Arch Chir 339:613, 1975
12. Malt RA, Harris WH: Replantation of limbs, in Najarian JS, Simmons RL, (Eds): Transplantation. Munich, Urban & Schwarzenberg, 1972, pp 711–719
13. Chen CW, Qian YQ, Yu ZJ: Extremity replantation. World J Surg 2:513, 1978
14. Balas P, Giannikas AC, Harto-Garofalides G, Plessas S: The present status of replantation of amputated extremities. Indications and technical considerations. Vasc Surg 4:190, 1970
15. Zwank L, Schweiberer L, Hertel P: Indikation, Technik und Ergebnisse bei Klein- und Grossreplantationen. Z Plast Chir 2:133, 1978
16. Zwank L, Hertel P, Schweiberer L: Replantationen—Funktion und soziale Aspekte. Deutsch Ärzteblatt H 45:2657, 1980
17. Peking Chishueit'an Hospital: Replantation of severed limbs: Analysis of 40 cases. Chin Med J 4:265, 1975
18. Tamai S, Hori Y, Tatsumi Y, et al: Major limb, hand, and digital replantation. World J Surg 3:17, 1979

19. Meyer VE, Chen ZE, Beasley RW: Basic technical considerations in reattachment surgery. Orthop Clin 12:871, 1981

20. Maurer PC, Hopfner R, Lange R, et al: Erfahrungen mit der Replantation grosser Gliedmassen. Fortschr Med 96:2181, 1978

21. Maurer PC, Heiss J, Bonke S, et al: Replantation von Gliedmassen—Erfahrungen, Technik, Ergebnisse. Unfallheilkunde 82:237–245, 1979

22. Maurer PC, Heiss J, Lange R, et al: Gliedmassen-replantation—Traum, Sensation, chirurgische Realität. Angio 4:51, 1982

23. Biemer E: Digital replantation, in Jackson IT (Ed): Recent Advances in Plastic Surgery. Edinburgh, Churchill Livingstone, 1981, pp 45–65

24. Sixth People's Hospital, Shanghai: Hyperbaric oxygen therapy in replantation of severed limbs: A report of 21 cases. Chin Med J 3:197, 1975

25. Buri P, Vogt ED: Traumatische Amputation und Gliedmassenverlust durch Gefässverletzungen. VASA 7:177, 1978

26. Hicks TE, Boswick JA, Solomons CC: The effect of perfusion on an amputated extremity. J Trauma 20:632, 1980

27. Steinau HU, Elert O, Schneider M: Prolongation of the ischemia tolerance of amputated extremities by a stroma-free hemoglobin solution. Thorac Cardiovasc Surg 28:35, 1980

28. Tauber A, Wendt P, Mittlmeier T, et al: Initial perfusion of extremities with Fluosol-43 prior to replantation—metabolic and hemodynamic investigations in rabbits, in Frey, Beisbarth, Stossek (Eds): Oxygen Carrying Colloidal Blood Substitutes. Proc 5th Internat Symposium Pefluorochem Blood Substitutes. Munich, Zuckschwerdt, 1982, pp 245–254

29. Larcan A, Matthieu P, Helmer J, Fieve G: Severe metabolic changes following delayed revascularization: Legrain-Cormier syndrome. J Cardiovasc Surg 14:609, 1973

30. Haimovici H: Muscular, renal, and metabolic complications of acute arterial occlusion: Myonephropathic-metabolic syndrome. Surgery 85:461, 1979

31. Kindhäuser V, Eigler FW: Das Postischämie—(Tourniquet)—Syndrom nach arterieller Gefässverletzung. Unfallheilkunde 82:275, 1979

32. Biemer E: Definitions and classifications in replantation surgery. Brit J Plast Surg 33:164, 1980

33. Biemer R: Replantationschirurgie in China. Deutsch Ärzteblatt H 45:2645, 1978

34. Chen ZE, Meyer VE, Kleinert HE, Beasley RW: Present indications and contraindications for replantation as reflected by long-term functional results. Orthop Clin 12:849, 1981

35. Maurer PC, Heiss J, Bonke S, et al: Experience with limb-replantation. Proc 5th Internat Congress, Internat Microsurgical Soc, Bonn, 1978. Amsterdam, Excerpta Medica, 1979, pp 33–35.

36. Malt RA, Rememsnyder JP, Harris WH: Long-term utility of replanted arms. Ann Surg 176:334, 1972

37. Millesi H: Microsurgery of peripheral nerves. World J Surg 3:67, 1979

38. Heiss J, Lange J, Maurer PC: The importance of vein reconstruction in replantation of upper limbs. Results of clinical and phlebographic follow-up in 22 cases. Thorac Cardiovasc Surg 30(Special Issue 1):40, 1982

PART V

Injury to the Venous System

F. William Blaisdell

Management of Injuries to the Vena Cava and Portal Veins

While the first anastomosis between two blood vessels was carried out between the portal vein and the inferior vena cava by Eck in 1877, and the technical challenge presented by arterial injuries has been quite satisfactorily resolved, the venous system still presents challenging technical problems that require solutions. In the recent Vietnam experience documented in the next chapter, vascular repair was extensively utilized but there were few venous injuries reported with venous repair performed in less than one-third. Ligation alone was done in the majority. Of the rare abdominal and pelvic venous injuries mentioned, repair was effected in only a handful.[1]

Early reports on the management of inferior vena cava injuries stressed the rarity of survival, particularly after suprarenal inferior vena cava and associated hepatic vein injuries. The first documented survivor of an inferior vena cava injury, from a bomb fragment, was reported in 1916 by Taylor.[2] The first series of any size was published in 1961 by Ochsner.[3] Until that time, only 19 survivors of inferior vena cava injuries had been documented in the literature, all but 3 as case reports. In Ochsner's series, 16 of 37 patients admitted alive to the hospital survived surgical treatment. Duke and others,[4] and Quast and others,[5] subsequently reported survival rates of 47 and 60 percent, respectively. Improved resuscitation techniques, better blood bank support, and more aggressive operative intervention all contributed to the survival rates reported in more recently published series. Technical advances permitted for the first time the isolation and repair of suprarenal vena cava and hepatic venous injuries.

Historical accounts of the management of portal and mesenteric vein injuries stress the importance of repair rather than ligation because ligation was considered to be incompatible with life, owing to massive visceral congestion and portal hypertension.[6] This dogma was based primarily on the results of canine experiments in which death invariably occurred after portal and superior mesenteric vein ligation. However, Robson, as early as 1897, and others subsequently reported cases in which the portal vein or superior mesenteric vein was ligated without adverse sequelae.[7] Child observed that acute portal vein ligation was possible in humans because of relatively good portal collateral flow.[8]

Vascular Surgical Emergencies
ISBN 0-8089-1843-5

Survival after abdominal venous injury depends upon the nature of the wounding agent, the presence or absence of shock at the time of hospital admission, the level of injury, and the number and type of associated vascular injuries. Most of the mortality occurs in those patients presenting in profound shock. Suprarenal and intrahepatic vena caval injuries carry a much higher mortality because of the increased difficulty in obtaining vascular control. In our previous experience, there was a mortality rate of 78 percent with suprarenal vena caval injuries as compared to 35 percent with infrarenal vena caval injuries.[9] The immediate cause of death in 90 percent of vena cava injuries was exsanguination. Late deaths are usually caused by multi-organ failure with sepsis. When there are associated aortic injuries, the mortality rates range between 57 and 100 percent.

For portal and mesenteric vein injuries, mortality rates average 60 percent with ranges between 53 and 71 percent.[10] In a collection of portal vein injuries, Busuttil and colleagues found that the death rate with lateral repair was 30 percent for portal and mesenteric vein injuries while that for ligation treatment was 78 percent.[11] Stone reported survival of 16 of 20 patients who required portal vein ligation for trauma.[12] He concluded, as did Child earlier, that portal collateral channels appear to be sufficient in most cases to prevent portal hypertension and splanchnic venous infarction after portal and superior mesenteric vein ligation. Portocaval shunting has rarely been used as a primary procedure because of the frequent development of encephalopathy in patients with previously normal hepatic blood flow.

DIAGNOSIS

Penetrating trauma is a far more common cause of major abdominal venous injury than blunt trauma. If the course of the penetrating object appears to pass in the vicinity of the major abdominal blood vessels, the likelihood of venous injury should be considered.

Blunt trauma, although it occurs much less commonly, is far more lethal than penetrating injury. Venous injury may be suspected when there is evidence of a major liver injury, particularly those associated with fall from heights. Under these circumstances, tears of hepatic veins and the suprarenal vena cava represent a distinct possibility. Direct blows to the center of the abdomen, which can produce avulsion injuries involving the renal pedicle, can result in tears of the renal veins at the insertion of the vena cava. Seat belt injuries may be associated with avulsion venous injuries at the level of the portal triad or the base of the mesentery. The vena cava is subject to injury during abdominal operations such as lumbar sympathectomy, nephrectomy, adrenalectomy, and aortic surgery. It can also be injured by trocars introduced for peritoneal dialysis or for lavage carried out for the diagnosis of hemoperitoneum. The portal vein may be injured during hepatic, biliary, or pancreatic surgery.

PATHOPHYSIOLOGY

Since the veins constitute a low pressure system, overlying tissues are capable of tamponading major lacerations. In order for major ongoing hemorrhage to occur, venous injuries must either decompress externally, into a body cavity or into the cavity produced by injury, such as that which occurs in association with pelvic fractures. Missed venous injuries, while they may be associated with massive bleeding initially, rarely produce secondary hemorrhage.

Normally, intrathoracic pressure is negative and the corresponding pressure in the abdominal veins in a supine position varies from slightly negative to slightly positive. As a result, there is a tendency for blood flow in lacerated veins to continue in normal channels. With the introduction of ventilatory support, however, particularly endotracheal intubation and mechanical ventilation as occurs with the induction of anesthesia, pressure within the chest is raised above atmospheric and with it there is a corresponding rise in venous pressure. This results in the potential for exsanguination into the abdominal cavity from previously partially tamponaded lesions. Therefore, sudden deterioration of a patient following initiation of positive pressure ventilation is a manifestation of major venous injury. A surgeon expecting to deal with trivial abdominal hemorrhage may, upon opening the abdomen, instead be confronted with massive venous hemorrhage, particularly, if or when the retroperitoneum is exposed. It is for this reason that patients with major trauma who present with evidence of major blood loss should have at least one cutdown placed during resuscitation.

PREOPERATIVE PREPARATION

The initial cutdown in reasonably stable patients is most easily accomplished on the saphenous vein at the ankle or on the antecubital or basilic vein at the elbow. The saphenous vein in the adult male usually accepts the entire cross-section of intravenous tubing. This can be supplemented by whatever percutaneous lines seem appropriate for the administration of drugs or withdrawal of blood specimens. Despite the fact that the cava is injured, administration of fluid via saphenous cutdown is just as effective in resuscitation as that administered through a jugular or subclavian catheter or cutdown; this, because the venous system constitutes one continuous pool of blood and raising the pressure in one portion raises the pressure in all portions of the thoracic and abdominal veins. Because of abundant collateral channels in the venous system, effective volume resuscitation can still be carried out with a saphenous cutdown even with the vena cava clamped. Were this not the case, it would be impossible to cross-clamp the inferior vena cava. Within a few minutes of caval occlusion, in the absence of collaterals, the entire blood volume would theoretically be trapped below the occluding clamp.

Preoperative evaluation should include chest and abdominal films, and, if there is any possibility of renal or renal pedicle injury, CT scan with contrast or intravenous pyelography should be performed. A bladder catheter is always indicated in the patient presenting with major injury and a nasogastric tube facilitates gastric decompression. As is true with most trauma cases, blood should be reserved for administration in the operating room since badly needed reserves can be depleted attempting to resuscitate the patient elsewhere. Patients can tolerate an hematocrit of 10 provided volume is maintained, and it is better to use balanced salt solution rather than red blood cells during resuscitation prior to vascular control. If the patient does not respond to rapid fluid infusion, operative control of the bleeding point should be utilized as part of the resuscitation process.

OPERATIVE PRINCIPLES

Trauma to the great intra-abdominal veins when associated with hemorrhage presents a far more difficult problem than that of corresponding arterial trauma for the following reasons:

1. Proximal control of arterial injuries usually stops hemorrhage, since with shock, distal collateral flow is relatively modest and back-bleeding is not a major problem. Venous injuries, conversely, require both proximal and distal control since distal pressure is raised, causing lacerations to bleed vigorously in both directions.
2. While cross-clamping of the artery during shock results in very little change in collateral flow, cross-clamping of veins results in marked increase in pressure and collateral bleeding is augmented dramatically in all branches entering the injured segment. Proximal and distal control therefore does not necessarily result in control of hemorrhage.
3. Arteries have integrity and hold sutures well. Veins often have the consistency of wet tissue paper and tear with the application of clamps or when sutured under tension.
4. Suture lines in large arteries rarely produce thrombotic problems, where suture lines in veins exposing raw surface produce a high risk of local thrombosis and embolism. Moreover, suture lines in veins tend to contract and obstruct flow with the passage of time whereas this is unusual in arteries.
5. Prosthetic substitutes work well within the major abdominal arteries and poorly or not at all in the venous system.

Abdominal venous injuries, like arterial injuries, are best exposed through a generous midline incision running from xiphoid to pubis. The bowel should be eviscerated, blood evacuated from the abdominal cavity, and any major bleeding controlled temporarily with packs while rapid assessment of the abdomen is carried out. Blood should be removed from all corners of the abdomen and these areas packed with laparotomy tapes to isolate bleeding. By doing so, there is less danger that the patient will exsanguinate from a second injury while the first is being treated.

When a venous injury is identified, hemorrhage can, in most cases, be controlled by the judicious application of pack and pressure. This permits volume restoration before attempts are made to expose the site of injury. The need for this relates to the fact that attempts to expose and control the area of injury result in further hemorrhage and, if the patient is hypovolemic, cardiac arrest may occur. Venous bleeding is also more subtle than arterial bleeding and the surgeon is often less aware of the magnitude of ongoing hemorrhage in venous injury as opposed to that of arterial injury. For this reason, continuous application of suction to the area of injury should not be allowed, since suction may remove blood so rapidly that the extent of the hemorrhage may not be appreciated by the surgeon. It is better to have the assistant aspirate for a few seconds, remove the sucker from the field, and then re-aspirate.

With the exception of the portal vein and the intrahepatic vena cava, exposure of the remaining intra-abdominal great veins is generally easier than the corresponding arteries. Local pressure can be used to control bleeding while proximal and distal dissection are carried out. In some instances, temporary intraluminal occlusion by balloon catheters can be used to control hemorrhage. The iliac veins are best exposed by severing the lateral attachments of the colon or cecum and retracting the large bowel medially. This permits exposure of the external and common iliac veins with the exception of that portion of the left common iliac vein underlying the aorta. With the exception of the ureter, all critical anatomy, including, most importantly the mesenteric circulation of the large intestine, is retracted away (Fig. 1).

The most difficult portion of the iliac system to isolate and control is the internal iliac vein or one of its major branches. This is particularly true when there are multiple injuries to the iliac venous system such as those that occur in association with major pelvic fractures. For this reason, venous hematomas in the vicinity of the pelvis are usually left alone unless there is an associated overlying laceration that results in free intraperitoneal bleeding. The problem with internal iliac vein injuries is that although proximal control is relatively easy to obtain, control of internal iliac vein tributaries can be exceedingly difficult as opening the hematoma results in extensive hemorrhage from the decompressed proximal smaller veins. Since both external iliac and common iliac veins have few, if any branches, the area of injury can be compressed with sponge sticks or fingers and direct repairs relatively easily carried out.

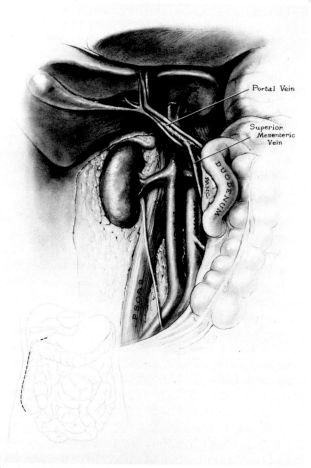

Fig. 1. Mobilization of entire right colon provides exposure of the iliac veins and vena cava. The portal vein is exposed by further mobilization of the duodenum and head of the pancreas.

Injuries to the extrahepatic suprarenal vena cava are readily exposed by a Kocher maneuver, mobilizing the duodenum and portal triad upward to the left. Those related to the intrahepatic cava and major hepatic veins are extremely difficult to expose and treat because massive hemorrhage usually is associated with any attempt to retract the liver upward. For this reason, a technique was developed for isolation of this portion of the vena cava utilizing an intracaval shunt.[13] Although it is possible to place a shunt from below the liver, this is actually more difficult than placing the shunt from above through the right atrium since excessive bleeding may occur while manipulating the vena cava as the catheter is inserted from below.

The best way to isolate the liver is to extend the midline abdominal incision upward as a median sternotomy incision. The pericardium is opened and the right atrial appendage exposed. A large bore catheter, 1 to 1.5 cm in diameter, can then be inserted through the atrial appendage while the intrapericardiac portion of the vena cava is palpated to ensure that the catheter passes into the inferior vena cava rather than into the right ventricle or coronary vein. The catheter should be manipulated gently since it may pass through a large laceration in the cava or may enter the right hepatic vein which is often 1.5 to 2 cm in diameter. If the catheter is curved, the curve should be directed to the right and posteriorly to ensure its unobstructed passage. Palpation of the catheter at the level of the renal veins verifies the proper location of the shunt. When the tip of the catheter has passed the level of the renal veins, it is cross-clamped at the level of the atrium and a side hole cut. The side hole is then advanced into the atrium as an atrial purse-string suture is tightened and the catheter secured. This side hole provides for the egress of blood into the atrium from the shunt that is left projecting from the atrial appendage (Fig. 2). Cutting the side hole after placement of the shunt ensures its proper location within the atrium. The end of the catheter projecting from the atrium can be used for rapidly infusing blood or crystalloid solutions. When exsanguinating injuries are present, an auto-transfusion device can be used to infuse crystalloid or blood. With this technique, 500 ml per minute can be infused. Crystalloid, consisting of balanced salt solution heated to 38° C, or warmed blood is used to prevent hypothermia.

With the catheter in place, the portal triad can be cross-clamped and umbilical tapes placed rapidly around the intrapericardial and suprarenal portion of the vena cava. When these are pulled up the caval segment isolation is complete.

Another method for those not comfortable with the transcardiac approach is to use the abdominal route, which constitutes a reasonable alternative. In this instance, it is better to sacrifice blood returning from below the renal veins. This constitutes about one-third of venous return and avoids extensive blood loss with manipulation of the catheter for placement. The cava is mobilized just below the renal veins and the lumbar veins in this segment clipped. The distal cava is occluded with an umbilical tape, a partial occluding clamp is placed across the vena cava just above this tape and below the renal veins, and a 34–36 Fr endotracheal or similar size plastic tube is advanced through a venotomy upward toward the atrium. As the tip of the catheter enters the atrium, a side hole is cut in the distal portion (which has still not entered the cava). The catheter is then advanced into the vena cava so that the side hole lies at the level of the renal veins with the end of the catheter projecting from the vena cava. Tapes are then pulled up around the catheter above the venotomy but below the renal veins, then above the renal veins resulting in diversion

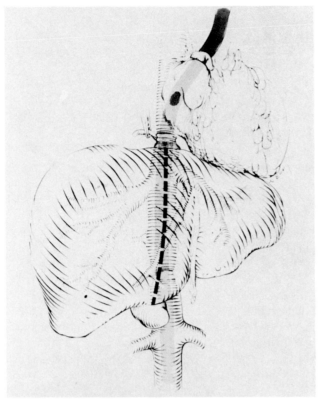

Fig. 2. Transatrial caval catheterization with the portal triad cross-clamped and tapes pulled up around the catheter, all interior caval flow is directed through the shunt.

of renal blood flow through the shunt into the atrium (Fig. 3). Another umbilical tape tied around the supradiaphragmatic portion of the vena cava completely isolates the intrahepatic portion of the vein with the exception of the adrenal and phrenic veins.

With the cava thus isolated and the portal triad cross-clamped, the liver can be rolled upward from the right by severing its attachments to the retroperitoneum and the cava exposed. Should major hepatic venous damage to the right or left lobe be involved, lobar hepatectomy may be required. This can be accomplished rapidly in a relatively avascular field when the caval isolation technique is used.

Injuries to the intrapericardial portion of the vena cava result in intrapericardial hemorrhage and pericardial tamponade. Isolation of this portion of the cava is difficult because of its close proximity to the atrium, but control can be obtained just as described for the intrahepatic portion of the vena cava.

If the patient has had blood volume restored, it is possible to occlude the vena cava return completely without shunting. This is accomplished by cross-clamping the cava just above or below the diaphragm and above the renal veins. Williams and Brenowitz[14] describe a technique of sequentially clamping the aorta at the diaphragmatic hiatus and the

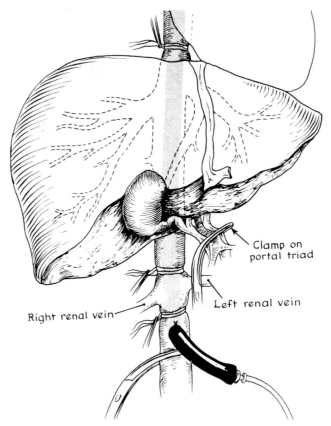

Fig. 3. Transcaval shunt permits isolation of the intrahepatic vena cava from the abdominal route.

vena cava within the pericardium to permit repair of the vena cava laceration at the diaphragm. This is usually not possible in patients who are not in shock who have high catecholamine levels in our experience.

As regards the portal vein, exposure can be difficult and in most instances the vein is best exposed posteriorly. This requires carrying out a generous Kocher maneuver with or without mobilization of the ascending colon and small bowel mesentery. Injuries to the junction of the splenic and mesenteric veins with the portal vein require extensive mesenteric mobilization with the entire bowel and mesentery retracted upward to the left. Injuries to the portal vein in the area of the portal triad can be approached with a combination of Kocher maneuver and the application of a vascular clamp across the proximal portal triad while the structures in the portal triad are dissected. Through and through injuries to the portal vein are best exposed posteriorly. The anterior opening if not bleeding actively can be ignored or the anterior opening can be exposed utilizing an extension of the posterior venotomy.

If there has been a penetrating injury to the pancreas that threatens the pancreatic duct, then distal pancreatic resection can be carried out and the splenic and mesenteric veins and/or the portal vein exposed anteriorly after removal of the distal pancreas. In certain complex injuries in which multiple associated injuries must be dealt with simultaneously, ligation of the portal vein can be utilized.

TECHNICAL CONSIDERATIONS

Definitive treatment of injured veins involves lateral repair, resection, and re-anastomosis, or ligation. Isolated injuries of the external, internal, or common iliac veins can be treated with ligation or repair. If the laceration is a simple one, meticulous repair with fine monofilament eversion sutures is usually associated with a good result (Fig. 4). However, complex injuries are difficult to repair without producing stenosis of the vein or leaving a raw surface of the vein exposed to the blood. This is thrombogenic and may result in complications of thrombosis, or worse yet, embolism. Therefore, complex injuries to the iliac veins and infrarenal vena cava are best treated by ligation of the injured segment. For complex vena caval injuries, the distal ligature is best placed at the level of the renal veins and the intervening lumbar veins ligated if necessary; this, because the segment above the ligature may be the source of thrombosis and subsequent embolism. If the injury is simple and can be cleanly repaired, this can be accomplished using partial occluding clamps or by trapping the vein with sponge sticks and packs (Fig. 5). Penetrating injuries involving both anterior and posterior walls of the vena cava can be managed either by suturing the posterior laceration through a widened anterior hole or alternatively ligating and dividing lumbar veins and rotating the cava for exposure and posterior repair (Fig. 6).

Ligation of the suprarenal vena cava is usually not compatible with survival since two-thirds of cardiac venous return is compromised. Severe injuries to this segment are usually incompatible with survival long enough to reach a point of definitive treatment. Prior to development of the intracaval shunt, there were no cases of successful repairs of the suprarenal vena cava reported in the literature. Occasionally, if vascular volume has been restored to normal, it may be possible to occlude this segment temporarily for repair as previously described.

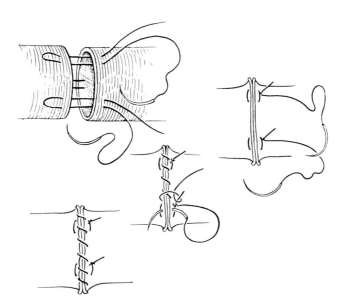

Fig. 4. Eversion of the intima is important when suturing a venous laceration or inserting a venous replacement graft.

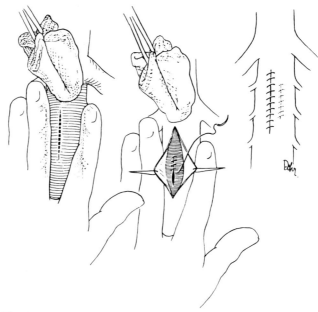

Fig. 5. Rather than attempt to clamp the vena cava, it is best trapped with sponge sticks and fingers.

There is no technical challenge quite as great as a complex injury of the infrarenal vena cava. There may be massive bleeding from lumbar veins and, as the injury is exposed, collateral bleeding can be such as to result in exsanguination. The assistant should control the vein from above with a sponge stick as the surgeon rolls a pack from above downwards so as to expose a small segment of the laceration. As the suture is initiated the pack can be rolled further downward as repair is carried out. As lumbar veins are identified, they are temporarily clipped.

Although the superior mesenteric vein can be ligated, thrombosis and loss of viability of bowel may result.[15,16] Therefore, this vein and the portal vein should be repaired if at all possible (Fig. 7). Portal triad injuries can be treated with the portocaval shunt. This is often difficult in unstable patients and, furthermore, is associated with severe morbidity due to protein intolerance. For these reasons, ligation is preferred if repair of the vein is not possible as this preserves collateral flow to the liver to a variable degree. Injuries to the junction of the portal and mesenteric veins can be treated with a venous patch if the injury is complex. Alternatively the splenic vein can be divided and used to reconstruct the superior mesenteric vein. The higher pressure portal system tolerates suture and repair on both an immediate and long-term basis better than lower pressure systemic veins. If an interposition graft is required, a segment of internal jugular vein, internal iliac vein, or external iliac or even saphenous vein is preferred. There has been some limited success using externally supported Gor-Tex grafts, but these represent a relatively poor alternative.

SUMMARY

Abdominal venous trauma carries a high mortality. The victims often present in shock and there are frequently other associated injuries. The inability to obtain vascular control

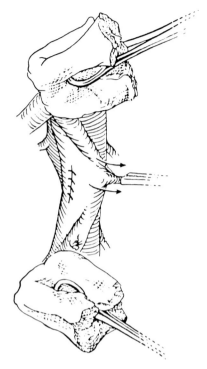

Fig. 6. Posterior lacerations require division of lumbar veins before the vena cava can be rotated for exposure of the laceration.

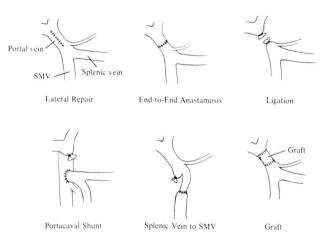

Portal vein

SMV   Splenic vein

Lateral Repair   End-to-End Anastamosis   Ligation

Graft

Portacaval Shunt   Splenic Vein to SMV   Graft

Fig. 7. Methods of reconstructing portal venous injuries.

273

rapidly results in death by exsanguination. Improved results can be expected if operative control of hemorrhage is carried out as part of the resuscitative process and large bore cutdowns are utilized in conjunction with resuscitation. Although repair by lateral suture grafting is the preferred treatment, in many cases ligation can be used to treat venous injuries with acceptable results.

REFERENCES

1. Rich NM, Spencer RC: Vascular Trauma. Philadelphia, WB Saunders, 1978
2. Taylor DC: Two cases of penetrating wounds of the abdomen involving the inferior vena cava. Lancet 2:60, 1916
3. Ochsner JL, Crawford ES, DeBakey ME: Injuries of the vena cava caused by external trauma. Surgery 49:397, 1961
4. Duke JH Jr, Jones RC, Shires GT: Management of injuries to the inferior vena cava. Am Surg 110:759, 1965
5. Quast DC, Shirkey AL, Fitzgerald JB, et al: Surgical correction of injuries of the vena cava: an analysis of sixty-one cases. J Trauma 5:1, 1965
6. Boyce FF, Lampert R, McFetridge EM: Occlusion of the portal vein. J Lab Clin Med 20:935, 1935
7. Robson AWM: Case of perforating wound of abdomen. Br Med J 2:77, 1897
8. Child CG III: The Hepatic Circulation and Portal Hypertension. Philadelphia, WB Saunders, 1954
9. Allen RE, Blaisdell FW: Injuries to the inferior vena cava. Surg Clin North Am 52:699, 1972
10. Peterson SR, Sheldon GF, Lim RC: Management of portal vein injuries. J Trauma 19:616, 1979
11. Busuttil RW, Kitahama A, Cerise E, et al: Management of blunt and penetrating injuries to the porta hepatis. Ann Surg 191:641, 1980
12. Stone HH: In discussion of Busuttil et al., Ann Surg 191:641, 1980
13. Schrock T, Blaisdell FW, Mathewson C: Management of blunt trauma to the liver and hepatic veins. Arch Surg 96:698, 1968
14. Williams CD, Brenowitz JB: Sequential aortic and inferior vena caval clamping for control of suprarenal vena caval injuries: case report. J Trauma 17:164, 1977
15. Schnug E: Ligation of the superior mesenteric vein. Surgery 14:610, 1973
16. Wilms EF, cited by Harsha WN, Orr TG: Ligation of superior mesenteric vein. Am J Surg 18:148, 1952

Norman M. Rich, James M. Salander
Paul M. Orecchia, Edward R. Gomez
Richard G. Kilfoyle, J. Leonel Villavicencio

Venous Injuries

Managing vascular emergencies due to venous injuries can be challenging, dramatic, and rewarding. While usually not as demanding as the initial management of hemorrhage from an arterial wound, bleeding from venous injuries can be more frustrating and difficult to control appropriately.[1] In addition to the initial management of venous injuries it is important to understand the pathophysiology that might result from interruption of a vein with the potential for acute venous hypertension and the potential for long-term sequelae associated with chronic venous insufficiency.[2] Statistically, the vast majority of injured veins that are treated are in the extremities. While some controversy persists there is increasing acceptance of the validity of a more aggressive approach to repairing larger caliber lower extremity veins.

The American military experience in the Vietnam War, particularly during the years 1965–1971, documented the importance of a more aggressive approach to the repair of lower extremity veins that were injured.[1] As had been documented repeatedly in many wars prior to the Vietnam War, large numbers of casualties with similar injuries treated over a relatively short period of time provided a unique opportunity for the evaluation of this new approach. Similar to the emphasis during the Korean Conflict in the early 1950s that arterial repairs could be performed successfully even under less than ideal conditions, the United States military surgical experience in Vietnam established the principles for repairing traumatized veins and provided successful results. The long-term clinical follow-up complemented by experimental research to better understand the pathophysiology associated with acute venous interruption was corroborative.[1,2]

In 1966 the Vietnam Vascular Registry was established at Walter Reed Army Medical Center to document the vascular injuries from the Vietnam War and to attempt to provide the long-term follow-up of patients who sustained vascular trauma among the American military.[3] Although there was some question about the true incidence of venous injuries and although there was more general interest in documenting the incidence of arterial injuries, the initial report from the Vietnam Vascular Registry included 718 vascular injuries with 194 venous injuries or 27 percent of the total. It was recognized that the figure was undoubtedly lower than the true incidence of venous injuries because many surgeons relegated venous injuries to minor significance. In an interim report from the Vietnam Vascular Registry in 1970 reviewing 1000 acute major arterial injuries in Vietnam, the incidence of concomitant venous injuries approached 38 percent.[4] The experience in Vietnam[3-8] as well as the follow-up efforts through the Vietnam Vascular Registry at Walter Reed Army Medical Center stimulated an additional study and report in 1974 that emphasized the need for a more aggressive approach to the repair of larger caliber lower extremity venous injuries.[9] This more aggressive approach was emphasized in an attempt to reduce the incidence of acute venous hypertension and to prevent the long-term sequelae associated with chronic venous hypertension. Corroborative evidence was documented in a subsequent report in 1976 involving 110 isolated popliteal venous injuries[10] and in 1977.[11,12] The Israel Military reported similar experience.[13]

After the initial civilian experience documented by Gaspar and Treiman in 1960,[14] there were sporadic civilian reports involving venous injuries. Danza in Uruquay published a case report of an interesting patient with combined lower extremity arterial and venous injuries with repair of both injuries utilizing autogenous greater saphenous vein.[15] As a result of the publication of the Vietnam experience, surgeons in the civilian sector have had more interest in repairing venous injuries than in the past and there have been increasing reports documenting success with the venous repairs.[16-21]

HISTORICAL NOTES

The development of vascular surgery in general has been documented in a number of excellent reviews; however, a special emphasis has been outlined recently regarding the historical aspects of direct venous reconstruction.[22] Travers and Guthrie are credited for closing successfully small venous lacerations in the early 19th century. Schede in 1882 is credited with the first successful lateral suture repair of a venous laceration in a human when he repaired a laceration of a femoral vein. He advocated this procedure in similar clinical situations. Experimentally, Eck, a Russian surgeon, made an important contribution in 1877 with the first successful experimental anastomosis of two vessels with lateral communication between the portal vein and the inferior vena cava. Kümmel performed the first clinical end-to-end anastomosis of a vein in 1889 in repairing the femoral vein. When Murphy in 1897 documented the first successful clinical end-to-end anastomosis of an artery, he also documented that he repaired a laceration in the common femoral vein. He contended that similar approaches should be utilized in the repair of veins as well as in arteries. Carrel and Guthrie are recognized for many outstanding contributions involving the basic principles of vascular surgery. They included suture of venous lacerations with arterial reconstructions.

World War I had a paucity of reports of the repair of injured veins despite the documented clinical and experimental evidence that existed at that time.[1] Goodman in 1918 wrote about the clinical use of lateral suture repair of venous lacerations when he described five patients with vascular injuries. Four of his patients had lateral suture repair of popliteal and superficial femoral veins. In the British Army in 1917 Makins relegated the management of injured veins to ligation with minimal importance placed on venous repair. He also proposed that the associated vein, which was uninjured, should be ligated when an arterial injury required ligation. It was not until World War II that it was demonstrated that there was no benefit from ligation of the concomitant vein with injured arteries which required ligation. During the Korean Conflict, 1950–1953, repair of injured veins was utilized in select patients with lateral suture repair being utilized. Hughes noted that most venous injuries were managed by ligation of the injured vein with resulting varying degrees of venostasis. He emphasized that several patients had severe venostasis resulting in limb loss following ligation of major veins that had been injured. He also reported that two investigators began to repair major veins to avoid complications and limb loss. Even though thrombosis occurred in some of the repairs there seemed to be fewer complications. The experience in Korea created a favorable situation for the increased interest in repairing injured veins in Vietnam.

During the Vietnam War there were two clinical reports that substantiated the earlier observations during the Korean experience involving the popliteal artery and the popliteal vein. In a retrospective study that evaluated 125 popliteal arterial repair failures, acute venous hypertension was noted as a significant factor leading to amputation in at least 19 patients and concomitant venous injury was documented in approximately 78 percent of the patients in the series.[8] Experience at the 12th Evacuation Hospital in Vietnam emphasized the early influence of repair of injured popliteal veins in the overall treatment of popliteal vascular injuries.[6] These two reports and the subsequent follow-up through the Vietnam Vascular Registry provided early clinical evidence of the value of repairing injured lower extremity veins.[1-12]

INCIDENCE AND ETIOLOGY

There is an increasing incidence of recognition and documentation of venous injuries, both in civilian experience and in military experience. Gaspar and Treiman in 1960 in Los Angeles were the first to document the civilian experience in management of a relatively large number of venous injuries.[14] In their experience in managing 228 patients with vascular injuries at the Los Angeles County General Hospital over a 10 year period, 22 percent, or 51 patients, had venous injuries. The superficial femoral vein was the most frequently injured vein (9 injuries) and the inferior vena cava and the internal jugular vein were each injured eight times. A representative example of more recent civilian experience comes from Hobson and co-workers in 1983 from Newark.[19] Among 262 major vascular injuries treated at the New Jersey University Hospital between January 1979 and February 1983, 31 percent of the injuries were venous (81 venous injuries). The femoral venous system was the most frequently injured: 30 percent of the total. Nine injuries involved the common femoral vein and 15 involved the superficial femoral vein. The mechanisms of injury involved gunshot wounds in 16 incidences, shotgun injuries in 4, blunt trauma in 2, a stab wound in 1 and a sharp object in 1. Agarwal and colleagues documented their experience in managing 115 civilian venous injuries at the Lincoln Hospital in New York City over a 7 year period between 1974 and 1980.[18] The internal and external jugular veins, femoral and iliac veins, and inferior vena cava accounted for 75 percent of the venous injuries. Gunshot wounds were responsible for 52 percent, stab wounds 36 percent, blunt trauma 7 percent, and shotgun wounds 5 percent of the venous injuries. In addition there are an increasing number of iatrogenic injuries to the venous system associated with invasive diagnostic and therapeutic techniques.

The incidence of venous injuries during armed conflict has been significant enough to warrant special attention.[1-12] Etiologic factors in armed conflicts include a variety of missile injuries involving bullets and fragments from a variety of exploding devices.

DIAGNOSIS

Frequently, arterial injury is more obvious than venous injury. Bright, red spurting blood from a wound, the presence or absence of distal pulses, warmth of an extremity, and developing neurological deficits all herald the possibility of arterial injury. Clinical detection of venous injury, however, may be more difficult to determine. Massive venous hemorrhage and massive hematomas associated with venous hemorrhage may be dramatic. There may be a steady flow of dark blood from a wound associated with venous injury or there may be relatively slow development of massive hematoma. Shock is common with major venous injuries. It should always be remembered that concomminant arterial injury may be part of the multiple injury complex and can contribute to exsanguinating hemorrhage.

Roentgenograms used routinely in evaluating injured patients have been of value in identifying offending missiles and/or associated fractures that may have caused venous trauma. Venography or phlebography remains the ultimate diagnostic tool in determining the location and the extent of venous injury with or without associated thrombus formation. Gerlock and associates provided appropriate emphasis and valuable information regarding phlebograms in patients with venous injuries in their civilian experience approximately 10 years ago.[23] Doppler ultrasonography has been useful and a practical diagnostic tool in evaluating patients with interrupted veins whether the cause was by trauma and/or thrombus formation. In acutely injured patients, however, the practical application of Doppler ultrasonography is limited. Impedance plethysmography, phleborrheography, and radionuclide studies all have similar limiting value in managing patients with multiple injuries; however, these modalities have been successful in diagnosing venous occlusions and they are particularly valuable in the long-term follow-up evaluations of patients with previous venous injuries.

PATHOPHYSIOLOGY

Pertinent experimental research deserves special notation because of the importance of understanding the pathophysiology associated with acute venous interruption as well as the long-term problems that can develop associated with chronic venous insufficiency. Haimovici and coworkers provided an excellent review in 1970 of the experimental and clinical evaluation of grafts in the venous system.[24] Investigators at Walter Reed Army Institute of Research augmented the information and emphasized the immediate decrease in femoral arterial flow as part of the evaluation of hemodynamics of acute venous occlusion in the experimental model. Femoral venous ligation in the canine hindlimb resulted in 50 percent to 75 percent reduction in femoral arterial flow with marked increases in femoral venous pressure and peripheral resistance. Hobson and coworkers provided extremely important additional information that these abnormal changes returned to baseline within approximately 72 hours.[25] Hiratzka and Wright in 1978 provided an additional current review of the experimental and clinical results of grafts in the venous system.[26] Numerous clinical observations were corroborated by valuable experimental information.

MANAGEMENT

Management of injured veins usually requires surgical intervention. Initially, control of hemorrhage from injured veins can be obtained by digital pressure or compressive bandages. This temporary control can also help prevent air from entering the venous system. General principles in managing patients with multiple injuries must be employed with appropriate supportive measures including infusion of whole blood and appropriate electrolyte solutions, and use of antibiotics. Patients with venous trauma should be treated by the principles of elective surgery to include the use of longitudinal incisions along the course of the injured vein that will provide adequate exposure for proximal and distal control of the vein to control the venous hemorrhage. Stabilization of fractures when associated with the injury must be obtained.

Recognizing the relatively high incidence of associated arterial injury with the injured vein, there is a frequent question regarding which vessel should be repaired initially. In the effort to minimize anoxia in a distal extremity, it is important to repair the injured artery as soon as possible. Nevertheless, in some instances, it may be more expeditious to repair the venous injury first, usually by lateral suture, to establish hemostasis and provide better exposure of the arterial injury. Copious irrigation with saline solution is helpful for both visualization and removal of foreign material. Adequate debridement is essential to remove nonviable tissue and remaining foreign material that might be a future nidus for infection. Digital pressure can be augmented by stick sponges to control venous bleeding. A proximal temporary tourniquet can provide simple, atraumatic control of hemorrhage. Vascular tapes encircling the vein both proximal and distal to the area of injury and partial occluding vascular clamps can be particularly useful in controlling hemorrhage from venous lacerations; the latter technique is particularly valuable in managing tangential injuries in large caliber veins.

Thrombus must be removed from the injured vein both proximally and distally prior to repair. Gentle pressure peripherally toward the area of venous injury can lead to the extrusion of thrombus. Utilization of a balloon catheter with gentle manipulation can also be helpful. There may be difficulty encountered with the balloon catheter during retrograde insertion because of competent venous valves and these valves should be protected. Heparin can be utilized, either locally or systemically to prevent additional propagation of thrombus, particularly if thrombus is present or if the venous occlusion is over a period of hours.

Meticulous surgical technique is mandatory during venous reconstruction.[27] Experimental and clinical experience have demonstrated repeatedly that meticulous technique is more critical in the management of injured veins than in the management of injured arteries. Fine synthetic suture on small needles minimizes bleeding from the repair site. If a continuous suture line is used, less tension is applied than in arterial anastomoses to prevent circular constriction. Leaving loops of a continuous line somewhat loose in venous repair may create a few leaks; however, bleeding usually stops with mild pressure for several minutes. Interrupted sutures may be preferred to continuous sutures. Autogenous venous patch grafts may be useful on occasion in preventing constriction at the repair site. If the venous repair cannot be accomplished by lateral suture, with or without patch, or by reconstruction with end-to-end venous anastomosis, the insertion of a vascular graft can be considered if the patient's condition is stable. Autogenous venous grafts, to date, are the only satisfactory grafts for the venous system.[1,2] The use of compilation grafts to create comparable diameter to the injured vein has been employed with increasing frequency and success.[19]

Completion venography in the operating room is an important adjunctive measure that should be utilized following venous reconstruction. Repeated venograms (phlebograms) are mandatory in the early post-operative period to determine the success of the repair. Adjunctive measures ranging from anticoagulants to temporary arteriovenous fistulas to sympathectomy have been advocated and utilized; however, additional experimental and clinical data will be required to determine the true efficacy of these various approaches.

RESULTS

The initial clinical evaluation of casualties in the Vietnam War provided data that supported the more aggressive approach in repairing injured lower extremity veins. First, the concerns about an increasing incidence of thrombophlebitis and pulmonary emboli were refuted.[1,5] Extensive experimental work at Walter Reed Army Institute of Research provided supporting evidence with a better understanding of the associated pathophysiology resulting from acute venous interruption. Additional clinical research was stimulated in turn to provide adequate clinical statistics. There was a unique opportunity that developed in the long-term follow-up of the Vietnam casualties through the Vietnam Vascular Registry involving 110 isolated popliteal venous injuries.[10] This important study emphasized that there was not an increased incidence of thrombophlebitis nor pulmonary emboli with attempted venous repair. Also, it demonstrated that there was significant edema in 51 percent of the patients who had ligation of the injured popliteal vein contrasted by only 13 percent of the patients with residual edema who had attempted venous repair of the popliteal vein. There was an additional favorable experience involving the 10 year follow-up of 51 Vietnam casualties who had larger caliber lower extremity venous injuries repaired with autogenous interposition venous grafts.[12] There was only one patient who developed transitory thrombophlebitis and no patients developed pulmonary emboli that could be detected clinically. A relatively low residual edema in approximately 12 percent of the patients existed following the attempted venous repairs.

Mullens and coworkers from Detroit in 1980 challenged the more aggressive approach in repairing injured veins.[28] Feliciano and colleagues from Houston in 1985 also emphasized that polytetrafluoroethylene (PTFE) grafts had limited value in repairing venous injuries.[29] Nevertheless, there are increasing reports of success in managing venous injuries by repair including those of Agarwal and colleagues,[18] Hardin and coworkers,[17] Hobson and colleagues,[19] and Jurkowich and coworkers.[30] Phifer and coworkers have documented extremely important long-term patency of venous repairs by venography as reported in 1985.[21]

FUTURE PROJECTIONS

Successful venous reconstruction remains an interesting and rewarding challenge in the management of injured veins, particularly those in the lower extremities. Despite the remaining controversy there is increasing evidence that the long-term sequelae frequently associated with chronic venous hypertension that may develop years after the initial venous interruption can be avoided by a more aggressive approach to repair of lower extremity venous injuries. Similar evidence does not exist in the upper extremity veins to the extent that has been documented in the lower extremities. Continued documentation of the management of venous injuries from various centers is essential as well as increased efforts to provide long-term follow-up for patients treated both by ligation of injured veins as well by venous repair. Additional information is needed to help guide future efforts in managing venous injuries.

REFERENCES

1. Rich NM, Spencer FC: Vascular Trauma. Philadelphia, WB Saunders Co., 1978
2. Hobson RW II, Rich NM, Wright CB (eds): Venous Trauma—Pathophysiology, Diagnosis and Surgical Management. Mount Kisco, Futura Publishing Company, Inc. 1983
3. Rich NM, Hughes CW: Vietnam Vascular Registry: A preliminary report. Surgery 62:218, 1969
4. Rich NM, Baugh JH, Hughes CW: Acute arterial injuries in Vietnam: 1,000 cases. J Trauma 10:359, 1970
5. Rich NM, Hughes CS, Baugh JH: Management of venous injuries. Ann Surg 171:724, 1970
6. Sullivan WG, Thornton FH, Baker LH, et al: Early influence of popliteal vein repair in the treatment of popliteal vessel injuries. Am J Surg 122:528, 1971
7. Rich NM, Sullivan WG: Clinical recanalization of an autogenous vein graft in the popliteal vein. J Trauma 12:919, 1972
8. Rich NM, Jarstfer BS, Geer RM: Popliteal artery repair failure: Causes and possible prevention. J Cardiovasc Surg 15:340, 1974
9. Rich, NM, Hobson RW II, Wright CB, Fedde CW: Repair of lower extremity venous trauma: A more aggressive approach required. J Trauma 14:639, 1974
10. Rich NM, Hobson RW, Collins GJ Jr, Andersen CA: The effect of acute popliteal venous interruption. Ann Surg 183:365, 1976
11. Rich NM, Collins GJ Jr, Andersen CA, et al: Venous trauma: Successful venous reconstruction remains an interesting challenge. Am J Surg 134:226, 1977
12. Rich NM, Collins GJ Jr., Andersen CA, McDonald PT: Autogenous venous interposition grafts in repair of major venous injuries. J Trauma 17:512, 1977
13. Schramek A, Hashmonai M, Farbstein J, Adler O: Reconstructive surgery in major vein injuries in the extremities. J Trauma 15:816, 1975
14. Gaspar MR, Treiman RL: The management of injuries to major veins. Am J Surg 100:171, 1960
15. Danza R, Mauro L, Arias J, et al: Reconstruction of the femoral–popliteal vessels with a double graft (arterial and venous) in severe injury of the limb. J Cardiovasc Surg 11:60, 1970
16. Blumoff RL, Proctor HJ, Johnson G: Recanalization of a saphenous vein interposition venous graft. J Trauma 21:407, 1981
17. Hardin WD, Adinolfi MF, O'Connell RC, Kerstein MD: Management of traumatic peripheral vein injuries, primary repair or vein ligation. Am J Surg 144:235, 1982
18. Agarwal N, Shah PM, Clauss RH, et al: Experience with 115 civilian venous injuries. J Trauma 22:827, 1982
19. Hobson RW II, Yeager RA, Lynch TG, et al: Femoral venous trauma: Techniques for surgical management and early results. Am J Surg 146:220, 1983
20. Brigham RA, Eddleman WL, Clagett GP, Rich NM: Isolated venous injury produced by penetrating trauma to the lower extremity. J Trauma 23:255, 1983
21. Phifer TJ, Gerlock AJ, Rich NM, McDonald JC: Long-term patency of venous repairs demonstrated by venography. J Trauma 25:342, 1985

22. Rich NM, Hobson RW II, Wright CB: Historical aspects of direct venous reconstruction, in Bergan JJ, Yao JTS (eds): Venous Problems. Chicago, Year Book Medical Publishers, 1978 pp 441–449
23. Gerlock AJ, Thal ER, Snyder WH III: Venography in penetrating injuries of the extremities. Am J Roentgenol 126:1023, 1976
24. Haimovici H, Hoffert PW, Zinicola N, et al: An experimental and clinical evaluation of grafts in the venous system. Surg Gynecol Obstet 131:1172, 1970
25. Hobson RW, Howard EW, Wright CB, et al: Hemodynamics of canine femoral venous ligation: Significance in combined arterial and venous injuries. Surgery 74:824, 1973
26. Hiratzka LF, Wright CB: Experimental and clinical results of grafts in the venous system: A current review. J Surg Res 25:542, 1978
27. Rich NM, Hobson RW II, Wright CB, Swan KG: Techniques of venous repair, in Swan KG, Hobson RW II, Reynolds DG, et al (eds): Venous Surgery in the Lower Extremities. St. Louis, Warren H Green, Inc, 1975
28. Mullins RJ, Lucas CE, Ledgerwood AM: The natural history following venous ligation for civilian injuries. J Trauma 20:737, 1980
29. Feliciano DV, Mattox KL, Graham JM, et al: Five-year experience with PTFE grafts in vascular wounds. J Trauma 25:75, 1985
30. Richardson JB Jr, Jurkovich GJ, Walker GT, et al: A temporary arteriovenous shunt (Scribner) in the management of traumatic venous injuries of the lower extremity. J Trauma 26:503, 1986

PART V I

Emergency Surgery in Arterial Aneurysm

Jesse E. Thompson
John J. Bergan

The Ruptured Abdominal Aortic Aneurysm

Management of the ruptured abdominal aortic aneurysm is emblematic of vascular emergencies and is the first procedure that comes to mind when physicians think of any vascular emergency. It is the hallmark of crisis management and is an important subject in education of emergency room physicians.

It is now just over 30 years since the first successful operations upon ruptured aneurysms were carried out by Bahnson, by Brock, by DeBakey and Cooley, and by Gerbode. Since that time, ruptured aneurysms have been treated more or less successfully on a wide scale.

It is recognized that aneurysms greater than 6 cm in diameter rupture more frequently than those that are smaller, but that small aneurysms do rupture.[1,2] While the age of the patient is an isolated consideration in management, it is never a contraindication to operation by itself. Emergency operation can be carried out with the expectation of success because of the acknowledged infrarenal location of more than 90 percent of ruptured aortic aneurysms. All of this is established and well known.

In the earliest days of aortic reconstruction, Cooley and DeBakey reported a survival time of between 10 hours and 9 days for patients with rupturing aneurysm.[3] Estes, writing from the Mayo Clinic just before the era of modern vascular surgery, found a survival time of 24 hours to as long as 6 months, acknowledging that all patients died because of rupture of the aneurysm.[4] Those observations by early workers have been corroborated by more modern observations using sophisticated techniques, including computed tomography. It is this latter technique that has allowed the observation of at least one aortic aneurysm that ruptured and spontaneously healed. The author of that article wondered, "Whether it is correct to operate upon a patient of this age who has concomitant disease or whether these patients should be allowed to live the last days of their life in more peaceful surroundings than an intensive care unit."[5]

Techniques of aortic imaging have allowed a definition of the expansion rate of abdominal aortic aneurysms. This varies somewhat according to the method used, but ranges around 5 mm per year. Thus, that aspect of the natural history of aortic aneurysms has been defined. On the other hand, all such studies show wide variation in expansion

Vascular Surgical Emergencies
ISBN 0-8089-1843-5

285

rates among the various aneurysms, with individual unpredictability in expansion to rupture occurring in each of the series.[6,7] This has led to universal advocacy of elective operation for aortic aneurysm.[8] As the mortality for elective operations has decreased, there has been increased justification for this approach. Thus, in the Dallas experience, the mortality in 432 patients operated upon from 1954 to 1961 was 17 percent but, in the next 5 years, the mortality was more than halved, to 7.4 percent, while in the next 10 years, it dropped to 6.4 percent despite increasing liberalization of indications for operation, especially in the elderly atherosclerotic patient.[9] Deaths in the early experience were due to technical complications, including intestinal gangrene, anastomotic leaks, and renal failure, whereas recent deaths have been largely cardiac and pulmonary, with the marked drop in mortality since 1978 occurring because of better knowledge of intensive care medicine.

Recent experience at the Massachusetts General Hospital suggests that patients under 70 years of age operated upon electively have a greater than 99 percent expectation of survival (2 deaths in 242 patients). Also, no deaths were noted in 67 patients with aneurysms measuring 5 cm or less in diameter.[10] Unfortunately, emergency operations for ruptured aneurysm remain a world-wide problem. The smaller aneurysms are not being diagnosed or, when noted, are simply observed. Surgery for ruptured aneurysms, which should be decreasing in frequency, continues to be an important part of the activities of every vascular service. For example, in a report from Milan, Italy, the very active vascular group there described experience with 832 patients with abdominal aortic aneurysms operated upon since 1965 and pointed out that the percent of ruptured aneurysms in each year's experience remained relatively uniform, ranging from 11 to 41 percent. In the most recent 5 years, this was still true (range, 15 to 39 percent).[11] Similarly, the report of Hernando et al from Madrid suggested that from 30 to 40 percent of their aortic aneurysm operations were performed on an emergency basis.[12] In an epidemiologic report on aortic aneurysms in Western Australia, it was noted that the diagnosis of abdominal aortic aneurysm had increased from 74.8 per 100,000 patients to 117.2 per 100,000 for men over 55 years of age, which was an increase of 56.7 percent.[13] Even more surprising was the increase in women from 17.5 per 100,000 to 33.9 per l00,000 for those over 55 years of age. During the 10 year period prior to that report, 478 patients had surgery for abdominal aortic aneurysms, 225 of which were elective with a 4.0 percent mortality, and 253 of which were emergency operations with a 31.2 percent mortality. Thus, the depressing theme of a continuing large proportion of ruptured aneurysms in a total aneurysm experience remains common.[14]

THE SYMPTOMATIC AORTIC ANEURYSM

The syndrome of expansion or rupture of an abdominal aortic aneurysm is similar to that of a renal stone. The patient will in general be a man of greater than average bodily habitus, complaining of back pain and flank pain radiating into the groin (Fig. 1). He may or may not give a history of syncope, but will show signs of decreased circulating blood volume, manifested by low blood pressure, tachycardia, and sweating. Johnson et al have pointed out that a decreased blood pressure or hematocrit reading suggest a decrease in blood volume and help to define a difference between expanding aneurysms and those that are ruptured.[15]

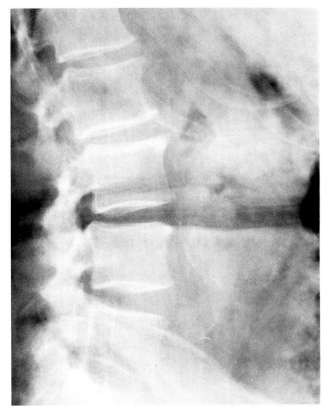

Fig. 1. In the emergency room, a lateral film of the abdomen as shown here may reveal the presence of a calcified aortic aneurysm wall and confirm the suspected diagnosis of ruptured aortic aneurysm.

Atypical presentations of rupture of abdominal aortic aneurysms are frequent. Among such atypical syndromes is acute femoral neuropathy with or without thigh ecchymosis. This signals the presence of a previously unsuspected ruptured aortic aneurysm.[16] Recognition of such femoral neuropathy caused by blood extravasation from the aneurysm rupture provides an opportunity for early exploration (Fig. 2). The neuropathy may manifest itself as pain in the hip, groin, or anterior thigh. Evidence of quadriceps weakness may be present. Sensation to pinprick is diminished over the anteromedial thigh. This neuropathy is due to compression of the femoral nerve between the iliacus and psoas muscles posteriorly as blood dissects inferiorly between those muscles and the fascial pockets overlying them. The nerve is compressed maximally as it passes under the inguinal ligament.[17]

Another atypical presentation is the association of ruptured abdominal aortic aneurysms with incarcerated inguinal hernia. This has been suggested by several observers, including Louras and Welch[18] and Merchant, Cafferata, and DePalma,[19] who correctly implicated cigarette smoking, increased collagenolytic activity, and decreased collagen strength in the aging population. This, combined with Busuttil, Abou-Zamzam, and

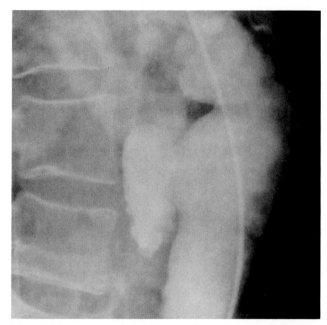

Fig. 2. Aortography is rarely done in patients with suspected rupture of an abdominal aortic aneurysm. This photograph of such an aortogram shows the retroperitoneal extravasation of contrast media from the aneurysm in its usual location below the renal arteries.

Machleder's observation of increased collagenase in the aortic wall in patients with large aneurysms, suggests that aortic wall dissolution in the face of aneurysm disease is more than just a mechanical stress/strain problem.[20]

CT SCANNING IN RUPTURED ANEURYSMS

Fortunately, typical or atypical presentation by patients with aortic aneurysms does allow accurate evaluation of the status of the aortic aneurysm by CT scanning. Only stable patients should be taken to the CT scanner for emergency evaluation. Patients who are hemodynamically unstable should not be subjected to such an examination but should, instead, be taken to the operating room. Nevertheless, a CT scan, when it can be done, may show an aortic aneurysm with a normally calcified wall, with or without concentric intraluminal thrombus. The images may show no extraaortic extravasation or a hyperlucent, thickened area of soft tissue anterior to the aneurysm, typical of an inflammatory aneurysm. A ruptured aortic aneurysm will show a soft tissue density outside the aortic wall (Fig. 3A), fracture of the calcified aortic wall, extravasation of contrast media outside the aortic wall, or penetration of the extraaortic hematoma into the leaves of the mesentery or retroaortic soft tissue (Fig. 3B).[21,22]

Visualization of the aorta and other abdominal structures by the CT allows accurate planning for surgical intervention. The CT scan may exclude the aneurysm as a source of the patient's complaint, or it may be possible to convert an emergency operation to an elective procedure, which will markedly decrease the operative risk.

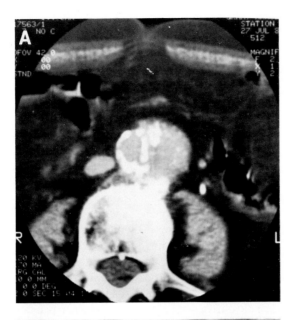

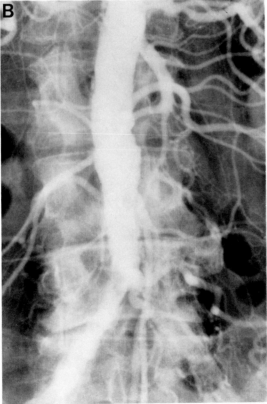

Fig. 3. (A) This CT scan shows the extraaortic soft tissue density that was found to be a hematoma from an extremely small aortic aneurysm. (B) The aortogram done in the patient with chronic contained rupture of an aortic aneurysm revealed only a small amount of dilation of the aorta and failed entirely to show the extraaortic hematoma.

289

EMERGENCY MANAGEMENT OF AORTIC RUPTURE

Typically, one-half of patients presenting to an emergency room with a ruptured aortic aneurysm have had back or flank pain symptoms for greater than six hours, and one-half of these will be in shock on arrival. Because this is true, it is necessary to have a prearranged plan of action. At least one, and preferably two, large intravenous cannulas should be placed in the upper extremities for immediate administration of crystalloid, blood, and medications. A central venous cannula should be inserted into the internal jugular or subclavian vein. The first blood sample should be sent to the laboratory for hematocrit and, more importantly, type and crossmatch for whole blood. While this is being done, the patient can be questioned and examined, the blood pressure recorded, and an estimation made of his cardiac performance and history. Next, a radial artery cannula should be placed for baseline blood gases and an electrocardiogram obtained from electrodes glued to the skin. Then, an indwelling Foley catheter should be inserted.

The typing and screening for major antibodies can be accomplished within 5 minutes and whole blood infused as necessary. If possible, however, it is best to wait the 1 hour required in most laboratories for specific crossmatching. Later, as specific transfusion products are used, the ratio of five units of packed cells accompanied by two units of fresh frozen plasma should be remembered to avoid coagulopathy. Should massive transfusion be required, a platelet count below 25,000/mm^3 should be accompanied by six packs of platelet transfusion.

As indicated above, the stable patient can be examined by computed tomography with an enormous amount of information being obtained from that study. However, the unstable patient must go directly to the operating theater.

OPERATIVE THERAPY

The surgical team must in every instance remind the anesthesiologist that the patient's condition will deteriorate with induction of general anesthesia. The skin preparation and draping must be done before induction of anesthesia and, with intravenous blood being infused, the midline abdominal incision can be made from xiphoid to pubis immediately after induction of the anesthesia. No attempt is made to control bleeding from the skin wound. Instead, the wound edges are packed with laparotomy pads and dry towels while a large, self-retaining retractor is inserted.

Over the years, as surgeons have become increasingly experienced at management of ruptured abdominal aortic aneurysms, control of the aorta proximal to the aneurysm has moved closer and closer to the lesion itself. Formerly, thoracotomy and control of the descending thoracic aorta was done. After 1960, Szilagyi's technique of control of the aorta inferior to the liver and medial to the stomach through an opening in the lesser sac was practiced. This approach is still used by some, who enlarge the exposure to the aorta by cutting the right crus of the diaphragm. However, proximal control of the aorta can be attained simply by reflecting the transverse colon and small bowel superiorly and to the right, opening the retroperitoneum by dividing the attachments of the third and fourth portions of the duodenum, carefully avoiding the inferior mesenteric vein but staying as high as possible above the retroperitoneal hematoma so as to enter the retroperitoneal space just below the left renal vein as it crosses the aorta. At this point, an infrarenal clamp can be placed in most instances. The distal iliac arteries are then clamped. With bleeding under control, the anesthesiologist can then proceed with the necessary further resuscitative measures.

There are alternative techniques that can be used occasionally. For example, a mechanical occluder can be placed on the aorta in the lesser sac or above the renal vein until a vascular clamp can be placed proximal to the site of the rupture.[23] In the usual situation of retroperitoneal contained hematoma, the aorta proximal to the aneurysm may be identified as being normal and can be encircled bluntly with a finger before being transversely crossclamped.

Adjuncts to successful aortic surgery in the emergency situation include autotransfusion devices, such as the cell saver, and systemic heparinization administered by the anesthesiologist prior to crossclamping of the aorta. Some surgeons, notably Crawford, avoid systemic heparinization to reduce bleeding, while others use local injection of heparin into the distal iliac arteries during occlusion. Should it be possible in a well-controlled situation, identification of the iliac arteries can be done and the distal arteries crossclamped before manipulation of the aorta and aneurysm. This maneuver will decrease the tendency for atheroembolization to occur.

Once proximal and distal control are obtained, the operation proceeds much as in an elective procedure. The aorta is incised, intrasaccular thrombus evacuated, and lumbar vessels suture-ligated. Careful attention is paid to the inferior mesenteric artery, which may be seen to be backbleeding in the aortic sac; if so, the orifice of this vessel is suture-ligated. Graft replacement by tube or Y-grafting is then accomplished. Should massive pelvic aneurysms be present involving the internal iliac arteries, with or without common iliac aneurysms, it may be necessary to take the reconstruction distally to the femoral arteries, and if this is done with proximal pelvic arteries excluded, the inferior mesenteric artery should be implanted on the Dacron tube.

Woven Dacron grafts are favored in the emergency situation over knitted grafts because they are less porous. Should there be concern about bleeding through the interstices of the graft, a woven graft can be preclotted and then flashed in an autoclave for 3 minutes. The resulting charred graft is esthetically unappealing but water-tight.

Declamping to restore distal circulation is done carefully, opening each of the vascular beds in concert with the anesthesiologist so that no hypotension occurs during this time. Crystalloid requirements during this procedure range around 2000 ml and should be supplemented by replacement of colloids, ml for ml.

ATYPICAL SITES OF RUPTURE

While rupture of an abdominal aortic aneurysm is catastrophic, an even more dangerous situation occurs when the confined retroperitoneal rupture perforates freely into the peritoneal cavity. In such a situation, the mortality of surgical treatment approaches 75 percent. It is in such a desperate situation of free intraperitoneal blood loss, profound shock, and a totally obscured retroperitoneum that the aorta must be controlled remote from the retroperitoneal hematoma. In this situation, it is wise to reflect the liver upward, the stomach downward, and enter the lesser omental sac directly over the pulsating aorta, compressing it vigorously against the spinal column until appropriate control of the aorta can be gained. When this is done and the small bowel and colon reflected upward, the aortic aneurysm can be entered directly and an intraluminal balloon inflated to obtain proximal control. A 30 ml Fogarty catheter has been used in such a situation effectively.[24,25] Once proximal control of the hemorrhage is assured, then the aortic wall can be dissected cleanly inferior to the renal arteries and an infrarenal clamp placed so as to resume renal artery perfusion.

Conversely, rupture of the aortic aneurysm into the inferior vena cava drops the mortality appreciably and provides the safest situation in which emergency aortic aneurysm surgery can be performed. When an aortic aneurysm ruptures into the vena cava, 90 percent of the patients will present a picture of high output cardiac failure combined with distension of thigh and leg veins and edema of the lower extremities bilaterally. Priapism has also been an astounding feature of this condition, as has a machinery murmur noted on auscultation of the abdomen. A widened pulse pressure and reduced diastolic pressure are seen in more than one-half of the cases. The decompensated congestive failure must be treated rapidly, and one should not be surprised to find hematuria, rectal bleeding, and even renal failure. Despite the severity of these findings, effective early treatment of such aortocaval fistulas is very rewarding, with a return of renal function to normal and a cure of the congestive cardiac failure in most cases.[26-29]

There are several precautions to be exercised in treating aortocaval fistulas. The first is prevention of pulmonary embolization from intrasaccular thrombi. Thus, the aorta is clamped proximally and distally. With the patient heparinized, the aortic aneurysmal sac is entered directly and its contents evacuated prior to manipulation of the cava. Frequently, there are multiple fistulas present in the thinned-out aortic wall, and each of these must be controlled from within the aortic aneurysm. Occasionally, a vena cava fistula will be noted in elective aortic aneurysm resection without any prior symptoms being present.[30]

When the University of Milan experience with ruptured aortic aneurysms was reviewed, the site of rupture of 226 abdominal aortic aneurysms was recorded. Retroperitoneal rupture occurred in 85.3 percent. Caval ruptures occurred in 5.7 percent and produced the lowest mortality of surgical reconstruction. Although enteric rupture of the aneurysm occurred in only 1.7 percent, it was associated with a 50 percent mortality.[31]

The enteric rupture of an aortic aneurysm is referred to as a primary aortoduodenal fistula, despite the fact that the vascular-enteric communication is clearly secondary to an aortic aneurysm. The term secondary aortoenteric fistula has been reserved for instances of erosion of an aortic graft into the intestine. Contrary to the left posterior rupture of aortic aneurysms into the retroperitoneum, it seems that primary aortoenteric fistulas occur anteriorly and on the right side of the aneurysm. Early in the development of this syndrome, patients will experience small amounts of gastrointestinal bleeding. These herald bleeds are followed by a more massive bleeding episode. Early, it is thought that there is an erosion of the intestinal mucosa without penetration of the aortic stream into the intestinal wall. Later, as infection supervenes, the aortic wall will undergo dissolution, and free rupture of the aneurysm into the intestine with fatal exsanguination will occur. Nearly all patients with primary aortoenteric fistula will have hematemesis or melena, but only an occasional patient will have flank pain or renal colic.

In the situation of primary aortoenteric fistula, it is perfectly acceptable to detach the duodenum surgically, repair the hole in the duodenum by transverse suture or even Roux-en-Y anastomosis if the hole is large, and then turn to reconstitution of the aortic stream with a Dacron graft. According to Sweeney and Gadacz's 1983 review, 21 of 33 patients reported in the literature survived such a repair of the intestinal tract with aortic reconstruction.[32] Alternatively, some authors have suggested an extraanatomic reconstruction of the aorta. However, effective retroperitoneal irrigation of antibiotic solution and administration of intravenous antibiotics for a period of time should succeed in allowing successful, one-stage operation for the primary aortoenteric fistula.

RESULTS OF TREATMENT OF RUPTURED ABDOMINAL AORTIC ANEURYSMS

While it is appropriate to discuss the mortality of most surgical operations, it may be that with ruptured abdominal aortic aneurysms one should speak of survival rather than mortality. During the early years or aortic surgery, operative mortality rates for ruptured aneurysms averaged well above 50 percent in most reported series. In the last 10 years, results have generally improved, ranging from 15 percent to 68 percent with a number of series reporting operative mortality in the 30–40 percent range.[33] In a series from Dallas, operative mortality for the first 25 years (92 cases) was 52.2 percent or a survival rate of 47.8 percent. In the last 4 years (22 cases) mortality has been 31.8 percent, or a survival of 68.2 percent.[34]

Recent reports have attempted to identify those factors that affected the outcome of surgical treatment of ruptured abdominal aortic aneurysm. In a review of the Cleveland Metropolitan experience, it was found that when only a small intramural hemorrhage or hematoma was present, the mortality was 17 percent; when the retroperitoneal hematoma was more extensive, the mortality rate was 43 percent; and if an incorrect diagnosis was made and a cardiopulmonary or cerebral event was suspected, the mortality was 75 percent.[33] Such an incorrect initial diagnosis led to delay of as much as 2½ days from admission to the hospital to operation. It is clear that success of operation is inversely related to the time interval between onset of symptoms and performance of surgery.

In another report, the University of Michigan group identified lengthy operation ($>$ 400 minutes), 100 percent mortality; persistent hypotension ($>$ 110 minutes), 88 percent mortality; blood loss $>$ 11,000 ml, 75 percent mortality; blood transfusions $>$ 17 units, 68 percent mortality; fluid administration $>$ 7,000 ml, 70 percent mortality; and a blood pressure $<$ 100 mmHg at the conclusion of the operation, 88 percent mortality.[35] Those authors arrived at the depressing conclusion that, "In general, these factors cannot be controlled by the surgeon and future significant reduction in the operative mortality rate may not be possible."

In taking a different approach to the problem, however, the Michigan group looked for factors that were associated with the rupture of small aortic aneurysms and identified some surprising elements. They observed that obstructive pulmonary disease, aneurysm size, and diastolic hypertension suggested early rupture of small aortic aneurysms.[36] They pointed out that 5-year rupture rates of small aneurysms varied from 2 percent when these risk factors were absent to 100 percent when all 3 factors were present.

Scobie and Masters' experience at Ottawa is typical of the application of early operation to elective aneurysm resection. They reported a decrease in their elective aneurysm mortality from 12 percent to 1.8 percent, but also indicated that for ruptured aneurysms, the mortality remained at an unfortunate rate of 45 to 52 percent.[37] Other reports from the community experience in Youngstown, Ohio,[38] Harlingen, Texas,[39] and Tacoma, Washington[40] also point out the need to avoid delay in operation, avoid allowing the patient to proceed into a shock state, and the dangers of an erroneous diagnosis.

A report from Manchester, U.K., detailed causes of death in 180 cases of ruptured aneurysm.[41] Eighteen percent died before operation could be carried out, 8 percent proved inoperable, and a further 10.5 percent died before operation could be completed. Overall mortality was 75 percent while operative mortality for those in whom a graft was completed was 60 percent. The most significant preoperative features influencing survival were a systolic BP < 80 mmHg on admission and a history of hypertension, angina or myocardial infarct. Mortality increased with increasing age. Administration of fresh frozen plasma preoperatively significantly increased survival.

With these facts in mind, it is not surprising to note the suggestions of the UCLA vascular group, which identified four problems associated with treatment of ruptured abdominal aortic aneurysms.[42] These were failure to proceed with elective aneurysmorrhaphy in patients with known abdominal aortic aneurysms, error in diagnosis of aortic rupture that led to delay in moving the patient from the admitting room to the operating room, intraoperative technical error that produced venous injury, and undue delay in anesthetic induction.

RENAL VEIN DIVISION ASSOCIATED WITH AORTIC ANEURYSM RUPTURE

Because of the difficulties in exposing the proximal aorta above a massive retroperitoneal hematoma, it is tempting to divide the renal vein with impunity. In the elective situation, it is clearly possible to divide the renal vein without deterioration of renal function. This was shown by the Chaim Sheba Medical Center group, which compared 15 patients with left renal vein division to 28 patients in whom the left renal vein was not ligated.[43] In these two groups of patients, there was no difference in postoperative complications, highest postoperative and predischarge levels of plasma urea and creatinine. On the other hand, the Uppsala group found that postoperative renal complications were frequent after left renal ligation.[44] A sustained increase in postoperative serum creatinine was found in six patients, one of whom had a total loss of left kidney function. Left nephrectomy was necessary in two other patients to control bleeding from the kidney. Two other patients had subinfarction or acute hemorrhagic infarction of the kidney. That group suggested that a restricted application of left renal vein ligation during aortic surgery should be recommended.

ISCHEMIC COLITIS AFTER RUPTURED ABDOMINAL AORTIC ANEURYSM RESECTION

Because patients with ruptured aortic aneurysms are those with prolonged tissue hypoperfusion and because prevention of atheromatous distal embolization to extremities or intestine may be incomplete, the colon becomes especially vulnerable to ischemic necrosis. Thrombosis of collateral colonic vessels may occur during the hypotensive event, and the ischemic mucosa produced by such clotting may be susceptible to bacterial penetration from intestinal flora. Reimplantation of the inferior mesenteric artery is increasingly encouraged in cases of elective aneurysm repair, and similarly, this problem is obtaining increased attention among surgeons interested in perfecting aortic surgery.

Postoperative ischemic colitis may be manifest by abdominal sepsis or by diarrhea, which may be either frankly bloody or produce guaiac-positive stools. Diarrhea, fever, increased abdominal girth, and septicemia are the findings that should alert the surgeon to immediate fiberoptic endoscopy. The suspected diagnosis can be confirmed if an ischemic, ulcerated, edematous mucosa is seen. Computed tomography can be used to demonstrate submucosal thickening and irregular narrowing of the colonic lumen. If a barium enema is obtained at this time, characteristic "thumb-printing" of the colonic margins, the classic sign of ischemic colitis, will be seen.[45] Necrotic colon should be resected immediately in order to prevent development of multiple-organ failure from associated sepsis. Antibiotic therapy is crucial, and the previously-placed aortic graft should not be exposed during the colonic operation.

CONCLUSION

Although the success of elective operation for abdominal aortic aneurysm has been proven and it has been shown clearly that such operation extends an individual's life expectancy, the problem of rupture of a neglected or missed abdominal aortic aneurysm remains with us in vascular surgery. Paradoxically, in highly-developed medical centers, where vascular surgery is practiced under almost ideal circumstances, the number of ruptured aneurysms seen per year has gradually diminished. In less medically-sophisticated surroundings, such as nonteaching hospitals in small communities, the ruptured abdominal aortic aneurysm remains a significant emergency problem. Because this is true, a surgical plan of action must be formulated before the emergencies occur, and this plan must be upgraded periodically to incorporate technical advances in clinical medicine. With regard to the ruptured aortic aneurysm, these include the liberal use of CT scanning of the abdomen, the application of cell-saving autotransfusion devices in surgery, and practice of the best possible intensive care medicine in the postoperative period. However, the problems surrounding the ruptured aortic aneurysm will not be solved until physicians taking care of an aging population recognize that prevention of aortic aneurysm rupture can be accomplished by early prescription of elective aneurysm resection.

REFERENCES

1. Darling RC: Ruptured arteriosclerotic abdominal aortic aneurysms—A pathologic and clinical study. Amer J Surg 188:404, 1978
2. Gore I, Hirst AE Jr: Arteriosclerotic aneurysms of the abdominal aorta: A review. Progr Cardiovasc Dis 26:113, 1973
3. Cooley DA, DeBakey ME: Ruptured aneurysm of the abdominal aorta. Excision and homograft replacement. Postgrad Med 16:334, 1954
4. Estes DE: Abdominal aortic aneurysm: A study of 102 cases. Circulation 2:258, 1950
5. Christenson JT, Norgren L, Ribbe E, et al: A ruptured aortic aneurysm that "spontaneously healed." J Cardiovasc Surg 25:571, 1984
6. Delin A, Ohlsen H, Swedenborg J: Growth rate of abdominal aortic aneurysms as measured by computed tomography. Br J Surg 72:530, 1985
7. Bernstein EF, Chan EL: Abdominal aortic aneurysm in high-risk patients: Outcome of selective management based on size and expansion rate. Ann Surg 200:255, 1984
8. Darling RC, Brewster DC: Elective treatment of abdominal aortic aneurysms. World J Surg 4:661, 1980
9. Thompson JE, Hollier LH, Patman RD, et al: Surgical management of abdominal aortic aneurysms. Factors influencing mortality and morbidity—A 20 year experience. Ann Surg 181:654,1975

10. McCabe CJ, Coleman WS, Brewster DC: The advantage of early operation for abdominal aortic aneurysm. Arch Surg 116:1025, 1981

11. Ruberti U, Scorza R, Biasi G, Odero A: Nineteen year experience on the treatment of aneurysms of the abdominal aorta: A survey of 832 consecutive cases. J Cardiovasc Surg 26:547, 1985

12. Serrano Hernando FJ, Martin Paredero VM, Del Rio A, et al: Abdominal aortic aneurysms. Results of surgical treatment. J Cardiovasc Surg 26:539, 1985

13. Castleden WM, Mercer JC, Paton R, et al: Abdominal aortic aneurysms in Western Australia: Descriptive epidemiology and patterns of rupture. Br J Surg 72:109, 1985

14. Crowson M, Fielding JWL, Black J, et al: Acute gastrointestinal complications of infrarenal aortic aneurysm repair. Br J Surg 71:825, 1984

15. Johnson G Jr, McDevitt NB, Proctor HJ, et al: Emergent or elective operation for symptomatic abdominal aortic aneurysm. Arch Surg 115:51, 1980

16. Merchant RF Jr, Cafferata HT, DePalma RG: Ruptured aortic aneurysm seen initially as acute femoral neuropathy. Arch Surg 117:811, 1982

17. Owens ML: Psoas weakness and femoral neuropathy: Neglected signs of retroperitoneal hemorrhage from ruptured aneurysm. Surgery 91:363, 1982

18. Louras JC, Welch JP: Masking of ruptured abdominal aortic aneurysm by incarcerated inguinal hernia. Arch Surg 119:331, 1984

19. Merchant RF Jr, Cafferata HT, DePalma RG: Pitfalls in the diagnosis of abdominal aortic aneurysm. Amer J Surg 142:756, 1981

20. Busuttil RW, Abou-Zamzam AM, Machleder HI: Collagenase activity of the human aorta: A comparison of patients with and without abdominal aortic aneurysms. Arch Surg 115:1373, 1980

21. Johnson WC, Gale ME, Gerzof SG, et al: The role of computed tomography in symptomatic aortic aneurysms. Surg Gynecol Obstet 162:49, 1986

22. Gomes MN, Wallace RB: Present status of abdominal aorta imaging by computed tomography. J Cardiovas Surg 26:1, 1985

23. Conn J Jr, Trippel OH, Bergan JJ: A new atraumatic aortic occluder. Surgery 64:1158, 1968

24. Hyde GL, Sullivan DM: Fogarty catheter tamponade of ruptured abdominal aortic aneurysms. Surg Gynecol Obstet 154:197, 1982

25. Hardy JD, Williamson JW: Management of the ruptured abdominal aortic aneurysm—Immediate control of the proximal aorta. World J Surg 5:553, 1981

26. Clowes AW, DePalma RG, Botti RE, et al: Management of aortocaval fistula due to abdominal aortic aneurysm. Amer J Surg 137:807, 1979

27. Nennhaus HP, Javid H: The distinct syndrome of spontaneous abdominal aorta-caval fistula. Amer J Med 44:464, 1968

28. Reckless JPD, McCall I, Taylor GW: Aorto-caval fistulae: An uncommon complication of abdominal aortic aneurysms. Br J Surg 59:461, 1972

29. Vanderveer JB, Robinson HJ, Blake AD: Abdominal aortic aneurysm with vena caval fistula. Arch Intern Med 114:551, 1974

30. Weinbaum FI, Riles TS, Imparato AM: Asymptomatic vena caval fistulization complicating abdominal aortic aneurysm. Surgery 96:126, 1984

31. Miani S, Mingazzini P, Piglionica R, et al: Influence of the rupture site of abdominal aortic aneurysms with regard to postoperative survival rate. J Cardiovasc Surg 25:414, 1984

32. Sweeney MS, Gadacz TR: Primary aortoduodenal fistula: Manifestation, diagnosis, and treatment. Surgery 96:492, 1984

33. Hoffman M, Avellone JC, Plecha FR, et al: Operation for ruptured abdominal aortic aneurysms: A community-wide experience. Surgery 91:597, 1982

34. Thompson JE, Talkington CM, Garrett WV, Smith BL: Unpublished data, 1986

35. Wakefield TW, Whitehouse WM Jr, Wu SC, et al: Abdominal aortic aneurysm rupture: Statistical analysis of factors affecting outcome of surgical treatment. Surgery 91:586, 1982

36. Cronenwett JL, Murphy TF, Zelenock GB, et al: Actuarial analysis of variables associated with rupture of small abdominal aortic aneurysms. Surgery 98:472, 1985

37. Scobie TK, Masters RG: Changing factors influencing abdominal aortic aneurysm repair. J Cardiovasc Surg 23:309, 1982

38. Vidal J, Hennessy VL Jr, Turner JJ: Results of operations upon abdominal aortic aneurysms at a community hospital. Surg Gynecol Obstet 153:363, 1981

39. Lawler M Jr: Aggressive treatment of ruptured abdominal aortic aneurysm in a community hospital. Surgery 95:38, 1984

40. Bodily KC, Buttorff JD: Ruptured abdominal aortic aneurysm. The Tacoma experience. Amer J Surg 149:580, 1985

41. Lambert ME, Baguley P, Charlesworth D: Ruptured abdominal aortic aneurysms. J Cardiovasc Surg 27:256, 1986

42. Hiatt JCG, Barker WF, Machleder HI, et al: Determinants of failure in the treatment of ruptured abdominal aortic aneurysm. Arch Surg 119:1264, 1984

43. Adar R, Rabbi I, Bass A, et al: Left renal vein division in abdominal aortic aneurysm operations. Effect on renal function. Arch Surg 120:1033, 1985

44. Rastad J, Almgren B, Bowald S, et al: Renal complications to left renal vein ligation in abdominal aortic surgery. J Cardiovasc Surg 25:432, 1984

45. Welling RE, Roedersheimer LR, Arbaugh JJ, Cranley JJ: Ischemic colitis following repair of ruptured abdominal aortic aneurysm. Arch Surg 120:1368, 1985

Walter J. McCarthy, John J. Bergan
James S.T. Yao, William R. Flinn

Rapidly Expanding Anastomotic Aneurysms

Aneurysms were not only known to Antyllus in the First Century BC, but he also correctly differentiated the characteristics of true and false aneurysms. Furthermore, Hippocrates recognized that false aneurysms could be iatrogenic as a consequence of blood letting. In the modern era, iatrogenic vascular injury is also common as is the appearance of anastomotic false aneurysm following arterial reconstruction. These are caused by failure of bonding of a vascular prosthesis to the arterial wall.

Rapidly expanding anastomotic aneurysms form a small, but important, subset of such anastomotic aneurysms. Most occur in the femoral position following aortofemoral bypass. Characteristically, these appear years after the operative event. Typically, they increase in size slowly and this allows elective repair. They are usually not septic in origin but are related to degeneration of the host artery, which becomes unable to prevent the vascular suture from cutting through its wall. Occasionally, however, a rapidly expanding anastomotic false aneurysm develops. This becomes a surgical emergency, especially in the early postoperative period when it is most commonly related to suture failure or wound sepsis. Similarly, sudden, rather than gradual expansion of an anastomotic aneurysm in the late postoperative course may occur. This chapter discusses the causes of stable and rapidly expanding anastomotic aneurysms and highlights the surgical approach to those that are rapidly expanding.

MECHANISMS OF ANEURYSM FORMATION

Expanding or ruptured anastomotic aneurysms and chronic stable anastomotic enlargements share the same etiology but have differing rates of progression and natural history.

Chronic Stable Anastomotic Aneurysms

Relatively stable anastomotic aneurysms are most frequently noticed 2 to 6 years following aortobifemoral prosthetic reconstruction and are usually related to degeneration of the host arterial tissue.[1] The concept of arterial degeneration is somewhat circumstantial in that disruption of a prosthetic arterial anastomosis implies either a defect of the suture, a failure of the prosthetic material, or a weakness in the native artery.[3] Several carefully reported series suggest that with most modern era (post silk) sutures, the anastomotic suture line remains intact, the prosthetic material is not dilated, but a portion of the affected anastomosis has separated from the host artery. Gaylis suggests that in 23 of his 25 cases, arterial degeneration was the implicated etiology with only 2 suture failures being detected.[3] McCabe noticed that of 69 femoral anastomotic aneurysms repaired, 10 recurred once and 1 recurred twice.[4] Furthermore, it is known that patients with one femoral aneurysm are likely to develop a femoral aneurysm in the contralateral groin or at the proximal aortic anastomosis. A recent report of anastomotic aneurysms in 36 patients identified 12 individuals with 2 aneurysms related to their aortobifemoral graft and 2 patients with aneurysms at all 3 anastomoses.[1] All were noninfected grafts. This evidence supports, but does not prove, the concept of arterial degeneration as the cause of most anastomotic false aneurysms. The exact etiopathology has yet to be fully clarified.

It is well known that the femoral anastomosis of an aortofemoral bypass is the most common site of anastomotic false aneurysm formation. These occur following 1–3 percent of all aortofemoral procedures.[5] Other anastomotic sites, including the proximal and distal anastomoses of femoropopliteal bypasses, only rarely develop anastomotic aneurysms.[1] Mechanical tension on the femoral anastomosis with chronic intermittent hyperextension of the thigh may contribute to the eventual suture line disruption. It has also been suggested that femoral endarterectomy at the time of initial aortofemoral bypass predisposes to anastomotic false aneurysm.[4] The different tissue bonding characteristics of woven and knitted Dacron grafts have prompted comparison of their aneurysm formation potential. Although there is some controversy, Christensen and Bernatz found a similar incidence of false aneurysm when they compared knitted and woven grafts.[8]

Suture disruption is often mentioned as a cause of false aneurysm formation but actually plays a minor role since the abandonment of silk and polyethylene suture in vascular surgery. Recent reports of aortobifemoral grafts sutured with braided Dacron or polypropylene indicate only a 4–10 percent incidence of suture-related mishaps in all anastomotic false aneurysms.[1] In contrast, evaluation of femoral anastomoses constructed with silk suture or polyethylene suture placed before 1970 emphasized suture failure as an important factor. In one series, 24 of 34 false aneurysms were related to suture failure.[7] Fortunately, neither silk nor polyethylene suture are commonly employed in modern vascular surgery.

Anastomotic sepsis must always be considered at the site of a suture line disruption. Intraoperative cultures for aerobic and anaerobic bacteria are mandatory at the time of all anastomotic false aneurysm repairs. Even chronic, apparently sterile false aneurysms may harbor indolent bacteria. Recent series suggest between 3 and 10 percent of chronic anastomotic aneurysms are septic.[1] Towne suggests that Staphylococcus epidermidis is an organism of particular importance to the development of anastomotic aneurysms. Positive intraoperative cultures mandate extended antibiotic therapy and may necessitate graft removal.

Rapidly Expanding Anastomotic False Aneurysms

Rapidly expanding false aneurysms constitute a surgical emergency. Immediately postoperatively rapid formation of a tense hematoma in a groin or neck incision implies suture failure until proven otherwise. Although monofilament polypropylene suture is generally durable, direct manipulation with surgical instruments can initiate suture fracture with great loss of tensile strength. Suture failure in the early postoperative period requires a prompt return to the operating room to staunch the hemorrhage. Suture failure after carotid endarterectomy is a particular example. The combination of airway compression, lost cerebral perfusion and hypovolemic shock may produce neurologic deficit.

Early anastomotic separation related to sepsis usually occurs between the first and fourth postoperative weeks. Actual suture line dehiscence is usually heralded by wound erythema or disruption, with purulent drainage or lymphatic discharge. Often wounds are known or suspected to be infected based on intraoperative cultures. Potentially exsanguinating hemorrhage is usually preceded by a relatively innocuous herald bleed. Arterial bleeding or sudden hematoma formation from a wound suspected to be infected demands operative exploration.

Septic anastomotic aneurysms are managed with the same principles as septic grafts. All foreign body must be removed and revascularization, if required, must not transgress the infected field.

Extreme mechanical tension on the arterial graft anastomoses occasionally precipitates anastomotic dehiscence in the early postoperative patient.[9] Individuals with aortofemoral reconstructions rarely hyperextend their grafts in the first few weeks postoperatively due to relative immobility. Dacron grafts exhibit some elasticity and if properly placed, automatically limit anastomotic tension. In contrast, axillofemoral reconstructions, using relatively nonelastic PTFE graft material, are uniquely susceptible to extreme positional tension. A graft length that seems adequate intraoperatively may be restricting with the patient's shoulder in a hyperabducted position.[9] The Northwestern University experience includes two axillary anastomotic disruptions in the early postoperative period under these circumstances. In one case, the PTFE anastomosis was simply separated at the axillary artery. In another, the PTFE graft material was severed across the anastomotic hood by a patient performing chinning exercises in bed postoperatively. Both these disruptions produced a rapidly expanding hematoma that was contained by the skin closure and could be repaired directly. Adequate graft length with enough redundancy to allow full shoulder motion seems mandatory to prevent this early complication. Placing the axillary anastomosis in the extreme medial position also limits the graft motion.[10]

Rapid expansion of an anastomotic dehiscence is less likely in the late postoperative period because the normal surrounding fibrous capsule temporarily contains any hematoma.[11] Nevertheless, occasionally a chronic stable anastomotic false aneurysm expands rapidly in the femoral area causing skin erosion leading to infection and/or external rupture and exsanguination. A sudden increase in size of an anastomotic aneurysm in the late postoperative period may suggest sepsis at the suture line. Infected false aneurysms tend to occur proximal to the time of operation, usually occurring between 4 and 8 months.[12]

Primary arteriopathy may also be responsible for delayed rapid expansion of an anastomotic aneurysm. This is generally reported after the repair of atherosclerotic artery but arterial disruption in Marfan's disease[14] and also in Behçet's arteritis has been described.[15]

The proximal anastomosis of an aortofemoral reconstruction only occasionally becomes aneurysmal in the late postoperative period. The mass effect may cause symptoms similiar to a rupturing abdominal aortic aneurysm or, more commonly, the lesion is asymptomatic. Knox reports six of eight proximal anastomotic aneurysms presenting with aortoenteric fistula without previous symptoms. All six of those patients died of the condition.[2] Olson reports four cases of proximal aortic anastomotic aneurysm presenting with upper GI bleeding all of whom also died.[17] These reports and others emphasize the need to investigate diagnostically the proximal aorta whenever femoral false aneurysms are detected.

DIAGNOSIS OF ANASTOMOTIC ANEURYSMS

A palpable mass is the hallmark of anastomotic aneurysms and was detected in 87 percent of patients with chronic, stable anastomotic false aneurysms in one large series.[1] The detection of a rapidly expanding anastomotic aneurysm is usually not subtle. Such expanding aneurysms in the femoral triangle often cause nerve compression with femoral radiation down the anterior thigh (Fig. 1). Occasionally, common femoral vein compression supervenes and a deep venous thrombosis is suspected. Proximal aortic anastomotic aneurysms may cause massive upper or lower GI bleeding as indicated above. Such intestinal bleeding after aortobifemoral graft placement must always be considered an anastomotic complication until proven otherwise.[17]

Objective diagnostic evaluation of anastomotic false aneurysms should include an arteriogram if the patient is stable (Fig. 2). This may demonstrate additional anastomotic false aneurysms and helps to define the proximal and distal native arterial anatomy. Infusion CT scanning has considerable utility and will detect anastomotic aneurysms unnoticed by arteriography (Fig. 3). It cannot be too strongly emphasized that the proximal anastomosis of an aortofemoral graft must be examined after the detection of a femoral false aneurysm.

B-mode scanning, though less precise than CT, is useful to differentiate small anastomotic false aneurysms from lymph collections and hematomas in the postoperative period following aortofemoral bypass. Scanning, however, is of little value in the face of rapid aneurysm expansion. B-mode scanning is also useful following sudden aortofemoral graft limb occlusion and will identify femoral false aneurysm formation as the cause of graft failure.

SURGICAL APPROACH TO RAPIDLY EXPANDING ANASTOMOTIC FALSE ANEURYSMS

Early Occurrence

In the immediate postoperative period, rapid hematoma formation usually implies suture failure and requires an immediate return to the operating room as suggested above. Rapid proximal and distal arterial control will allow primary repair of the failed anastomosis either by reestablishing the suture line or by adding additional graft length to correct an early inadequacy. Dehiscence of a septic anastomosis in the early postoperative period presents a more difficult problem. The prosthetic graft must be removed and the ischemic region reperfused if necessary by extraanatomic bypass.

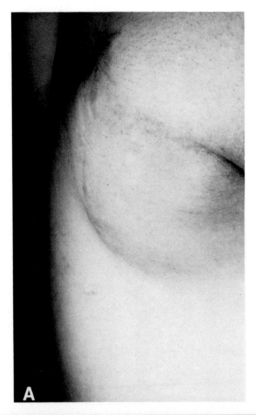

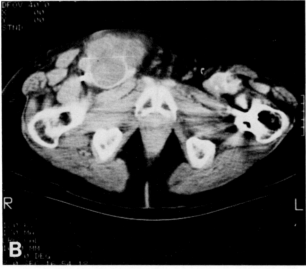

Fig. 1. (A) This photograph of a right groin mass shows its sub-inguinal prominence with tendency toward lateral expansion. Such a mass, lateral to the healed linear incision used for graft to femoral artery bypass strongly suggests the presence of an anastomotic aneurysm. When distal neuropathic radiation of pain occurs, an expansile change is suspected and this is confirmed by development of cutaneous ecchymotic changes. (B) The CT scan serves to confirm the presence of the right femoral anastomotic aneurysm and clearly demonstrates the extraaneurysmal hematoma. Note the very thin skin covering of this acutely symptomatic aneurysm. This converts what would have been a chronic problem to be dealt with electively into an acute surgical emergency.

303

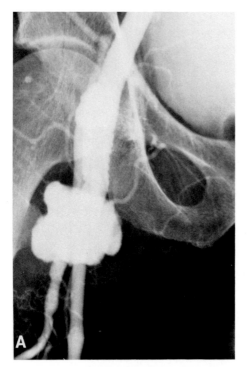 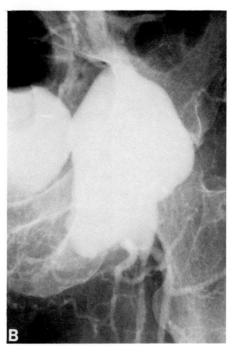

Fig. 2. (A&B) These photographs of an aortogram performed on a 71-year-old man with an aortofemoral graft in residence for 6 years show many characteristics of chronic, stable, and acutely expanding anastomotic aneurysms. Note, in the right femoral area, the ridges of the knitted Dacron graft limb, the disruption of the toe of the anastomosis and the well-defined margins of the chronic, stable aneurysm. On the femoral exposure taken at a later phase in the contrast study the aneurysm is larger, its margins are more indistinct and the lesion is extending above the inguinal ligament. The history of rapid change in size of the mass coupled with observation of acute femoral neuropathic pain confirms the angiographic impression of recent activity in a previously stable anastomotic false aneurysm.

Delayed Occurrence

The operative approach to expanding anastomotic aneurysms in the more delayed postoperative period allows for more formal proximal and distal control.

Aorta

Proximal abdominal aortic false aneurysms are approached by first gaining aortic control intraabdominally at the diaphragm. Control of the graft body and native iliac arteries is then obtained. The aortic reconstruction often necessitates converting an end-to-side anastomosis to an end-to-end anastomosis and placing an extension from the native aorta to the existing graft.

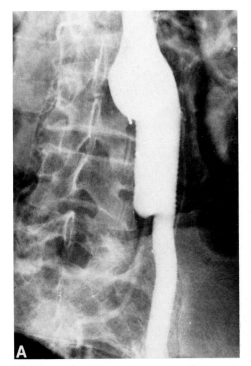
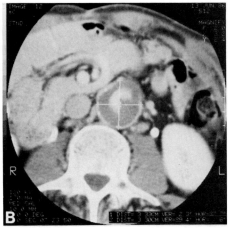

Fig. 3. (A&B) These photographs illustrate the complementary information afforded by aortography and CT scanning in definition of anastomotic aneurysm. The aortogram suggests presence of the proximal anastomotic disruption and confirms the right graft limb occlusion caused by the femoral anastomotic aneurysm thrombosis. The CT scan shows clearly the aortic aneurysm and suggests its stability with no extension of the extraaortic mass into psoas muscles.

Iliac

Iliac artery anastomotic aneurysms are complicated by the proximity of the ureter. An intravenous pyelogram and a CT scan should be obtained. The placement of ureteral stents before laparotomy considerably facilitates the aneurysmal isolation and reduces likelihood of ureteral injury. Stent placement can be accomplished after anesthetic induction and adds little time to the operative procedure. The value of ureteral stents can hardly be overemphasized. In simplifying the approach to iliac false aneurysms, one usually needs only to oversew the iliac artery and extend the graft to the femoral artery.

Femoral

Large or rapidly expanding femoral false aneurysms are best approached with preliminary control of the graft and the native external iliac artery. A standard transplant incision affords rapid and reliable exposure of these structures. Once proximal control is achieved, the false aneurysm may be safely entered directly and distal control achieved using balloon occlusion catheters.[8] Dissection of the femoral system can then proceed with resection of diseased native artery and removal of thrombotic debris. An extension of prosthetic material can then be fashioned from the existing graft limb to the distal femoral system. Consideration should always be given to performing a profundaplasty especially if profunda femoral stensois exists.[1] Some authors advocate converting the existing end-to-side femoral anastomosis to an end-to-end reconstruction hoping to prevent future false aneurysm formation.[11] Cultures must always be obtained even in the face of the most benign appearing nonseptic false aneurysm.

CONCLUSION

Rapidly expanding anastomotic aneurysms should be differentiated as a special category of false aneurysms of iatrogenic origin. This is true because of the very real possibility of their rupturing externally, producing an infected arteriocutaneous fistula at best and lethal exsanguinating hemorrhage at worst. Observation of chronic anastomotic aneurysms reveals that not all are stable, but some that follow the law of aneurysms, the law of LaPlace, continually expand to rupture through the scar, organized hematoma, and the fascia that initially restricts their growth. Rapid expansion may be heralded by lancinating neuropathic pain radiating in the distribution of perianeurysmal nerves. The patient may note increase in size of a previous mass or development of pulsatile swelling where none was present before. The physician may note skin changes, indicating subcutaneous tension and extravasation of blood. B-mode imaging or CT scanning confirms the diagnosis and defines prognosis, as indicated by proximity of the expanding hematoma to skin. Such information in turn dictates need for emergency, urgent, or elective intervention.

REFERENCES

1. Dennis JW, Littooy FN, Greisler HP, et al: Anastomotic pseudoaneurysms. Arch Surg 121:314, 1986
2. Knox WG: Peripheral vascular anastomotic aneurysms. Ann Surg 183:120, 1976
3. Gaylis H: Pathogenesis of anastomotic aneurysms. Surgery 90:509, 1981
4. McCabe CJ, Moncure AC, Malt RA: Host-artery weakness in the etiology of femoral anastomotic false aneurysms. Surgery 95:150, 1984
5. Haimovici H: False aneurysms, in Haimovici H, (ed.): Vascular Surgery: Principles and Techniques. New York, McGraw-Hill, 1976, pp. 522–532
6. Satiani B, Kazmers M, Evans WE: Anastomotic arterial aneurysms. Ann Surg 192:674, 1980
7. Starr DS, Weatherford C, Lawrie GM, et al: Suture material as a factor in the occurrence of anastomotic false aneurysms: An analysis of 26 cases. Arch Surg 114:412, 1979
8. Christenson RD, Bernatz PE: Anastomotic aneurysms involving the femoral artery. Mayo Clinic Proc 47:313, 1972
9. Daar AS, Finch DRA: Graft avulsion: An unreported complication of axillofemoral bypass grafts. Br J Surg 65:442, 1978
10. Ward RE, Holcroft JW, Conti S, et al: New concepts in the use of axillofemoral bypass grafts. Arch Surg 118:573, 1983
11. Moore WS: Anastomotic false aneurysm, in Moore WS (ed.): Vascular Surgery: A Comprehensive Review. New York, Grune & Stratton, 1983, pp. 768–774

12. Nunn DB, Rao N, Renard A: Anastomotic aneurysms. Am Surg 41:281, 1975
13. Sawyers JL, Jacobs JR, Sutton JP: Peripheral anastomotic aneurysms: Development following arterial reconstruction with prosthetic grafts. Arch Surg 95:802, 1967
14. Crawford ES: Marfan's syndrome: Broad spectral surgical treatment of cardiovascular manifestations. Ann Surg 198:487, 1983
15. Jenkins AA, MacPherson AS, Nolan B, et al: Peripheral aneurysms in Behçet's disease. Br J Surg 63:199, 1976
16. Clinicopathologic Conference: Oro-genital ulceration with phlebo-thrombosis (Behçet's syndrome) complicated by osteomyelitis of lumbar spine and ruptured aorta. Br Med J 1:357, 1965
17. Olsen WR, DeWeese M, Fry WJ: False aneurysm of abdominal aorta. Arch Surg 92:123, 1966

Ramon Berguer
Pamela Benitez

Surgical Emergencies from Intravascular Injection of Drugs

Serious complications of intravascular drug abuse are seen with increasing frequency in urban hospitals.[1] Approximately 40 cases per year are seen at Detroit Receiving Hospital. Since 1980 a several-fold increase has been encountered over the number seen during the previous decade.[2] Since 1980 we have noted new patterns of presentation with a higher incidence of upper extremity complications, the use of newer combinations of drugs, and a prevalence of methicillin-resistant Staphylococcus aureus as the infecting pathogen.

In 1981, we reported our experience with 53 infected femoral aneurysms from heroin injection.[3] Since then 172 additional drug abuse vascular complications in 162 patients have been seen at our institution. This report analyzes the clinical course of the more recent group of patients stressing their characteristic presentation and the emergency management.

MATERIALS AND METHODS

We reviewed all records of patients discharged from Detroit Receiving Hospital from July 1980 to March 1985 with a discharge diagnosis of vascular injury secondary to drug abuse. Clinical and laboratory data were recorded. Excluded from this series were intra-cerebral, pulmonary, cardiac valvular, and abdominal vascular complications as well as septic thrombophlebitis. After these exclusions, we were left with 162 patients who had 172 occurrences of acute vascular injury from drug abuse. There were 118 males and 44 females. Ages ranged from 19 to 54. The vascular complication was located in the neck in 4 cases, in the arm in 32 and in the leg in 136 (Table 1).

The drugs were pentazocine, heroin, tripelennamine, barbiturates, "mixed jive," cocaine and propoxyphene. Table 1 specifies the type of lesions found. By far the most common lesion was an infected arterial pseudoaneurysm.

Table 1
Types of Injury

Upper Extremity	(all arterial)
Aneurysm	20
Distal Ischemia	12
Lower Extremity	
Aneurysm	
Arterial	112
Venous	10
AVF	6
Arterial Laceration	1
Venous Necrosis	5
Venocutaneous Fistula	2
Carotids	
Aneurysm	2
AVF	1
Arterial Necrosis	1

NECK COMPLICATIONS

There were four instances of vascular complication in the neck, all involving the common carotid artery. Three patients presented with a pulsatile mass and one with neck pain and dysphagia. All three pulsatile masses had bruits. Three patients were correctly diagnosed clinically and underwent preoperative angiography. The fourth patient was misdiagnosed as an abscess and an arteriogram was not obtained. No patient presented with systemic signs of infection (fever $> 100°$ F and leukocytosis $> 10^3$ WBC/mm^3) or bacteremia. The patient who was misdiagnosed as an abscess had it drained and the proper diagnosis was made 5 days later when he had a hemorrhage from a necrotic carotid artery wall. The other three patients who had been correctly diagnosed clinically were found at arteriography to have two common carotid artery aneurysms and one common carotid to internal jugular vein arteriovenous fistula. All four patients had ligation of their common carotid arteries. In two a median sternotomy was necessary. There were no neurological deficits. The most common finding in this group was the presence of a mass in the neck with some degree of induration and cellulitis.

UPPER EXTREMITY COMPLICATIONS

Although aneurysm and abscess formation characterize cervical vascular complications of drug abuse, in the upper extremity, distal (hand) ischemia is a common complication in addition to pseudoaneurysm. Patients with hand ischemia from drug abuse appeared in the emergency room shortly after injection because of immediate, severe pain in the distribution of the involved artery. Following drug injection the first manifestation was a hyperemic flush, which progressed to edema, rubor, and finally to cyanosis and gangrene depending on the severity of the injury. There were 12 cases presenting with distal ischemia and 20 cases presenting with an infected aneurysm. Location of the injury is shown in Table 2.

Table 2
Location of Injury (Vessels)

Upper Extremity	Aneurysm	Ischemia	Total
Subclavian	0	1	1
Axillary	1	0	1
Brachial	12	1	13
Radial	6	6	12
Digital	1	4	5
	20	12	32

By far the most common complaint was pain generally associated with cellulitis (Table 3) but severe ischemia was present in 31 percent of the patients. The infection was generally local. Only a minority of patients presented with evidence of systemic sepsis as shown on blood cultures which were positive in only 12 percent of the cases. Only 10 of the 32 patients underwent arteriography. Eight of the 10 arteriograms defined the arterial abnormality. There were two false–negative studies.

In eight patients with distal ischemia, conservative treatment consisting of heparin, reserpine, dextran, and/or streptokinase was tried without any improvement. Stellate ganglion blocks were not successful in three additional patients. All patients with infected aneurysms underwent surgery. Mycotic aneurysms were treated by ligation and excision. Gangrenous digits were amputated in seven patients with digital ischemia. One patient required wrist disarticulation for gangrene of the hand. There were no arterial reconstructions done and no complications were noted from ligation of the involved artery in patients with infected pseudoaneurysms.

LOWER EXTREMITY COMPLICATIONS

Aneurysms, abscess formation, and ischemia are typical of cervical and upper extremity complications of drug abuse. Lower extremity complications are characterized by delay in presentation for treatment. All patients gave a history of injection in the groin area usually one to two weeks prior to their arrival in the emergency room. The shortest

Table 3
Upper Extremity—32 Occurrences

Presenting Signs and Symptoms	Aneurysms	Ischemia	Total
Pain	15	11	26
Cellulitis	16	5	21
Ischemia/Gangrene	0	10	10
Mass			
Pulsatile	9	0	9
Nonpulsatile	4	0	4
Neuromuscular Deficit	2	7	9
Decreased or Absent Pulses	4	5	9
Hx of or Presently Bleeding	4	0	4
Cardiac Murmur	0	2	2
Bruit	4	0	4

interval between injection and appearance was 3 days; the longest 3 months. The immediate, shearing pain described by patients with hand ischemia was not observed in this group. The classic presentation was pain, cellulitis or abscess, and a pulsatile mass. Pus, blood, and a pulsatile mass provided an unforgettable triad. In contrast to upper extremity cases, ischemia and gangrene were seen only in 3 percent of the cases (Table 4). Also in contrast to those patients with hand ischemia, those with leg complications often had systemic sepsis. Table 5 compares the clinical presentation of patients with arm and leg vascular injury.

An arteriogram was performed in 102 patients (75 percent) and an ultrasound scan was obtained in 27 patients (20 percent). The arteriogram was very useful for delineation of the lesion, identifying the vessels involved and in planning the operative approach. The ultrasound on the contrary had an unacceptable incidence of false–positive and false–negative results and did not help in planning treatment (Table 6). The location and type of lesions found in the lower extremity group are listed in Table 7. The common femoral artery was the vessel most frequently involved. In addition to 112 mycotic aneurysms that were the most common lesion (82 percent) we found also 6 arteriovenous fistulae in conjunction with aneurysmal disease of the artery and of the vein. There were also two venocutaneous fistulae, five patients with necrosis of the vein wall and one laceration of the common femoral artery.

All 118 patients presenting with an arterial mycotic aneurysm or arteriovenous fistula of the leg had ligation and excision of the infected vessel(s). Of the 102 patients who had simple ligation and excision of the groin vessels involved, 13 percent underwent amputation, 2 percent died, and 74 percent had no postoperative ischemia. Of the 47 patients who had triple ligation and excision (common, deep and superficial femoral arteries), 19 percent had an amputation, compared to 6 percent in those who had only one vessel ligated.

Thirteen patients had triple vessel ligation and excision and arterial reconstruction by means of a bypass graft: 8/13 had immediate grafting (< 6 hours postop) and had no amputation although one had his infected graft removed at a later date without complications. Five of 13 patients had delayed (> 6 hours) grafting and 3/5 had an amputation. One patient in this subgroup had his infected graft removed at a later date.

Table 4
Lower Extremity—136 Occurrences

Presenting Signs and Symptoms	Arterial Aneurysm	Venous Aneurysm	Other	AVF	Total
Pain	74	6	5	6	91
Cellulitis	46	5	4	1	56
Ischemia/gangrene	4	0	0	0	4
Mass					
pulsatile	61	2	1	3	67
nonpulsatile	19	3	1	0	23
Neuromuscular deficit	4	0	0	0	4
Decreased or absent pulses	23	0	1	0	24
Hx of or presently bleeding	18	3	7	1	29
Cardiac murmur	25	2	1	0	28
Bruit	58	0	0	3	61

Table 5
Comparison Upper and Lower Extremity Arterial Injuries

Presenting Signs and Symptoms	UE (N = 32)	LE (N = 136)
Ischemia/gangrene	10/32 = 31%	4/136 = 3%
Neuromuscular deficit	9/32 = 28%	4/136 = 3%
Fever (> 100° F)	9/32 = 28%	53/118 = 45%
Increased WBC (> 10,000 mm³)	11/32 = 34%	86/118 = 73%
Bacteremia	44%*	60%*

*Percent of blood cultures drawn

Table 6
Lower Extremity Diagnostic Studies

	Angiogram (102 done)	Ultrasound (27 done)
True positive	86	8
True negative	10	0
False positive	2	15
False negative	4	4

Table 7
Location of Injury

Lower Extremity—Arterial

	Aneurysm (112)	AVF (6)	Laceration (1)	= 119
Common femoral	42			
Superficial femoral	14			
Deep femoral	24			
Superficial & deep	3			
Common & deep	1			
Common, deep & superficial	29			
External iliac	2			
Lateral circumflex	3			
Anterior tibial	1			
	119			

(all AVF's were with common femoral vein)

Lower Extremity—Venous

	Aneurysm (10)	Necrosis (5)	Venocutaneous Fistula (2)	=17
Common femoral	8	5	2	
Deep femoral	1	0	0	
Common iliac	1	0	0	

313

Table 8
Results of Blood Cultures Drawn on Admission

Positive cultures			52	(50%)
Meth-resistant Staph aureus	28	(54%)		
Meth-sensitive Staph aureus	13	(25%)		
Streptococcus (includes anaerobic)	11	(21%)		
Gram negative rods	10	(19%)		
Negative cultures			51	(50%)
Total blood cultures drawn*			103	

*not done in 73 patients

Half of the patients who had blood cultures drawn on admission had positive cultures. The predominant organism (54 percent) was methicillin-resistant Staph aureus. The results of the blood cultures on admission are shown in Table 8. The abscesses were cultured during the operation in 81 percent of the cases and of those cultured 92 percent grew bacteria. Here too the most common organism was methicillin-resistant Staph aureus. Antibiotic therapy was intravenous vancomycin for a mean of 18 days in those patients who had methicillin-resistant Staph aureus cultured from either blood or abscess. In the other patients nafcillin or nafcillin plus an aminoglycoside were used for an average of 6 days.

DISCUSSION

A number of mechanisms may singly or in combination result in infection and destruction of the arterial wall. These include puncture with contaminated needles, development of an intimal flap, chemical injury of the arterial wall from direct or perivascular injections, and secondary infection of a perivascular hematoma caused by repeated injections. Embolization of particulate matter may cause digital ischemia or gangrene. In our series, the most important mechanisms involved were (1) a groin infection spreading to the artery or (2) a direct arterial injury associated with hematoma and subsequent infection. Embolization from an underlying bacterial endocarditis was rare. Only seven patients were found to have valvular involvement either before, during, or following hospitalization.

The diagnosis of an ischemic complication in the hand from drug injection is easy because the patient usually presents to the emergency room with severe pain and/or ischemia shortly after having injected the drug.

In patients presenting with infected aneurysms in the arm or leg the delay between injection and presentation with an infected aneurysm may be several weeks. The presentation of a patient with a tender pulsatile mass who has fever and leukocytosis should arouse the suspicion of a mycotic aneurysm and prompt an arteriogram.

False venous aneurysms were not diagnosed preoperatively in any of the 10 patients who had them and the arteriogram, when performed, was negative. These patients were treated for a presumed diagnosis of abscess and during drainage, disruption of the venous wall and a large hematoma was found. In none of them was there extensive blood loss or any complication that could be related to the incorrect preoperative diagnosis.

In patients with hand ischemia the use of medical therapy (heparin, dextran, vasodilators) did not improve results. The incidence and type of amputation was the same in those patients who had medical therapy intraarterially or intravenously as in those who did not. Although patients with arm complications tend to present to the hospital shortly after injection a delay of several hours is not uncommon and this is perhaps the reason why systemic medications do not improve the outcome. In some patients with poorly defined digital ischemia the definitive amputation was delayed until demarcation had occurred.

The basic principle for the treatment of a mycotic aneurysm has been clearly established in previous reports[3-5]: the involved vessels must be ligated and excised. Ligation must be done to healthy, noninfected artery lest delayed hemorrhage ensue. Conservative techniques of local repair such as patch or direct suture have no place in infected aneurysms secondary to drug injection.[5] Different strategies have been proposed to deal with the aneurysm, namely: (1) obtaining proximal and distal control before entering the aneurysm, (2) obtaining distal control of the superficial femoral artery followed by proximal dissection to the aneurysm, (3) gaining proximal control first by means of a separate retroperitoneal approach to the external iliac artery, and (4) entering the aneurysm directly and getting proximal and distal control by intravascular occlusion of the vessel openings with a finger. As Johnson has previously reported from our institution,[4] and this review confirms, the method used to approach the aneurysm has no effect on the outcome. We prefer, however, obtaining proximal control prior to entering the aneurysmal sac.

The question of simultaneous revascularization has been debated in the literature. The important objections against simultaneous revascularization are the frequent lack of peripheral veins for grafting (from previous injections and infections) and the threat of bacteremia (present in 50 percent of the patients) to the prosthetic graft. Ischemia following ligation and excision is assessed in the recovery room after the patient awakens from anesthesia. The absence of pulses, of course, does not indicate ischemia. If the patient has severe constant pain upon awakening and has clinical and noninvasive findings indicative of severe ischemia consideration can be given to a remote bypass provided that the proposed path for the graft is free of inflammation and infection. It is to be noted that even though bypass grafts can be placed, it can be expected that 14 percent of all patients with infected aneurysms end up having an amputation.

Delayed revascularization (> 6 hours) is obviously useless at least in the group with 3-vessel ligation where 3 of 5 patients ended up with amputation. As for immediate (< 6 hours) revascularization in patients with 3-vessel ligation our numbers (8 patients) are too few to unequivocally endorse it. Even though no amputation was done in this small subgroup, 1/8 patients developed chronic ischemia, 2/8 patients had neuromuscular deficits, and 1/8 patients underwent late removal of an infected graft, without complications; a matter that puts into question the original need for it.

In order to revascularize the leg through a pathway different than the anatomic course of the vessels, two operations have been proposed: bypass through the obturator foramen and the lateral circumflex bypass. The pros and cons of these two procedures have been discussed elsewhere.[3]

After ligation and excision the drained areas are left open to heal by secondary intention. The high incidence of methicillin-resistant Staph poses special problems. Thirty percent of our patients had bought "street" cephalosporin to self-treat their abscesses prior to hospitalization. In addition a number of patients also grew gram negative rods that had been very rare in previous reports. Patients with methicillin-resistant Staph were given vancomycin generally for 2 weeks. Only one patient in this entire series was readmitted later because of bacterial endocarditis. If the patient presents with marked cellulitis and bacteremia, it seems sensible to start treatment with vancomycin and an aminoglycoside until bacterial cultures and identification are completed. We saw three patients who returned with infected grafts following extraanatomic bypass. All three had had methicillin-resistant Staph at their first and subsequent operations. Patients with moderate cellulitis without bacteremia are given nafcillin. Whatever the organism, antibiotic therapy is given until cellulitis and/or sepsis abate. We no longer endorse the previously recommended 6 weeks course of antibiotics.

SUMMARY

We report here 162 patients presenting with 172 vascular complications from drug abuse seen from July 1980 to March 1985. The lesions found were arterial and venous aneurysms, peripheral ischemia or gangrene, and arteriovenous fistula. The different presentation of the vascular complications in the neck, arm, and leg are discussed. Arteriography is the diagnostic test of choice. Intravascular medical therapy did not influence results.

Patients with gangrenous lesions or advanced ischemia had amputations performed immediately. Mycotic aneurysms were managed primarily by ligation, excision, and drainage. Our data do not support delayed ($>$ 6 hours) revascularization and are inconclusive though suggestive that immediate ($<$ 6 hours) revascularization may have a place in selected cases. The predominant organism found in blood and in abscesses was methicillin-resistant Staph aureus.

REFERENCES

1. Wallace JR, Lucas CE, Ledgerwood AM: Social, economic and surgical anatomy of a drug related abscess. Am Surg 52:398, 1936
2. Fromm SH, Lucas CE: Obturator bypass for mycotic aneurysm in the drug addict. Arch Surg 100:82, 1970
3. Berguer R, Feldman AJ: Infected groin aneurysms from heroin addiction, in Bergan JJ, Yao JST, (eds): Aneurysms: Their Diagnosis and Treatment. New York, Grune and Stratton, 1982
4. Johnson J, Ledgerwood AM, Lucas CE: Mycotic aneurysm—New concepts in therapy. Arch Surg 118:577, 1983
5. Anderson CB, Butcher HR, Ballinger WF: Mycotic aneurysms. Arch Surg 109:712, 1974

PART VII

Emergency Aortic Surgery

D. Craig Miller

Surgical Emergencies of the Thoracic Aorta

Since acute traumatic tears of the thoracic aorta due to deceleration injury and aortoenteric fistulae (in this case, aortoesophageal and aortobronchial fistulae) are covered elsewhere in this monograph, this chapter will focus on the most common naturally-occurring catastrophic events that mandate emergency surgical intervention on the thoracic and thoracoabdominal aorta: *acute aortic dissection and ruptured thoracic aortic aneurysm.* Penetrating traumatic injuries of the thoracic aorta will also not be discussed in this essay as the principles of surgical treatment of such injuries are common to those outlined in the section of this book dedicated to Arterial Injuries.

ACUTE AORTIC DISSECTION

The pathological entity termed aortic dissection, improperly called "dissecting aortic aneurysm" in the past, has evolved over the last three decades from the niche of an incidental autopsy curiosity to become one of the most challenging diseases that the cardiovascular surgeon faces today.[1] The signs and symptoms of acute aortic dissection are truly protean and can mimic those of essentially all other acute medical or surgical illness; for this and other reasons, it is sobering to realize that even today substantial proportions of patients who sustain an acute aortic dissection and are admitted to hospital continue to die either misdiagnosed or undiagnosed.[2-4]

Furthermore, acute aortic dissection is the most common clinical catastrophe involving the aorta (occurring at least 50 percent more frequently than ruptured atherosclerotic *abdominal* aortic aneurysm and many times more frequently than ruptured atherosclerotic *thoracic* aortic aneurysm[5]). The fact that ruptured abdominal aortic aneurysm is widely perceived to occur more frequently than acute aortic dissection only reflects the limitations of our current clinical and diagnostic skills. It is also important to recognize that the incidence of acute aortic dissection may be increasing in the industrialized world—possibly today exceeding 10–20 cases per million population per year[6] or even higher.[7]

Vascular Surgical Emergencies
ISBN 0-8089-1843-5

319

Although the overall salvage rate for patients with acute aortic dissection has improved dramatically over the last 20 years,[1,8-10] our current diagnostic and therapeutic efforts remain suboptimal; this is due, in part, to the well-appreciated clinical diagnostic difficulties,[11] a generally low index of clinical suspicion,[11] delay and technical difficulty in confirming the diagnosis, continuing debate pertaining to whether *medical* or *surgical plus medical* treatment is the optimal management strategy (at least for patients with descending thoracic aortic dissections), formidable technical difficulties encountered in the past by the cardiovascular surgeon,[8] and ongoing confusion regarding classification of the various types of aortic dissection.[1,4] Notwithstanding the substantial improvements in surgical results and diagnostic accuracy that have been accomplished, the fundamental keys to future progress pivot almost exclusively on: (1) increased clinical suspicion; (2) more prompt diagnosis; and, (3) earlier institution of definitive therapy. There exists a compelling need to recognize the possibility of acute aortic dissection as quickly as possible so that a definitive diagnostic examination can be performed rapidly—during the first 48 hours the mortality rate for patients with undiagnosed or untreated acute type A dissections is approximately *1 percent per hour.*[1,2,4,9,10] This dismal natural history of the disease explains why upwards of 35 percent of hospitalized patients (and fully 55 percent of patients in the acute type A subgroup) in a recent report from Vancouver, British Columbia[2] and 11 percent of patients in the Massachusetts General Hospital series[3] died without a correct antemortem diagnosis. Furthermore, these sobering figures must be considered to be under-estimates, since outpatients were not considered nor were hospitalized patients who died without a postmortem examination being conducted.

Classification Systems

An important consensus has been established recently concerning the descriptive classification of aortic dissections, albeit a variety of different terms are used. Arbitrarily, dissections are considered to be *acute* if they are less than 14 days old, but this acuity threshold is obviously not absolute. The cardinal feature of all classification systems is currently predicated solely upon whether or not the ascending aorta is involved by the dissecting process (irrespective of the site of primary intimal tear and regardless of the distal extent of the dissecting hematoma). Such is the principal determinant of the pathophysiology and expected biological behavior of the dissection; hence, ascending aortic involvement determines the patient's prognosis and modulates therapeutic management. If the ascending aorta is involved, the dissection is termed "type A" (Stanford[1]), "proximal" (Massachusetts General Hospital[3]), "ascending" (University of Alabama[12]), or "type I" (De Bakey)[4,13]. If the ascending aorta is not involved (the tear being located either in the aortic arch or the descending thoracic aorta and, again, regardless of the distal extent of the dissection), then it is called "type B," "distal," "descending," or "type III" (Fig. 1).

Practical advantages of such a simplified classification concept include: (1) Determination of whether or not the ascending aorta is involved (using angiography, computerized tomographic [CT] scanning, magnetic resonance imaging [MRI], or digital subtraction angiography [DSA]) is relatively easy compared to determining exactly where the primary tear is located and the distal extent of the dissection; (2) Ascending aortic involvement should prompt consideration of emergency surgical treatment in essentially all patients, whereas type B acute dissections can be treated either surgically or medically; (3) Patients

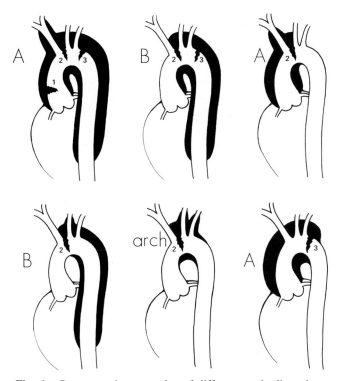

Fig. 1. Representative examples of different aortic dissections classified according to the Stanford type A (A) and type B (B) nomenclature system, which is predicated upon whether or not the ascending aorta is involved. Isolated arch dissections (bottom middle panel) are rare, usually extending either retrograde to involve the ascending aorta or distally to involve the descending aorta or both. Patients with a type A dissection where the intimal tear is located beyond the left subclavian artery (bottom right panel) are troublesome; they must be approached via a median sternotomy as would any patient with a type A acute dissection. Site of primary intimal tear: 1 = ascending aorta, 2 = transverse aortic arch, 3 = descending thoracic aorta. (From Miller DC: Surgical management of aortic dissections: Indications, perioperative management, and long-term results, in Doroghazi RM, Slater EE (eds): Aortic Dissection. New York, McGraw-Hill Book Company, 1983. With permission.)

with type A dissections are approached through a median sternotomy incision using total cardiopulmonary bypass in contrast to a left thoracotomy and partial (femoral-femoral) cardiopulmonary bypass for patients with type B dissections; and, (4) The most common causes of death and the most frequent complications in medically-treated patients with acute dissections differ markedly according to whether or not the ascending aorta is involved.

Diagnostic Difficulties

Acute aortic dissection is uncommon, but not rare. Patients dying of acute aortic dissection have been misdiagnosed as having a myriad of other diseases,[2,11] many of which prompt emergency consultation with a general or vascular surgeon. Included in this long list are acute myocardial infarction (MI), unstable angina, pericarditis, aortic (and/or mitral) valve disease, congestive heart failure, heart block, acute hypertensive crisis, pulmonary embolism, pneumothorax, pleurodynia, lymphoma, bronchogenic carcinoma, esophageal spasm and/or reflux, peptic ulcer disease, ureteral colic, acute cholecystitis, appendicitis, biliary colic, "acute surgical abdomen," bowel infarction, incarcerated hernia, sigmoid volvulus, diverticulitis, pyelonephritis, acute renal failure, pancreatitis, musculoskeletal back pain, sciatica, stroke, syncope, paraplegia, transient ischemic attacks, vertebrobasilar insufficiency, occlusive peripheral vascular disease, and acute arterial thromboembolism. This diversity of symptoms and physical signs is due in part to the rather unpredictable alterations in end-organ blood supply that can occur as the dissecting process propagates distally resulting in variable pathoanatomic consequences at each important aortic tributary.[1,9] For the subspecialist who is consulted, whether he or she be a vascular surgeon, neurologist, urologist, cardiologist, general surgeon, neurosurgeon, pulmonary specialist, gastroenterologist, or orthopedic surgeon, it is obviously important not to focus solely on the subsystem that initiated the consultation. For example, the sudden onset of unilateral lower limb ischemia in a patient with an acute aortic dissection should be an opportunity for the peripheral vascular surgeon to help the attending physician confirm the correct diagnosis expeditiously and thereby institute early definitive therapy; to proceed first with a local revascularization procedure or embolectomy (having missed the central, life threatening problem) only causes more delay and is frequently futile anyway. Additionally, intravenous streptokinase is now being used widely for patients with suspected acute MI (without coronary angiographic confirmation); clearly, such thrombolytic therapy can rapidly prove to be fatal if the patient has an acute dissection or the MI is due to a dissection.[14]

The cardinal symptom of acute dissection is the sudden onset of severe, lancinating pain, often starting in the anterior chest or interscapular region with later migration[11]; however, the acute pain can be located in essentially any portion of the body. Indeed, some patients present months or years later with chronic aortic dissections without any recall of an acute event. Obviously, a high index of clinical suspicion is necessary to differentiate acute aortic dissection from this host of other acute illnesses in the first few hours; it is helpful to consider the diagnosis of aortic dissection when the constellation of clinical signs and symptoms simply do not lend themselves to a single diagnosis, i.e., when simultaneous involvement of multiple, diverse organ systems does not appear to have any common explanation.

Although acute aortic dissection occurs most often in middle-aged and elderly men, women (especially those in the third trimester of pregnancy) and children are also affected.[11] It is especially tragic in these young patients to have the correct diagnosis confirmed only when it is too late, e.g., after a child with abdominal pain is found to have infarction of the entire small and large bowel or when aortic rupture results in the death of both the mother and her fetus. Younger individuals with degenerative *elastic degeneration* in the aortic media (including those with Marfan's syndrome, Ehlers-Danlos syndrome, or annulo-aortic ectasia) are prone to develop type A dissections; in contrast, the older, hypertensive population with *muscular degenerative* changes in the aortic media (a normal function of the aging process) are at highest risk for type B dissections.[1,11]

Perioperative Medical Management

Patients with suspected acute aortic dissection should initially receive intensive medical therapy (aimed at reducing blood pressure and cardiac inotropic state[1,3,15]). Such treatment is implemented immediately and continued throughout the time period when the diagnostic tests are being performed. The preferred drugs are intravenous propranolol or metaprolol combined with a continuous infusion of sodium nitroprusside. Beta blockade is essential in that it compensates for the actual increase in *aortic* dP/dt caused by the arteriolar vasodilatation effect of the nitroprusside. Mean, peak systolic, and diastolic recoil aortic pressures are maintained at the lowest possible level consistent with adequate perfusion to the heart, brain, and kidneys. The patient should be monitored in an intensive care unit, preferably under the direction of a cardiovascular surgeon. Level of consciousness and ECG should be monitored continuously; urine output, central venous (and/or pulmonary artery) pressure, and arterial pressure should be measured directly. The mean arterial pressure should be lowered to the 60–70 mm Hg range, assuming that such controlled hypotension does not result in oliguria, myocardial ischemia, or obtundention.

Definitive Diagnostic Methods

Major diagnostic advances have been made recently. The wide availability of CT scanning has markedly enhanced the rapidity and ease of ruling out or confirming the diagnosis of acute aortic dissection,[1,4,16] even in small community hospitals without angiography or open heart surgery facilities (Fig. 2A and 2B). CT scanning (with intravenous contrast infusion) for the diagnosis of aortic dissection is rapid, accurate, and enables the astute clinician to exercise clinical suspicions more freely; it should be utilized as the first step on an emergency basis. Conventional aortography remains the diagnostic benchmark, but angiography is not totally specific, especially in the rare circumstance when the false lumen is thrombosed. Although much more time consuming than CT scanning and not as widely available today, magnetic resonance imaging (MRI) produces precise images of the aorta and its major branches (Fig. 2C and 2D) and can be used for patients with aortic dissections, assuming that using MRI does not result in inordinate time delays. Another useful diagnostic technique is biplane cineangiography of the thoracic aorta, which can demonstrate the blood flow dynamics of the dissection in the ascending aorta, aortic arch, and the brachiocephalic branches. Intravenous or (preferably) intra-arterial DSA can also be employed with satisfactory diagnostic accuracy. Two-dimensional echocardiography is helpful on occasion (particularly in patients with type A dissections), but is not sensitive or specific enough to be used as a definitive diagnostic test. Irrespective of which imaging modality is utilized, the key is *rapid diagnosis* such that the patient can receive appropriate treatment as soon as possible. To reiterate, the

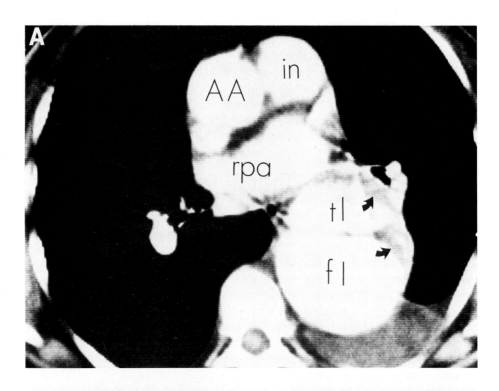

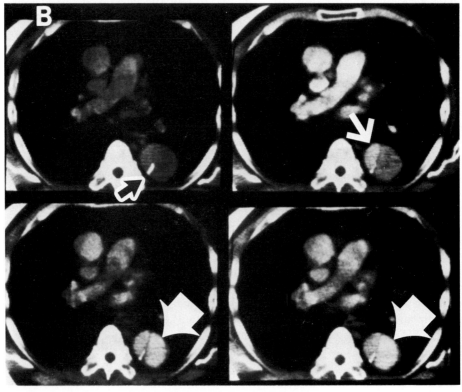

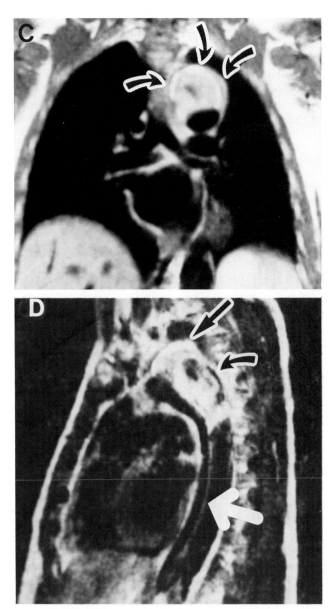

Fig. 2. (A) CT scan (with contrast) demonstrating a normal ascending aorta (AA) and a large dissection involving the descending aorta, with a relatively small true lumen (tl) and a larger false lumen (fl). The linear lucency between the true and false lumens represents the "intimal flap" and is characteristic. A small amount of thrombus is seen in both lumens (arrows). In= right ventricular infundibulum; rpa= right pulmonary artery. (B) Four dynamic CT scans (with contrast) in a patient with a type B dissection showing early and progressive filling of the true lumen (arrow, top right panel) followed by later washout with nonopacified blood (bottom right panel) and slower, more stagnant filling of the false lumen (large arrowheads, bottom panels). Part of the calcified intimal flap between the two lumens is well demonstrated in the earliest image (top left panel) before the injection of contrast (black arrow). (C and D) Anteroposterior (AP) and lateral (LAT) MRI scans of a patient with an aortic dissection. A large false lumen filled mostly by thrombus (black arrows) involving the distal aortic arch and proximal descending aorta is well demonstrated in the AP image; the LAT scan nicely shows a longitudinal intimal flap (arrow) separating the two lumens for the entire length of the descending aorta and the large, saccular false aneurysmal component at the level of the distal arch (black arrows).

mortality rate for undiagnosed and/or untreated patients with acute aortic dissections during the first 2 days is approximately 1 percent per hour. Procrastination and delay simply can not be tolerated or accepted. Indeed, if the patient is moribund or exceedingly unstable hemodynamically, it is necessary on some occasions to proceed directly to the operating room without the luxury of a definitive diagnostic study.

Indications for Operation

The indications for operation are clear for patients with acute type A dissections, but remain somewhat controversial for those with acute type B dissections. The optimal definitive treatment for patients with acute type A aortic dissections is emergency surgical intervention.[1-4,8-10,13] This should be considered for essentially all patients; however, individual judgment is necessary in cases where coexistent chronic, progressive systemic diseases, neoplasm, far advanced (physiological) age, or pre-existent multiorgan failure otherwise limit the patient's life expectancy.[1,9] Furthermore, rare cases of complicated acute dissection in which the false lumen is already thrombosed (does not opacify with contrast during CT or angiography) can probably also be managed with medical therapy alone due to the excellent prognosis of this small subgroup of patients.[1,3,9,15] On the other hand, the decision-making process in patients with *acute type B dissections* remains controversial.[1,3,8-10,13,15] The principal reasons for this debate pertain to the relatively good (compared to those with acute type A dissections) prognosis of these patients when treated medically[3,15] and the historically high surgical mortality rates (averaging 38 percent in the 1960s and 1970s[8]). Therapeutic policies that reserve surgical treatment only for those patients who fail medical management, however, have been associated with operative mortality rates as high as 75–100 percent[1,8,9] in experienced cardiovascular surgical referral centers; moreover, 2 of the 3 strongest independent risk factors portending an increased likelihood of operative death in the Stanford surgical experience (rupture and renal and/or visceral ischemia or infarction[9] [*vida infra*]) represented complications that occur commonly when medical management fails. Thus, such therapeutic protocols result in a paradoxical situation where the indications for surgical intervention are identical to the factors known to increase the operative mortality risk. Guided by the hypothesis that the overall salvage rate for patients with acute type B dissections might be optimized by routine, early surgical intervention, we implemented such a management policy in 1977 (if the false lumen was not thrombosed and major contraindications to operation did not exist).

Operative Techniques

Either total (type A patients) or partial (type B patients) cardiopulmonary bypass (CPB) is used for patients with aortic dissections at Stanford University Medical Center (Fig. 3). Femoral-femoral partial CPB remains our preferred method for patients with type B dissections (Fig. 3B). A fairly uniform operative approach has been employed over the last 25 years, which has been reported in detail previously.[1,8-10] In brief, a limited segment of ascending or descending thoracic aorta (containing the primary intimal tear, if it is exposed) is resected (Fig. 4). For patients with acute type B dissections, the aortic segment to be resected is dictated by the area containing the most severe degree of injury; this usually is the proximal 5–15 cm of the descending thoracic aorta (Fig. 5). Using partial CPB, the incidence of new paraplegia following resection of acute type B dissec-

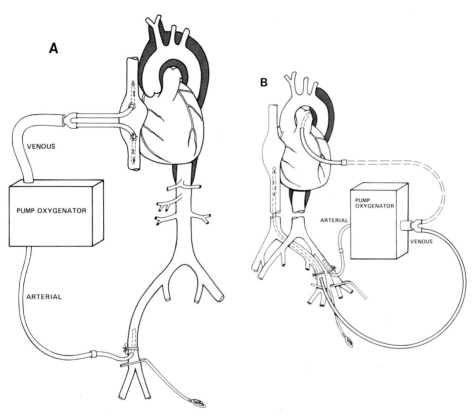

Fig. 3. Schematic representation of total cardiopulmonary bypass (CPB) used for repair of type A dissections (A) and partial (femoral-femoral) CPB used at Stanford for repair of type B dissections (B). If the long venous cannula can not be advanced into the right atrium, then additional venous return can be achieved by means of a second cannula inserted into the main pulmonary artery. As described in the text, use of a guidewire from the femoral vein has eliminated the need for this extra venous cannula. (From Miller DC: Surgical management of aortic dissections: Indications, perioperative management, and long-term results, in Doroghazi RM, Slater EE (eds): Aortic Dissection. New York, McGraw-Hill Book Company, 1983. With permission.)

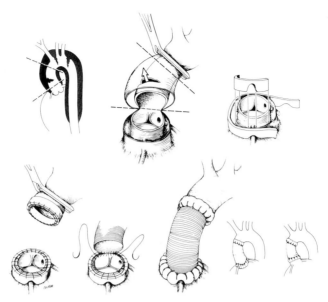

Fig. 4. Operative technique for repair of acute type A aortic dissections. When the native aortic valve is preserved, a careful and complete reconstruction of the aortic root is imperative, as illustrated in the upper right panel. See text for details. (From Miller DC: Surgical management of aortic dissections: Indications, perioperative management, and long-term results, in Doroghazi RM, Slater EE (eds): Aortic Dissection. New York, McGraw-Hill Book Company, 1983. With permission.)

tions has been 4 percent at Stanford; however, 17 percent of patients required postoperative hemodialysis,[9] some of whom were also on dialysis preoperatively. Although no method offers complete protection from paraplegia and renal failure, partial CPB has yielded satisfactory results in our hands and has not generated excessive complications of its own. A small proportion of patients also require arch replacement concomitant with resection of either the ascending or descending thoracic aorta.

The aorta is transected circumferentially both distally and proximally, the false lumen is obliterated using one or more strips of Teflon felt (usually one layer in the false lumen and another outside the adventitia) and a separate whip stitch of 4-0 SH-1 polypropylene (Prolene, Ethicon, Inc., Somerville, N.J.), and a tubular low porosity, woven Dacron graft (Meadox Medicals Inc., Oakland, N.J.) is interposed using a continuous 54 ″ 3-0 SH Prolene suture. Primary or plastic repair techniques and ringed intraluminal prostheses are not used, nor are "graft inclusion" or wrapping techniques. The aortic valve can be preserved in upwards of 82 percent of patients with acute type A dissections using various reconstructive techniques,[1,9] but is *universally* replaced if the patient has Marfan's syndrome or annulo–aortic ectasia.[1,6,7,17,18] An elaborate and careful aortic root reconstruction is required if the aortic valve is preserved in order to guarantee long-term durability of the valve reconstruction and to eliminate the occurrence of late false aneurysms or redissections involving the sinuses of Valsalva; these reconstructive methods usually include insertion of a custom-tailored piece of Teflon felt into the remaining false lumen (down to the aortic valve annulus) to obliterate completely any remaining patent false lumen and to

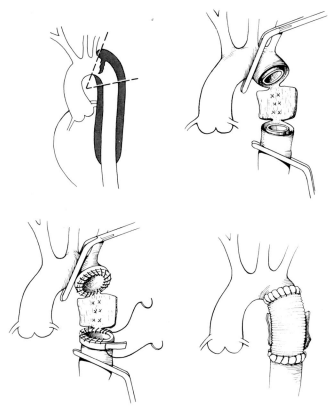

Fig. 5. Operative technique for repair of acute type B aortic dissections. See text for details. (From Miller DC: Surgical management of aortic dissections: Indications, perioperative management, and long-term results, in Doroghazi RM, Slater EE (eds): Aortic Dissection. New York, McGraw-Hill Book Company, 1983. With permission.)

buttress the aortic root repair (Fig. 4).[1] If the coronary ostia are markedly displaced cephalad away from the aortic annulus (most commonly, the right coronary in patients with Marfan's syndrome), then they are reimplanted into the Dacron graft as *full thickness, end-to-side* Carrel patches, whether or not a "composite" graft is used for combined aortic valve and ascending aortic replacement.[1]

Although resection of the primary intimal tear is performed if it is exposed in the segment of the aorta that is isolated, this was successfully accomplished in only 85 percent (148/175) of patients for various reasons (82 percent of acute type A, 89 percent of chronic type A, 92 percent of acute type B, and 79 percent of chronic type B).[9] The tear could conceivably have been resected—but was not—in 21 cases (12 percent); the tear was located in the transverse aortic arch in 16 of these 21 patients (76 percent) who underwent only replacement of the ascending aorta (n=9) or the descending aorta (n=7). Thus, the tear was not resected in only 9 percent (16/175) of patients because concomitant aortic arch replacement was deferred. As discussed below, whether or not the primary intimal tear was able to be resected had no important statistical bearing on the risk of operative death, late death, or late reoperation.[9,10]

Surgical Results

The operative mortality rates for patients with acute aortic dissections have fallen dramatically over the last 10 years in certain centers, in part due to earlier clinical diagnosis and more prompt institution of definitive therapy.[9,17,18] As illustrated in Figure 6, the contemporary (1977–1982) operative risk at Stanford is now 7 ± 5 percent (plus or minus 70 percent confidence limits) for patients with acute type A dissections and 13 ± 12 percent for those with acute type B dissections.[9] Multivariate statistical analysis using a logistic regression equation revealed that only (earlier) operative date (p= 0.02), renal dysfunction (p= 0.01), cardiac tamponade (p= 0.0124), and renal/visceral ischemia and/or infarction (p= 0.0173) were significant, *independent* incremental risk factors predicting an increased likelihood of operative death in the type A subgroup. In the type B subgroup, (older) age (p= 0.05), rupture (p= 0.0166), and renal/visceral ischemia and/or infarction were the only determinants. When all patients were considered, chronic pulmonary disease (p= 0.0349) and site of tear (p= 0.0068) (arch > descending > ascending) emerged as predictors of operative mortality in addition to operative date, renal failure, tamponade, and renal/visceral ischemia and/or infarction. It is interesting that several covariates did not attain statistical predictive significance, including type (A versus B), acuity (acute versus chronic), age (except for type B subset), previous operation, stroke, paraplegia, tear resection, concomitant AVR or coronary bypass grafting, emergency operation, and Marfan's syndrome.

The long-term outlook for patients who were discharged from hospital has also been recently analyzed using Cox model linear regression techniques.[10] As shown in Figure 7A, the 5 year actuarial survival estimate was 78 ± 6 percent for discharged patients with

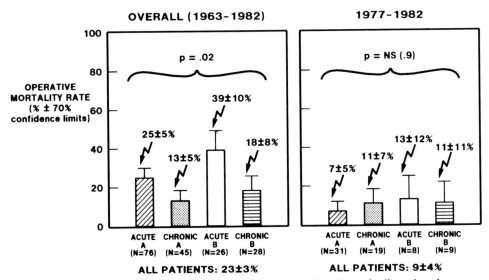

Fig. 6. Operative mortality rates for patients with acute and chronic aortic dissections between 1963 and 1982. As shown in the right panel, the results have improved rapidly in the recent time frame, with the current operative risk being 7 ± 5 percent (plus or minus 70 percent confidence limits) for patients with acute type A dissections and 13 ± 12 percent for those with acute type B dissections. Before 1976 the overall mortality rate was 31 ± 5 percent (34/108) compared to the current (1977–1982) overall risk of 9 ± 4 percent. (From Miller DC, Mitchell RS, Oyer PE, et al: Independent determinants of operative mortality for patients with aortic dissections. Circulation 70 (Suppl I): I-153, 1984. With permission of the American Heart Association.)

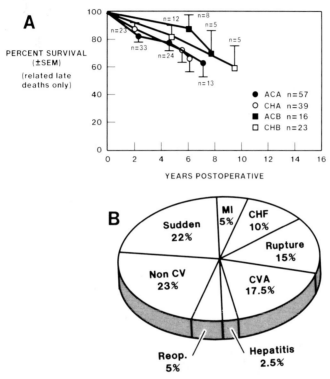

Fig. 7. (A) Actuarial survival curves for discharged patients with acute type A (ACA), acute type B (ACB), chronic type A (CHA), and chronic type B (CHB) aortic dissections after surgical treatment. (From Haverich A, Miller DC, Scott WC, et al: Acute and chronic aortic dissections—Determinants of long-term outcome for operative survivors. Circulation 72 (Suppl II): II-2, 1985. With permission.) (B) Cause of late deaths following surgical repair of aortic dissections, with particular emphasis on the 15 percent of deaths that were due to rupture of another aortic aneurysm or false aneurysm due to the dissection.

acute type A dissections and 88 ± 12 percent for those with acute type B dissections. Significant, independent risk factors for late death included stroke (p= 0.0005), remote MI (p= 0.0218), renal dysfunction (p= 0.0068), and (earlier) operative date (p= 0.0142). It should be emphasized that 15 percent of all late deaths were due to rupture of a contiguous or remote portion of the aorta (Fig. 7B), usually confined to a localized segment; although clearly not optimal, this figure compares favorably with the 29 percent proportion observed in the long-term follow-up study from Baylor.[13] The entire aorta must be followed closely on an indefinite basis with serial CT or MRI scans to detect enlargement of a localized false aneurysmal segment (*all* dissections, to be semantically correct, are false aneurysms) prior to rupture; furthermore, careful medical management with antihypertensive and negative inotropic (beta blockade) drugs is also imperative indefinitely. In our experience, late reoperation related to the dissection was necessary in 13 ± 4 percent of patients after 5 years and 23 ± 6 percent after 10 years (Fig. 8). Independent incremental risk factors for late reoperation included (younger) age (p= 0.0009), and site of tear (p= 0.0196) (arch > descending > ascending). Neither tear resection nor whether or not the aortic valve was preserved had any important statistical bearing on the probability of late death or reoperation.[10] Some of these reoperations were related to the original repair, and, as such, represent "treatment failures"; improved operative methods and a better understanding of the pathophysiology and pathologic anatomy of the disease should reduce the incidence of these late complications to a very low level. On the other hand, the majority were operations directed at other portions of the thoracic or abdominal aorta to correct new problems arising in the remaining dissected aorta, either proximal or distal to the site of the original repair; such simply represents good medical/surgical care and pivots on surveillance of the entire aorta indefinitely using CT and MRI scans.[1,10]

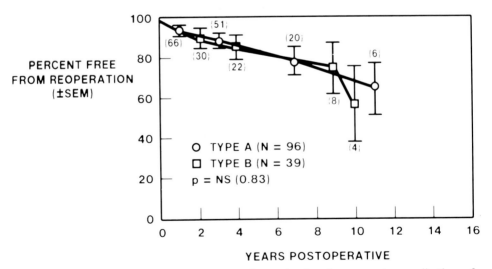

Fig. 8. Actuarial incidence of reoperation (procedures related to the aorta or to complications of the dissection) after surgical repair of aortic dissections. Reproduced from Haverich A, Miller DC, Scott WC, et al: Acute and chronic aortic dissections—Determinants of long-term outcome for operative survivors. Circulation 72 (Suppl II): II-2, 1985. With permission.)

RUPTURED THORACIC AORTIC ANEURYSM

The other major thoracic aortic surgical emergency to be discussed in this essay is rupture of atherosclerotic or degenerative aneurysms. While it had been believed that the incidence of ruptured thoracic aortic aneurysm was lower than that of ruptured *abdominal* aortic aneurysm (based on Danish autopsy studies[5]), this may not be the case today. A recent epidemiological study (1951–1980) from Olmsted County, Minnesota (a rural Midwestern location with a unique capability to gather data for population-based studies) suggests that the incidence of thoracic aortic aneurysm (dissections, atherosclerotic, and other etiologies) in the United States may actually be as high as 59 cases per million population per year (or, expressed differently, 5.9 cases per 100,000 person-years of observation).[7] These authors observed that the natural history of patients with thoracic aortic aneurysms (excluding dissections) who did not undergo surgical treatment was actually worse than that for similar patients with abdominal aortic aneurysms (1 and 3 year actuarial survival estimates of 58 percent and 26 percent compared to 69 percent and 56 percent, respectively).

This Mayo Clinic report by Bickerstaff et al[7] also emphasized the critical importance of making the diagnosis earlier, the extremely high incidence of rupture (which occurred in 74 percent of patients with a 94 percent death rate), and the relatively frequent (25 percent) finding of an associated abdominal aortic aneurysm. The diagnosis of thoracic aortic aneurysm was not previously suspected in 70 percent of the patients who presented with aneurysm rupture; the diagnosis had been known in the other 16 patients prior to aneurysm rupture, but only for an average of 2 years. The actuarial survival estimates after the diagnosis was made were only 39 percent at 1 year and 13 percent at 5 years. The etiology of these aneurysms, however, was varied: dissection—51 percent, atherosclerotic—29 percent, and other—20 percent. Ninety-five percent of the dissections ruptured, compared to 51 percent of the nondissections; similarly, the 1 and 5 year survival rates were less favorable for patients with dissections: 22 percent and 7 percent versus 57 percent and 19 percent, respectively. Nevertheless, atherosclerotic and degenerative thoracic aortic aneurysms are more common and rupture more frequently than generally appreciated. For example, the earlier 1964 Mayo Clinic "pre-surgical era" reported by Joyce et al on 107 patients with thoracic aortic aneurysms (73 percent atherosclerotic and 19 percent luetic) found rupture to account for only 32 percent of deaths and the 10 year survival rate (untreated) was 30 percent.[19]

McNamara and Pressler[20,21] have also contributed to our knowledge of the natural history of patients with thoracic aneurysms. Among 22 nonsurgically treated patients with atherosclerotic descending thoracic aneurysms, 40 percent of all deaths were due to rupture; all aneurysms except one were larger than 10 cm in diameter.[20] In their subsequent report, rupture was the cause of death in 44 percent of patients with atherosclerotic ascending or descending aneurysms, compared to 77 percent of patients with aortic dissections.[21] The survival rate for all patients with atherosclerotic thoracic aortic aneurysms was only 20 percent at 5 years.

The cardinal and most important management guideline for patients with ruptured thoracic aortic aneurysms is to proceed to the operating room as expeditiously as possible.[22] Delaying operation in order to perform a thoracentesis or other diagnostic procedures is usually counter-productive. The clinical history, physical examination, and chest x-ray are usually sufficient to make the diagnosis. Even if the hemothorax is located in the right chest, a left posterolateral thoracotomy should be undertaken with dispatch. Type specific whole blood is available almost immediately in most hospitals, and waiting until many units of blood are typed and cross matched is not generally prudent. If the patient is hemodynamically stable and the diagnosis is not clear, then an emergency CT scan (with IV contrast) can be performed rapidly in most hospitals without precipitating inordinate delay. In my opinion, proceeding with a formal thoracic aortogram is usually not necessary and only results in excessive delay in getting the patient to the operating room.

Most ruptured thoracic aneurysms involve the descending aorta since ascending atherosclerotic aneurysms are relatively rare.[22] Ruptured ascending aneurysms are repaired using a median sternotomy, total CPB, and techniques similar to those outlined above for patients with acute type A dissections. The preferred method of visceral, renal, and spinal cord protection at Stanford continues to be partial (femoral-femoral) CPB for resection of descending thoracic aortic aneurysms, including ruptured aneurysms. In most cases the rupture is contained within the mediastinal pleura and not freely communicating with the pleural space; such allows time for one surgical team to be opening the left chest while another surgeon is rapidly isolating the left (or right) common femoral vein and artery. Cannulation (a short 16–22 French Bardic catheter for arterial inflow and a long 28 French cannula advanced up into the right atrium) is accomplished after systemic heparinization before dissection begins in the mediastinal hematoma, such that CPB can be instituted immediately should massive bleeding be encountered; furthermore, shed blood can be retrieved using the cardiotomy suckers and instantaneously reinfused from the pump. One "trick" that works well if the venous cannula cannot be passed beyond the junction of the iliac vein and inferior vena cava is to thread a 0.038 inch guidewire to the atrium and advance the cannula up over the wire. Bypass flow is gradually increased to 1,500–2,000 ml/min keeping the left ventricular filling pressure (pulmonary capillary wedge pressure) constant; proximal hypertension is controlled with sodium nitroprusside. Additionally, single lung ventilation with an endobronchial tube markedly facilitates these procedures and minimizes trauma to the left lung. Although no method proffers complete immunity from paraplegia and acute renal failure (clamp only, TDMAC [Gott] shunt, CPB, or one of the latter techniques based on monitoring of somatosensory potentials), partial CPB has been associated with a 2 percent incidence of paraplegia and a 14 percent incidence of renal failure (medically treated or requiring dialysis) over the last 20 years at Stanford in 51 patients with degenerative or atherosclerotic descending thoracic aneurysms.[22] The ruptured segment is isolated (usually with the proximal cross clamp placed between the left carotid and subclavian arteries) taking care not to exclude excessively long lengths of normal aorta on either side of the aneurysm, opened, and replaced with a low porosity, woven tubular Dacron graft (Meadox Medicals, Oakland, N.J.).

Results

As intuition would predict, the results of surgical intervention for ruptured thoracic aortic aneurysms are not optimal.[22] This is due, in part, to the acute insult and resulting hypotension, which all too often leads to preoperative multisystem failure, e.g., renal failure, acute MI, and stroke. A comprehensive analysis of the incremental risk factors surrounding resection of degenerative and atherosclerotic aneurysms was recently completed at Stanford.[22] Between 1962 and 1982 175 consecutive patients underwent operation for ascending (n=124) or descending (n=51) thoracic aneurysms (excluding dissections and syphilitic, traumatic, false, arch, and thoracoabdominal aneurysms). The operative mortality rate was 4 percent for the *elective* ascending subgroup and 6.5 percent overall; for the descending subgroup, the overall operative mortality rate was 18 percent (50 percent [4/8] for patients requiring emergency operations and 12 percent for elective cases).[22] Multivariate discriminant analysis revealed that the only significant, independent predictors of an increased likelihood of operative death in the ascending subgroup were emergency operation (p= 0.001) and (older) age (p= 0.031). In the descending subgroup these determinants were emergency operation (p= 0.008) and congestive heart failure (CHF) (p= 0.009). When all patients were analyzed, emergency operation (p= 0.0001), renal dysfunction (p= 0.019), and (older) age predicted a higher operative risk (Fig. 9A). The adverse influence of aneurysm rupture was subsumed by the covariate "Emergency Operation." Translated into actual mortality rates, the adverse impact of these risk factors was clearly evident, as illustrated in Figure 9B. Emergency operation for ascending aneurysm was associated with a 60 percent mortality (versus 4 percent for urgent or elective cases); the risk was 15 percent for patients greater than 62 years old (versus 3 percent for younger patients). In the descending subgroup, the operative mortality rate was 50 percent for emergency cases (versus 12 percent for elective cases) and 60 percent for patients with CHF (versus 14 percent for those without cardiac failure). For all patients, emergency operation carried a 54 percent mortality rate (versus 6.2 percent), age greater than 75 years was associated with a 50 percent mortality rate (versus 7.3 percent in patients younger than 75 years), and the operative mortality rate was 66 percent in patients with renal dysfunction (versus 9 percent for those with normal renal function). This analysis confirmed that it is imperative to avoid emergency procedures (usually for ruptured aneurysms) if at all possible; however, such can be accomplished only if the diagnosis is made earlier and the appropriate surgical procedure performed electively. Given the coupling of emergency operation and advanced age as strong incremental risk factors, it is specious reasoning to defer elective resection of a thoracic aortic aneurysm simply because the patient is "too old." *Res ipsa loquitur.* If a rational decision not to consider elective operative intervention is reached (hopefully in concert with the cardiovascular surgeon, the primary care physician, and the patient's family) on the basis of ongoing illness, far advanced age, or other medical or social reason, however, then it should be understood by all concerned parties that it is not really logical nor realistic to plan to proceed with an emergency surgical procedure should frank aneurysm rupture occur.

Follow-up out to 19 years (cumulative follow-up totaled 860 patient-years) allowed determinants of late death to be analyzed, as graphically shown in Figure 10.[22] In the ascending subgroup, only older age (p= 0.014) was found to portend strongly a statistically significant less favorable prognosis. In the descending subgroup, hypertension (p= 0.002) and CHF (p= 0.055) were weak determinants of late death. When all 175 patients were considered, advanced age (p= 0.009) and male gender (p= 0.042) strongly predicted more attrition over time. Nevertheless, the overall actuarial survival estimates for discharged patients were 78±4 percent at 5 years and 53±6 percent at 10 years (Fig. 11). These long-term survival rates represent dramatic improvement over the dismal natural history of this disease, at least as informally inferred indirectly from the data in the studies cited above.[7,19-21] It must be noted, however, that 13 percent of all late deaths (Fig. 12) were due to rupture of other aortic aneurysms, underscoring the need for indefinite close medical and surgical follow-up and continuous vigilance.

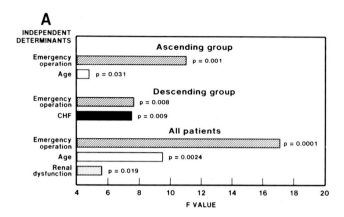

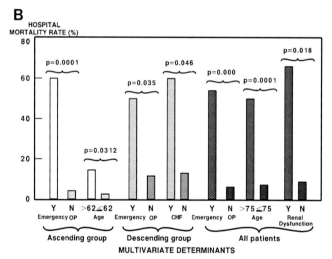

Fig. 9. (A) Independent, significant determinants of an increased likelihood of operative death in patients with atherosclerotic or degenerative thoracic aortic aneurysms. The relative predictive strength of each covariate is graphically shown by the F value on the abscissa. (B) Predicted operative mortality estimates (extrapolated from the logistic regression equation) according to specific independent, significant determinants. (From Moreno-Cabral CE, Miller DC, Mitchell RS, et al: Degenerative and atherosclerotic aneurysms of the thoracic aorta. J Thorac Cardiovasc Surg 88:1020, 1984. With permission.)

336

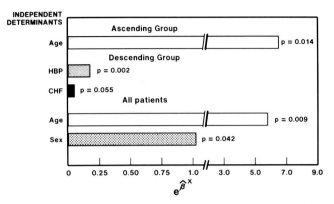

Fig. 10. Independent, statistically significant (multivariate analysis) determinants of late death in patients with atherosclerotic or degenerative thoracic aortic aneurysms. The relative statistical predictive power of each covariate is graphically shown represented by the regression coefficient on the abscissa, $e\hat{\beta}^{x}$.(From Moreno-Cabral CE, Miller DC, Mitchell RS, et al: Degenerative and atherosclerotic aneurysms of the thoracic aorta. J Thorac Cardiovasc Surg 88:1020, 1984. With permission.)

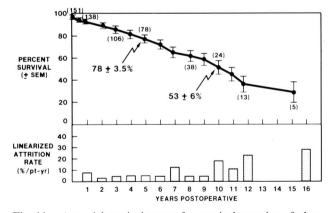

Fig. 11. Actuarial survival curve after surgical resection of atherosclerotic or degenerative thoracic aortic aneurysms. (From Moreno-Cabral CE, Miller DC, Mitchell RS, et al: Degenerative and atherosclerotic aneurysms of the thoracic aorta. J Thorac Cardiovasc Surg 88:1020, 1984. With permission.)

337

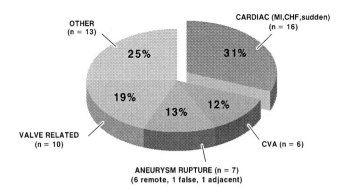

Fig. 12. Cause of late deaths among patients with atherosclerotic or degenerative thoracic aortic aneurysms. Note particularly that 13 percent of all late deaths were due to rupture of another aortic aneurysm.

REFERENCES

1. Miller DC: Surgical management of aortic dissections: Indications, perioperative management, and long-term results, in Doroghazi RM, Slater EE (eds): Aortic Dissection. New York, McGraw-Hill Book Company, 1983, pp 193–243
2. Jamieson WRE, Munro AI, Miyagishima RT, et al: Aortic dissections: Early diagnosis and surgical management are the keys to survival. Can J Surg 25:145, 1982
3. Doroghazi RM, Slater EE, DeSanctis RW, et al: Long-term survival of patients with treated aortic dissections. J Am Coll Cardiol 3:1026, 1984
4. Miller DC: When to suspect aortic dissection: What treatment? Cardiovasc Med 9:811, 1984
5. Sorenson HR, Olsen H: Ruptured and dissecting aneurysms of the aorta. Incidence and prospects of surgery. Acta Chir Scand 128:644, 1964
6. Pate JW, Richardson RL, Eastridge CE: Acute aortic dissections. Am Surgeon 42:395, 1976
7. Bickerstaff LK, Pairolero PC, Hollier LH, et al: Thoracic aortic aneurysms: A population-based study. Surgery 92:1103, 1982
8. Miller DC, Stinson EB, Oyer PE, et al: Operative treatment of aortic dissections. J Thorac Cardiovasc Surg 78:365, 1979
9. Miller DC, Mitchell RS, Oyer PE, et al: Independent determinants of operative mortality for patients with aortic dissections. Circulation 70 (Suppl I):I-153, 1984
10. Haverich A, Miller DC, Scott WC, et al: Acute and chronic aortic dissections—Determinants of long-term outcome for operative survivors. Circulation 72 (Suppl II):II-22, 1985
11. Slater EE: Aortic dissection: presentation and diagnosis, in Doroghazi RM, Slater EE (eds): Aortic Dissection. New York, McGraw-Hill Book Company, 1983, pp 61–70
12. Applebaum A, Karp RB, Kirklin JW: Ascending vs. descending aortic dissections. Ann Surg 183:296, 1976
13. DeBakey ME, McCollum CH, Crawford ES, et al: Dissection and dissecting aneurysms of the aorta: Twenty-year follow-up of five hundred twenty-seven patients treated surgically. Surgery 92:1118, 1982
14. Satler LF, Levine S, Kent KM, et al: Aortic dissection masquerading as acute myocardial infarction: Implication for thrombolytic therapy without cardiac catheterization. Am J Cardiol 54:1134, 1984
15. Wheat MW Jr: Intensive drug therapy, in Doroghazi RM, Slater EE (eds): Aortic Dissection. New York, McGraw-Hill Book Company, 1983, pp 165–192

16. Perez JE: Noninvasive diagnosis: computed tomography and ultrasound, in Doroghazi RM, Slater EE (eds): Aortic Dissection. New York, McGraw-Hill Book Company, 1983, pp 133–148

17. Wolfe WG, Oldham HN, Rankin JS, et al: Surgical treatment of acute ascending aortic dissection. Ann Surg 197:738, 1983

18. Meng RL, Najafi H, Javid H, et al: Acute ascending aortic dissection: Surgical management. Circulation 64 (Suppl II):II-231, 1981

19. Joyce J, Fairbain J, Kincaid O, et al: Aneurysms of the thoracic aorta: A clinical study with special reference to prognosis. Circulation 29:176, 1964

20. McNamara JJ, Pressler VM: Natural history of atherosclerotic thoracic aortic aneurysms. Ann Thorac Surg 26:468, 1978

21. Pressler VM, McNamara JJ: Thoracic aortic aneurysm. Natural history and treatment. J Thorac Cardiovasc Surg 79:489, 1980

22. Moreno-Cabral CE, Miller DC, Mitchell RS, et al: Degenerative and atherosclerotic aneurysms of the thoracic aorta. J Thorac Cardiovasc Surg 88:1020, 1984

Kenneth L. Mattox

Decelerating Aortic Injury

HISTORICAL PERSPECTIVES

Vesalius[1] was the first to report this interesting type of aortic tear in 1557 in a patient who fell from a horse. Subsequent autopsy series reported by Hawkes in 1935[2] and Strassman in 1947[3] have included a combined total of 16,600 autopsies with only 138 cases of traumatic aortic rupture. Symbas, in 1972, summarized the historical aspects of blunt injury to the thoracic aorta.[4]

The modern era of decelerating injury to the thoracic aorta began with the increase in high speed motor vehicle accidents. Parmley's early report in 1958[5] focused attention on the incidence and nature of these injuries. Then, reports during the 1960s established that this injury could be successfully managed by simple clamp repair or using the newly developed cardiopulmonary bypass equipment.[6-8] During the 1970s several temporary bypass shunts, some using a heparinless centrifugal pump, were developed to decrease the complications seen with classic cardiopulmonary bypass.[9,10] During the 1980s debates centered on the determinants of the dread complication of paraplegia, timing of operation and which specific operative approaches resulted in the best chance for survival with lowest overall complications. Preventive social issues have been addressed.[11,12]

ISSUES

Blunt injury to the thoracic aorta has been the subject of numerous articles and book chapters during the past 30 years. These publications address a variety of issues and, at times, even "mix" pathologic conditions of the aorta, including traumatic, degenerative, atherosclerotic, and metabolic conditions. The issues involved in analysis of deceleration injury to the thoracic aorta include:

Vascular Surgical Emergencies
ISBN 0-8089-1843-5

1. Mechanism of injury-pathophysiology
2. Natural history-incidence
3. Pre-hospital management
4. Clinical history, physical findings and radiographic findings
5. Techniques to confirm the diagnosis
6. Timing of operation(s)
7. Early pharmacologic treatment
8. Anesthetic management
9. Technique of operation
10. Distal organ protection
11. Length of cross clamp time
12. Use of the pump, temporary bypass shunt, or simple clamping and repair techniques
13. Determinants of paraplegia and other complications
14. Intraoperative monitoring techniques
15. Perioperative adjuncts
16. Socio/legal issues

MECHANISM OF INJURY

Healthy aortas rupture at pressures between 580 mm Hg and 2500 mm Hg.[13] Deceleration during an automobile accident at 30 mph may exceed 172 Gs.[14] This force is combined with a tearing force on the points of aortic attachment caused by the oblique position of the aorta and the tendency for the fluid filled column to remain in motion when the chest wall abruptly stops.[15] At the thoracic outlet the deceleration may be combined with a pinching of the aorta, innominate artery, trachea, esophagus, and innominate vein between the manubrium and vertebral bodies. At other points of tension during deceleration the aorta may "rupture" or the intima, media and even the adventitia may be partially or completely torn throughout the circumference of the aorta.

INCIDENCE OF INJURY

Parmley's report cited almost uniformly fatal injuries in all locations of the thoracic aorta, especially the proximal descending, just above the aortic annulus, at the diaphragmatic hiatus, and the aortic arch.[5] In civilian series, patients having aortic injury and arriving alive at a treatment facility almost always have injuries involving the thoracic aorta just distal to the left subclavian artery, with the tear beginning at the ligamentum arteriosum. The second most common site of injury is the aortic arch at the take off of the innominate artery. Blunt injuries to the ascending aorta and vertically at the aortic arch are so very rare as to warrant a case report each time they are encountered in a live patient.

In the United States, more than 8000 persons annually will have traumatic aortic rupture. Eighty to 93 percent of all decelerative injuries occur in occupants of automobiles involved in accidents.[1,16,17] Six percent of deceleration aortic injury patients are pedestrians struck by automobiles.[1] Among fatalities following auto accidents, up to 18 percent of the victims will have an injured thoracic aorta.[5,18-23] Greendyke[20] reported a 12 percent incidence of aortic rupture among fatalities not ejected from the automobile, and a 27 percent incidence among fatalities who were ejected. In aircraft accident victims, bursting and tearing of the aorta are commonly seen along with many other nonsurvivable evidences of massive deceleration.

Aortic deceleration injury is extremely rare in patients less than 12 years of age or older than 65 years. Most victims are between 20 and 30 years old, and this injury occurs 9 times more often in men than women. It is estimated that 1.5–7.0 percent of patients with blunt chest injury admitted to a surgical unit will have an aortic injury.[24,25]

NATURAL HISTORY

In at least four studies, 80–85 percent of patients found to have blunt thoracic aortic injury were dead prior to arrival at a medical treatment facility.[5,23,26,27] Many of these patients had massive decelerative injuries, and the aortic transection was merely part of that constellation of nonsurvivable injuries. Of the 15–20 percent of patients arriving alive at an emergency facility with this injury, the mortality rate if untreated is 30 percent at 6 hours, 49 percent at 24 hours, 72 percent at 8 days, 82 percent at 3 weeks, and 90 percent at 16 weeks.[5] Untreated, only 5 percent of patients with this injury will survive to develop chronic traumatic aneurysms.[5,28]

PATHOPHYSIOLOGY OF THE SPINAL CORD AS IT RELATES TO THE INJURED THORACIC AORTA

The spinal cord may be subject to altered function from both anatomic and physiologic variables when the aorta is injured. The arterial supply to the spinal cord is via paired posterior spinal arteries and a single anterior spinal artery. The anterior spinal artery is the more primitive and the more variable with regard to anatomy. Arterial trunks to the anterior spinal artery are extremely variable and arise from the vertebral/basilar system, the subclavian artery, the intercostal arteries, the lumbar segmental arteries and, at times, branches from the iliac arteries. Some of the segmental branches may not even have a connection to the anterior spinal artery. One or more large branches may supply the major truncal component to this spinal circulation, and this large contributor has been named the arteria radicularis anterior magna or the artery of Adamkiewicz. From the medulla to the cauda equina, the anterior spinal artery may be a continuous and substantial patent vessel. It may, however, be interrupted and/or segmented numerous times or have small tenuous connecting collaterals between segmental arteries. This variable anatomy is extremely difficult to determine preautopsy (Fig. 1).

Ischemia, reperfusion, chemical injury, direct contusion, and other conditions may result in spinal canal pressure increases. Increased pressures may be due to a spinal cord swelling, analogous to brain swelling in cerebral contusion. In such instances, compromise of both the venous and arterial blood flow in the spinal cord occurs. Various spinal segments, especially the anterior tracts, may be compromised since the circulation to this area is the most primitive and the more tenuous. In these situations, the surgeon might consider using drugs to reduce cord swelling. If increased intracranial pressure is present,

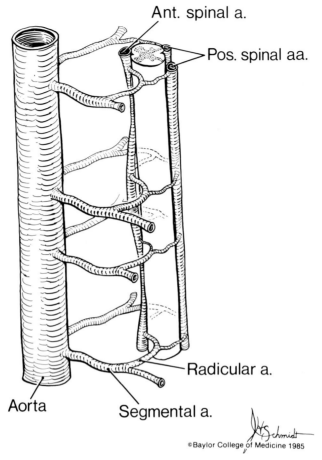

Fig. 1. Drawing depicting the variable anatomy of the segmental arteries off the aorta, the anterior radicular artery, and the anterior spinal artery.

remove spinal fluid from the lumbar spinal canal to reduce increased cord compartment syndrome.

PREHOSPITAL ISSUES

Patients with decelerative injuries require careful extrication, basic life support, and expedient transport to a treatment facility. The ambulance attendant should document the cardiovascular and neurologic status and seek interventions directed by his local EMS medical control. Starting intravenous fluids and applying pneumatic antishock garments to patients with suspected thoracic aortic injury can be seriously questioned and may even compound the injury.[29,30] There is no question that such a patient should be taken to a regional facility (trauma center) that has the capability to resuscitate the patient as well as the ability to recognize and treat complex vascular and associated injuries. Stopping at the nearest nontrauma center emergency room for "stabilization" cannot be justified.

CLINICAL ISSUES

Suggestive Clues from Patient History

A few nonspecific suggestive clues gleaned from the patient's history might cause the initial examining physician to suspect the presence of a decleration aortic injury. Such clues are:

Another person killed in the same accident
Marked deformity of the vehicle cockpit area
Head-on collision
Fall of more than 2 floors
Fall from mountain or "ski lift" type equipment
Aircraft crash
History of paresis or paraplegia

Suggestive Clues from Physical Examination

Nonspecific suggestive clues found on physical examination and associated with blunt aortic injury include:

Steering wheel imprint on chest
Palpable fracture of the sternum
Palpable clavicular fracture
Palpable multiple left rib fractures
Intrascapular murmur
Upper extremity hypertension
Decreased or absent femoral pulses
Paraplegia or lower extremity paresis on admission
Anuria or decreased urine output

It must be noted that 50 percent of patients subsequently found to have deceleration aortic injury will have no external sign of trauma.

Suggestive Clues Found on X-Ray Studies

The greatest factors eliciting the awareness or suspicion of blunt aortic injury are those found on the initial routine chest x-ray.[31] Debate exists as to whether the 72″ EPA or the 36″ supine or portable chest x-ray is the more appropriate. However, a high level of suspicion can be achieved with either, and the patient's condition should determine which is performed. The 72″ EPA roentgenogram is the preferred if it can be achieved. Chest x-ray clues that should cause the initial examining physician to consult a surgeon and consider anteriography include:

Widening of the upper mediastinum greater than 8 cm. (Fig. 2)
Loss of aortic knob contour (Fig. 3)
Left apical pleural hematoma cap (Fig. 4)
Fractured sternum
Fractured 1st and/or 2nd rib
Fractured scapula

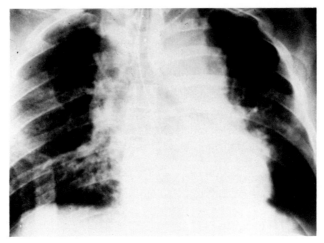

Fig. 2. Anterior posterior (36″) chest x-ray demonstrating a widened mediastinum, nasogastric deviation to the right, and depression of the left main stem bronchus in a patient with a decelerative aortic injury.

Hematoma of the thoracic outlet
Massive left hemothorax
Depression of the left main stem bronchus greater than 140° from the trachea
Calcium layering in the aortic knob (double shadow sign)
Loss of aortic knob contour on lateral chest x-ray
Anterior displacement of the trachea on the lateral chest x-ray

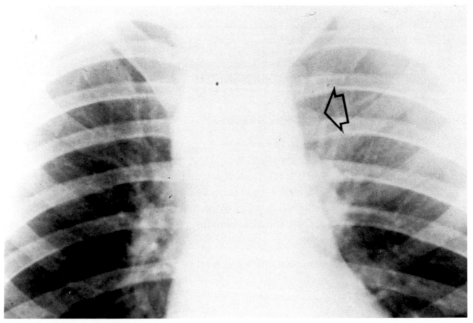

Fig. 3. Chest x-ray demonstrating obliteration of the aortic knob without mediastinal widening in a patient with blunt aortic injury.

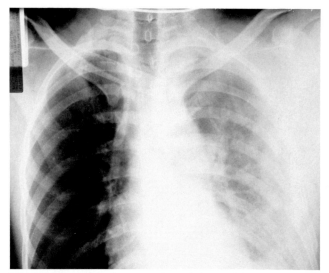

Fig. 4. Chest x-ray demonstrating a left apical hematoma, a left hemothorax, tracheal deviation to the right and depression of the left main stem bronchus in a patient with an aortic injury.

Fracture dislocation of the thoracic spine on lateral chest x-ray
Deviation of the trachea to the side opposite the mediastinal hematoma
Deviation of the nasogastric tube in the esophagus away from the midline
Obliteration of the aortopulmonary window on lateral chest x-ray

Radiographic Imaging

Thoracic aortography is performed via a retrograde femoral route. At least two projections of the entire thoracic aorta are obtained. Specifically, the ascending aorta, innominate artery, thoracic aorta at the ligamentum arteriosum, and the thoracic aorta at the diaphragm are examined for subtle signs of intimal disruption. No attempt is made to cannulate the intercostal arteries, as this procedure has a small incidence of paraplegia complications. On occasion, combined thoracic, cerebral, or abdominal arteriography might be indicated. The arteriogram catheter is withdrawn to the abdominal aorta and left in place as an extraarterial monitor during the induction of anesthesia and during the clamp time of the operation.

Should difficulty in passing the arteriogram catheter from the retrograde femoral route be encountered, especially resistance to passage when the tip of the catheter is at the aortic isthmus, other techniques are available. The catheter may be passed from a right brachial artery cut down into the ascending aorta. Even without digital subtraction equipment, a transvenous injection of dye demonstrates the thoracic aorta on the recirculation phase.

Numerous new imaging techniques might seem indicated in blunt thoracic aortic injury. However, such tests are confusing and are not recommended. The time lost in obtaining computed tomography (CT) scans in addition to the standard contrast arteriogram is not justified. Digital subtraction angiography, CT, and magnetic resonance do not

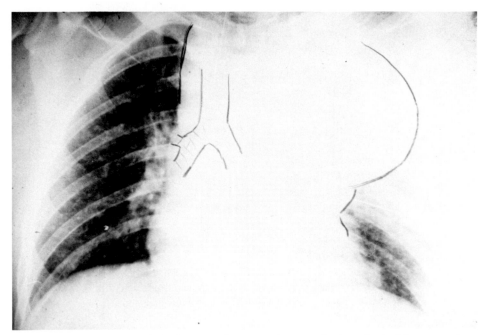

Fig. 5. Chest x-ray (retouched) demonstrating a massive contained mediastinal hematoma in a patient with blunt aortic injury.

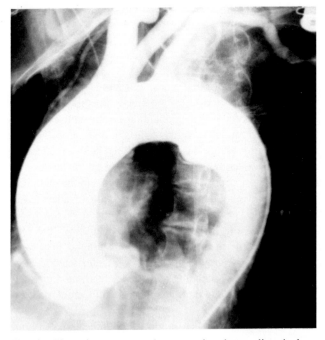

Fig. 6. Thoracic aortogram demonstrating ductus diverticulum, which is sometimes mistaken for an aortic decelerative injury.

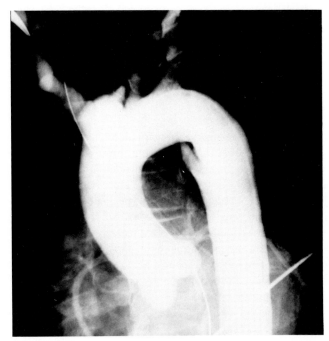

Fig. 7. Thoracic aortogram in a 78-year-old woman demonstrating a residual of a vascular ring originally thought to be an aortic tear.

add to information already provided by classic aortography but may yield misleading data.[19,32]

On rare occasion, the hematoma may be expanding so rapidly that exsanguinating rupture appears to be imminent (Fig. 5). In such instances thoracotomy is performed without arteriography.

The arteriogram may disclose anatomy or pathology that is not an acute or chronic traumatic injury. Such confusing conditions include a ductus diverticulum (Fig. 6), a vascular ring (Fig. 7), or even a dissecting aneurysm. In such lesions an operation may not be indicated at all or require an alternate operative approach.

Associated Injuries

As with any deceleration injury, multisystem trauma is common. Depending on the vector of the deceleration, virtually any organ system can be significantly injured. The most common associated injuries are to the central nervous system, the skeletal system, and to intraabdominal organs. A careful and sequential initial and secondary survey for injury must be carried out.

Presented with a patient with polytrauma and an injury to the thoracic aorta, the surgeon is faced with a decision with regard to operative priorities. For the patient in shock with a stable, nonexpanding thoracic hematoma and a positive peritoneal lavage, an abdominal incision precedes the thoracic procedure.[33] In the patient with a very large expanding mediastinal hematoma, the thoracic procedure is first priority. On rare occasion a two team approach (even involving neurosurgical or orthopedic surgeons) might be indicted.

OPERATION

Timing

Although delayed operative intervention for deceleration injury of the descending thoracic aorta has been suggested in the literature, most authors recommend immediate operation once the diagnosis is made and a competent surgical team is available.[11,12,34] Transfer of patients with lesions at the innominate artery is less risky than for those with injury to the ascending or descending thoracic aorta. With injuries at the take off of the innominate artery, the hematoma is virtually contained and does not rupture preoperatively among those patients arriving alive at a trauma center. For injuries to the ascending or descending thoracic aorta, free rupture into the pericardial or pleural cavities results in almost immediate death from exsanguinating hemorrhage. With all aortic decelerative injuries one may consider the prearteriography and preoperative use of drugs such as propanilol or even nitroprusside to alter the wall sheer forces (decrease the dP/dt) and thereby decrease the chance of a rupture.

Preparation

Multiple intravenous portals should be secured prior to the skin incision. At least four large bore intravenous catheters allow for massive fluid administration whenever it is needed. These fluids should be kept at a minimal flow rate prior to need.

Numerous physiologic parameters may require monitoring. Depending on the clinical status of the patient, the surgeon and the anesthesiologist may choose to monitor just a few or even all of the following parameters:

> EEG tracings
> Preoperative cerebral acuity and neurologic status
> Continuous intraarterial blood pressure
> Digital read out of blood pressure and the mean arterial pressure
> Central venous pressure
> Mean pulmonary artery diastolic pressure and pulmonary capillary wedge pressure
> Pulmonary artery pressures
> Thermal dilution cardiac outputs
> Urinary output
> Pulse rate
> Respiratory rate
> Arterial blood gases
> Measured fluid and blood losses and gains
> Blood hematocrit levels
> Sensory evoked potentials
> Motor evoked potentials

Both the patient and his or her family must be told of the serious, life-threatening nature of this injury as well as the greater than 6 percent chance of lower extremity paralysis and the 10–30 percent chance of dying. A signed and witnessed informed consent must be obtained. The hospital records should contain all pertinent clinical and laboratory information and a written preoperative statement of the extent of the injury and the specifics of the discussion with the patient and the family.

The anesthesiologist may choose to use a double lumen endotracheal tube if it can be used with safety. Autotransfusion equipment, if available, is brought into the operating room. Medications such as nitroprusside, nitroglycerine, dopamine, etc., which might be needed urgently are premixed and hung prior to induction of anesthesia. Any special equipment or devices that might be needed are brought into the operating room, and prior to skin incision all operating room supportive personnel are told of the planned operative procedure.

Technique

Initial Technique

For documented injuries to the ascending aorta, the aortic arch (and the proximal innominate artery), the patient is placed in the supine position, and the incision is a median sternotomy with right neck extension. For injuries from the distal arch to the aorta at the diaphragm, the patient is placed in a right lateral recumbent position. The incision is in the fourth left interspace for injuries at the usual location, the fifth interspace for double injuries, and the seventh interspace for isolated injuries to the distal descending thoracic aorta. After entering the pleural space the left lung is deflated and one lung anesthesia begun if a double lumen endotracheal tube was used. The hemithorax is explored and the extent of the hematoma(s) assessed. Plans are made for the positioning of the anticipated proximal and distal occluding vascular clamps. Communication of the specifics of this plan, especially to the anesthesiologist, is mandatory. Should use of a temporary bypass shunt or a bypass pump be considered, the necessary equipment should be readied at this point.

Approaches

Using traditional cardiopulmonary pump bypass equipment, a variety of techniques have been used to decrease "strain" on the left heart and to provide controlled perfusion to the lower body. These techniques include:

> Femoral vein to femoral artery bypass
> Left atrium to femoral artery bypass
> Left ventricle to femoral artery bypass
> Left heart to distal descending thoracic aortic bypass

In all but the first of these options the oxygenator does not need to be utilized, as the technique does not even partially bypass the lungs.

Temporary heparin coated bypass shunts have been developed by Gott[9] and Wakabashi.[10] These shunts do not require total body heparinization with its inherent problems. The shunts are usually inserted in the ascending aorta or the aortic arch, although at times they may be inserted via purse string into the apex of the left ventricle. The distal cannula is usually inserted in either the distal thoracic aorta or the left femoral artery. At least one or both of these cannulas is thus inserted in a portion of the aorta that already contains an adventitial hematoma. A variation of this shunt is to add an in line centrifugal pump to assure a controlled lower extremity perfusion.[35]

As success with clamp/repair techniques (without heparin, pumps, or temporary shunts) was reported for elective atherosclerotic and degenerative aneurysms of the descending thoracic aorta, it was logical to apply this technique to acute traumatic injuries to the aorta.[16] Furthermore, in some of the early reports (1960s), this technique was as successful as was the use of the pump. Among busy trauma centers this technique is now the option most often used.

For documented complex injuries of the ascending aorta and aortic arch, cardiopulmonary bypass is mandatory for complete repair.[36] For injuries to the proximal innominate artery at the aortic arch, simple bypass grafting without shunts (extraluminal or intraluminal), heparin, pumps, hypothermia, or other complex adjuncts is possible with a high degree of success (Fig. 8).

Specific Technique

For complex injuries of the ascending aorta and arch, innovative planning for customized reconstruction is individually tailored to each extremely rare lesion,[36] the specifics of which are beyond the scope of this chapter. For simple blunt injuries to the aortic arch at the innominate artery, the proximal ascending aorta and the proximal innominate artery

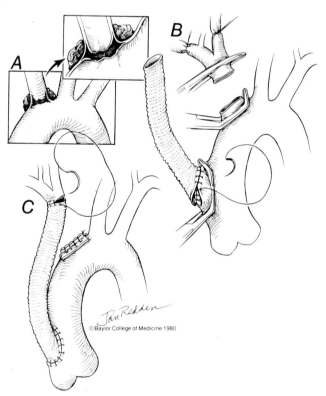

Fig. 8. Drawing depicting technique of approach and repair of blunt injury to the aortic arch at the takeoff of the innominate artery.

are exposed prior to entering the hematoma.[37,38] A 10–14 mm prosthetic graft is sutured to the side of the ascending aorta (Fig. 8). The distal innominate artery is clamped proximal to the subclavian/carotid bifurcation to allow for cerebral perfusion via collaterals. An end-to-end graft to distal innominate artery anastomosis is accomplished taking care to adequately flush the graft when suturing has been completed and prior to reestablishment of flow. The hematoma is now entered, dividing the left innominate vein if necessary for exposure. A partially occluding clamp is placed across the proximal aortic arch, taking care not to occlude the left common carotid artery. The aortic injury is closed with the aid of prosthetic pledgets. On rare occasions a similar technique, even using a bifurcated graft must be used if a concomitant left carotid artery injury is present.

Blunt injury to the descending thoracic aorta just distal to the left subclavian artery requires a deliberate, specific plan of action. After exploration, the aorta distal to the hematoma and the left subclavian artery are encircled with tapes. With gentle blunt and sharp dissection the aortic arch is encircled between the left carotid and subclavian arteries. Care is taken to identify and protect the vagus and phrenic nerves, which are frequently hidden in the hematoma. Care must also be taken in separating the undersurface of the aortic arch from the pulmonary artery, as the hematoma may have distorted the anatomy and entry into the aortic or pulmonary lumen presents control and repair difficulties. If, at this point, the injury appears to extend to the undersurface area of the aortic arch (a rare occurrence), cardiopulmonary bypass should be considered since repair of such an injury is virtually impossible without use of the pump.

With the anesthesiologist prepared to pharmacodynamically alter the cardiac workload and arterial resistance as well as maintain the mean arterial blood pressure above 80 torr, the vascular occluding clamps are applied to the aortic arch, the subclavian artery, and the distal descending thoracic aorta. The pleura over the most prominent portion of the hematoma is then entered. The area of intimal, medial, and even adventitial damage is assessed. The aorta is entered transversely beginning at the medial side of the tear, and the degree of tear is determined. The distal clamp is moved closer to the injury to prevent nonperfusion to as few intercostal arteries as possible. No intercostals are ligated unless they are involved in the tear and are injured. Replantation of injured intercostal arteries is not possible. If the tear is partial, a lateral aortorrhaphy using 4-0 polypropylene suture is performed. If complete transection has occurred, a prosthetic graft may be required. A running suture line beginning medially in the area of the ligamentum arteriosum allows the surgeon to sew in the graft (or at times to perform an end-to-end anastomosis) while sewing toward himself. Following completion of both suture lines, the distal aorta is "flushed" and the surgeon prepares to slowly (*repeat: slowly*) remove the clamps. Communication between the anesthesiologist and the surgeon is mandatory at this point. Afterload reducing agents are stopped and fluid is given at an increased rate. Vasopressors may be temporarily indicated. It may take as long as 15–30 minutes to slowly release the ratchets on the clamp to assure that the mean arterial pressure does not go below 80 torr. Hemostasis at the suture lines is assured, the left lung is reexpanded, and the chest is closed in a routine manner.

A large number of adjuncts may be considered and used by the surgeon if deemed helpful in any phase of the management. The pump is indicated if the proximal extent of the tear is in a position that prohibits accurate suturing in the distal aortic arch. When the tear extends to the ascending aorta, multiple perfusion catheters or even deep hypothermia and circulatory arrest might be needed for precise repair. Temporary bypass shunts are preferred by some thoracic surgeons to reduce the reliance on pharmacologic control.

Neither the use of the pump or a shunt protects the spinal cord circulation served by the intercostal arteries between the clamps. Autotransfusion devices, especially those such as the BRAT* or the Haemonetics Cell Saver,† which allow rapid processing in the operating room, are an indispensable aid in vascular trauma. Such devices reduce the reliance on banked blood and may even be used postoperatively in the intensive care unit. Successful use of the sutureless intraluminal graft in acute blunt thoracic aortic injury has not been reported. Sensory and motor evoked potentials to assess spinal cord function during the clamp time have received variable acceptance by thoracic and trauma surgeons, as the variable loss and reappearance of the potential tracing spikes are difficult to interpret. Furthermore, regardless of the technique initially chosen by the surgeon, to change an approach in the middle of the operative procedure would add significantly to the clamp time. Various neuroplegic solutions are being investigated but have not been adapted clinically.

RESULTS

Operative Survival/Mortality

Depending on the year of the report, the survival of patients arriving alive in the operating room ranges from 20 to 100 percent in selected cases. Analyzing large series of all patients presenting to a trauma center alive, the current mortality rates range between 2 and 30 percent. Most deaths are secondary to two separate processes: (1) Death may result from exsanguinating hemorrhage before operative control of the proximal and distal aorta has been achieved. Once the protective pleura surrounding the aorta ruptures, survival is less than 3 percent. (2) Death may result from the effects of polytrauma, especially injury to the lungs, central nervous system, and the abdominal organs. Although these two separate and distinct mechanisms are responsible for some of the deaths in all reported series, determining just which is the major contributing factor to the death in any particular reported case is extremely important. The mortality when the pump and its accompanying heparinization are used averages more than 30 percent.[12] The mortality following repair with either clamp/repair or shunt techniques is approximately 15 percent.[15]

Complications

Complications are seen among survivors in any polytraumatized patient. When decelerative aortic injury is present, complications usually are a reflection of severe and always multisystem injury. Complications are to be expected, not only because of the multisystem trauma and significant deceleration, but also because of the nature of the surgery required to treat these multiorgan injuries. Although reported variably, the incidence of complications seen in the patient with decelerative aortic injury are discussed in the order of their prevalence.

Pulmonary complications of atelectasis, pneumonia, and/or empyema are the most common following any trauma. Early mobilization, bronchopulmonary toilet, incentive

---

*Cardiovascular Systems Inc., 2408 Timberloch, Suite B-11, The Woodlands, Texas 77380.
† Haemonetics, 17 Erie Drive, Natick, Mass. 01760

spyrometry, and other techniques will aid to reduce these complications. Broad spectrum antibiotics are usually given following both thoracic and vascular surgical procedures and continued until the chest tubes are removed.

Posttraumatic respiratory insufficiency can occur following blunt trauma to the chest, aspiration, postoperative infection, and many other etiologies associated with trauma. Respiratory insufficiency requiring prolonged intubation occurs in more than 30 percent of patients with aortic decelerative injury.

Temporary or permanent hoarseness may occur in as many as 10–25 percent of patients undergoing repair of descending thoracic aortic lesions of any nature. With extensive acute hematoma obliterating normal landmarks and with a stretching of either the vagus or the left recurrent laryngeal nerve, temporary hoarseness might occur. At times, the tear is in close juxtaposition to these nerves and to accomplish repair of the aortic injury a nerve may be stretched during the retraction or encircled inadvertently during suture repair. The surgeon should seek to avoid this complication by attempting to identify and protect all nerves. The postoperative occurrence of hoarseness does not imply a breach of surgical technique, but rather more often is a reflection of the complexity of the repair. If the hoarseness does not disappear in 6 to 15 weeks, Teflon injection of the immobile vocal cord aids in voice rehabilitation.

Paraplegia is the most dreaded complication following acute aortic deceleration injury. For the patient, the family, the surgeon, and the health team, postoperative paralysis and sensory loss cause disappointment, frustration, anger, introspection, and accusations. Multiple factors may contribute to paraplegia and each of these may act singularly or together:

> The extremely variable anatomy of the anterior spinal artery distribution and anatomy
> The severity of the original injury
> The extent and duration of the prehospital hypotension
> Possibly the extent and level of alcohol consumption prior to the accident
> The length of time before arrival at the trauma center
> The presence of a pseudocoarctation syndrome
> The timing of the operation
> Possibly the length of cross clamp time (open to debate)
> The extent of intercostal artery injury found at the time of aortic opening and the number of intercostal arteries which must be ligated because they were injured at the site of the transection
> Hypotension at the time of the release of the cross clamp at the end of the operation
> "Spinal canal compartment syndrome"
> Other as of yet undetermined factors

Paraplegia may be present at the time of presentation and even reverse following successful repair (even in clamp times up to 62 minutes without "protective" shunts or pumps). Paraplegia may be discovered immediately after arteriography, after surgery, or may even develop 1–5 days postoperatively. Although a few authors have suggested that a clamp time of 30 minutes or less is required to protect a patient from developing paraplegia, close analysis of large series does not substantiate this time limit. Paraplegia has occurred in patients with extremely short clamp times and failed to occur in patients with clamp times exceeding 45 minutes. When large series of acute and chronic traumatic aortic injury repairs are compared, no significant difference in the rate of paraplegia between clamp/repair and shunt techniques can be discerned.[12] It appears that a paraplegia rate of 7–10 percent occurs regardless of the technique for repair of acute traumatic aortic transection, whereas paraplegia is seen in approximately 3 percent of repairs for chronic traumatic aneurysm.[29] The occurrence of paraplegia alone does not in any way imply that the surgeon did not use prudent judgment and good operative technique. Regardless of the technique used, the intercostal arteries and the spinal cord between the isolating clamps are at risk for ischemia if that particular portion of the cord is supplied only by arteries from that location.

Postoperative hemorrhage may stem from many sources. It uncommonly occurs from the suture line. Postoperative hemorrhage requiring reoperation usually occurs from the cannulation sites for tubing for bypass pumps or bypass shunts. Late reoperation may be required because of a false aneurysm at the site of cannulation.

Cerebral insufficiency was seen more commonly when pumps (with required heparinization) were routinely used for aortic repair following trauma. Many patients with blunt thoracic aortic injury also have concomitant head injury, and the cerebral insufficiency is secondary to the original injury rather than a complication of the surgery.

Renal insufficiency as a direct result of aortic cross clamping or shunt perfusion during repair of aortic injuries is extremely rare. Renal insufficiency, be it in the form of renal failure or a temporary rise in the BUN and creatinine, is more often associated with preoperative shock and/or the use of nephrotoxic antibiotics and other drugs, rather than from the technique of aortic repair.

Other complications less frequently encountered include infection of aortic grafts, recurrent false aneurysms, peptic ulceration, Clostridia difficile infections, wound infections, myocardial infarction, and pulmonary embolism.

SOCIAL ISSUES

Preventive Measures

Patients with decelerative injuries to the thoracic aorta almost always present to the hospital after 10 PM at night. Blood alcohol levels are elevated in more than 50 percent of patients. When the patient is a victim of an automobile–pedestrian/bicycle etc. accident the driver of the automobile is often legally intoxicated. Any prevention technique *must* include reducing simultaneously mixing driving and consuming alcohol or other drugs.

Since 85 percent of patients who have aortic decelerative injury die before reaching a hospital, preventive strategies are imperative. Some preventive measures that might be taken include:

> Control of the drunk driver
> Active restraints in automobiles (such as seat belts)
> Passive restraints in automobiles (such as air bags)
> Air bags in aircraft
> Separation of pedestrian, bicycle, and motor vehicular traffic

Medical–Legal Issues

In a litigious society it is often assumed that an undesirable result implies malpractice. If such is the case, 50 percent of lawyers in all lawsuits would be guilty. Death and complications are known to occur. The specific complication of paraplegia is mentioned and recognized as a potential problem in virtually every article on aortic decelerative injury. Since no technique assures protection from the complication of paraplegia and since the time needed to perform the repair is determined by the extent of the injury, neither clamp time nor the technique (clamp/repair or shunt) should imply that the surgeon is either imprudent or technically inept. If a legal responsibility exists, it is for governmental agencies to assure that victims of trauma be taken to the closest appropriate facility for managing major trauma, rather than to the closest emergency room for stabilization and later transfer.

REFERENCES

1. Vesalius A: in Bonetus T, Sepulchretaum sive Anataomia Practica ex Cadaveribus Morbo Denatis, Geneva, 1700, sec. 2, p 290
2. Hawkes SZ: Traumatic rupture of the heart and intrapericardial structures. Amer J Surg 37:503, 1935
3. Strassman G: Traumatic rupture of the Aorta. Amer Heart J 22:458, 1947
4. Symbas PN: Traumatic injuries of the heart and great vessels. Springfield, IL, Charles C. Thomas, 1972, p 148
5. Parmley LF, Mattingly TW, Manion WC, et al: Nonpenetrating injury of the aorta. Circulation 17:1086, 1958
6. Beall AC, Arbegast NR, Ripepi AC, et al: Aortic laceration due to rapid deceleration. Arch Surg 98:595, 1969
7. Spencer FC, Guerin PF, Blake HA, et al: A report of fifteen patients with traumatic rupture of the thoracic aorta. J Thorac Cardiovasc Surg 41:1, 1961
8. Grover LK: Traumatic aneurysm of the thoracic aorta. N Engl J Med 270:220, 1964
9. Donahoo JS, Brawley RK, Gott VL: The heparin-coated vascular shunt for thoracic aortic and great vessel procedures: A ten-year experience. Ann Thorac Surg 23:507, 1977
10. Wakabayashi A, Connolly JE, Stemmer EA, et al: Heparinless left heart bypass for resection of thoracic aneurysms. Am J Surg 130:212, 1975
11. Williams TE, Vasko JS, Kakos GS, et al: Treatment of acute and chronic traumatic rupture of the descending thoracic aorta. World J Surg 4:545,1980
12. Mattox KL, Bickell WH, Pepe PE, et al: Prospective randomized evaluation of MAST in post traumatic hypotension. J Trauma (In press), 1986
13. Oppenheim FG: Gibt es eine Sportanruptur der gesdunden Aorta und wie kommit sie zustande? Munchen Med Wschr 65:1234, 1918
14. Marsh CL, Moore RC: Deceleration trauma. Amer J Surg 93:623, 1957
15. Jackson FF, Berkas EM, Roberts VL: Traumatic aortic rupture after blunt trauma. Dis Chest 53:577, 1968
16. Symbas PN, Tyras DH, Ware RE: Traumatic rupture of the aorta. Ann Surg 178:6, 1973
17. Spencer FC, Guerin PF, Clake HA, et al: A report of fifteen patients with traumatic rupture of the thoracic aorta. J Thorac Cardiovasc Surg 41:1, 1961
18. Zeldenrust J, Aarts JH: Traumatische Aorta-ruptuur bij Verkeersongevallen. Ned Tiyschr Geneeskd 106:464, 1962
19. Egan TJ, Neiman HL, Herman RJ, et al: Computed tomography in the diagnosis of aortic aneurysm dissection or traumatic injury. Radiology 136:141, 1980
20. Greendyke RM: Traumatic rupture of the aorta: Special reference to automobile accidents. JAMA 195:527, 1966
21. Kirsh MM, Kahn DR, Crane JD: Repair of acute traumatic rupture of the aorta without extracorporeal circulation. Ann Thorac Surg 10:227, 1970

22. Kirsh MM, Behrendt DM, Orringer MB: The treatment of acute traumatic rupture of the aorta: A 10 year experience. Ann Surg 184:308, 1976

23. Sutorius DJ, Schreiber JT, Helmsworth JA: Traumatic disruption of the thoracic aorta. J Trauma 13:583, 1973

24. Bross W: Injuries of the thoracic aorta. J Cardiovasc Surg 12:95, 1962

25. Heberer G: Ruptures and aneurysms of the thoracic aorta after blunt chest trauma. J Cardiovasc Surg 12:115, 1971

26. Mattox, KL: Invited commentary on blunt injury to the descending thoracic aorta. World J Surgery 4:551, 1980

27. Hartford JM, Fayer RL, Shaver TE, et al: Transection of the thoracic aorta: Assessment of a trauma system. Amer J Surg 151:224, 1986

28. McCollum CH, Graham JM, Noon GP, et al: Chronic traumatic aneurysms of the thoracic aorta: An analysis of 50 patients. J Trauma 19:248, 1979

29. Mattox KL, Holzman M, Pickard LR, et al: Clamp/repair: a safe technique for treatment of blunt injury to the descending thoracic aorta. Ann Thorac Surg 40:456, 1985

30. Lewis FR: Prehospital intravenous fluid therapy: Physiologic computer modeling. J Trauma 25:699, 1985

31. Fisher RG, Hadlock F, Ben-Menachem Y: Laceration of the thoracic aorta and brachiocephalic arteries by blunt trauma. Rad Clin North Am 19:91, 1981

32. Heiberg E, Wolverson MK, Sundaram M, et al: CT in aortic trauma. AJR 140:1119, 1983

33. Borman KR, Aurbakken CM, Weigelt JA: Treatment priorities in combined blunt abdominal and aortic trauma. Amer J Surg 144:728, 1982

34. Akins CW, Buckley MJ, Daggett W, et al: Acute traumatic disruption of the thoracic aorta: A ten-year experience. Ann Thorac Surg 31:305, 1980

35. Oliver HF, Maher TD, Liebler GA, et al: Use of the Biomedicus centrifugal pump in traumatic tears of the thoracic aorta. Ann Thor Surg 38:586, 1984

36. Reyes LH, Rubio PA, Korompai FL, et al: Successful treatment of transection of aortic arch and innominate artery. Ann Thorac Surg 19:468, 1975

37. Graham JM, Feliciano DV, Mattox KL, et al: Innominate vascular injury. J Trauma 22:647, 1982

38. Richardson JD, Smith JM, Grover FL, et al: Management of subclavian and innominate artery injuries. Amer J Surg 134:780, 1977

Alexander D. Shepard
Calvin B. Ernst

Aortoenteric and Aortocaval Fistulae

Aortoenteric and aortocaval fistulae represent two unusual, highly lethal complications of atherosclerotic disease of the abdominal aorta. Diagnosis can be difficult and surgical correction taxing even to the experienced vascular surgeon. Successful management is dependent upon prompt recognition and early, aggressive operative intervention. Without operation patients with aortoenteric fistulae will succumb to massive gastrointestinal bleeding or sepsis while patients with aortocaval fistulae will die from cardiac decompensation.

AORTOENTERIC FISTULAE

Classification and Incidence

There are two types of aortoenteric fistulae—primary and secondary. Primary fistulae result from erosion of the abdominal aorta into an adjacent segment of the gastrointestinal tract. Most commonly an abdominal aortic aneurysm ruptures into the overlying third or fourth portion of the duodenum (Fig. 1). However, arterial wall degeneration from a variety of causes including infection, irradiation, pancreatitis, and neoplastic involvement can lead to enteric communication with bleeding.[1,2] Primary aortoenteric fistulae are exceedingly rare with only 189 cases reported in the world's literature.[3]

Secondary aortoenteric fistulae follow abdominal aortic reconstruction with synthetic vascular prostheses and are of two varieties. The more common type (approximately 90 percent), graft enteric or anastomotic enteric fistula, is a direct communication between the aortic lumen at a suture line and bowel (Fig. 2).[4] The second type, graft enteric erosion or paraprosthetic enteric sinus, is considerably less frequent and results from prosthetic graft erosion into the bowel lumen some distance from an anastomosis (Fig. 3).[4,5] A graft enteric erosion may eventually evolve into a graft enteric fistula if local infection spreads to an adjacent suture line with subsequent breakdown. Secondary aortoenteric fistulae are much more common than primary aortoenteric fistulae and represent

Vascular Surgical Emergencies
ISBN 0-8089-1843-5

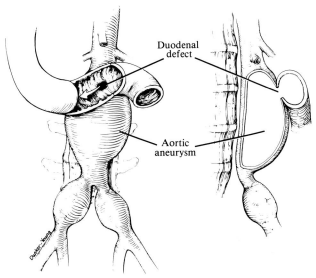

Fig. 1. Primary aortoduodenal fistula secondary to abdominal aortic aneurysm. (Reprinted from Ernst CB: Aortoenteric fistulas, in Haimovici H (ed.): Vascular Emergencies. E. Norwalk, CT, Appleton-Century-Crofts, 1982. With permission.)

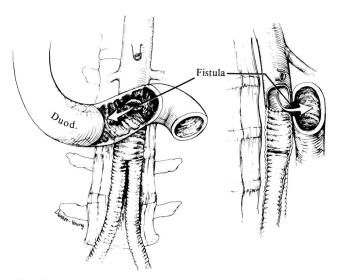

Fig. 2. Secondary aortoduodenal fistula. (Reprinted from Ernst CB: Aortoenteric fistulas, in Haimovici H (ed.): Vascular Emergencies. E. Norwalk, CT, Appleton-Century-Crofts, 1982. With permission.)

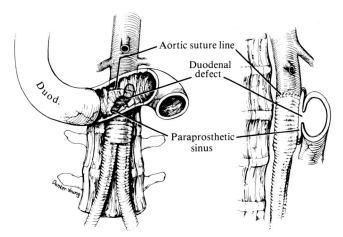

Fig. 3. Aorto paraprosthetic sinus. The prosthesis is seen through the duodenal defect (left). The paraprosthetic sinus extends up to the proximal anastomosis, which is intact (right). (Reprinted from Ernst CB: Aortoenteric fistulas, in Haimovici H (ed.): Vascular Emergencies. E. Norwalk, CT, Appleton-Century-Crofts, 1982. With permission.)

a greater technical challenge because of prior surgical procedures. With improved operative technique the incidence of this complication has decreased from 4–10 percent of aortic reconstructions in the 1960s to current estimates of 1–2 percent.[5,6]

Pathogenesis

Aortoenteric fistulae involve any segment of the gastrointestinal tract but most commonly occur between the infrarenal aorta and the overlying relatively fixed distal duodenum. In a recent study Bunt noted that 85 percent of secondary aortoenteric fistulae involved the duodenum, 8 percent the jejunum, and 5 percent the ileum.[4] Isolated instances of colonic, gastric, and esophageal involvement have also been reported.

Primary aortoenteric fistulae usually result from direct erosion of an abdominal aortic aneurysm into the duodenum. With aneurysmal expansion the duodenum is stretched out with focal wall ischemia and thinning. Anterior rupture into the duodenum may, thus, represent the path of least resistance for an expanding aneurysm. Less than 20 percent of primary aortoenteric fistulae involve other segments of the gastrointestinal tract.[3]

Two major mechanisms have been implicated in the pathogenesis of secondary aortoenteric fistulae, mechanical bowel erosion or aortic anastomotic dehiscence. Purely mechanical factors may lead to progressive bowel erosion by the pulsatile noncompliant aortic prosthesis.[5,7,8] The third and fourth portions of the duodenum, already relatively fixed in the retroperitoneum, can be further tethered to the graft by scarring and foreign body reaction. Local damage or ischemia of the duodenal wall at the time of the initial procedure may also be a contributing factor.[5] Pulsatile pressure necrosis of the adherent bowel wall causes slow erosion and eventual perforation. Duodenal contents including bacteria and digestive enzymes then bathe the graft and surrounding area leading to retroperitoneal infection and tissue destruction. As this process dissects locally, the proximal anastomotic suture line becomes involved with ultimate disruption. Assuming this mechanism, graft enteric erosions may represent a first stage in the development of aortoenteric or anastomotic enteric fistulae. Accordingly, proper separation of the graft from bowel at the time of the initial aortic procedure should be of paramount importance in avoiding fistulization. The significant decrease in the incidence of this complication in recent series stressing this surgical principle lends support to this theory.

The second mechanism of aortoenteric fistulization holds that aortic graft suture line disruption is the primary event with secondary pseudoaneurysm formation and eventual bowel erosion.[9] Anastomotic disruption may result from suture material fatigue, aortic wall degeneration, or local infection. Two recent reports of secondary aortoenteric fistulae with high incidences of proximal anastomotic pseudoaneurysms have emphasized the possible importance of suture line infection.[10,11] Such infection may result from operative contamination or bacteremic seeding following graft implantation. The well documented presence of bacteria in aneurysm wall cultures represents an important potential source for inoculation.[12,13] The higher incidence of positive wall cultures from ruptured aneurysms than from elective aneurysms correlates with the higher incidence of aortoenteric fistulae following emergent aneurysm repair than after elective repair, which is greater still than the incidence following grafting for occlusive disease. The exact role of primary suture line infection in the genesis of aortoenteric fistulae is impossible to determine because of the high incidence of positive cultures found at the time of repair. Whether such infection is a primary or secondary process is unknown. Undoubtedly both mechanical and infectious factors play a role in the development of aortoenteric fistulae but most authors seem to favor a primary erosive process followed by secondary infection.[7,8]

Presentation

The symptom complex of gastrointestinal bleeding, sepsis, and abdominal pain classically associated with aortoenteric fistulae is rarely present in any one patient. The mode of presentation depends on the type of aortoenteric fistula. For primary fistulae and secondary graft enteric fistulae where the aortic lumen communicates with the bowel, gastrointestinal bleeding predominates. Sixty-four percent of patients with primary aortoenteric fistulae and 75 percent with graft enteric fistulae present with gastrointestinal bleeding.[3,4] Such bleeding in graft enteric fistulae occurs as hematemesis (35 percent), melena (32 percent), or hematochezia (8 percent).[4] Bleeding is rarely massive at onset and is usually intermittent ("herald" hemorrhages) over several hours or days and occasionally months as the fistula spontaneously seals with thrombus. Recognition and surgical correction at this stage offer the best chance for survival. Without intervention the fistula slowly enlarges, inevitably resulting in sudden and fatal exsanguination. Hemorrhage from graft enteric erosions or paraprosthetic sinuses is less common than from direct communications and usually presents as chronic, small volume, lower gastrointestinal bleeding.[4,14] In this situation, bleeding occurs from the eroded edges of the bowel wall or through the graft interstices following lysis of the fibrin pseudointima by digestive enzymes.[8,15]

Systemic infection is most common with graft enteric erosions (60 percent) where a fistulous communication with the aortic lumen is absent.[4,14,15] Signs and symptoms range from low grade fevers and malaise with leukocytosis to bacteremia with septic shock.[4,14,15] Patients can present with groin masses, often with spontaneous drainage as in synthetic graft infections without enteric communication.[14] Blood cultures when positive usually grow enteric organisms with *E. coli* predominating.[15] Hypertrophic osteoarthropathy and septic emboli limited to the lower extremities with localized cellulitis or septic arthritis have been reported but are unusual as initial symptoms.[5,14] Signs of systemic infection occur less commonly with graft enteric fistulae (14 percent) and not at all with primary aortoenteric fistulae, again, supporting a primarily erosive mechanism for fistula formation.

Abdominal pain is the least frequent symptom of the classic triad. It is most common with primary aortoenteric fistulae (32 percent) secondary to an acutely expanding aneurysm.[3] Only 20 percent of patients with graft enteric erosions and 11 percent with graft enteric fistulae present with abdominal pain.[4] A pulsatile abdominal aneurysm may be palpable in patients with primary aortoenteric fistulae or pseudoaneurysms of the proximal suture line but is an inconsistent finding.[3,8] In a recent review of primary aortoduodenal fistulae only 25 percent of patients had a palpable aneurysm.[3]

The interval from initial aortic reconstruction to presentation with symptoms in secondary fistulization is variable ranging from 2 days to 14 years with an average of 3–5 years.[8,11,16] The variable nature of the clinical presentation precludes easy diagnosis and emphasizes the importance of a high index of suspicion when any patient with an abdominal aortic aneurysm or a history of aortic reconstruction presents with these symptoms.

Diagnosis

Any patient with an abdominal aortic aneurysm or a history of aortic reconstruction who develops gastrointestinal bleeding should be considered to have an aortoenteric fistula until proven otherwise. Aggressive diagnostic evaluation should be launched immediately and not ended until a source of bleeding has been identified. The high mortality associated with delay in diagnosis and treatment is well documented.[16-18] Most patients present early in the course of fistulization with intermittent bleeding or signs of infection and can, therefore, undergo a rapid but deliberate workup.[8] Unfortunately, no currently available diagnostic test, or combination of tests, is sufficiently accurate to consistently detect aortoenteric communications. Correct preoperative diagnosis, while not always possible, is very helpful in planning surgical intervention. For those patients in whom the diagnosis is still in question despite a complete workup, diagnostic celiotomy is the only alternative. Similarly, in patients who present with exsanguinating hemorrhage or hemodynamic instability, emergency operation must be undertaken as the definitive diagnostic test.

Of the various diagnostic modalities available, upper gastrointestinal endoscopy may be the most helpful and is usually the first study performed. The procedure must be carried out by an experienced endoscopist with a fiberoptic endoscope long enough to reach the third and fourth portions of the duodenum. Only with careful examination of the distal duodenum can a definitive diagnosis be made. In only 6 instances of 20 endoscopically documented aortoenteric fistulae reported in the literature has the synthetic graft been seen protruding through the duodenal wall.[19] Other findings highly suggestive of the diagnosis include an extrinsic pulsatile mass compressing the distal duodenum, a punctate ulceration in the third or fourth portion of the duodenum, and hemorrhage emanating from the distal duodenum.[19] In several early studies endoscopy suggested the diagnosis in less than 10 percent of cases and was, therefore, felt to be of limited value.[8,10,11] In more recent reviews, however, where repeat endoscopy is aggressively utilized, the diagnostic rate approaches 50 percent.[14,16,18] Even when negative for fistula identification, endoscopy can be helpful by documenting presence of other gastrointestinal tract lesions. It is important to remember, however, that the discovery of such lesions, even if bleeding, does not always exclude an aortoenteric fistula.[8,14,16] Endoscopy can be dangerous and a patient may suddenly exsanguinate during endoscopic manipulation of the distal duodenum. Unstable patients should therefore only be endoscoped in the operating room.[8]

CT scanning has only recently been accepted as an important test in diagnosis of suspected aortoenteric communications. Rarely such scans can be diagnostic of aortoenteric fistulae by documenting intraluminal aortic gas or a perigraft leak of oral contrast material.[20] More frequently, CT scanning may document signs of aortic graft infection including periprosthetic gas and/or fluid collections.[21] The presence of periprosthetic gas later than 6 weeks after operation is virtually pathognomonic of infection while the presence of fluid after 6 weeks is highly suspicious.[22] Upon identifying periprosthetic fluid, CT-guided needle aspiration can be confirmatory.[23] The accuracy of these findings in diagnosing aortoenteric fistulae and/or aortic graft infection was recently confirmed in a series where aortoenteric fistulae were identified in six of six patients and excluded in four others.[21] It has been suggested that CT scanning be the initial diagnostic study in stable patients with suspected fistulae. Endoscopy is then reserved for those patients with negative CT scans.

Nuclear imaging techniques have also been proposed for diagnosing graft infection. Gallium scanning, popular over the last decade, has been supplanted by the more accurate and convenient indium-labeled white cell study.[24,25] The overall accuracy of these techniques in detecting aortoenteric fistulae has not been specifically addressed although the sensitivity of these tests for excluding aortic graft infection has been reported to be excellent.[25] Other investigators maintain that CT scanning is still more accurate.[22] Both modalities, however, are dependent upon the presence of graft infection to support a diagnosis of aortoenteric fistulae and, hence, may be negative in those instances where associated infection is minimal or absent.

Barium contrast studies and aortography have a low yield in the evaluation of suspected fistulae.[5,8,26] Helpful findings on upper gastrointestinal series include presence of contrast material around the graft ("coiled spring sign"), compression of the distal duodenum, duodenal erosion, and opacification of an extraluminal sinus tract.[17,27] Aortography may document a pseudoaneurysm or, rarely, extravasation of contrast material through the fistula.[27] Such findings are infrequent and a negative study does not exclude the diagnosis. Despite its limited diagnostic potential, aortography is helpful in planning operation by delineating the anatomy of the proximal anastomosis and distal run-off vessels. Other diagnostic studies described include positive blood cultures for enteric organisms particularly when drawn from the femoral artery with concomitant negative arm venous blood cultures, and tagged red cell scans positive for a distal duodenal bleeding site.[5] Though these techniques may be helpful in individual cases, low sensitivity limits their usefulness and widespread application.

In summary, diagnostic evaluation of patients with suspected aortoenteric fistulae is dictated by their clinical presentation. A small number of individuals with a history of previous aortic reconstruction or a known abdominal aortic aneurysm who present with massive gastrointestinal bleeding are best managed by prompt celiotomy. The majority of patients will present with low volume gastrointestinal bleeding and/or signs of graft infection and can undergo a rapid evaluation that should include CT scanning and upper gastrointestinal endoscopy. If either study is positive, aortography should be obtained to plan surgical intervention. If both CT scanning and endoscopy are negative and the patient remains stable, a period of careful observation may be warranted.[14] Occasionally, such patients will require a diagnostic celiotomy to establish or exclude the diagnosis.

Treatment

Operation represents the only treatment option for aortoenteric fistulae; left untreated, patients will invariably succumb to sepsis or exsanguinating gastrointestinal hemorrhage. The objectives of operation are: (1) control of bleeding, (2) closure of the bowel defect, (3) eradication of associated infection, and (4) selective restoration of distal circulation. The operative approach for accomplishing these objectives varies with the type of fistula.

Primary aortoenteric fistulae appear to be different from secondary fistulae in that infection plays a limited role. Unless there is extensive associated infection or contamination most authorities have adopted Daugherty and his colleagues' recommendation to proceed with bowel closure and standard aneurysm repair with placement of an in situ prosthetic graft.[28] A recent review has documented the safety of this approach with only 1 episode of graft infection and death (5 percent) occurring in 19 patients so treated.[3] Intraoperative cultures of the aortic wall should be obtained to guide postoperative antibiotic coverage; if negative, a prolonged course of antibiotic therapy is unnecessary. In the event that associated sepsis is obvious and extensive or duodenal spillage significant, this treatment plan should be abandoned for the approach described below for secondary aortoenteric fistulae.

Several treatment options exist for dealing with secondary aortoenteric fistulae: (1) local treatment, (2) graft excision without revascularization, (3) graft excision with in situ prosthetic revascularization, (4) graft excision with autogenous in situ revascularization, and (5) graft excision with selective extraanatomic revascularization. In selected patients, successful outcome can be achieved with each of these. Graft excision without revascularization may prove successful for patients with previous lower extremity amputations or those initially operated upon for occlusive disease with reasonable compensating collateral development. Similarly, in rare instances with minimal or no local sepsis, simple closure of the bowel and vascular defects or replacement with a second prosthetic graft has been successful. However, when analyzing studies from centers most experienced in managing this complication it is clear that graft excision with restoration of distal circulation by extraanatomic bypass or autogenous reconstruction produces the best results. Lesser procedures have a high incidence of fistula recurrence and death. Mortality for local treatment alone was 85 percent, for graft excision without revascularization 73 percent, for graft excision with in situ prosthetic revascularization 53 percent, and for graft excision with extraanatomic bypass 37 percent.[4]

Given that total graft excision, closure of the bowel defect, and remote bypass is the best treatment option in these patients the proper sequence and timing of these procedures depends upon the mode of presentation. In patients with active or continuous bleeding or in patients in whom celiotomy is performed for diagnosis, graft excision *must* precede extraanatomic bypass. With this operative sequence the major risks are associated with the metabolic consequences of prolonged distal ischemia and the increase in cardiac afterload attendant with aortic closure. Occasionally, patients will not require immediate lower extremity revascularization but it is often difficult to determine this on clinical grounds.[8] It is, therefore, better to proceed with immediate axillobifemoral bypass in the majority of cases. Such combined procedures are unquestionably taxing for both the patient and surgeon but represent the safest course.

In patients in whom a preoperative diagnosis has been firmly established the question arises as to whether extraanatomic bypass should precede graft excision. Arguments against preliminary remote bypass include the possibility that the new graft will become infected prior to removal of the old infected graft, fear that competitive flow will cause thrombosis of the extraanatomic bypass, and concern that a few patients will be subjected to unnecessary revascularization. While occasional instances of secondary infection of extraanatomic bypasses have been reported, the number is small and their management relatively easy.[29] Competitive flow causing extraanatomic graft thrombosis does not appear to be a problem, and the number of patients who will not require revascularization following graft excision is very small.[30] Results with preliminary remote bypass recently documented a 17 percent mortality among patients who underwent extraanatomic bypass prior to aortic graft excision, and a 53 percent mortality when graft excision was performed first.[31] A staged approach with two separate operative procedures may represent the best treatment. Reilly and her colleagues reported a mortality of 26 percent when the 2 operations were performed at the same sitting and a reduced mortality of 13 percent when remote bypass preceded graft excision by 4–6 days.[29]

Operative Technique

Once the diagnosis has been confirmed or efforts at diagnosis are unfruitful despite strong suspicions, prompt operation is mandatory to avoid the increased mortality associated with delay in treatment.[8,16,17] With an established diagnosis of aortoenteric fistula preliminary axillobifemoral bypass should be performed in the stable patient, preferably several days prior to abdominal exploration. In patients with aortic tube or aortoiliac grafts and virgin groins, extraanatomic bypass is straightforward and follows established guidelines. Patients with previous femoral anastomoses, however, require bypass through fresh tissue planes separate from old incisions to avoid potential contamination. In this setting, distal anastomoses to the deep femoral, superficial femoral, or proximal popliteal arteries may be necessary. Cross femoral extensions must also avoid previous groin incisions, although use of autogenous vein may allow bypass through or into a potentially contaminated field. Broad spectrum antibiotics are administered preoperatively and continued through the postoperative period. Length and specificity of antibiotic therapy is determined by operative findings and organisms identified.

Ideally, abdominal exploration should follow remote bypass after a recovery period of several days. In unstable patients or individuals in whom diagnosis is not firmly established, celiotomy becomes the first procedure. Swan-Ganz monitoring and autotransfusion are invaluable aids during the procedure. A long midline incision offers adequate exposure and avoids contamination of extraanatomic grafts or potential tunnels in the flanks and suprapubic region. Prior to abdominal exploration the supraceliac aorta should be dissected to allow expeditious occlusion should sudden uncontrolled hemorrhage be encountered during dissection of the infrarenal aorta. Occlusion at this level is also the best approach for controlling ongoing massive gastrointestinal bleeding. If possible, an attempt should next be made to obtain infrarenal control to avoid prolonged suprarenal occlusion during subsequent fistula division. If the fistula is divided during infrarenal dissection, digital compression or balloon catheter tamponade can be used in conjunction with supraceliac cross clamp to control bleeding while infrarenal occlusion is obtained.

In cases of primary aortoenteric fistulae aneurysmal enlargement should be obvious. Proximal and distal arterial control allow safe dissection of the duodenum off the aneurysm with a minimum of bleeding. With secondary aortoenteric fistulae, the duodenum is carefully dissected away from the prosthesis using a scalpel. If no communication is found at this level, thorough examination of the entire length of the prosthesis must be undertaken. All loops of adherent small bowel and colon must be mobilized off the graft to identify fistulae at other sites. There is often no associated inflammatory mass so that a careful inspection is the only acceptable means for excluding or establishing the diagnosis.

After identifying and dividing the fistulous tract, the enteric defect, if small, can be closed primarily with a few simple sutures. Larger holes may require bowel resection with end-to-end anastomosis or closure of the proximal end of the bowel with anastomosis of the jejunum to the second portion of the duodenum.

Since there is no associated infection in most primary aortoenteric fistulae, it is safe to proceed with standard aortic reconstruction. Aortic wall cultures should be taken to rule out infection and guide possible postoperative antibiotic therapy. Prior to graft placement the retroperitoneum and debrided aneurysm sac are thoroughly irrigated with antibiotic solution to minimize contamination and potential graft sepsis. Graft coverage with viable retroperitoneal tissue, residual aortic wall, and/or omentum is important in the prevention of secondary aortoenteric fistulae. If operative cultures ultimately yield bacterial growth, organism specific long-term oral antibiotic therapy must be maintained.

Since with secondary aortoenteric fistulae infection is nearly always present, even if there is no obvious purulence or surrounding inflammatory response, the entire prosthesis must be excised. Distal anastomoses are dismantled and the involved arteries closed. Iliac vessels can be closed with a mechanical stapler or monofilament synthetic suture. Aorto-femoral graft excision requires reopening the old groin incisions, taking care not to contaminate recently placed extraanatomic grafts. Femoral artery closure with a vein patch may sometimes be necessary to preserve perfusion of the pelvic vessels.

The Achilles heel of treatment of secondary aortoenteric fistulae is the proximal aortic stump. Stump disruption from inadequate closure or residual infection may occur in up to one third of patients both early and late and is almost always fatal.[29,32] To minimize this complication some have advocated preserving aortic continuity whenever possible.[29] With end-to-side proximal anastomoses this can sometimes be accomplished by lateral aortorrhaphy or vein patching. End-to-end anastomoses can occasionally be managed with autogenous tissue reconstruction, but because of the high incidence of infection at the level of the proximal suture line this option is usually not possible.

It is mandatory that all infected retroperitoneal tissue including aortic wall be debrided back to healthy noninfected planes. In rare circumstances, this may require transposition of the renal arteries to a higher level or hepato/spleno–renal anastomoses to allow closure of noninfected aorta.[29] The aortic stump can be closed in a number of ways but most commonly by two rows of monofilament synthetic suture using a horizontal mattress stitch for the proximal row and a running over and over stitch for the distal row. Reinforcement of the stump with viable tissue is also important and can be accomplished with prevertebral fascia, omentum, or a seromuscular patch of jejunum.[33-35] Additional coverage with viable tissue is important to assure complete separation of bowel and aorta. Some authors have advocated placement of irrigating and drainage catheters in the retroperitoneal bed to allow postoperative irrigation with povidone-iodine or antibiotic solution.[36] High dose antibiotics are continued postoperatively and altered on the basis of operative cultures. When graft excision precedes remote bypass for emergency or diagnostic purposes, extraanatomic bypass should follow celiotomy with reprepping and draping and a new operative setup. Occasionally, such bypass will not be needed, as in individuals with bilateral amputations or large preexisting collaterals, but such patients are the exception rather than the rule.

Results

Primary aortoenteric fistulae are so rare that only case reports have appeared in the literature. In a review of 118 cases of primary aortoduodenal fistula reported over the last 30–40 years, a mortality rate of 35 percent was noted among the 34 patients undergoing operation.[3] Of the 22 survivors, 19 underwent primary duodenal repair and standard prosthetic aortic reconstruction. Three patients treated in this fashion had positive aortic wall cultures, 2 are long-term survivors and the third died 5 months postoperatively from an anastomotic disruption. Graft related complications were not identified in 95 percent of long-term survivors supporting the safety of this approach. Survival of patients with secondary aortoenteric fistulae depends upon prompt recognition and early operation. Without operation death is a universal outcome.[4] Delay in operation until recurrent massive hemorrhage or advanced sepsis intervenes results in a death rate of 75–100 percent.[16-18] While anecdotal reports of success with local repair or graft replacement have been recorded, the best results, 63 percent survival, are obtained with total graft excision and extraanatomic bypass.[4] When local closure of the fistulous communication was employed, survival was 15 percent. Graft excision without revascularization resulted in 27 percent survival while graft excision followed by in situ prosthetic replacement had a 47 percent survival. Improved results with graft excision and selective remote bypass in one recent report resulted in a survival of 90 percent.[26]

Aortic stump disruption is the leading cause of both perioperative and late deaths, emphasizing the importance of adequate aortic wall debridement and closure as well as careful long-term follow-up.[29] Myocardial infarction, renal failure, and multiorgan failure are other important causes of perioperative mortality.

Prevention

Given the grave prognosis of aortoenteric fistulae, prevention assumes paramount importance. Adherence to established surgical techniques at the time of initial aortic reconstruction should minimize the occurrence of this dreaded complication. Prophylactic antibiotics and/or antibiotic irrigation should always be used. Gentle dissection of the duodenum is necessary to prevent ischemic injury or microperforation that can lead to graft contamination. When the aorta is densely adherent to the duodenum, as when managing an inflammatory aneurysm, aneurysm wall should be left attached to the bowel rather than attempting complete separation. Recognition of the high incidence of bacterial growth from aneurysmal contents, particularly from ruptured aneurysms, emphasizes the need for operative cultures.[12,13] Positive cultures suggest long-term antibiotic therapy, though there is no firm clinical evidence to support this recommendation.

Every attempt should be made to minimize the erosion potential of the implanted prosthesis. Care should be taken in trimming the graft to a proper length to avoid both undue tension on suture lines and redundancy with resultant kinking and buckling, which may predispose to erosion. Although on theoretic grounds end-to-end proximal anastomosis seems less prone to enteric erosion than an end-to-side configuration, there are no convincing data to support this impression. Adequate separation of the graft from the duodenum with viable tissue is the most important technical point for prevention of this complication. There is usually sufficient retroperitoneal tissue to interpose two layers between the prosthesis and adjacent bowel. The debrided aneurysm sac can be closed around the prosthesis to provide another layer of protection. Occasionally, in very thin individuals or in redo aortic operations there is insufficient retroperitoneal tissue for adequate coverage. In this situation a pedicle of omentum can be passed through the transverse mesocolon and sutured over the graft (Fig. 4).[34]

Adoption of these principles over the last 2 decades has probably been responsible for the steady decline in the incidence of secondary aortoenteric fistulae. Continued adherence to these practices may lead to the eventual eradication of this devastating complication.

AORTOCAVAL FISTULAE

Etiology and Incidence

Aortocaval fistulization is a rare but well recognized complication of aortic aneurysmal disease and trauma. Prompt diagnosis and early surgical intervention are usually necessary for successful management.

Aortocaval fistulae are of two types—spontaneous and posttraumatic.[37] Spontaneous fistulae, the more common of the two, result from aneurysmal degeneration of the abdom-

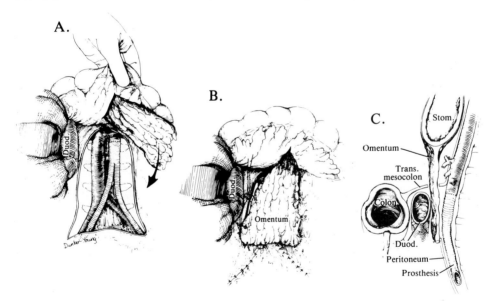

Fig. 4. (A) Omentum passed through an incision in the transverse mesocolon. (B) Omentum sutured to the retroperitoneal tissues covers the prosthesis, separating the prosthesis from the duodenum. (C) Sagittal view, showing omentum passed through the transverse mesocolon and interposed between the prosthesis and bowel. (Reprinted from Ernst CB: Aortoenteric fistulas, in Haimovici H (ed.): Vascular Emergencies. E. Norwalk, CT, Appleton-Century-Crofts, 1982. With permission.)

inal aorta with rupture into the inferior vena cava. Syphilis, infection, connective tissue disorders, and neoplasms have also been noted to cause aortocaval fistulae. The incidence of spontaneous aortocaval fistula is low, ranging from 0.3 to 3.0 percent of unruptured aneurysms and 3 to 4 percent of ruptured aneurysms.[38,39] These fistulae are usually located between the right posterolateral wall of the distal aorta and the adjacent anterior wall of the lower inferior vena cava.[40,41] Here the bulge of the aneurysm comes into direct contact with the unprotected vena cava causing compression and eventual erosion. Less commonly, spontaneous fistulae develop from aneurysmal degeneration of the iliac arteries. Fistulization into the left renal vein has also been reported, usually when the vein follows an anomalous retro-aortic course.[42] With this anatomic variant, the vein is positioned more caudal than usual coming into contact with the posterior bulge of the aneurysm.

Posttraumatic fistulae are either secondary to penetrating abdominal trauma or iatrogenic injury during lumbar disc excision. Fistulae secondary to penetrating trauma are uncommon because of the relatively protected retroperitoneal position of the aorta and cava and the highly lethal nature of most injuries in this region.[43] When present, such fistulae are usually secondary to stab wounds or low velocity gunshot wounds that were inadequately explored and hence unrecognized at the time of initial presentation (Fig. 5).

Postlaminectomy fistulae are caused by penetration of the anterior spinous ligament during lumbar discectomy, usually with pituitary rongeurs.[44] Simultaneous injury of the closely approximated and relatively fixed aorta/iliac arteries and cava/iliac veins results in fistula formation. The location of the fistula is dependent upon the site of disc excision,

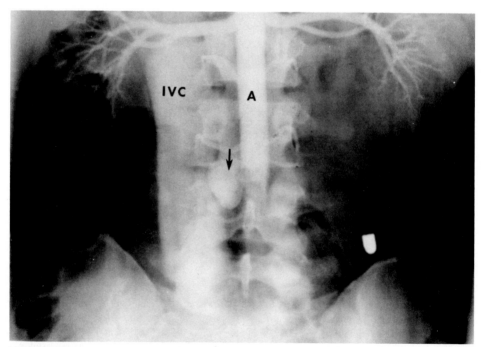

Fig. 5. Posttraumatic aortocaval fistula. Pseudoaneurysm appears between the aorta and inferior vena cava (arrow). The .22 caliber bullet appears in the left lower quadrant. A = aorta, IVC = inferior vena cava.

most commonly the L4–L5 or L5–S1 interspaces with resultant injuries to the iliac vessels. Fistulization between the aorta and vena cava usually occurs only after L3–L4 interspace excisions. Surprisingly, massive bleeding is rarely encountered during these procedures and fistulization is only recognized during the postoperative course or in long-term follow-up. Such fistulae are relatively rare with less than 100 reported in a review of the world's literature through 1976.[44]

Pathophysiology

The natural history of aortocaval fistulae depends on both the hemodynamic alterations induced by arteriovenous shunting and the etiology of the fistula. The pathophysiologic response to arteriovenous shunting is a decline in mean arterial pressure with a concomitant decrease in peripheral perfusion. To maintain adequate tissue perfusion the heart compensates with an increase in rate, stroke volume, and output.[45,46] The overall hemodynamic effects on the heart and peripheral circulation depend on the size and location of the arteriovenous shunt. The larger the fistula, the greater the shunt and the more work demands placed on the heart. Proximal fistulae have greater flow than distal fistulae because of the lower resistance of the involved vessels (larger diameter and shorter distance from the heart equals lower resistance).[45] With large proximal communications such as spontaneous aortocaval fistulae, cardiac compensation may not be enough to maintain adequate peripheral perfusion. Renal hypoperfusion results in activation of the renin-angiotensin-aldosterone system with salt and water retention.[47] An increase in plasma volume produces a dilutional anemia. In severe cases oliguria and azotemia occur. Renal dysfunction is further exacerbated by the presence of renal venous hypertension.

Decreased perfusion of the lower extremities is another consequence of aortocaval fistulae. In fact, if the fistula is large enough, it may induce retrograde flow in the iliac arteries and distal aorta, in effect stealing blood from the periphery. Distal perfusion is further compromised by the presence of venous hypertension and concomitant arterial occlusive disease. Diminished peripheral circulation is manifest by decreased pedal pulses and cool, mottled, cyanotic legs and feet. Elevated venous pressure in the pelvis and lower extremities leads to regional edema of the buttocks, hips, and legs with prominent varicosities. Venous congestion of the kidneys and bladder may result in hematuria in up to 30 percent of patients with aortocaval fistulae.[48,49]

With spontaneous aortocaval fistulae the arteriovenous communication is usually large or rapidly becomes so because of the friable nature of the diseased aortic wall. Hemodynamic aberrations can, therefore, begin abruptly and quickly lead to cardiac decompensation and death as the fistula enlarges. Traumatic and postlaminectomy fistulae, on the other hand, are usually small and fixed in size. Cardiac decompensation in this setting is gradual in onset and less severe than the often sudden and rapidly progressive failure seen with aortocaval fistulae of aneurysmal origin.

Clinical Presentation

Because of the rarity of the diagnosis and the wide variety of clinical presentations, aortocaval fistulae are correctly diagnosed preoperatively only 50 percent of the time.[49] Spontaneous fistulae usually present with signs and symptoms of a ruptured abdominal aortic aneurysm. Ninety to 95 percent of patients will complain of abdominal or back pain secondary to retroperitoneal hemorrhage and/or caval engorgement and 30 percent will be hypotensive.[37,41] Following decompression into the vena cava, the clinical picture of a large arteriovenous fistula rapidly becomes apparent, with tachycardia and widened pulse pressure. Eighty percent of patients will have a palpable aneurysm and 75 percent an audible abdominal bruit.[49] The classical continuous or machinery-like bruit may not be present because of intermittently occluding thrombus. With rapid enlargement of the arteriovenous communication, signs and symptoms of cardiac decompensation occur. Although only 40 percent of patients will develop overt heart failure, approximately two-thirds will have some signs of cardiac compromise with shortness of breath, cardiomegaly, or tachycardia.[37,41,49] Renal insufficiency with oliguria and azotemia occurs in 27 percent and hematuria in 32 percent. Rectal bleeding, which occurs occasionally, and some cases of hematuria are thought to be caused by acute congestion and rupture of submucosal veins within the rectum and bladder.[48] Regional edema of the buttocks and lower extremities secondary to both heart failure and venous hypertension is seen in 40–50 percent of patients.[37,41] Pulmonary embolization of aortic mural thrombus is a rare event.[38] Ischemia of the lower extremities is a variable but significant finding. Aortocaval fistulae are sometimes asymptomatic and discovered only at the time of aneurysm repair when the surgeon is surprised by massive venous hemorrhage following removal of intraaortic thrombus.[38,39]

Patients with spontaneous aortocaval fistulae tend to be older like other patients with aneurysmal disease of the aorta.[37] Because of coexisting coronary arterial disease and other degenerative conditions associated with advanced age, they tolerate the sudden onset and rapid progression of hemodynamic changes poorly. In contrast, patients with posttraumatic fistulae are usually young, healthy individuals with small arteriovenous communications that produce hemodynamic alterations slowly. These patients usually present weeks, months, or even years after the episode of trauma or iatrogenic injury with the gradual onset of congestive heart failure and local signs of arteriovenous fistulae.[44]

Diagnosis

Diagnosis of aortocaval fistula is usually based on a thorough history and physical examination but the diagnosis is often missed because of the variable clinical presentation and a low index of suspicion.[49] The presence of abdominal or back pain, a pulsatile abdominal mass with associated bruit, and signs and symptoms of congestive failure are sufficient evidence in most cases to make the diagnosis. Confirmatory studies such as CT scan or ultrasound are unnecessary although they may be useful as part of the routine evaluation of any patient with an abdominal aortic aneurysm. Aortography helps in planning the operative approach and may localize the exact site of the fistula, although rapid flow may preclude fistula site identification. In patients with equivocal findings or posttraumatic fistulae, angiography is especially valuable (Fig. 5). Other studies including isotope angiography and transfemoral Swan-Ganz catheter insertion have been described in the literature but have limited clinical practicality. In patients with posttraumatic fistulae a history of penetrating trauma or lumbar disc excision should be carefully sought.

Treatment

Successful treatment of spontaneous aortocaval fistulae requires operation. Without operative intervention, progressive cardiac decompensation and death are inevitable.

Most patients will benefit from a short period of preoperative resuscitation with diuresis, and use of inotropic agents.[46] Patients with severe pulmonary edema and massive fluid overload may require up to 12–24 hours of such therapy prior to urgent operation. Prolonged efforts at medical control of heart failure, however, are inappropriate and dangerous. It is impossible to control the increased cardiac preload by any means other than fistula interruption. With delay there is risk of enlargement of the hole in the friable aortic wall with accelerated clinical deterioration. Swan-Ganz monitoring is mandatory and intravenous fluids and transfusions should be limited until the fistula is closed. Anemia in most cases is secondary to hemodilution and not retroperitoneal hemorrhage.

The surgical approach to aortocaval fistula is similar to standard abdominal aortic aneurysm repair. Proximal and distal arterial control are obtained away from the site of the presumed arteriovenous communication. Dissection and manipulation of the aneurysm should be minimized to avoid dislodging aortic mural thrombus that can pass through the fistula and result in pulmonary embolization. To decrease the risks of embolization and to minimize venous back bleeding following aneurysmotomy, proximal and distal venous control has been suggested.[50] Most surgeons, however, feel such dissection is dangerous and unnecessary and rely on venous control from within the aneurysm using direct digital occlusion of the fistula, caval compression with sponge sticks, or insertion of balloon occlusion catheters through the fistula into the vena cava.[38,40] No attempt should be made to separate the aneurysm from the vena cava by external division of the fistula. It is easier and safer to oversew the caval communication from within the aneurysm (Fig. 6). In a recent review this approach was accompanied by an 84 percent survival while with all other techniques operative mortality approached 50 percent.[49] Application of the aortic cross clamp should be gradual as rapid aortic occlusion may precipitate cardiac arrest secondary to a sudden reduction in venous return. After opening the aneurysm care should be exercised in removing the laminated thrombus to prevent caval embolization. Because the aortic wall can be friable it is usually best to take large bites, utilizing felt pledgets if necessary. Following closure of the caval defect, aneurysm repair proceeds routinely with prosthetic graft placement. Blood loss during such procedures can be substantial and autotransfusion has proven useful.

Repair of posttraumatic aortocaval fistulae is necessary to prevent both progressive cardiac decompensation and rupture of possible associated pseudoaneurysms, but it need not be performed urgently as with spontaneous fistulae.[51] Cardiac failure should be aggressively treated preoperatively and medical management maximized prior to operative intervention. Surgical repair is usually best accomplished with proximal and distal control of all involved arteries and veins. As with spontaneous fistulae, direct division of the arteriovenous communication should be avoided. Closure can usually be obtained from within the arterial lumen or through a separate venotomy. If a portion of arterial wall requires resection because of extensive damage and/or pseudoaneurysm formation, continuity can be restored by patch angioplasty, end-to-end anastomosis, or interposition grafting.

Results

The mortality rate of spontaneous aortocaval fistulae is high. Review of the English litrature through 1975 documented an immediate postoperative survival rate of only 55 percent.[40] All patients not undergoing operation died. With the advent of autotransfusion and improvements in anesthetic technique and postoperative care, results have improved.

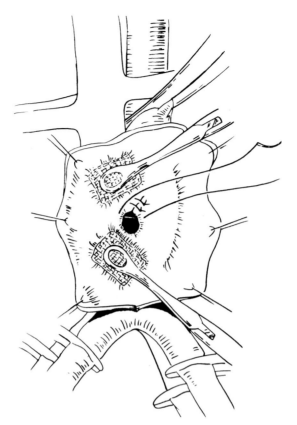

Fig. 6. Technique of repair of aortocaval fistula. The fistula is
sutured through the opened aneurysmal sac.

Analysis of 46 patients reported between 1975 and 1982 documented an increase in
immediate postoperative survival to nearly 90 percent with an overall survival of 70
percent.[52] As might be expected, the primary causes of death in this elderly, high risk
group were myocardial infarction and renal failure. Patients with posttraumatic fistulae
fared better, largely because they are younger and healthier, and have less cardiac compromise. Mortality for postlaminectomy fistulae was 7 percent while for aortoiliac arteriovenous fistulae secondary to trauma, the mortality was less than 10 percent.[44,51] Morbidity
in these patients largely results from failure to restore arterial and/or venous continuity.

REFERENCES

1. Estrada FP, Tachoysky TJ, Orr RM Jr, et al: Primary aortoduodenal fistula following radio-
    therapy. Surg Gynecol Obstet 156:646, 1983
2. Geary SR, Walworth EZ: Aortoduodenal fistula secondary to metastatic carcinoma. JAMA
    235:2520, 1976
3. Sweeney MS, Gadacz TR: Primary aortoduodenal fistula: Manifestation, diagnosis, and treat-
    ment. Surgery 96:492, 1984
4. Bunt TJ: Synthetic vascular graft infections. II. Graft-enteric erosions and graft-enteric fistu-
    las. Surgery 94:1, 1983

5. Elliott JP, Smith RF, Szilagyi DE: Aortoenteric and paraprosthetic-enteric fistulas. Arch Surg 108:479, 1974

6. Donovan TJ, Bucknam CA: Aortoenteric fistula. Arch Surg 95:810,1967

7. DeWeese MS, Fry WJ: Small bowel erosion following aortic resection. JAMA 179:882, 1962

8. Kleinman LH, Towne JB, Bernhard VM: A diagnostic and therapeutic approach to aortoenteric fistulas: Clinical experience with twenty patients. Surgery 86:868, 1979

9. Humphries AW, Young JR, deWolfe VG, et al: Complications of abdominal aortic surgery. Arch Surg 86:43, 1963

10. Buchbinder D, Leather R, Shah D, et al: Pathologic interactions between prosthetic aortic grafts and the gastrointestinal tract. Amer J Surg 140:192, 1980

11. Busuttil RW, Reese W, Baker JD, et al: Pathogenesis of aortoduodenal fistula: Experimental and clinical correlates. Surgery 85:1, 1979

12. Ernst CB, Campbell HC Jr, Daugherty ME, et al: Incidence and significance of intraoperative bacterial cultures during abdominal aortic aneurysmectomy. Ann Surg 185:626, 1977

13. Macbeth GA, Rubin JR, McIntyre KE, et al: The relevance of arterial wall microbiology to the treatment of prosthetic graft infections: Graft infection vs. arterial infection. J Vasc Surg 1:750, 1984

14. Reilly LM, Ehrenfeld WK, Goldstone J, et al: Gastrointestinal tract involvement by prosthetic graft infection. Ann Surg 202:342, 1985

15. O'Mara C, Imbembo AL: Paraprosthetic-enteric fistula. Surgery 81:556, 1977

16. Champion MC, Sullivan SN, Coles JC, et al: Aortoenteric fistula—Incidence, presentation, recognition, and management. Ann Surg 195:314, 1982

17. Frye MW, Thompson WM: Aortic graft-enteric and paraprosthetic-enteric fistulas. Amer J Surg 146:183, 1983

18. O'Donnell TF, Scott G, Shepard A, et al: Improvements in the diagnosis and management of aortoenteric fistula. Amer J Surg 149:480, 1985

19. Bunt TJ, Doerhoff CR: Endoscopic visualization of an intraluminal Dacron graft: Definitive diagnosis of aortoduodenal fistula. Southern Med J 77:86, 1984

20. Kukora JS, Rushton FW, Cranston PE: New computed tomographic signs of aortoenteric fistula. Arch Surg 119:1073, 1984

21. Mark AS, Moss AA, McCarthy S, et al: CT of aortoenteric fistulas. Invest Radiol 20:272, 1985

22. Mark AS, McCarthy SM, Moss AA, et al: Detection of abdominal aortic graft infection: Comparison of CT and In-labeled white blood cell scans. AJR 144:315, 1985

23. Cunat JS, Haaga JR, Rhodes R, et al: Periaortic fluid aspiration for recognition of infected graft: Preliminary report. AJR 139:251, 1982

24. Lawrence PF, Dries DJ, Alazraki N, et al: Indium 111-labeled leukocyte scanning for detection of prosthetic vascular graft infection. J Vasc Surg 2:165, 1985

25. Brunner MC, Mitchell RS, Baldwin JC, et al: Prosthetic graft infection: Limitations of indium white blood cell scanning. J Vasc Surg 3:42, 1986

26. Perdue GD, Smith RB, Ansley JD, et al: Impending aortoenteric hemorrhage—The effect of early recognition on improved outcome. Ann Surg 192:237, 1980

27. Thompson WM, Jackson DC, et al: Aortoenteric and paraprosthetic-enteric fistulas: Radiologic findings. Am J Roentgenol 127:235, 1976

28. Daugherty M, Shearer GR, Ernst CB: Primary aortoduodenal fistula: Extraanatomic vascular reconstruction not required for successful management. Surgery 86:399, 1979

29. Reilly LM, Altman H, Lusby RJ, et al: Late results following surgical management of vascular graft infection. J Vasc Surg 1:36, 1984

30. Ernst CB: Axillary-femoral bypass graft patency without aortofemoral pressure differential. Ann Surg 181:424, 1975

31. Trout HH, Kozloff L, Giordano JM: Priority of revascularization in patients with graft enteric fistulas, infected arteries, or infected arterial prostheses. Ann Surg 199:669, 1984

32. Kiernan PD, Pairolero PC, Hubert JP Jr, et al: Aortic graft-enteric fistula. Mayo Clin Proc 55:731, 1980

33. Fry WJ, Lindenauer SM: Infection complicating the use of plastic arterial implants. Arch Surg 94:600, 1967

34. Goldsmith HS, de los Santos R, Vanamee P, et al: Experimental protection of vascular prosthesis by omentum. Arch Surg 97:872, 1968

35. Shah DM, Buchbinder D, Leather RP, et al: Clinical use of the seromuscular jejunal patch for protection of the infected aortic stump. Amer J Surg 146:198, 1983

36. Connolly JE, Kwaan JH, McCart PM, et al: Aortoenteric fistula. Ann Surg 194:402, 1982

37. Nennhaus HP, Javid H: The distinct syndrome of spontaneous abdominal aortocaval fistula. Am J Med 44:464, 1968

38. Baker WH, Sharzer LA, Ehrenhaft JL: Aortocaval fistula as a complication of abdominal aortic aneurysms. Surgery 72:933, 1972

39. Dardik H, Dardik I, Strom MG: Intravenous rupture of arteriosclerotic aneurysms of the abdominal aorta. Surgery 80:647, 1976

40. Mohr LL, Smith LL: Arteriovenous fistula from rupture of abdominal aortic aneurysm. Arch Surg 110:806, 1975

41. Reckless JPD, McColl I, Taylor GW: Aorto-caval fistulae: An unknown complication of abdominal aortic aneurysms. Br J Surg 59:461, 1972

42. Suzuki M, Collins GM, Bassinger GT, et al: Aorto-left renal vein fistula: An unusual complication of abdominal aortic aneurysm. Ann Surg 184:31, 1975

43. Mattox KL, Whisennand HH, Espada, R, et al: Management of acute combined injuries of the aorta and inferior vena cava. Amer J Surg 130:720, 1975

44. Jarstfer BS, Rich NM: The challenge of arteriovenous fistula formation following disc surgery: A collective review. J Trauma 16:726, 1976

45. Strandness DE Jr, Sumner DS: Arteriovenous fistula. Hemodynamics for Surgeons. New York, Grune & Stratton, Inc, 1975, pp 621-623

46. Merrill WH, Ernst CB: Aorta-left renal vein fistula: Hemodynamic monitoring and timing of operation. Surgery 89:678, 1981

47. Davis JO, Urguhart J, Higgins JT, et al: Hypersecretion of aldosterone in dogs with a chronic aortic-caval fistula and high output heart failure. Circ Res 14:471, 1964

48. Brewster DC, Ottinger LW, Darling RC: Hematuria as a sign of aorto-caval fistula. Ann Surg 186:766, 1977

49. Astarita D, Filippone DR, Cohn JD: Spontaneous major intra-abdominal arteriovenous fistulas: A report of several cases. Angiology 36:656, 1985

50. Hafner CD, Cranley JJ, Krause RJ, et al: Acute abdominal aortal-vena cava fistula. Vasc Surg 3:149, 1969

51. Symes JM, Eadie DGA, Maclean ADW: Traumatic aorto-caval fistula associated with a horseshoe kidney. J Trauma 14:402, 1974

52. McDonald GR, Graham KJ, Barratt-Boyes BG: Aortocaval fistulae: An occasional cause of congestive cardiac failure. Aust N Z J Surg 52:573, 1982

PART VIII

Visceral Arteries

Fred A. Weaver
Patrick W. Meacham
Richard H. Dean

Acute Renal Artery Occlusion

Surgical intervention for renovascular disease is most frequently employed for elective management of renovascular hypertension. However, a spectrum of conditions does present acutely and several require urgent or emergency intervention. The more common of these conditions are:

Trauma
Embolism
Acute dissection
Spontaneous thrombosis
Iatrogenic injury
Aneurysm rupture

In some, urgent management may be directed toward prevention of loss or retrieval of renal function. In others, intervention is required to prevent death.

Since each of these conditions is distinct from the others, they will be addressed individually. Common to all of them is the pathophysiology of renal ischemia. As it impacts on management decisions in each of the entities, it will be discussed first.

EFFECT OF ISCHEMIA ON RENAL FUNCTION

Because instantaneous renal revascularization of the acutely ischemic kidney is clinically impossible, the value of renal revascularization is dependent both on the severity and the duration of renal ischemia. Alteration of metabolic pathways begins almost immediately after the onset of total ischemia, for available levels of renal cortical adenosine triphosphate (ATP) drop to less than 50 percent of normal after only 1 minute.[1] Although short periods of ischemia are well tolerated, renal excretory dysfunction can be demonstrated after only 30 minutes of warm ischemia time.[2] Further, increasing amounts of permanent loss of renal function occur after only 1 hour of warm ischemia, and minimal, if any, function is retrievable after 6 hours of total ischemia.

When renal perfusion is acutely reduced but not totally interrupted, the effect on the renal parenchyma and renal function is more variable. Subcritical reductions in perfusion

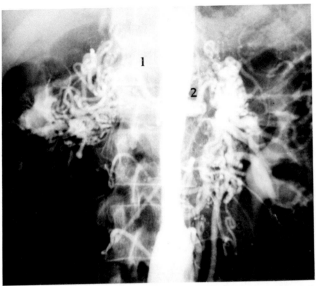

Fig. 1. Arteriogram of a 32-year-old male with chronic bilateral renal artery occlusions and massive network of perinephric collaterals (1—lumbar, 2—adrenal, 3—gonadal, ureteral).

produce a diminution in renal plasma flow available for filtration and an increased tubular reabsorption of such filtered water. This homeostatic mechanism may result in a virtual cessation of urine flow during the period of ischemia, yet reestablishment of urine flow and normal renal function may immediately follow revascularization. Since functional studies such as the intravenous pyelogram may demonstrate no observable function during periods of subcritical ischemia, their use in the preoperative assessment to gauge the value of revascularization versus primary nephrectomy in patients with acute renal ischemia is limited.

The extent of renal ischemia produced by acute renal artery occlusion is variable and primarily dependent on the magnitude of available collateral pathways of renal perfusion. Potentially important donors of collateral flow include the adrenal, ureteral, lumbar, and gonadal arteries. Although these vessels may provide no clinically important collateral flow in the young patient with acute traumatic disruption of the renal artery, they may have developed to such an extent that relatively normal excretory function may be maintained after total occlusion occurs in a previously stenotic renal artery (Fig. 1). Indeed, variation in the availability of collateral flow is frequent and thus the period of ischemia consistent with retrieval of useful renal function inconstant. Therefore, decisions regarding the management of these patients must be individualized, both in regard to the underlying cause and its clinical presentation.

RENAL ARTERY TRAUMA

Traumatic injury of the renal artery is an uncommon clinical problem occurring in only 7 percent of penetrating and 4 percent of blunt abdominal and back injuries.[3,4]

Associated injuries to other organs are present in 75 percent of patients with blunt renal artery trauma and virtually all patients with penetrating injuries.[3,4]

Signs and symptoms of renal trauma include flank pain and tenderness and microscopic or gross hematuria. Hematuria in any form, however, is absent in approximately 20 percent of patients with significant renal injury. Oliguria or anuria is uncommon and reflects the presence of severe bilateral injury or occlusion to a solitary kidney.

Although life-threatening hypotension secondary to profound hypovolemic shock may abort the appropriateness of preoperative diagnostic studies, a bolus injection of contrast material and a "one-shot" intravenous pyelogram is valuable in massive abdominal trauma. The utility of such a study is primarily to exclude the presence of major renal trauma and to prove the presence of a normally functioning contralateral kidney when renal injury is suspected.

When the hemodynamic status allows preoperative assessment, a more standard intravenous pyelogram is indicated whenever major intraabdominal blunt or penetrating trauma is present. If discrepancy between the function of the two kidneys is identified, angiographic study of the renal anatomy is indicated. This empiric approach to exclusion of renovascular injuries is particularly useful in blunt abdominal trauma, for as many as 25 percent of renal injuries are not readily apparent at operation.[5]

Operative management of trauma to the renal vasculature is dependent on several factors. Among these are the extent and site of the renovascular injury, the degree of associated renal parenchymal and renal pelvic trauma and the magnitude of associated nonrenal injuries. In patients with abdominal trauma, associated renovascular lesions most commonly require nephrectomy.[4,6] The frequent occurrence of extensive damage to the renal parenchyma and associated other injuries requiring emergency management necessitate this approach. Certainly, the patient's overall hemodynamic status and the magnitude of other procedures required frequently lead to primary nephrectomy of a theoretically salvageable kidney. Needless to say, sacrifice of the injured kidney while managing other complicated, potentially lethal injuries, when a normal contralateral kidney is present, is not only appropriate but also preferential. Occasionally, however, the renal artery lesion is the only major injury and revascularization is imminently feasible (Fig. 2).

Associated injuries to the renal venous system are common and may require simultaneous management. In this regard, one should remember that renal artery branches are "end arteries" and segmental severe ischemia or infarction accompanies their sacrifice. Renal vein branches have many collaterals and branch renal veins do not require repair. Instead, they can be ligated without significant compromise to renal venous drainage.

In patients with main renal artery or extrarenal branch renal artery injuries in whom the added risk and duration of operation are not a practical concern, operative management of the injured artery usually requires aortorenal bypass. Rarely, reapproximation of the injured vessel can be performed. Nevertheless, the proven predictability of success of saphenous vein aortorenal bypass argues for its preferential use.

Proximal control of the aorta and, if possible, the proximal renal artery are achieved prior to entering the hematoma. After isolation of the proximal and distal vessel, and debridement of the area of trauma, the reversed saphenous vein is anastomosed "end-to-end" as described elsewhere.[7] If clinically important, even multiple branch injuries may require revascularization. In this circumstance, the use of ex vivo repair is appropriate, for the kidney can be cooled with a renal preservative solution and repair of multiple branches performed in a more controlled environment.

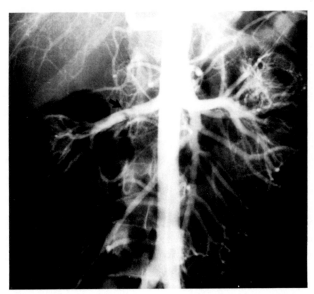

Fig. 2. Arteriogram demonstrating intimal flap (arrow) with near occlusion and thrombus in main renal artery following motor vehicle accident.

The results of renal revascularization in both blunt and penetrating trauma are disappointing. In the review by Clark et al,[5] only 2 of 12 kidneys (17 percent) that underwent successful revascularization had reestablishment of clinically significant renal function. In all of these instances revascularization was performed between 3 and 18 hours after injury. This pessimistic view regarding the frequency of retrieval of preoperatively absent function is mimicked in our experience and tempers enthusiasm for the value of revascularization after several hours of warm, total ischemia.

EMBOLIC RENAL ARTERY OCCLUSION

Embolic renal artery occlusion and secondary renal infarction was first described by Traube in 1856.[8] Such emboli gained little attention until Hoxie and Coggin's 1940 review of 205 patients who were found to have renal artery emboli and infarction at autopsy. The uncommon nature of this event is stressed in their report, however, for these patients were collected from a total autopsied population of 14,411. Interestingly only 2 of the 205 patients had the correct diagnosis made ante mortem. Nevertheless, their report summarized the salient clinical features of embolic occlusion of the renal artery.[9] These features include acute onset of back or flank pain, costovertebral angle tenderness, nausea and vomiting, and hematuria. Unfortunately, these symptoms reflect the consequences of acute renal infarction and do not appear early when the effects of the renal ischemia are reversible.

Over 90 percent of major renal artery emboli are cardiac in origin, and up to 30 percent may be bilateral.[10] The frequency of bilaterality may be less; however, for unilateral emboli that do not cause symptoms of renal infarction may remain unrecognized. In contrast, major bilateral emboli will acutely affect total excretory function and promptly lead to profound azotemia.

Initial evaluation to identify acute renal ischemia secondary to renal artery embolization includes either intravenous pyelography or isotope renography. Renal angiography is performed if either of these studies suggest impaired renal perfusion. Characteristically, renal angiography will demonstrate the proximal stump of the renal artery without visualization of the distal vessel or branches (Fig. 3). If the embolus is small or fragments on impact, similar segmental branch occlusions may be seen.

Unfortunately, a variety of disorders imitate acute embolic occlusion in their presentation and the correct diagnosis is rarely made in the first few hours after occlusion. In the 1984 literature review by Nicholas and DeMuth,[11] a mean delay of 4.3 days elapsed between the onset of symptoms and surgical intervention. This delay may not play a dominant role in the results of attempted revascularization, because the initial symptoms of pain and tenderness probably reflect infarction of at least a portion of the renal parenchyma. Nevertheless, an unknown yet potentially important component of the renal parenchyma may remain intact and retrievable.

The decision for operative intervention and removal of renal artery emboli is dependent on the degree of associated excretory dysfunction, the site of the embolus, and the overall status of the patient. Nonoperative management with anticoagulant therapy may be preferable in the patient with distal branch emboli and in the patient with severe cardiac disease or other severe risk factors in whom contralateral renal function is satisfactory. In contrast, urgent intervention with embolectomy is preferential when the embolus is only partially occlusive or when overall renal function is threatened by bilateral emboli or embolism to a solitary kidney. Although urgent intervention is important for reestablishment of renal perfusion, operation should be undertaken only after the patient is stabilized and significant abnormalities in cardiac performance, fluid, and electrolyte imbalances or uremic acidosis are corrected. Since many hours or even days may transpire between the embolic event and its recognition, most retrievable renal function has been lost by the time

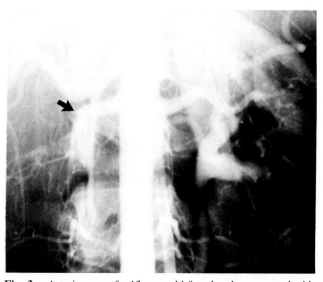

Fig. 3. Arteriogram of a 13-year-old female who presented with abrupt onset of flank pain, nausea and vomiting. Right main renal artery is totally occluded by embolus (arrow); echocardiogram later demonstrated aortic and mitral valve vegetations.

of diagnosis. The added time consumed by correcting such risk factors minimally increases the extent of irreversibly lost function while significantly improving the patient's probability of survival.

Operation usually employs a midline xiphoid to pubis incision with exposure of the renal artery and aorta as described elsewhere.[7] Additional proximal aortic exposure for crossclamping above the superior mesenteric artery is achieved by partial division of the right and left diaphragmatic crura. After mannitol (12.5 g) and heparin (7500 units) has been administered, the aorta is crossclamped above the superior mesenteric artery and below the renal arteries. A transverse aortotomy is performed at the level of the renal artery and an embolectomy catheter is used to retrieve the embolus. Primary closure of the aortotomy without a patch usually is possible. If associated atherosclerotic disease of the renal artery is identified, the incision is carried across the ostium and endarterectomy is performed. Following such endarterectomy, the incision commonly is closed with a patch to insure maintenance of a widely patent vessel.

Results of revascularization for embolic renal artery occlusion are distinctly superior to results of similar revascularization for traumatic occlusions. In a review of collected cases, Lacombe[12] reported that 23 of 33 kidneys (70 percent) submitted to embolectomy had salvage of renal function. In contrast to most traumatic occlusions, he found many renal artery emboli to be nonocclusive. In these instances, the residual patency allows sufficient parenchymal perfusion to maintain cellular structure and thus the return of function following revascularization.

Finally, recent experience with local intraarterial infusion of fibrinolytic agents suggests it may have a role in the management of some patients with renal artery emboli.[13] Its potential clinical utility is in patients with distal, branch emboli and in patients considered unacceptable operative risks. Success of fibrinolytic therapy, however, is limited to patients with emboli composed of relatively immature clot. Embolized valvular vegetations, portions of mature organized thrombi, or atheromatous debris will not respond to such therapy. For this reason, operative intervention and embolectomy is superior when operative risk is acceptable and the embolus is situated in a retrievable location.

RENAL ARTERY DISSECTIONS

Renal artery dissections may produce clinically insignificant disturbances in renal perfusion, create a hemodynamically important stenosis and secondary renovascular hypertension, or present acutely with signs of renal infarction. When a dissection does not produce acute clinical symptoms, it goes unrecognized until angiographic evaluation for renovascular hypertension is performed. Although such chronic dissections may require elective operative management, they will not be discussed further in this text.

Acute spontaneous renal artery dissections usually occur as a complication of underlying atherosclerotic or fibromuscular dysplastic renovascular disease. In the review by Smith et al,[14] they found that upper abdominal or flank pain with radiation to the epigastrium was the most common associated complaint (92 percent). Hematuria was present in 33 percent. All patients had onset of severe hypertension, and acceleration of preexisting hypertension occurred in 40 percent.

Initial diagnostic evaluation of these complaints includes intravenous pyelography or isotope renography. Once an abnormality of renal function is noted by these studies, angiographic definition of the lesion is required.

Angiography usually demonstrates an irregular contour to the arterial lumen with alcoves of contrast in the dissected false lumen and double densities reflecting opacification of the true and false lumen (Fig. 4). Branch vessels may have stenotic origins or be totally occluded by the intramural hematoma. In the review by Smith et al,[14] there was branch renal artery involvement in 33 percent and bilateral dissection in 25 percent.

Since spontaneous acute dissections are recognized by their production of acute local symptoms of renal ischemia, progression of the dissection to total occlusion and permanent loss of renal function is threatened unless intervention and revascularization is performed. Similar to the approach for management of other acute renal artery pathologies, one should intervene urgently after controlling any associated conditions that might accelerate the risk of intervention.

Operative intervention usually requires a branch renal artery repair. When the distal end of the dissection is limited to the main renal artery this may entail only extension of the arteriotomy onto an appropriate branch. Nevertheless, if the dissection has extended distally to involve the origin of branches, ex vivo preservation of the kidney during multiple branch repairs is preferable. For this reason, preparation for ex vivo reconstruction should be undertaken in each instance. Details of this technique are described elsewhere.[15]

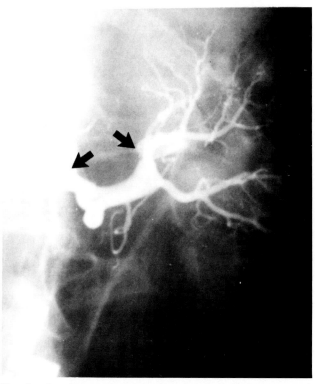

Fig. 4. Arteriogram demonstrating extensive spontaneous renal artery dissection with double density of the main renal artery and extension into branches of the renal artery.

ACUTE RENAL ARTERY THROMBOSIS

Acute thrombosis of a previously stenotic renal artery is usually silent and simply a manifestation of progression of the underlying atherosclerotic lesion. Similar to acute thrombosis of arteries at other sites, it may be due to the deposition of clot on the thrombogenic surface of the stenotic atherosclerotic lesion or hemorrhage into the plaque with acute progression of the lesion to total occlusion. In most instances, collateral perfusion to the kidney has developed to such an extent that the event is totally silent and goes unrecognized. Occasionally, however, such an event is recognized acutely due to its adverse effect on excretory function in a solitary kidney (Fig. 5) or in the only kidney with previously significant residual function. Although all such patients will exhibit a history of antecedent hypertension, the cause for their acute presentation is acceleration of hypertension and the development of oliguric acute renal failure.

Diagnostic evaluation of any patient presenting with such a constellation of symptoms should include angiography. In prior years, reticence to perform angiography was based on the nephrotoxic effect of the large amount of contrast material necessary for such an evaluation. With the introduction of digital subtraction angiography, however, such a

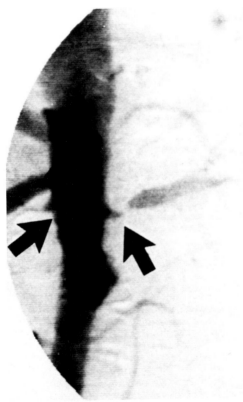

Fig. 5. Intraarterial digital subtraction arteriogram showing stump of previously removed right kidney (arrow) and total occlusion (arrow) with late visualization of the distal left renal artery in a 65-year-old female with acute onset of anuria and severe hypertension.

study employs as little as 6 ml of contrast and has no significant detrimental effect on residual renal function.

Although many physicians are tempted to react to the clinical presentation with immediate operation and attempted revascularization, a more planned approach is superior. Since the acute event is usually more than 24 hours old and primarily represents a reduction in perfusion to a point below the critical level for maintenance of urinary output, attention to correction of metabolic derangements prior to intervention is of utmost importance in controlling the risk of such an intervention. In this manner, the patient may require several days of dialysis or even correction of other more lethal cardiac derangements prior to renal revascularization. In any event, one should adopt the premise that the amount of retrievable renal function is not dependent on the timing of intervention and that renal failure can be controlled by hemodialysis while malignant hypertension and cardiac risk factors are improved.

Prediction of a salutary effect of revascularization is predicated on the demonstration of distally patent vessels beyond the occlusions and the bilateral nature of the disease. In a recent review of our experience,[16] no patient had a significant response in excretory function when only a unilateral lesion was present. In contrast, patients with bilateral reconstructable lesions or an occlusion to a solitary kidney had a dramatic response to intervention. In these patients reinstitution of urine flow was almost instantaneous after completion of revascularization, and the majority required no further dialysis in the immediate postoperative period.

IATROGENIC RENAL ARTERY TRAUMA

Iatrogenic renal artery injury may occur from a spectrum of causes, yet most notable are injuries after diagnostic or interventional radiologic procedures. Although diagnostic renal angiography may cause acute dissection or perforations (Fig. 6), these events are rare in experienced hands. Of more practical concern is the risk of trauma requiring operative intervention in association with attempted percutaneous transluminal angioplasty (PTA) of renal artery lesions. Since the mechanism of PTA is the use of controlled fracture of the stenotic lesion, one might expect a frequent occurrence of complications requiring surgical intervention. Certainly the immediate postdilatation arteriogram frequently demonstrates worrisome dissections or clefts, yet most of these induced lesions remodel and lead to at least temporary benefit in renal perfusion and hypertension (Fig. 7).

In experienced centers, complications of PTA that require urgent intervention occur in less than 10 percent of cases[17] and include acute thrombosis, perforation, and clinically significant dissections of the vessel. Minor guide wire perforations and minor dissections without associated symptoms are usually well tolerated and can be monitored closely with follow-up angiography alone. Acute thrombosis or major dissections producing acceleration in renal ischemia with associated symptoms of pain, tenderness, hypertension, and hematuria require urgent operative management to salvage threatened renal function. Although nephrectomy may be required, most such injuries can be successfully managed by revascularization with salvage of the kidney.

In this setting, the operative field frequently is complicated by the presence of hematoma and periadventitial inflammation. Revascularization, therefore, usually requires a more complicated reconstruction than would have been needed to manage the

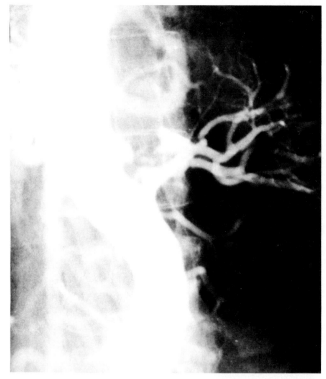

Fig. 6. Postoperative renal arteriogram demonstrating disruption
of aortorenal bypass suture line immediately following inadvertent
pressure contrast injection at the anastomotic site.

initial lesion. Due to the potential need for such intervention, close coordination between
the interventional radiologist and the surgeon must be maintained when PTA is employed.

RUPTURED RENAL ARTERY ANEURYSMS

Renal artery aneurysms are relatively uncommon and may be present in only 0.3–0.7
percent of the population.[18] Although concern over potential rupture of such aneurysms
has prompted their prophylactic repair, the risk of rupture is unknown. Certainly, diameters greater than 2 cm, presence in females of childbearing age, and evidence of increasing
size on serial studies are recognized factors potentially increasing risk of rupture. Of
greatest concern, however, is their increased potential for rupture during pregnancy.

Elective management of clinically silent aneurysms may require complex branch
repairs using ex vivo techniques. The results of such interventions, however, should be
predictably successful. Operations for rupture of renal artery aneurysms are more appropriately concerned with patient survival since most present with profound hypotension
secondary to retroperitoneal hemorrhage. In these circumstances, attempted dissection of
the renal arteries and revascularization frequently is an unrealistic goal. Instead, control of
the point of hemorrhage and primary nephrectomy usually is required. Finally, follow-up
angiography to exclude the potential presence of contralateral renal artery fibromuscular

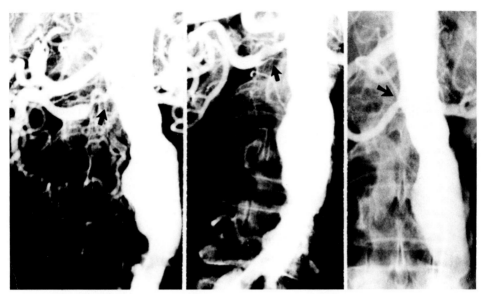

Fig. 7. Preinterventional arteriogram (left), obtained immediately after percutaneous transluminal angioplasty (middle), and one year follow-up arteriogram (right) showing remodeling of an initially worrisome intimal dissection. The patient has remained normotensive on no medications for 2 years after treatment.

disease or aneurysms is important in the overall management of these patients, since subsequent elective, prophylactic management of such disease may be necessary.

ACKNOWLEDGEMENT

Supported in part by NIH Grant #14192-13, Specialized Center of Research in Hypertension, Vanderbilt University Medical Center, Nashville, Tennessee.

REFERENCES

1. Collste H, Bergström J, Hultman E, et al: ATP in cortex of canine kidneys undergoing hypothermic storage. Life Sci 10:1201, 1971
2. Ward JP: Determination of the optimum temperature for regional renal hypothermia during temporary renal ischemia. Br J Urol 47:17, 1975
3. Lock JS, Carraway RP, Hudson HC Jr, et al: Proper management of renal artery injury from blunt trauma. South Med J 78:406, 1985
4. Brown MF, Graham JM, Mattox KL, et al: Renovascular trauma. Am J Surg 140:802, 1980
5. Clark DE, Georgitis JW, Ray FS: Renal arterial injuries caused by blunt trauma. Surgery 90:87, 1981
6. Turner WW Jr, Snyder WH III, Fry WJ: Mortality and renal salvage after renovascular trauma: review of 95 patients treated in a 20 year period. Am J Surg 146:848, 1983
7. Dean RH: Surgery for renovascular hypertension, in Bergan JJ, Yao JST (eds.): Operative Techniques in Vascular Surgery. New York, Grune & Stratton, 1980, pp 81–87

8. Traube L: Über den Zusammenhang von Herz und Nieren krankhiten. Berlin, A. Hirschwald, 1856, p 77

9. Hoxie HJ, Coggin CB: Renal infarction: Statistical study of two hundred and five cases and detailed report of an unusual case. Arch Intern Med 65:587, 1940

10. Lessman RK, Johnson SF, Coburn JW, et al: Renal artery embolism: Clinical features and long-term follow-up of 17 cases. Ann Intern Med 89:477, 1978

11. Nicholas GG, DeMuth WE Jr: Treatment of renal artery embolism. Arch Surg 119:278, 1984

12. Lacombe M: Surgical versus medical treatment of renal artery embolism. J Cardiovasc Surg 18:281, 1977

13. Fischer CP, Konnak JW, Cho KJ, et al: Renal artery embolism: Therapy with intra-arterial streptokinase infusion. J Urol 125:402, 1981

14. Smith BM, Holcomb GW III, Richie RE, et al: Renal artery dissection. Ann Surg 200:134, 1984

15. Dean RH: Renovascular hypertension. Curr Probl Surg 22:1, 1985

16. Dean RH, Englund R, Dupont WD, et al: Retrieval of renal function by revascularization: study of preoperative outcome predictors. Ann Surg 202:367, 1985

17. Tegtmeyer CJ, Kofler TJ, Ayers CA: Renal angioplasty: Current status. AJR 142:17, 1984

18. Tham G, Ekelund L, Herrlin K, et al: Renal artery aneurysms: Natural history and prognosis. Ann Surg 197:348, 1983

James C. Stanley, Thomas W. Wakefield
Linda M. Graham, Gerald B. Zelenock

Ruptured Splanchnic Artery Aneurysms

Splanchnic artery aneurysms are unusual vascular lesions, but nearly 22 percent present first as emergencies and 8.5 percent are fatal.[1] The vessels involved in decreasing order of frequency, include: the splenic, hepatic, superior mesenteric, celiac, gastric-gastroepiploic, jejunal-ileal-colic, pancreaticoduodenal-pancreatic, and gastroduodenal arteries (Table 1). Today, the natural history of splanchnic artery aneurysms is becoming better defined because they have been increasingly recognized by abdominal arteriography and computerized tomography (CT).[2-5] Rupture of such aneurysms, especially those having an inflammatory cause, is the most common life or organ-threatening emergency produced by splanchnic artery aneurysms. Aneurysm thrombosis is less often an emergency. The various splanchnic aneurysms produce unique syndromes as emergencies, and discussion about them must be individualized.

SPLENIC ARTERY ANEURYSM

Splenic artery aneurysms account for approximately 60 percent of all splanchnic artery aneurysms.[5-7] Incidental demonstration of these lesions in 0.78 percent of nearly 3600 consecutive abdominal arteriographic studies performed at the University of Michigan perhaps reflects their true frequency in the general population.[6]

Females are four times more likely than males to develop these aneurysms. Three distinct conditions may weaken the splenic artery and contribute to the formation of these aneurysms: (1) arterial fibrodysplasia, (2) repeated pregnancies, with 40 percent of women harboring these lesions being grand multiparous, and (3) portal hypertension with splenomegaly. Although some splenic aneurysms are due to arteriosclerotic disease, calcific changes in the aneurysm without similar involvement of the adjacent vessels suggest arteriosclerosis is a secondary event rather than a primary pathologic process. Most splenic artery aneurysms are saccular, occur at branchings, and in 20 percent of patients are multiple. Inflammatory disease, such as chronic pancreatitis, and trauma are less common causes of these aneurysms, although they are more apt to present as emer-

Vascular Surgical Emergencies
ISBN 0-8089-1843-5

Table 1
Ruptured Splanchnic Artery Aneurysms

Aneurysm Location	Frequency Within Splanchnic Circulation (%)	Frequency of Rupture (%)	Site of Rupture	Mortality With Rupture (%)
Splenic artery	60	<2	Intraperitoneal within lesser sac; Intragastric with pancreatitis-related inflammatory aneurysms	25, 70 During pregnancy
Hepatic artery	20	20	Intraperitoneal and biliary tract with equal frequency	35
Superior mesenteric artery	5.5	Uncommon (Thrombosis more common)	Intraperitoneal and retroperitoneum	50
Celiac artery	4	13	Intraperitoneal	50
Gastric and gastroepiploic arteries	4	90	Intraperitoneal (30%); Intestinal tract (70%)	70
Pancreaticoduodenal, pancreatic, and gastroduodenal arteries	3.5	75 Inflammatory; 50 Noninflammatory	Intestinal tract common; Intraperitoneal and biliary tract less common	50
Jejunal, ileal, and colic arteries	3	30	Intestinal tract common; Intraperitoneal uncommon	20

gencies. Microaneurysms within the spleen are usually associated with connective tissue disorders and are of less clinical importance.

Signet-ring calcifications in the left upper quadrant noted on plain abdominal radiographs are often the first indication of splenic artery aneurysms. However, diagnosis is usually made after angiography performed for some other disease state (Fig. 1). Ultrasonography, CT scanning, and magnetic resonance imaging are useful diagnostic studies, and are of particular value in identifying bleeding aneurysms. Symptoms of left upper quadrant or epigastric pain have been ascribed to these aneurysms in up to 20 percent of cases, although it is unlikely that such are always due to the aneurysm.

Ruptured splenic artery aneurysms are usually associated with bleeding that is initially contained within the lesser sac. Occasionally, blood may exit through the foramen of Winslow, collecting along the right paravertebral gutter with production of right lower quadrant pain. Containment of bleeding within the lesser space allows many patients to be treated before free bleeding into the peritoneal cavity and vascular collapse occur. Intraperitoneal hemorrhage, whether part of such a "double rupture" phenomenon or not, represents a life-threatening complication of these aneurysms. Pancreatitis-related aneurysms are often a source of intestinal hemorrhage, with aneurysmal erosions usually occurring into the stomach or pancreatic ductal system.[8-12] Arteriovenous fistula formation from rupture of a splenic artery aneurysm into the splenic vein is a rare, but recognized cause of portal hypertension and gastrointestinal hemorrhage.[13]

The risk of splenic artery aneurysm rupture depends to some extent upon the etiology of these lesions, with rupture of bland aneurysms occurring in less than 2 percent of cases.[6] Among patients with these aneurysms, rupture has been just as likely to occur when the aneurysm is calcified, resides in a normotensive patient, or in individuals older than 60 years. In contrast to this relatively benign bland aneurysm, rupture has occurred in more than 95 percent of those associated with pregnancy.[6,14,15] Maternal mortality in these cases approaches 70 percent, and fetal mortality exceeds 75 percent. Thus, splenic artery aneurysms recognized during pregnancy, even though asymptomatic, should be considered a serious health hazard.

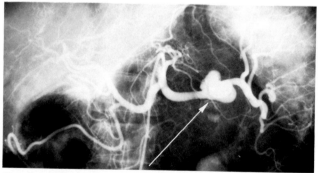

Fig. 1. Selective celiac arteriogram confirming presence of a splenic artery aneurysm (arrow) associated with erosion of a pancreatic pseudocyst into midsplenic artery. (Reproduced from Stanley JC, Frey CF, Miller TA, et al: Major arterial hemorrhage: A complication of pancreatic pseudocysts and chronic pancreatitis. Arch Surg 111:435, 1976. ©American Medical Association. With permission.)

Operative mortality with ruptured splenic artery aneurysms reported during the decade from 1960 to 1970 was 25 percent.[4] Given the 2 percent incidence of rupture, it would seem ill-advised to undertake elective operative intervention for an asymptomatic splenic artery aneurysm in any patient where the risk of operative death might predictably be greater than 0.5 percent. For example, in patients with aneurysms associated with portal hypertension, operative intervention certainly carries a mortality greater than 0.5 percent. Percutaneous transcatheter embolization of aneurysms may be appropriate in such higher-risk patients.[16,17]

Operative intervention for expanding or ruptured splenic artery aneurysms in the past usually entailed splenectomy. With increasing success in splenic salvage for trauma and a recognition of the immunologic importance of splenic preservation, simple obliteration or excision of distal aneurysms has become preferable to splenectomy. Clearly, treatment of most proximal splenic artery aneurysms should not require removal of the spleen. Exclusion of proximal lesions, especially those inflammatory aneurysms embedded within the pancreas, is preferred to aneurysmectomy. Certain of the latter aneurysms may be best treated by distal pancreatectomy if they are expanding or ruptured. Other aneurysms, especially those associated with pancreatic pseudocysts, are most easily treated by incising the aneurysmal sac and ligating entering and exiting vessels from within.

HEPATIC ARTERY ANEURYSM

Hepatic artery aneurysms account for nearly 20 percent of all splanchnic artery aneurysms.[5,18,19] Males are affected twice as often as females. Nontraumatic aneurysms have usually been discovered during the sixth decade of life. Causes of these lesions have been attributed to: atherosclerosis (32 percent), medial degeneration (24 percent), trauma (22 percent), and infection associated with illicit drug use (10 percent). Connective tissue arteriopathies have also been incriminated as a less common cause of these lesions. Aneurysms of the hepatic artery are usually solitary, being extrahepatic in nearly 80 percent of cases and intrahepatic in 20 percent. In general, these aneurysms are fusiform when less than 2 cm in size.

Symptomatic hepatic artery aneurysms are unusual, but when such is the case, they characteristically present with right upper quadrant and epigastric pain. Acute expansion of hepatic artery aneurysms may cause severe upper abdominal discomfort similar to that of pancreatitis. Although large aneurysms may cause obstructive jaundice, the presence of a pulsatile mass is uncommon.

Hepatic artery aneurysm rupture was reported in 44 percent of cases described in the literature from 1960 to 1970.[4] The incidence of rupture in contemporary series is closer to 20 percent, and the true frequency may be considerably less. Mortality attending rupture continues to be approximately 35 percent. Hemorrhage from ruptured hepatic artery aneurysms occurs equally into the biliary tract and the peritoneal cavity. Hemobilia, manifest by biliary colic, hematemesis, and jaundice often accompany this bleeding.[20] Chronic melena is a less common sequela of aneurysm rupture. Intraperitoneal bleeding is most often associated with inflammatory aneurysms.

Common hepatic artery aneurysms, located proximal to the gastroduodenal and right gastric vessels, can usually be treated by aneurysmectomy or aneurysmal exclusion, without arterial reconstruction. The extensive hepatic collateral circulation usually ensures adequate liver blood flow despite interruption of the proximal hepatic artery. Hepatic arterial insufficiency is more likely to accompany treatment of aneurysms involving the more distal hepatic artery and its extrahepatic branches. In the absence of coexisting liver disease, complex arterial reconstructions should be avoided and simple ligation undertaken if temporary operative occlusion of the aneurysmal artery does not cause obvious hepatic ischemia. Direct vascular reconstruction must be undertaken with either prosthetic or autologous grafts if compromised liver blood flow becomes apparent. Ligation of extrahepatic branches to control bleeding from intrahepatic aneurysms may be useful; however, irreparable liver ischemia and necrosis may accompany such treatment.[19] On such occasions, hepatic resection for intrahepatic aneurysms may prove to be the safest form of therapy. In select cases of hepatic artery aneurysms, percutaneous transcatheter obliteration of the aneurysm may be an acceptable alternative to surgical intervention.[21-23]

SUPERIOR MESENTERIC ARTERY ANEURYSM

Aneurysms of the proximal superior mesenteric artery account for 5.5 percent of all reported splanchnic artery aneurysms.[5] Infection has been the etiology in nearly 60 percent of reported cases. The frequency of these aneurysms in contemporary times appears to be less. This may be a consequence of fewer mycotic lesions, although mycotic aneurysms secondary to nonhemolytic streptococci from left-sided bacterial endocarditis involve this vessel more frequently than any other muscular artery. Males and females are affected equally. Superior mesenteric artery aneurysms have also been associated with medial degeneration, atherosclerosis, and trauma.

Superior mesenteric artery aneurysms are currently diagnosed most often during arteriographic studies performed for nonvascular disease. In symptomatic patients, abdominal discomfort is common, varying from mild to persistent severe pain that is often suggestive of intestinal angina.

Rupture of superior mesenteric aneurysms into the peritoneal cavity is unusual,[24] and gastrointestinal hemorrhage associated with these aneurysms usually reflects thrombosis and subsequent intestinal infarction.[4] The critical location of these aneurysms near origins of the inferior pancreaticoduodenal and middle colic arteries causes early isolation of the mesenteric circulation with aneurysmal dissection or occlusion by aneurysmal thrombus. In such circumstances obstruction of the superior mesenteric artery produces intestinal ischemia untempered by the usual collateral network from the adjacent celiac and inferior mesenteric arterial circulations.

Surgical intervention in these cases often involves management of significant intestinal ischemia. In this clinical setting aneurysmectomy or simple ligation of vessels entering and exiting the aneurysm without arterial reconstruction would prove catastrophic. Intestinal revascularization by means of an aortomesenteric graft or some other bypass is often necessary, but has been accomplished infrequently. Because of the potential for infection, autologous vein or arterial grafts are favored over prosthetic conduits.

Aneurysmal obliteration without arterial reconstruction may prove the simplest manner of treatment in select cases not presenting as emergencies. Surprisingly, ligation and aneurysmorrhaphy have been the most commonly reported means of managing these lesions.[5,25,26] Temporary clamping of the superior mesenteric artery and assessment of Doppler signals along the intestine's antimesenteric border assists in defining the adequacy of collateral vessels in maintaining intestinal viability.

CELIAC ARTERY ANEURYSM

Celiac artery aneurysms represent 4 percent of splanchnic artery aneurysms.[5] Important clinical differences exist among cases reported before and after 1950.[27] Recently no sex predilection has been noted. In the earlier time-period, half the lesions had infectious etiologies. In the latter time-period most aneurysms have been associated with medial defects or atherosclerosis. Most contemporary cases have been asymptomatic or have been associated with vague abdominal discomfort.

Rupture rates approach 13 percent, with an attendant mortality of 50 percent. This is in contrast with previously published rupture rates greater than 80 percent.[28] Aneurysmal disruption usually causes bleeding into the peritoneal cavity by way of the lesser space. Gastrointestinal bleeding with direct rupture into the stomach, or by indirect communication through the pancreatic ducts, is exceedingly uncommon.

Celiac artery aneurysms, in the presence of acute expansion or rupture, are best exposed by a thoracoabdominal incision extending from the left midaxillary line within the seventh intercostal space across the costal margin inferiorly in a midline or a right subcostal route. Exploration of the abdomen prior to entering the chest is reasonable, in that most intact aneurysms may be treated using only an abdominal approach.

Aneurysmectomy with arterial reconstruction of the celiac trunk is the preferred treatment for most celiac artery aneurysms, although simple ligation of the celiac artery has been advocated in select patients.[27,29] If the latter course is undertaken, foregut collateral blood flow must be documented to be sufficient to prevent hepatic necrosis. If inadequate blood flow to the liver is evident, hepatic revascularization becomes necessary. Revascularization procedures under those circumstances are usually performed with autologous vein or prosthetic grafts from the thoracic or infrarenal aorta to the distal common hepatic or proper hepatic arteries. Successful outcomes in contemporary times occur in greater than 90 percent of celiac artery aneurysms treated with elective operation.

GASTRIC AND GASTROEPIPLOIC ARTERY ANEURYSMS

Aneurysms of the gastric and gastroepiploic arteries account for 4 percent of all splanchnic artery aneurysms.[5] Males outnumber females 3 to 1, with the majority of these lesions affecting patients over 50 years of age. Most of these aneurysms are solitary. Perigastric aneurysms are usually acquired, either as a result of medial degeneration or periarterial inflammation. Secondary atherosclerosis is a common accompaniment of these lesions. Gastric artery aneurysms are ten times more common than gastroepiploic artery aneurysms.

Perigastric aneurysms often present as vascular emergencies without preceding symptoms. Rupture has been reported in greater than 90 percent of the cases, with gastrointestinal bleeding occurring nearly twice as often as intraperitoneal hemorrhage. That these events are catastrophic is emphasized by a mortality attending rupture approaching 70 percent.[4]

Treatment of gastric and gastroepiploic artery aneurysms does not involve reconstructive arterial surgery. Intramural gastric lesions should be excised with appropriate portions of the stomach. Extramural aneurysms may often be treated by arterial ligation alone, with or without aneurysm excision. Many of these aneurysms are small and a diligent search for them is often tedious if preoperative localization has not been established by arteriographic studies.

JEJUNAL, ILEAL, AND COLIC ARTERY ANEURYSMS

Intestinal branch aneurysms account for 3 percent of all splanchnic artery aneurysms.[5,30] These aneurysms usually occur after 60 years of age, with no sex predilection noted. Solitary aneurysms have been reported in 90 percent of cases. Congenital or acquired medial defects are responsible for most lesions. Atherosclerosis affects 20 percent of these aneurysms, usually as a secondary process. Occasional aneurysms occur as sequelae of endarteritis from septic cardiac emboli.

Most reported cases of jejunal, ileal, and colic artery aneurysms have been associated with rupture. This event carries an attendant mortality of approximately 20 percent.[4] Discovery of increasing numbers of intact intestinal aneurysms during arteriographic studies for nonvascular disease suggests that contemporary rupture rates are close to 30 percent. Ruptured aneurysms are often associated with gastrointestinal hemorrhage. Rupture into the leaves of the mesentery or the free peritoneal cavity is uncommon, although small mesenteric branch aneurysms are more apt to be the source of bleeding with abdominal apoplexy than any other splanchnic aneurysm.

Surgical therapy of intestinal aneurysms requires their careful localization, which is best accomplished by preoperative arteriographic studies. Operative localization without the latter studies may be exceedingly time-consuming and difficult. Arterial ligation, with or without aneurysmectomy, is usually sufficient therapy. Clearly, if bowel infarction or intramural hemorrhage has occurred, resection of the involved segment of intestine should be undertaken. Aneurysms of the inferior mesenteric artery are quite rare, with data regarding their clinical significance being anecdotal at best.[31]

PANCREATICODUODENAL, PANCREATIC, AND GASTRODUODENAL ARTERY ANEURYSMS

Aneurysms of the pancreatic and pancreaticoduodenal arteries account for 2 percent of all splanchnic artery aneurysms. Gastroduodenal artery aneurysms represent an additional 1.5 percent of these aneurysms. Males are four times as likely to exhibit these lesions compared to females, with most patients being older than 50 years of age. These peripancreatic lesions are the most life-threatening of all splanchnic artery aneurysms.[5,32-34] The most serious of these aneurysms are caused by pancreatitis with vascular necrosis or vessel erosion by adjacent pseudocysts. Congenital, arteriosclerotic, and traumatic lesions are less common.

Most patients with these peripancreatic aneurysms experience symptoms of epigastric pain and discomfort, perhaps a reflection of the fact that approximately 60 percent of gastroduodenal and 30 percent of pancreaticoduodenal artery aneurysms are pancreatitis-related. Asymptomatic aneurysms of these arteries, regardless of etiology, are unusual.

Rupture of gastroduodenal and pancreaticoduodenal aneurysms into the intestinal tract occurs in 75 percent of inflammatory and 50 percent of noninflammatory lesions. Bleeding may occur into the stomach as well as the biliary or pancreatic ductal system. Arteriography is essential to confirm the presence of these lesions, although CT scanning and magnetic resonance imaging are of increasing importance in recognizing these lesions (Fig. 2). Mortality rates with rupture approach 50 percent.

Operative intervention is appropriate in all but the poorest risk patient with gastroduodenal, pancreaticoduodenal, or pancreatic arterial aneurysms.[32,34] In general, pancreaticoduodenal and pancreatic artery aneurysms are more difficult to manage than gastroduode-

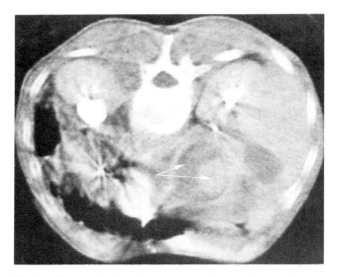

Fig. 2. Computerized axial tomogram of a gastroduodenal artery aneurysm (long arrow) contained within a pancreatic pseudocyst (short arrow). (Reproduced from Eckhauser FE, Stanley JC, Zelenock GB, et al: Gastroduodenal and pancreaticoduodenal artery aneurysms: A complication of pancreatitis causing spontaneous gastrointestinal hemorrhage. Surgery 88:335, 1980. With permission.)

nal artery aneurysms.[32,35] Treatment is often best accomplished by ligation from within the aneurysmal sac rather than extraaneurysmal dissection and arterial ligation. Because of dense inflammatory adhesions associated with pancreatitis, extensive mobilization of this gland and the duodenum may prove hazardous. If aneurysm rupture has occurred into a pancreatic pseudocyst or abscess, some form of drainage procedure should accompany control of the aneurysmal vessel. Pancreatic resections, ranging from distal pancreatectomy to pancreaticoduodenectomy, may be appropriate therapy in select patients. Transcatheter embolization and electrocoagulation also have been employed to ablate certain aneurysms,[36-38] although frequent rebleeding and rupture with such therapy precludes it from becoming standard treatment.[39]

REFERENCES

1. Stanley JC: Abdominal visceral aneurysms, in Haimovici H (ed.): Vascular Emergencies, New York, Appleton-Century-Crofts, 1981, pp 387–397
2. Busuttil RW, Brin BJ: The diagnosis and management of visceral artery aneurysms. Surgery 88:619, 1980
3. Graham JM, McCollum CH, DeBakey ME: Aneurysms of the splanchnic arteries. Am J Surg 140:797, 1980
4. Stanley JC, Thompson NW, Fry WJ: Splanchnic artery aneurysms. Arch Surg 101:689, 1970
5. Stanley JC, Whitehouse WM Jr: Splanchnic artery aneurysms, in Rutherford RB (ed.): Vascular Surgery (2d Ed), Philadelphia, W.B. Saunders, 1984, pp 798–813

6. Stanley JC, Fry WJ: Pathogenesis and clinical significance of splenic artery aneurysms. Surgery 76:889, 1974

7. Trastek VF, Pairolero PC, Joyce JW, et al: Splenic artery aneurysms. Surgery 91:694, 1982

8. Clay RP, Farnell MB, Lancester JR, et al: Hemosuccus pancreaticus. An unusual cause of upper gastrointestinal bleeding. Ann Surg 202:75, 1985

9. deVries JE, Schattenkerk ME, Malt RA: Complications of splenic artery aneurysm other than intraperitoneal rupture. Surgery 91:200, 1982

10. Harper PC, Gamelli RL, Kaye MD: Recurrent hemorrhage into the pancreatic duct from a splenic artery aneurysm. Gastroenterology 87:417, 1984

11. Stabile BE, Wilson SE, Debas HT: Reduced mortality from bleeding pseudocysts and pseudoaneurysms caused by pancreatitis. Arch Surg 118:45, 1983

12. Stanley JC, Frey CF, Miller TA, et al: Major arterial hemorrhage: A complication of pancreatic pseudocysts and chronic pancreatitis. Arch Surg 111:435, 1976

13. Williams DB, Payne SP, Foulk WT, et al: Case report: Splenic arteriovenous fistula. Mayo Clin Proc 55:383, 1980

14. MacFarlane JR, Thorbjarnason B: Rupture of splenic artery aneurysm during pregnancy. Am J Obstet Gynecol 95:1025, 1966

15. O'Grady JP, Day EJ, Toole AL, et al: Splenic artery aneurysm rupture in pregnancy: A review and case report. Obstet Gynecol 50:627, 1977

16. Probst P, Castaneda-Zuniga WR, Gomes AS, et al: Nonsurgical treatment of splenic-artery aneurysms. Radiology 128:619, 1978

17. Waltman AC, Luers PR, Athanasoulis CA, et al: Massive arterial hemorrhage in patients with pancreatitis. Complementary roles of surgery and transcatheter occlusive techniques. Arch Surg 121:439, 1986

18. Guida PM, Moore SW: Aneurysm of the hepatic artery. Report of five cases with a brief review of the previously reported cases. Surgery 60:299, 1966

19. Iseki J, Tada Y, Wada T, et al: Hepatic artery aneurysm. Report of a case and review of the literature. Gastroenterol Jpn 18:84, 1983

20. Harlaftis NN, Akin JT: Hemobilia from ruptured hepatic artery aneurysm: Report of a case and review of the literature. Am J Surg 133:229, 1977

21. Goldblatt M, Goldin AR, Shaff MI: Percutaneous embolization for the management of hepatic artery aneurysms. Gastroenterology 73:1142, 1977

22. Jonsson K, Bjernstad A, Eriksson B: Treatment of a hepatic artery aneurysm by coil occlusion of the hepatic artery. Am J Roentgenol 134:1245, 1980

23. Kadir S, Athansoulis CA, Ring EJ, et al: Transcatheter embolization of intrahepatic arterial aneurysms. Radiology 134:335, 1980

24. Blumenberg RM, David D, Skovak J: Abdominal apoplexy due to rupture of a superior mesenteric artery aneurysm: Clip aneurysmorrhaphy with survival. Arch Surg 108:223, 1974

25. DeBakey ME, Cooley DA: Successful resection of mycotic aneurysm of superior mesenteric artery: Case report and review of the literature. Am Surg 19:202, 1953

26. Olcott C, Ehrenfeld WK: Endoaneurysmorrhaphy for visceral artery aneurysms. Am J Surg 133:636, 1977

27. Graham LM, Stanley JC, Whitehouse WM Jr, et al: Celiac artery aneurysms: Historical (1745-1949) versus contemporary (1950-1984) differences in etiology and clinical importance. J Vasc Surg 2:757, 1985

28. Shumacker HB Jr, Siderys H: Excisional treatment of aneurysm of celiac artery. Ann Surg 148:885, 1958

29. Hertzer NR, Mullally PH: Celiac artery aneurysmectomy with hepatic artery ligation. Arch Surg 104:337, 1972

30. McNamara MF, Griska LB: Superior mesenteric artery branch aneurysms. Surgery 88:625, 1980

31. Graham LM, Hay MR, Cho KJ, et al: Inferior mesenteric artery aneurysms. Surgery 97:158, 1985

32. Eckhauser FE, Stanley JC, Zelenock GB, et al: Gastroduodenal and pancreaticoduodenal artery aneurysms: A complication of pancreatitis causing spontaneous gastrointestinal hemorrhage. Surgery 88:335, 1980

33. Gadacz TR, Trunkey D, Kieffer RF: Visceral vessel erosion associated with pancreatitis. Case reports and a review of the literature. Arch Surg 113:1438, 1978

34. Verta MJ Jr, Dean RH, Yao JST, et al: Pancreaticoduodenal artery aneurysms. Ann Surg 186:111, 1977

35. Spanos PK, Kloppedal EA, Murray CA: Aneurysms of the gastroduodenal and pancreaticoduodenal arteries. Am J Surg 127:345, 1974

36. Prasad JK, Chatterjee KS, Jonston DWB: Unusual case of massive gastrointestinal bleeding-pseudoaneurysm of the head of the pancreas. Can J Surg 18:490, 1975

37. Thakker RV, Gajjar B, Wilkins RA, et al: Embolisation of gastroduodenal artery aneurysm caused by chronic pancreatitis. Gut 24:1094, 1983

38. Vujic I, Anderson MC, Meredith HC, et al: Successful embolization of the dorsal pancreatic artery to control massive upper gastrointestinal hemorrhage. Ann Surg 46:184, 1980

39. Lina JR, Jaques P, Mandell V: Aneurysm rupture secondary to transcatheter embolization. Am J Roentgenol 132:553, 1979

John J. Bergan, William R. Flinn
Walter J. McCarthy, III, James S. T. Yao

Acute Mesenteric Ischemia

"Acute occlusion of the mesenteric vessels results almost
invariably in intestinal gangrene and has, even if surgically
treated, an appalling mortality rate."[1]

It would be very pleasant to say in 1986 that the quotation above, expressed 10 years ago, could now be revised. Unfortunately, this is not true. Acute mesenteric ischemia still commands an astounding mortality. For example, in describing a 26-year experience with mesenteric vascular problems at the Baylor University Medical Center in Dallas, Rogers et al[2] pointed out that of 12 patients treated for acute mesenteric ischemia, 8 suffered embolic occlusion of the superior mesenteric artery, and the operative mortality was 62.5 percent. As mesenteric embolization represents the most favorable surgical situation encountered in treatment of acute mesenteric ischemia, this is a disappointing statistic. Similarly, in an experience with mesenteric ischemia described from the University of Rochester Medical Center, Sachs et al[3] pointed out an overall mortality rate of 65 percent over a 15-year period. The best record was obtained in patients without arterial occlusion but instead with venous thrombosis treated by simple intestinal resection. Indicating that the problem is not one of geography but transcends international boundaries, the experience of the Hospital de la Santa Cruz y San Pablo in Barcelona described by Rius et al[4] admits that the overall mortality rate was 84.7 in surgical treatment of mesenteric infarction.

The fact that the condition of acute mesenteric ischemia occurs in only 1 or 2 per 1000 surgical emergencies in Denmark to 0.38 percent of acute abdominal operations in Barcelona suggests that infrequency of occurrence contributes to the lack of success in treatment. Added to this fact is realization that surgical therapy will vary with the time delay in diagnosis and treatment and with the extent of metabolic derangement within a given patient. Nevertheless, the availability of methods to revascularize ischemic intestine prior to resection of necrotic bowel is tantalizing. An aggressive approach to the problem to increase the number of survivors of mesenteric infarction continues to seem justified. In order to ascertain exactly how much has been accomplished in this regard, the following review was undertaken.

Vascular Surgical Emergencies
ISBN 0-8089-1843-5

The Medical Records Department of the Northwestern Memorial Hospital provided charts of patients with mesenteric infarction encountered during the 40 month period starting January 1, 1983, and ending May 1, 1986. In all, 21 patients were identified, 6 with mesenteric artery embolization, 8 with mesenteric artery thrombosis, and 6 with nonorganic intestinal ischemia, and 1 unclassifiable. In this cohort, 10 were women and 11 were men. The main problems complicating the care of these patients were severe associated medical conditions, markedly advanced age, and delayed or uncertain diagnosis. Accurate identification of the lesions was difficult, and philosophical considerations regarding diagnostic decisions and therapeutic plans were of concern. Table 1 displays the age, sex, and associated medical conditions of the patients with acute mesenteric ischemia managed during this period of time. This tabulation shows the difficulty of initiating aggressive diagnostic and surgical therapy in this severely ill group of patients.

One example of difficulty in determining an accurate diagnosis of the cause of mesenteric infarction is illustrative. This patient, a 77-year-old woman with steroid dependency and atrial fibrillation, was under care for sternal dehiscence and infection following a coronary artery bypass graft when she became acutely acidotic, toxic, and died. Autopsy showed necrosis of small bowel and colon of undetermined cause. Thus, the clinical situation favored the diagnosis of both embolic occlusion of the superior mesenteric artery and nonocclusive ischemia. The patient's age and coronary atherosclerosis favored a diagnosis of atherosclerotic thrombosis. The pathologist failed to clarify the issue at autopsy.

Difficulty in determining the diagnosis in each of these patients was encountered. The experience of other centers in this regard was borne out by a review of the Northwestern experience. Surgeons, when consulted, did diagnose intestinal infarction. Medical colleagues were less specific in categorizing the acute abdomen in the aged. Buchardt Hansen and Christoffersen[1] also indicated that diagnostic difficulties caused 14 patients in their series of 56 to be admitted into the medical department. Three, when admitted to the surgical department, were moved to the medical department because of suspicion of a medical diagnosis, which was most commonly acute myocardial infarction. Because of this and other factors attending difficulty in diagnosis, only 19 percent of their surgically treated patients underwent operation in the first 24 hours. The experience was similar at the University of Rochester,[3] where the delay from onset of symptoms to operation ranged from 18 hours to 9 days.

A thoughtful analysis of the problem of diagnosis suggests that the main difficulties include failure to identify the patient at risk, insufficient appreciation of the nonspecific presentation of some patients, the lack of a reliable noninvasive diagnostic test, and erroneous diagnosis of more familiar medical or surgical conditions. At Northwestern, the current chart review showed that staff internists, cardiac and general surgeons, and general surgical residents were more aware of the possibilities of diagnosis of acute mesenteric ischemia than physicians in other centers publishing their experience.

Acute mesenteric ischemia caused by arterial occlusion will occur as frequently with embolic occlusion as with thrombotic occlusion, as is again shown in this review. It is a disease of patients with previous myocardial infarction, with or without cardiac failure and/or arrhythmia. These facts identify a particular group at high risk for mesenteric embolization. Also, the presence of obvious atherosclerotic stigmata, such as stroke, amputation, or previous arterial reconstruction, identifies further the patient with high risk for mesenteric thrombosis. Some internists will point out that bowel infarction and alcoholism are linked, but it is not appreciated by such experts that bowel infarction is chiefly

Table 1

Associated Conditions in Patients with Acute Mesenteric Ischemia

Age/Sex	Associated Conditions	Treatment	Result
Mesenteric Artery Thrombosis			
47/M	Acute myelogenous leukemia	Segmental resection	Survival
54/F	Severe inanition, cachexia	Mesenteric revascularization	Survival
65/M	Extremity gangrene, postop. total hip repair	None	Death
70/F	CVA, MI	Laparotomy	Death
75/F	Ovarian carcinoma, DIC, hemodialysis	Laparotomy	Death
79/F	Neutropenia, WBC 0.9×10^3	None	Death
82/M	Terminal COPD, abdominal a. aneurysm	None	Death
84/F	Congestive heart failure	None	Death
Mesenteric Embolization			
31/M	Thrombosed aortic graft, coagulopathy, lymphoma, bilateral lower extremity amputations	Embolectomy, intestinal resection, second look	Death
40/M	Cardiomyopathy, congestive heart failure	Exploratory laparotomy	Death
71/M	None	Heparin anticoagulation	Survival
81/M	Terminal COPD	None	Death
82/F	Pneumonia, acute MI, renal failure	None	Death
84/F	Atrial fibrillation, hemiplegia, TIA	None	Death
Nonocclusive Mesenteric Infarction			
69/M	CABG, dopamine infusion	Intraarterial papaverine	Death
73/F	Acute MI	Resection ileum and caecum	Death
75/M	Acute MI, CABG, IABP, renal failure	Laparotomy, colon resection	Death
78/F	CABG	Laparotomy, colon resection	Death
81/M	CHF, aortic & mitral valvular insufficiency, diabetes, pneumonia	None	Death
81/M	CHF, atrial fibrillation, inanition, weight loss	None	Death
Unclassifiable			
77/F	Steroid dependency, atrial fibrillation, sternal dehiscence and infection post CABG, acidosis	None	Death

due to venous thrombosis in that situation and that this occurs with or without cirrhosis and peritonitis.[5]

Given that patients with previous myocardial infarction harboring previous atherosclerotic stigmata are a high risk group, an additional fact can be added that frequently the patients at risk are those living in nursing homes or chronic care facilities. The presence of severe abdominal pain and abdominal distension in a nursing home inmate who is post-stroke, amputation, or myocardial infarction, should strongly suggest a diagnosis of acute mesenteric infarction.

Several other categories of patients represent high risk for mesenteric infarction. Those undergoing intraaortic balloon pumping or who are in severe cardiac failure following coronary artery bypass grafting and those receiving large dosage vasopressor therapy and/or dopamine represent an obvious category for nonorganic intestinal occlusion. It had been less appreciated by us that chronic obstructive pulmonary disease may also be a risk factor for mesenteric infarction.

An addition to the problem of diagnosis is the nonspecific presentation of some patients. Classically, acute mesenteric ischemia is characterized by severe abdominal pain, bowel emptying including both colon evacuation and vomiting, and leukocytosis. The abdominal pain is of sudden onset in patients with embolic occlusion of the mesenteric artery, but will be of more insidious onset in patients with thrombotic or nonorganic occlusion of the mesenteric vessels. The abdominal pain will be accompanied by cramping and bowel evacuation, but early in the development of the syndrome, there will be no blood in the stool and the patient may not even describe bowel emptying. Furthermore, the pain of mesenteric arterial thrombosis, developing more slowly, is often associated with abdominal distension, and as such, mimics bowel obstruction rather than mesenteric infarction.

Physical findings are nonspecific, as well. Abdominal tenderness is found but is not localized. If localized, however, it is right-sided and may be confused with a diagnosis of cholecystitis or appendicitis. Most commonly, hypotension with metabolic acidosis suggests mesenteric infarction. Therefore, these findings of nonspecific abdominal pain and tenderness associated with hypotension and acidosis present in a patient with arteriosclerotic stigmata or in an aged patient must strongly suggest the diagnosis of mesenteric infarction. Unfortunately, a combination of acidosis, hypotension, and general illness out of proportion to physical findings often leads the inexperienced clinician to suspect diverticulosis, hemorrhagic pancreatitis, or myocardial infarction. While a history of weight loss, with or without gastrointestinal distress, will be present in nearly all patients who have thrombotic occlusion of the mesenteric artery, such important history will be absent in the patients with mesenteric artery embolization. In many recorded experiences with mesenteric infarction, the embolization syndrome is more common than the syndrome of thrombosis of the mesenteric artery.

Surgeons are very much aware of the fact that no specific laboratory test will suggest, much less diagnose, mesenteric infarction. Hemoconcentration, hyperamylasemia, hyperphosphatemia, and metabolic acidosis are often seen in patients with mesenteric infarction, but these are nonspecific indicators. The most promising report of early diagnosis of intestinal infarction came from Jamieson et al,[6] who suggested a diagnostic triad of leukocytosis, acidosis, and elevated phosphate. They reported elevated inorganic phosphates in serum and peritoneal fluid in the early stages of mesenteric ischemia. Experience at Northwestern has not confirmed these observations, and in fact, hyperphosphatemia occurred only in the single patient with renal failure and mesenteric infarction. No other patient had elevated phosphorus.

In a series of 65 clinical cases reported by Gorey,[7] serum was available for analysis in 13 and serum phosphate was only elevated in 2. Graeber et al,[8] reporting on the Walter Reed Army Medical Center experience, described elevated serum CPK (especially the MM isoenzyme) and total LDH (particularly LDH III) in intestinal and colonic infarction. Gorey has found that LDH may or may not be elevated, and that serum CPK was elevated only early in the ischemic period. Both of these enzymes fluctuated widely.

With regard to the problem of metabolic acidosis, it is recognized that this problem may become more acute after relief of the occlusion and release of toxic agents of tissue origin and bacterial development. Such release of toxic agents is complicated by the fact that some of these may be cardiodepressant and vasoactive. These have been identified by Kobold and Thal[9] and by Parks et al.[10] Brooks and Carey[11] emphasized that metabolic acidosis in the absence of shock and hypotension should strongly suggest extensive intestinal ischemia, and when present, this is a helpful signal. However, absence of metabolic acidosis confuses the issue entirely.

Radiographs of the abdomen are obtained in nearly all acute abdominal conditions, but these films are no more sensitive than laboratory testing in acute mesenteric ischemia. Classic signs are described by radiologists. These include thickening of the bowel wall, separation of loops of bowel by edema, thickening of valvuli conniventes, and intramural or portal air. All of these are late findings and, especially the finding of portal air, preclude salvage of the patient, as was shown at Northwestern in the 40-year-old man with cardiomyopathy.

With regard to the problem of accurate identification of the diagnosis, only contrast arteriography is diagnostic. Recent explorations into the use of ultrasonic visualization of mesenteric vessels have been very informative with regard to the diagnosis of chronic intestinal ischemia.[12] In the situation of acute intestinal ischemia with bowel distension and gas-filled intestines, however, it is to be expected that ultrasound will have very little to contribute in the immediate future.

Taking these facts into consideration, high risk patients suspected of having mesenteric infarction should be considered for angiography in all instances in which the patient is thought to be salvageable.

ACUTE MESENTERIC ANGIOGRAPHY

Transfemoral aortography for visualization of the mesenteric vessels should be done in the anteroposterior and lateral positions in order to visualize the origins of the celiac axis, superior mesenteric artery, and inferior mesenteric artery. Characteristically, in mesenteric artery thrombosis, a total blockage of the contrast media in the main stem of the mesenteric artery will occur within 1 cm of its aortic origin. The celiac axis may be seen to be occluded simultaneously (Fig. 1). When the diagnosis is arterial thrombosis, both the celiac axis and the superior mesenteric artery will be expected to be involved. The inferior mesenteric artery may or may not be occluded. On the other hand, when angiography reveals a total blockage of contrast media in the main stem of an otherwise normal mesenteric artery, the diagnosis is mesenteric embolization (Fig. 2). The usual location of such an occlusion is proximal or distal to the origin of the middle colic artery,

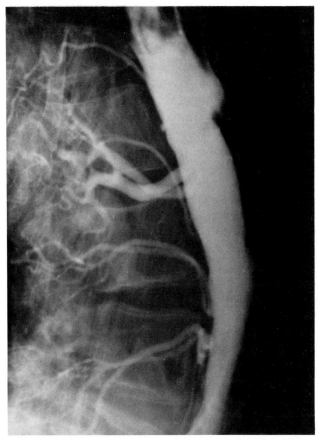

Fig. 1. Mesenteric infarction caused by atherosclerotic thrombosis of the mesenteric circulation will present this picture on aortography. The celiac axis, superior mesenteric artery, and inferior mesenteric vessels will fail to be visualized.

and the first branches of intestinal circulation to the jejunum will be seen to be spared. Nonocclusive mesenteric ischemia is demonstrated by mainstem vessel patency with segmental symmetric branch vessel stenosis.

LAPAROTOMY

Surgical exploration of the abdomen may occur under one of two circumstances in mesenteric infarction. The first, and most desirable, is when a preoperative diagnosis has been suspected and confirmed by angiography. In such a situation, a Swan-Ganz catheter can be placed for monitoring of afterload reduction, metabolic acidosis can be corrected, and fluid resuscitation accomplished. A less desirable situation occurs when surgical judgment calls for laparotomy for an acute abdomen, diagnosis unspecified. In this situation, the patient arrives with partial or no correction of acidosis, fluid loss, and cardiac decompensation. Revascularization of the ischemic gut in such a situation greatly

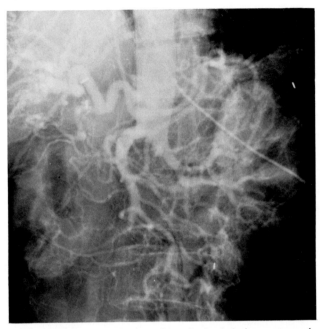

Fig. 2. This anteroposterior view obtained during aortography shows a normal mainstem mesenteric artery with an occlusion in its midportion. An incidental left renal artery embolus is also visualized.

increases the operative risk due to release of vasoactive peptides and unspecified cardiodepressant agents in the mesenteric vascular bed.

Recognition of the mesenteric infarction is not difficult, but the precise diagnosis of the condition causing the infarction may escape judgment of the most discerning and experienced surgeon. While resection of necrotic bowel will be necessary whether the diagnosis is embolic or thrombotic occlusion of the mesenteric artery, the actual method of revascularization will be different in each condition. Embolic occlusion can allow revascularization by simple mesenteric artery embolectomy, while thrombotic occlusion will demand a formal, full-scale revascularization, either by aortomesenteric bypass or by aortomesenteric endarterectomy.

SURGICAL VERIFICATION OF DIAGNOSIS

It has been found that embolic occlusion of the gut produces one of two characteristic patterns. The first, and most common, is ischemic compromise of the small bowel and variable portions of large bowel, with sparing of the proximal jejunum. This is the classic presentation of mainstem mesenteric artery embolization, in which the embolus has lodged distal to the jejunal branches of intestine. The second, and less well-recognized, pattern of intestinal ischemia is patchy, segmental ischemia occurring in several disparate loops of small bowel. This picture is caused by atheroembolic fragments in segmental and arcade branches. Whenever either of these patterns is present, intestinal embolization is the most likely diagnosis and should be assumed to be present.

Thrombotic occlusion of the mesenteric artery may produce a variable pattern of ischemia but usually involves the entire small bowel and variable amounts of large bowel. Specifically, the proximal portion of jejunum is compromised, as well as the central small bowel. When the celiac axis is also occluded, the duodenum may be ischemic, and when all three intestinal vessels are occluded by thrombosis, the descending colon and rectum may be ischemic also.

Unfortunately, the iliocolic arborization is the final common pathway of intestinal infarction. Both embolic and thrombotic ischemia may show only necrosis of this vulnerable bowel segment. Therefore, severe iliocolic ischemia as such does not aid in differentiating the various causes of the mesenteric infarction.

Confirmation of the diagnosis at laparotomy is obtained by passing the right hand of the surgeon behind the root of the mesentery and palpating the pulsations of the mesenteric artery. In embolic occlusion, the pulsations will stop abruptly at the site of the embolus. In thrombotic occlusion, there are no pulsations in the superior mesenteric artery and, of course, when the celiac axis is also occluded, there will be no pulsations in this anterior aortic branch, which can be visualized through the lesser omental bursa. Mainstem pulsations in the face of intestinal ischemia and/or necrosis connote nonocclusive infarction (Fig. 3).

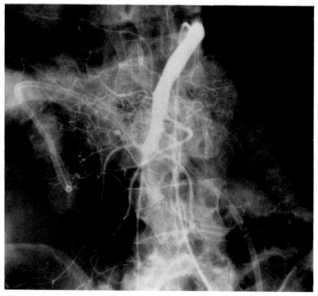

Fig. 3. When neither thrombotic nor embolic occlusion of the mesenteric artery is present, intestinal ischemia may be caused by nonorganic occlusion, as shown on this selective mesenteric arteriogram. Note sparsity of branch vessels and the small caliber of those visualized.

SURGICAL TREATMENT

Embolic occlusion of the superior mesenteric artery is the most common cause of intestinal infarction and is the easiest to disobliterate. The mesenteric artery is exposed between atraumatic slings exactly where the pulsation ceases. Branches from the artery are carefully preserved but overlying venous tributaries to the mesenteric vein are ligated with impunity. After a sufficient length of the artery is skeletonized, a transverse incision is made, and a #3 Fogarty catheter is introduced proximally and distally until clearing of the artery has been assured. Liberal irrigation of the distal artery with heparinized saline solution will aid in dislodging propagated thrombi. The embolus itself will be a characteristic reddish, granular, "hamburger-like" mass, whereas the propagated clot will be a maroon, tubular structure. The thrombus that caused the embolic occlusion can be readily distinguished from the clot that formed after mesenteric circulation became stagnant. Restitution of arterial flow can be obtained by transverse suture of the mesenteric artery with 6-0 monofilament suture.

Restoration of the mesenteric arterial stream in cases of mesenteric thrombosis is more difficult than simple embolectomy. A full-scale, formal vascular reconstruction will be required. No amount of Fogarty catheter manipulation of the thrombus will result in successful revascularization, simply because the atherosclerotic lesion at the aortic origin of the mesenteric artery cannot be removed with a Fogarty catheter. In order to perform the superior mesenteric bypass, it is necessary to detach the entire fourth portion of the duodenum from the ligament of Treitz, fully mobilizing the small bowel away from the aorta. This provides a very short distance between the aorta and the superior mesenteric artery, which can be bridged by a short, wide segment of proximal saphenous vein. If the infrarenal aorta is severely diseased and will not accept a graft, a retropancreatic tunnel allows proximal anastomosis to the supraceliac aorta. This is exposed by an incision in the crus of the diaphragm, as described below. Although prosthetic grafts have been used to revascularize mesenteric circulation in chronic situations, they are to be avoided in instances of acute intestinal infarction.

If the patient's condition allows celiac axis revascularization, this should be done after completing the superior mesenteric artery bypass. In the past, we have advocated saphenous vein grafts from the infrarenal aorta to the celiac axis. However, the increasing appreciation of transabdominal supraceliac aortic surgery during the latter part of 1985 has caused this to be the preferred avenue of approach. The lesser omental bursa is entered between hemostatic clamps, and the right crus of the diaphragm incised vertically so as to expose the aorta superior to the celiac axis. This can be encircled rapidly with a finger and then an atraumatic sling for cross-clamping. The celiac axis is covered by dense fibrous and nerve tissues that make up the solar plexus. This can be dissected free from above downward, maintaining the integrity of the celiac artery. Virtually always, the axis will be found to be patent distal to the proximal atherosclerotic plug. After aortic cross-clamping, a saphenous vein graft can be attached above the celiac axis and then to the celiac artery directly for an in-line bypass of the proximal celiac occlusion.

ASSESSMENT OF INTESTINAL VIABILITY

Tests of intestinal viability include clinical judgment,[13] fluorescein dye,[14] trypan blue, patent blue 5, the Doppler probe,[15,16] electromyography, pH recordings, bowel temperature, oxygen electrodes,[17] radionuclides,[18] and tetrazolium analysis of mucosa. Fortunately, clinical judgment has an overall accuracy of greater than 90 percent, which compares favorably to fluorescein-induced fluorescence, which is said to have an accuracy of 100 percent. Our own method of assessment involves irrigating the bowel with warm saline and packing it between pads for a 20-minute interval, during which time the Doppler probe is obtained. A gas-sterilized probe is kept available in our operating theater at all times, but cold sterilization of a probe can be used in an emergency when the gas-sterilized probe is not available.

The Doppler examination is sensitive and accurate. The probe is placed on the antimesenteric surface of the ischemic bowel over acoustic gel. The absence of arterial signals is certain evidence of irreversible ischemic damage even though revascularization has been done. The presence of arterial Doppler signals does not guarantee survival of the intestine, but strongly suggests that the bowel can be left in place, rather than resected.

When clinical judgment and/or Doppler studies suggest the presence of intestinal necrosis, that segment of intestine should be removed. While it is acknowledged that no surgeon can ascertain accurately the potential for intestinal viability before revascularization, it is likewise held that experienced surgeons are good judges of bowel viability after revascularization has taken place.

ANASTOMOSIS OR ENTEROSTOMY

After resection of necrotic bowel, the choice remains between anastomosis of the segments of remaining bowel or enterostomy. In the past, emphasis has been placed upon anastomosis, with or without a second-look procedure. An alternative to this is temporary enterostomy, which allows inspection of the mucosa of the bowel in the postoperative period. This may be an alternative to reexploration in an emergency situation, and should be considered whenever bowel is resected after revascularization for embolic or thrombotic occlusion of the mesenteric vessels. It may be the treatment of choice in mesenteric venous thrombosis.

SECOND LOOK

Judgment for performing the second-look procedure will derive from information obtained at the first operation. No analysis of the patient's postoperative course will allow determination of the need for a second-look procedure. This must be decided upon at the first laparotomy.

The second look may be just an open-and-close procedure or may require further resection of ischemic intestine. The time interval between the first and second operations will allow vigorous resuscitation of the patient, with correction of any residual acidosis, hypovolemia, and anemia. This interval is usually 18 to 24 hours.

PHILOSOPHICAL CONSIDERATIONS

This section of the discussion of occlusion of mesenteric vessels has been left to last because it is simply the most difficult. We as surgeons are trained in some measure in scientific thinking and to a great extent in technical decision-making and execution. We are not trained in philosophical judgment. Yet, clearly, every patient with mesenteric infarction should not be submitted to surgery. Each person will die ultimately, and for some mesenteric infarction will be their mode of exodus. A glance at Table 1 will show that acute mesenteric infarction is the mechanism of death in patients who are otherwise terminally ill. Three of these patients had been hospitalized in the terminal phases of COPD or malignancy and experienced mesenteric infarction while hospitalized. While it has been recognized in the past that nonorganic intestinal ischemia might be the cause of mesenteric infarction in such patients, this more recent review shows that both embolization and thrombosis can be the modus operandi for the acute intestinal ischemia. Consideration of the associated conditions was the most common cause for no treatment or delayed treatment in each of the patients seen in this review. Therefore, the diagnostic and therapeutic considerations discussed above apply to the salvageable patient and not to every aged, undernourished, acidotic, arteriosclerotic patient transferred from a chronic care facility to the acute hospital. While each surgeon makes up his or her own mind about the care of the individual patient, the surgeon must take into consideration the philosophical problems posed by mesenteric infarction.

PREVENTION OF INTESTINAL INFARCTION

Now that the diagnosis of nonocclusive mesenteric infarction is being clarified and treated by better cardiac management and proper control of cardiac afterload reduction, prevention of mesenteric infarction centers on correcting the two other causes of such intestinal arterial occlusion. Embolus remains the most dramatic cause of mesenteric artery occlusion leading to mesenteric infarction. Prevention of mesenteric embolization involves recognition of the cardiac source of such emboli. Proper anticoagulant management in the aged patient who may or may not be senile and confined to a chronic care facility is difficult or impossible. On the other hand, embolic occlusion of the mesenteric artery occurs in younger, active persons who have known cardiac arrhythmia or a history of recent myocardial infarction, with or without a ventricular aneurysm. Should a peripheral embolus have occurred, this should be a signal that a more important central embolus to the mesenteric bed or cerebral vasculature should be prevented by anticoagulant therapy or surgical removal of the source.

Mesenteric infarction resulting from chronic atherosclerotic occlusive disease of the mesenteric artery and celiac axis can be prevented. The survey by Kwaan and Connolly[19] of the experience at the Long Beach Veterans Administration Hospital showed that in 25 patients with acute intestinal ischemia resulting from arteriosclerotic mesenteric occlusion, symptoms including progressive loss of weight and digestive disturbances mimicking peptic ulcer disease or cholecystitis were consistent findings. Delay and mistakes in making the clinical diagnosis resulted in an 80 percent mortality in this group of patients. Awareness of possible mesenteric artery occlusive disease in patients with ill-defined gastrointestinal symptoms and weight loss is critical to diagnosis. Should the diagnosis be suspected, aortography can be done and effective surgical management applied.[20]

Experience at Northwestern with a 54-year-old woman who thrombosed her 90 percent occluded mesenteric artery while awaiting intestinal arterial bypass (Table 1) shows how dangerous chronic intestinal ischemia can be.

Visualization of mesenteric vessels by B-mode Doppler ultrasound is now possible, and quantitation of blood flow within these vessels is regularly done.[12,21] Turbulent flow can be detected by spectrum analysis, and if necessary, even provocative alimentation can be performed to confirm the diagnosis. Early suspicion of the diagnosis of mesenteric arterial insufficiency with confirmation by ultrasound scan will allow the prevention of mesenteric infarction in those individuals who are active, viable, and potentially salvageable. In contrast is the situation in which advanced bowel infarction with refractory shock, persistent acidemia, diffuse peritoneal signs are present, in which surgical exploration is ineffective even if infarction is found. When resection is the only form of therapy that can be applied, the course of advanced infarction is not altered by such surgical therapy.[5]

VENOUS THROMBOSIS

Acute intestinal venous thrombosis is not truly acute mesenteric ischemia, but in its advanced form, it mimics intestinal infarction. Acute mesenteric venous thrombosis requiring laparotomy and/or segmental resection of intestine was not encountered during the 40-month period of this review. In our past experience, it was noted that venous thrombosis produced profound edema of the bowel wall and obvious venous congestion. Confirmation of the diagnosis was made by transecting the small veins of the mesentery and extruding fresh clot from them. In the past, it was thought that mesenteric venous thrombosis was a coagulopathy, preceded or triggered by illness, stress, or viremia. It had been noted that thrombin antagonists, such as antitrypsin, alpha$_2$ macroglobulin, fibrin, or fibrin degradation products were associated with mesenteric venous thrombosis and conversely, antithrombin-III deficiency had been noted in some patients.

During the 24-month period from March, 1984 to March, 1986, a period encompassed by this review of mesenteric emergencies at the Northwestern University Medical Center, there were 16 patients with documented splanchnic venous thrombosis. The diagnosis was made by computed tomography and/or arteriography, with or without hepatic venography. The cause of the splanchnic venous thrombosis in this group of patients included coagulopathy (five), Budd-Chiari syndrome (four), pancreatic carcinoma (two), cirrhosis and portal hypertension (two), pancreatitis (one), and unknown cause (two). None of the patients experienced segmental bowel necrosis nor required laparotomy for intestinal resection. Therefore, it is clear that the syndrome of acute mesenteric venous thrombosis mimicking intestinal infarction is much rarer than the diagnosis of mesenteric venous thrombosis itself.

ACKNOWLEDGEMENT

This work was supported in part by the Conrad Jobst Foundation, the Seabury Foundation, and the Northwestern Vascular Research Foundation.

REFERENCES

1. Buchardt Hansen HJ, Christoffersen JK: Occlusive mesenteric infarction. A retrospective study of 83 cases. Acta Chir Scand Suppl 472:103, 1976

2. Rogers DM, Thompson JE, Garrett WV, et al: Mesenteric vascular problems. A 26-year experience. Ann Surg 195:554, 1982

3. Sachs SM, Morton JH, Schwartz SI: Acute mesenteric ischemia. Surgery 92:646, 1982

4. Rius X, Escalante JF, Llaurado JM, et al: Mesenteric infarction. World J Surg 3:489, 1979

5. Cooke M, Sande MA: Diagnosis and outcome of bowel infarction on an acute medical service. Amer J Med 75:984, 1983

6. Jamieson WG, Marchuk S, Rowsom J, et al: The early diagnosis of massive acute intestinal ischaemia. Br J Surg 69(Suppl):S52, 1982

7. Gorey TF: The outlook in mesenteric infarction. Terence Millin Lecture, Bicentenary International Surgical Conference, Royal College of Surgeons of Ireland, Sept 14, 1984

8. Graeber G, Cafferty T, Riordan M, et al: Changes in serum total creatinine phosphokinase (CPK) and its isoenzymes caused by experimental ligation of the superior mesenteric artery. Ann Surg 193:499, 1981

9. Kobold EE, Thal AP: Quantitation and identification of vasoactive substances liberated during various types of experimental and clinical intestinal ischemia. Surg Gynecol Obstet 117:315, 1963

10. Parks D, Bulkley G, Granger DN, et al: Ischemic injury in the cat small intestine: role of superoxide radicals. Gastroenterology 82:9, 1982

11. Brooks DM, Carey LD: Base deficit in superior mesenteric artery occlusion, an aid to early diagnosis. Ann Surg 122:352, 1973

12. Sandager G, Flinn WR, McCarthy WJ, et al: Assessment of visceral arterial reconstruction using duplex scan. Bruit (in press)

13. Bulkley GB, Zuidema GD, Hamilton SR, et al: Intraoperative determination of small intestinal viability following ischemic injury. A prospective, controlled trial of two adjuvant methods (Doppler and fluorescein) compared with standard clinical judgment. Ann Surg 193:628, 1981

14. Carter MS, Fantini GA, Sammartano RJ, et al: Qualitative and quantitative fluorescein fluorescence in determining intestinal viability. Amer J Surg 147:117, 1984

15. Hobson RW II, Wright CB, Rich NM, et al: Assessment of colonic ischemia during aortic surgery by Doppler ultrasound. J Surg Res 20:231, 1976

16. Cooperman M, Martin EW Jr, Carey LC: Determination of intestinal viability by Doppler ultrasonography in venous infarction. Ann Surg 191:57, 1980

17. Locke R, Hauser CJ, Shoemaker WC: The use of surface oximetry to assess bowel viability. Arch Surg 119:1252, 1984

18. Gharagozloo F, Bulkley GB, Zuidema GD, et al: The use of intraperitoneal xenon for early diagnosis of acute mesenteric ischemia. Surgery 95:404, 1984

19. Kwaan JHM, Connolly JE: Prevention of intestinal infarction resulting from mesenteric arterial occlusive disease. Surg Gynecol Obstet 157:321, 1983

20. Hollier LH, Bernatz PE, Pairolero PC, et al: Surgical management of chronic intestinal ischemia: A reappraisal. Surgery 90:940, 1981

21. Jäger KA, Fortner GS, Thiele BL, et al: Non-invasive diagnosis of intestinal angina. J Clin Ultrasound 12:588, 1984

Iatrogenic Vascular Emergencies

Robert B. Rutherford
William H. Pearce

Acute Problems Following Diagnostic and Interventional Radiologic Procedures

Angiography helped usher in the "Golden Era" of vascular surgery and, in its wake, we now see the rising tide of interventional radiology. Diagnostic procedures are often essential to the vascular surgeon, whereas therapeutic interventions by angiographers may be definitively therapeutic at best, helpful adjuncts, or frankly competitive and damaging at worst. In most instances the main justification for such interventional procedures as percutaneous transluminal angioplasty (PTA), thrombolytic therapy (SK/UK), and transcatheter therapeutic embolization (TE) in preference to an operative repair is a lesser morbidity and mortality. However, the improvement achieved may be significantly less, both in degree and duration, than the surgical alternative. Furthermore, serious complications of such intervention may occur. The vascular surgeon's concern with these procedures is not that of an interested competitor, but instead, as a consultant who ultimately approves of their application. This, within indications based on factual knowledge of risk and benefit—with full knowledge of his or her ability to recognize and deal with the complications as they arise.

The focus of this chapter is on *acute* problems following diagnostic or interventional radiologic procedures, particularly those requiring emergency intervention. Such complications as failure to complete the procedure successfully (technical failure) or failure to achieve its anticipated result (therapeutic failure) will not be discussed, nor will late complications such as postcatheterization stenoses or aneurysm.

Emergency complications may be categorized according to the procedure (e.g., PTA or SK/UK) or their manner of presentation (e.g., hemorrhage, necrosis, renal shutdown, etc.). However, many of these complications are common to all procedures because they each require arterial cannulation and catheter passage through the arterial tree to a preselected site with injection of contrast media. The general complications will be discussed first and then specific complications associated with selected procedures.

Vascular Surgical Emergencies
ISBN 0-8089-1843-5

PROBLEMS ASSOCIATED WITH ARTERIAL PUNCTURE

Although the direct needle approach is still used occasionally for simple femoral and brachial arteriography, it has been for the most part replaced by catheter techniques using a plastic sheath needle. For angiograms requiring contrast injection at or near the catheter introduction site, the plastic sheath can be advanced to the hilt after the needle has been withdrawn. The site of the arterial puncture (e.g., femoral, axillary) is merely a convenient point of access to the arterial tree and the Seldinger method[1] is then employed to place the catheter tip precisely. The exact site for the arterial puncture depends upon the patient's arterial anatomy and the procedure performed. In this technique, after the needle is withdrawn from its Teflon sleeve, a guide wire is introduced and its tip is advanced to the appropriate site. A longer plastic catheter replaces the outer sheath and is advanced over the guide wire to the desired location. Several problems can arise from these maneuvers. They are (1) concomitant puncture of the adjacent vein resulting in arteriovenous fistula formation; (2) dissection and false passage; (3) perforation of the vessel wall at a remote site from that of catheter introduction; (4) subintimal hemorrhage with luminal narrowing; (5) atheroembolism; (6) localized trauma leading to thrombosis; (7) thrombus formation around the catheter with secondary embolization; (8) bleeding from the catheter introduction site; (9) late stricture or false aneurysm. The incidence of these complications is directly related to the experience of the angiographer and the number of procedures performed per year.[2]

Arteriovenous Fistula

It is not always appreciated that the angiographers commonly also puncture the opposite wall of the artery at the time of catheter introduction. This is *deliberate* for it allows better placement of the needle and facilitates subsequent advancement of guide wires and catheters. Should the adjacent vein also be punctured in this maneuver, and especially if guide wires and/or catheter tips reenter this opening, an arteriovenous fistula can result. While this complication is rare (less than 1 percent), its early recognition and closure is desirable.[3] Therefore, puncture sites should routinely be auscultated for bruits. When a suspicious bruit is detected, especially when accompanied by a thrill, the diagnosis of A-V fistula can be readily confirmed by inspection of the analog-Doppler waveform recorded at or just proximal to the fistula.[4] Arteriography then is necessary to plan surgical closure.

Proximal control is rarely a problem because puncture usually has been made low where the femoral vein begins to shift from a medial to posterior position behind the artery or into the profunda femoris vein, which crosses behind the superficial femoral artery and in front of the profunda femoris artery. Dissection will be aided by study of the arteriogram, the location of the puncture wound, palpation of the thrill, or staining of the tissues. When the fistula is operated upon early, it will often "separate" during the dissection. Anyone who has witnessed the brisk hemorrhage that accompanies this event will understand the need for approaching and controlling the proximal and distal vessels prior to direct attack on the fistula.

Dissection and False Passage

Intimal flaps are easily raised and dissection can easily occur in the subintimal plane that is used in performing an endarterectomy. In the Seldinger technique, the guide wire may inadvertently be introduced under an intimal defect and advanced along the arterial wall easily in this false passage. Because the cleavage plane produced by degenerative changes in the outer media offers surprisingly little resistance, the guide wire and later the catheter may be easily advanced in this plane and will be seen to follow the same anatomic pathway as the artery. Blood may readily flow along this passage so that the angiographer may still obtain a backflow of blood through the catheter. However, if he performs a test injection, it will reveal a characteristic appearance of false passage (Fig. 1). The failure to use a test injection, or properly identify the dissection may result in a power injection of a full contrast load (30–70 ml) being made, often with disastrous consequences.

Localized dissections, without a significant degree of arterial occlusion, may be dealt with by continued observation, particularly if the patient is to undergo reconstruction

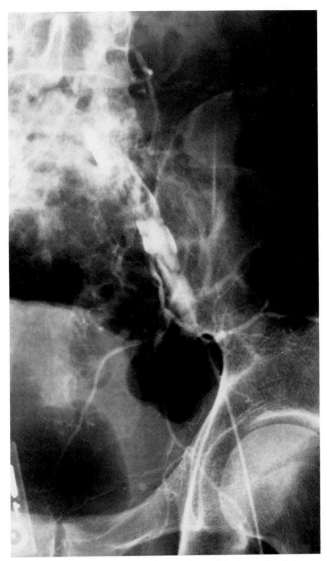

Fig. 1. Characteristic appearance of arterial dissection by contrast media injection shown here in the left iliac artery.

anyway. However, major degrees of dissection with occlusion of important arterial segments and branches require urgent surgical intervention. Particularly tragic are instances
in which renal dissection occurs with renal ischemia and shutdown. The extent of the
dissection can usually be gauged as occurring from the upper reaches of the contrast back
down to the site of catheter introduction. Techniques developed for the successful management of dissecting aortic aneurysms will need to be applied, usually combining graft
replacement of most of the involved segment and incorporating closure of the false
passage into the anastomotic suture lines. Attempts to restore or preserve flow through the
natural lumen by such maneuvers as cutting out distal "windows" are not advised for
major dissections. In addition, consideration must be given to reimplantation of any major
outflow branches (e.g., renal or mesenteric arteries). If the false passage has dissected up
into three branches, one might be tempted to perform an orificial endarterectomy, but this
blind procedure might ultimately result in distal occlusion. Dividing the vessel beyond the
point of dissection, or if this is not possible, suturing the two lumina together and either
reimplanting this opening or connecting it to the graft using an interposition vein graft, is
recommended.

Remote Perforation

Perforation and extraluminal contrast injection are also uncommon, occurring in 0.4–
1.75 percent of patients undergoing angiography.[3] Extraluminal contrast is most likely to
occur with translumbar arteriography. This complication is usually caused by the guide
wire and is quite rare except when attempting balloon dilation of irregular stenoses or
occlusions. Contained false passage is a more likely consequence. Sometimes, if it is
small and contained, dye extravasation can be treated expectantly. Free perforations with
extravasation usually do not result in massive exsanguinating hemorrhage because of
containment by surrounding tissue. Even the retroperitoneum offers sufficient resistance
that time is allowed for surgical intervention. Nevertheless, once such perforations become clinically manifest, because of local pain, hematoma formation, dropping hematocrit, or hemodynamic deterioration, they should be treated with the same aggressiveness
applied to other penetrating arterial injuries.

Subintimal Hematoma with Luminal Narrowing

Rarely at the time of forceful contrast injection, the catheter tip will "whip" or
"vibrate" striking the arterial wall and producing subintimal bleeding. Smooth defects of
this sort are quite characteristic (see Fig. 2). This complication is more common in the
carotid and renal arteries. A number of such subintimal or "mural" hematomas have been
reported in the carotid artery, and as threatening as they may appear, they do surprisingly
well when managed conservatively with and without heparinization. Follow-up arteriography usually shows complete resolution. Whether or not this becomes the site of future
degenerative changes is not known.

Atheroembolism

Dislodgement of atherosclerotic material during transfemoral arteriography is not a
common complication. The usual sequelae are transient livido reticularis or a frank "blue
toe" syndrome. Very infrequently, however, dislodgement of atherosclerotic debris in the

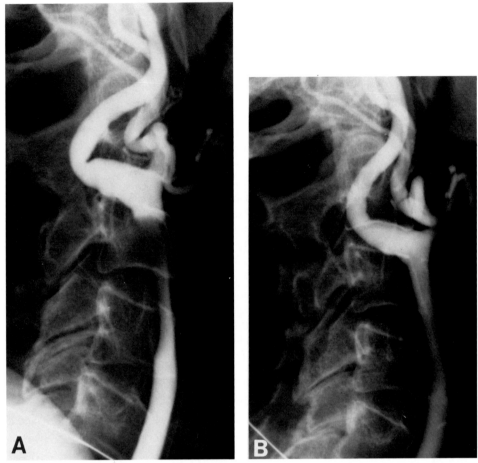

Fig. 2. Subintimal hematoma of the carotid artery produced by catheter tip trauma: (A) immediately after subintimal hemorrhage, (B) two weeks later with only heparin therapy.

visceral circulation may produce bowel ischemia. The possibility of intestinal infarction should be suspected when a patient complains of severe abdominal pain following arteriography. Immediate laparotomy is required with resection of the involved intestine. Although this complication is extremely unusual, the high mortality and morbidity associated with it warrants this aggressive approach.

Arterial Thrombosis

Arterial trauma at the site of catheter introduction leading to thrombosis is not uncommon, particularly in badly diseased arteries (0.14–0.7 percent)[4] and those of small children. This is usually associated with at least a limited false passage or intimal flap. However, since the initial procedure is often being performed for symptomatic occlusive disease, its worsening by another thrombotic occlusion normally creates a degree of ischemia requiring immediate intervention. Clearly audible flow through distal arteries with adequate perfusion pressures on Doppler examination, the lack of ischemic pain and a normal neurologic examination *may* warrant continued surveillance or proceeding with planned reconstruction on schedule. This must be recognized as a calculated risk. The femoral and axillary arteries are readily accessible and can be explored under local anesthesia, if necessary. The thrombotic occlusion is readily disobliterated and eventually will require correction. Therefore, there is usually little justification for delay. At the time of exploration it should be remembered that these catheter induced thromboses have a local cause that must be corrected rather than simply performing a thrombectomy. The lesion is usually at the puncture site or just proximal. A longitudinal arteriotomy is performed with repair of the intimal flap and occasionally patch closure.

Thrombus Formation Around the Catheter

With prolonged procedures, as in the case of thrombolytic therapy, the build-up of thrombus material around the catheter is a common occurrence. During prolonged infusion of SK/UK concomitant heparin is recommended. If the build-up of thrombotic material does not result in occlusion of the lumen, it often will be "stripped" when the catheter is removed and embolize. Nonthrombogenic catheters and guide wires have helped reduce this complication.[5] While the incidence of such emboli is higher than generally appreciated, many if not most of them are small and of little clinical importance. Sometimes this soft clot may lyse spontaneously or be lysed by continued infusion of thrombolytic agents. However, if a significant degree of ischemia is produced, surgical intervention with careful Fogarty catheter thromboembolectomy is mandatory. Occasionally incomplete removal of distal thrombus by balloon catheters will justify intraoperative instillation of urokinase or streptokinase.[6]

Hemorrhage from the Catheter Introduction Site

This is the most common complication associated with the introduction of angiographic catheters (.26–.53 percent).[3] The larger the catheter and the more frequent the catheters are exchanged, the larger the tear in the artery. Theoretically a 7 or 8 French catheter should leave a less than 3 mm puncture wound, but additional linear tears are common and the opening in the artery is usually 2–3 times this large. Indeed, it is surprising that the puncture sites do not bleed more often or result in more false aneurysms.

Minor extravasation is invariable at the puncture site. Clinically significant hematoma formation is relatively uncommon, and when reasonably well contained, is accepted as an almost routine consequence of arterial puncture. Hypertensive individuals are more prone to develop this complication. High diastolic pressure (>110) is a relative contraindication to angiography. Large hematomas should be surgically drained and the puncture wounds repaired. This not only reduces the risk and consequences of secondary infection and/or false aneurysm formation, but reduces the morbidity and, if this complication has been associated with a limited diagnostic or therapeutic procedure, often reduces hospital stay.

controlled by direct pressure. Since the catheter is usually directed upward, the arterial puncture is proximal to the point of skin entry, and not infrequently enters the external iliac at or above the inguinal ligament. The standard maneuver of groin compression employed at the time of catheter removal in this case may result in upward dissection of blood into the retroperitoneal space. Further dissection occurs easily and without any telltale expansion or discoloration in the groin. These patients present with back pain, a drop in hematocrit and, eventually, tachycardia and hypotension. A Gray-Turner sign (purplish discoloration on the side of the abdomen and flank) may not appear for many hours or days. Indications for exploration relate primarily to the degree of blood loss. An oblique lower quadrant incision with retroperitoneal approach provides proximal control and evacuation of the hematoma; repair is usually then effected through a high vertical groin incision with division of the inguinal ligament and upward retraction of the underlying muscle fibers.

Axillary hematomas are a treacherous complication of angiography when this route is utilized because of resulting axillary neuropathy. Direct nerve injury at the time of puncture is rare, but that occurs as a compressive neuropathy that results from extravasated blood accumulating within the confines of the axillary sheath (0.5 percent).[7] The resulting neuropathy is often persistent and disabling, and it is the main reason many angiographers avoid this route whenever possible. Close surveillance is indicated in patients undergoing transaxillary procedures. The patient should be recruited into this effort and instructed to insist upon immediate physician attention should any paresthesia, numbness, or weakness develop. Since the consequences of axillary neuropathy are so lasting and disabling, immediate evacuation of all axillary hematomas is indicated, even when signs and symptoms are not impressive.

Late Strictures and False Aneurysms

Delayed complications of arterial catheterization are probably more common than realized, and are common in children in whom serial surveillance by noninvasive methods is recommended for several years. However, by definition, these late appearing complications are beyond the scope of this chapter.

The foregoing discussion has focused on complications common to most invasive angiographic procedures. The remainder of this chapter will focus on those acute problems that are specific to the procedures carried out through the introduced catheter.

PROBLEMS RELATED TO THE INJECTION OF CONTRAST MEDIA

Although "reactions" to contrast media injections should decrease as nonionic solutions become more available, the vascular surgeon must continue to hold himself ready to respond to the serious problems that injections of contrast media can create; specifically, idiosyncratic reactions, adverse systemic hemodynamic responses, and renal and neurotoxicity.

Idiosyncratic Reactions

There are a number of unusual responses to the injection of contrast media, most of which are not truly allergic but rather idiosyncratic reactions. Although they are more likely to occur in "atopic" individuals than those with a history of previous reactions, they are also more likely in anxious or apprehensive patients. They are probably due to the media rather than the iodine, they are not dose related, and no sensitivity test is reliable in predicting their occurrence. Although patients of all ages can suffer major reactions from contrast media, most of the less serious reactions occur in those under 50, and most of the fatal reactions occur in those over 50 years of age.[8] Mild reactions that are self limited and require no treatment are nausea and vomiting, headache, chills, sweating, dizziness, itching and hives, and edema. Intermediate reactions are also transient but more serious and do require treatment. They include vasovagal hypotension, progressive edema and urticaria, and mild bronchospasm. Major reactions, which are life-threatening and require urgent treatment, are severe hypotension, convulsions, pulmonary edema, severe bronchospasm, laryngeal edema, and cardiac arrhythmias. These idiosyncratic reactions are at times difficult to distinguish from those due to cardiovascular or nervous system chemotoxicity, particularly at the outset (see below). Any serious reaction requires the administration of oxygen and 0.5 ml of 1:100 epinephrine HCL IM or slowly IV. Solucortef (100 mg) is indicated for a laryngeal edema and asthma, aminophylline (250 mg) for the latter and pulmonary edema, and sodium thiopental (200 mg) for neurologic convulsions. Cardiogenic shock will require pressor agents and cardiopulmonary arrests obviously require intubation and ventilation, external cardiac massage (with and without defibrillation), and full scale maintenance of an adequate circulatory volume and pH. The mortality following intravenous injection of contrast material for excretory urography is 1 in 50,000.[9] As infrequent as such reactions are, their potential seriousness dictates that angiographic suites be fully equipped to handle such emergencies, and angiographers and vascular surgeons be trained and current in advanced life support methods.

Chemotoxic Reactions

Cardiopulmonary

Contrast agents are hyperosmolar and have vasodilatory effects. These effects rarely result in hypotension in well hydrated patients, but vasovagal bradycardia can produce this effect as well. With injections close to the heart, a myocardial depressant effect can be seen, as well as arrhythmias. In addition, transient (3 seconds) rises in heart rate, stroke volume, and blood pressure can occur. Persistent and more serious rises in blood pressure, in fact a hypertensive crisis, can occur when angiography is carried out in the presence of an unsuspected pheochromocytoma. Severe pulmonary edema, presumed to be of neurogenic origin, is a rare sporadic occurrence.

Renal

Although contrast media are known to exert a direct toxic effect on endothelium, the mechanism of the renal damage induced is unknown. It is known to be related to dosage, concentration, and duration of exposure. Patients with preexisting renal disease, diabetes, and dehydration are at increased risk, and good hydration with a brisk diuresis is protective.[10] One should not be fooled by the initial diuresis caused by these hyperosmolar agents and fail to follow and maintain urinary output during the day following angiography.

Central Nervous System

Neurotoxicity depends not only on dose and osmolarity but the type of contrast agent. Sodium containing agents are more toxic than meglumine media, diatrizoate media are more toxic than iothalamates. Convulsions, cortical blindness, and stroke may result. Some other remote effects, e.g., pulmonary edema, hyperthermia, ventricular fibrillation, and the vasovagal effects are also central in origin.

ACUTE PROBLEMS CREATED BY THROMBOLYTIC THERAPY

Bleeding Complications

Systemic use of streptokinase or urokinase to lyse thrombi in the venous or arterial tree results in the significant incidence of bleeding complications, the most serious of which is fatal cerebral hemorrhage, which has been reported in one large series to occur in 3 percent of treated patients.[11] The direct infusion of these agents through an angiographic catheter placed in or near the thrombus allows a higher level to be achieved at the site of thrombus formation with a much lower systemic level. Even with this approach, systemic disturbances in coagulation mechanisms may occur, although they are less in degree and frequency than with systemic dosage. There is a general conviction that a grace or "golden" period of approximately 24 hours exists during which time serious hemorrhagic complications are rare. Many series confirm this impression but a period of complete immunity does not exist, particularly when higher doses of urokinase or streptokinase are used.[12] Streptokinase must bind with plasminogen to form a complex before it becomes active. Its thrombolytic effect, therefore, follows a rising and falling curve, and it is sometimes difficult to be sure of which slope of the curve the patient is on as the dose response is variable. Urokinase acts more directly and has a shorter half life than streptokinase. It is this rather than an overall greater effectiveness as a lytic agent that has been used to justify its use in the face of its much greater cost.

Serious bleeding complications can occur with both agents, even with "local infusions." However, they are more likely to occur with either high dose of infusions or prolonged administration, or when contraindications to the use of thrombolytic therapy have been ignored (see Table 1).

While close monitoring of the catheter entry site for bleeding and coagulation studies every 4–6 hours, with particular attention to the fibrinogen level, can minimize these hemorrhagic complications, they are not completely avoidable and the vascular surgeon must be prepared to deal with them promptly.

If a hemorrhagic diathesis has been produced, serious bleeding occurs, or one must intervene surgically for other complications in the face of active thrombolytic therapy, the following measures are recommended:

1. Discontinue the infusion of SK/UK (and heparin) and remove the infusion catheter. Ordinarily, this alone will suffice if one is responding to a dropping fibrinogen, oozing at the catheter site, or needs to intervene surgically, because the effect of these agents is short lived. The half life of urokinase is less than half that of streptokinase (80 minutes), although the latter's secondary effects on coagulation mechanisms may last much longer.

2. If further measures are needed because abnormal bleeding is encountered at the time of surgery, fresh frozen plasma should be administered to replace the deficient clotting factors and cryoprecipitate given to restore fibrinogen levels.

Table 1
Contraindications to Thrombolytic Therapy

Absolute contraindications
1. Current active bleeding
2. Intracranial disease or recent surgery
3. Limb threatening ischemia already exists

Relative contraindications
1. Major surgery or delivery within 10 days
2. Known hemorrhagic coagulopathy
3. Recent major trauma or cardiac massage
4. Uncontrolled hypertension
5. Severe hepatic or renal dysfunction
6. Pregnancy
7. Mural thrombus in the heart, cardiac valvular vegetation, mural thrombus in the proximal arterial tree (e.g., aortic aneurysm)
8. Diabetic hemorrhagic retinopathy or similar eye pathology

3. If there is serious active bleeding, epsilon aminocaproic acid (EACA) should also be given to stop active fibrinolysis.

Thromboembolic Complications

Indwelling catheters proximal to the point of infusion are prone to thrombus formation. This can be retarded by concomitant administration of heparin, either systemically or through a double lumen catheter. Even if local thrombosis is not induced, thrombus adhering to the catheter may embolize when it is withdrawn. Finally, the thrombus does not always lyse in an even and progressive fashion. Large segments of clot may be dislodged to embolize into the distal arterial tree. Either thrombosis or embolism can suddenly produce a limb threatening ischemia that did not exist previously.

In such an event, prompt action must be taken with exploration of the proximal artery and removal of clot proximally and distally with Fogarty balloon catheters. If significant bleeding is encountered during these efforts, the steps recommended above should be followed. Hopefully in the future, tissue plasminogen activator (TPA) will reduce the frequency and seriousness of the hemorrhagic complications, but it is not likely to reduce the thromboembolic complications unless its use significantly shortens the duration of thrombolytic therapy.

PROBLEMS ASSOCIATED WITH BALLOON CATHETER DILATION

Problems associated with catheter introduction and manipulation are identical to those previously described for angiography but, as with thrombolytic therapy, are much more frequent when balloon angioplasty is carried out because more contrast media and larger catheters tend to be used and catheter passage must often be made through irregularly narrowed or totally occluded arteries. Table 2 summarizes the incidences of these complications. While the list of complications is long, most are of minor consequence,

Table 2

Complications of Percutaneous Transluminal Angioplasty

Complications	Kumpe et al[24](%)	Glover et al[13](%)	Knight et al[18](%)	Sinning et al[25](%)	Campbell et al[26](%)	Johnston et al[27](%)	Jones et al[28](%)	Krepel et al[29](%)
Puncture Site								
Hematoma	3.8	5.5	22.0	18.0	15.0	6.5		1.8
Thrombosis			5.0				1.2	
False Aneurysm	1.5							
A-V Fistula						.3		
Arterial Perforation with Dye Extravasation			10.0		5.0			
Arterial Spasm								.6
Dilation Site								
Contained False Passage	4.5							
Intimal Dissection		4.5					1.2	
Intimal Flaps								
Thrombosis	4.5	6.4	5.5	4.5				1.2
Balloon Rupture or Failure	5.3	3.7						
Embolization	7.0	2.8	1.0	9.0	5.0	1.8		2.4
Other		2.8					2.4	
Overall Complication Rate	23.1	26.0	43.5	32.0	20.0	9.0	5.0	6.0
Complications Requiring								
Surgical Intervention	5.5	5.0	13.0		5.0	.8	.8	1.2
Technical Failure	8.1	22.0	13.0	4.0	23.0	7.0	7.0	16.0
Mortality (up to 1 mo)	0	0	0	9.0	0	1.0	2.0	0

and few require surgical intervention. Total complications in some high risk series are as high as 30–50 percent,[13,14] but they usually range below 20 percent.[15,16] Those requiring surgical intervention now rarely exceed 5 percent[17,18] but surgical intervention is required more frequently when PTA is unsuccessful[19] and the radiologist inexperienced.[17] In our series, as many complications occurred in the first 15 as the subsequent 95 dilations. Zeitler et al showed a progressive drop in the complication rate in their institution over 3 time periods from 14 percent to 4 percent, and of those requiring surgical intervention, from 2.3 percent to 0.45 percent.[20] Although one high risk series was reported with a 3 percent mortality,[14] deaths following peripheral arterial PTA are now extremely rare.

In 1985, Schubart and Porter[21] reviewed the complications in 10 reported series totaling 1711 attempted PTAs of lower extremity arteries and found an overall average complication rate of 11 percent; of these 29 percent were groin hematomas, 15 percent were vessel thromboses, 14 percent false passage, 14 percent distal embolization, 6 percent balloon rupture, and 6 percent dissection with collateral occlusion. Major arterial perforations constituted 5 percent of all complications, and bleeding at the catheter site, 4 percent. In terms of the frequency of such complications, groin hematomas led with just under 4 percent, and thrombosis, embolism, and false passage occurred in close to 2 percent each. The remainder of listed complications occurred between 0.5 and 1 percent. There were only 5 reported pseudoaneurysms (0.3 percent), 7 arteriovenous fistulas (0.4 percent), and 6 patients who went into renal shutdown (0.3 percent).

Groin hematomas, active bleeding at the catheter entry site, remote perforation, and other general complications related to catheter introduction have already been discussed and, although they occur more commonly than with simple angiographic procedures, their management does not differ in this setting. The same can be said for thromboembolic complications. Probably the only complication that is different and specific is that of balloon rupture. Balloon rupture occurs quite commonly, but with current fabrication methods, it usually occurs linearly rather than transversely and thus no longer requires surgical intervention. In the early days of the Grüntzig technique of balloon dilation, surgical extrication of transversely ruptured balloons was not an uncommon event.

Also worthy of comment are complications occurring with renal artery angioplasty. Arterial spasm is common during renal angioplasty, having been noted in 27 percent of dilations in one report.[22] It is related to catheter manipulation and, therefore, operator experience. Fortunately, it usually responds to vasodilators, particularly nitroglycerin. Some angiographers premedicate their patients before renal PTA with either nifedipine or sublingual nitroglycerin.

Clearly all the other complications described earlier can and do occur in renal artery balloon angioplasty, i.e., dissection, thrombosis, embolization, and arterial rupture. While the incidence of these complications is admittedly low, the results are catastrophic in this circumstance because the renal arterial tree consists of end arteries and renal tissue has a very limited tolerance to ischemia, leaving insufficient time for surgical intervention.

ACUTE PROBLEMS ENCOUNTERED AFTER THERAPEUTIC EMBOLIZATION

Embolization of most of the vessels of the body has been carried out for everything from malignant tumors to headaches, portal hypertension to varicoceles, and traumatic bleeding to congenital A-V malformations. In these efforts many strange objects have been introduced from coils to gelfoam to beads. In addition, concentrated alcohol, bucry-late, and detachable balloons are being employed. Judging from close to 50 articles on the adverse effects of therapeutic embolization published in 1984–1985, the list of organs and tissues suffering ischemic insult must now be close to complete.[23] Gallbladder and bile duct necrosis (with 9 deaths), bile duct stricture, emphysematous cholecystitis, liver necrosis, bleeding gastric ulcers, splenic infarcts and abscesses, renal infarcts with and without hypertension, hemorrhagic pancreatitis, small and large bowel ischemia, sciatic and other peripheral nerve palsies, spinal cord injury, bladder necrosis, impotence, adrenal crises, pulmonary embolism, ventricular fibrillation, and cerebral infarction were all reported at least once during this period. The incidence of each of these complications is unknown because the denominator is unknown, but it is presumed to be low. The vascular surgeon is most likely to invoke this therapeutic approach in the management of congenital arteriovenous fistulas, but since these malformations can occur anywhere, he needs to monitor his patients closely for ischemia, not only in the target area, if the approach is "too successful," but in nearby circulatory beds, if the embolization becomes misdirected. Furthermore, late secondary infection of occult infarcts with abscess formation must be kept in mind. Finally, although these catastrophic complications are less when therapeutic embolization is applied for AVMs than for some other indications, it should be kept in mind that therapeutic benefit is usually short lived and must be limited to specific indications such as bleeding, disseminated intravascular coagulation, systemic hemodynamic effects, and refractory painful ulcerations.

REFERENCES

1. Seldinger SI: Catheter replacement of needle in percutaneous arteriography. Acta Radiol 39:368, 1953
2. Adams DF, Fraser DB, Abrams HL: The complications of coronary arteriography. Circulation 48:609, 1973
3. Hessel SJ, Adams DF, Abrams HL: Complications of angiography. Radiology 138:272, 1981
4. Rutherford RB: Noninvasive testing in the diagnosis and assessment of arteriovenous fistulas, in Bernstein EF (ed.): Noninvasive Diagnostic Techniques in Vascular Disease. St. Louis, C.V. Mosby Co., 1984
5. Cramer R, Moore R, Amplatz K: Reduction of the surgical complication rate by the use of a hypothrombogenic catheter coating. Radiology 109:585, 1973
6. Quinones-Baldrich WJ, Zierler RE, Hiatt JC: Intraoperative fibrinolytic therapy: an adjunct to catheter thromboembolectomy. J Vasc Surg 2:319, 1985
7. Molnar W, Paul DJ: Complications of axillary arteriotomies. Radiology 104:269, 1972
8. Rose JS: Contrast media, complications and preparation of the patient, in Rutherford RB (ed.): Vascular Surgery, 2nd edition. Philadelphia, WB Saunders Co., 1984
9. Fischer H: Choices for intravascular contrast agents. Curr Probl in Diagnost Radiol 6:3012, 1976
10. Martin-Paredero W, Dixon SM, Baker JD, et al: Risk of renal failure after major angiography. Arch Surg 118:1417, 1983
11. Fiessinger JN, Alach M, Lagneau P, et al: Indications de la streptokinase dans les oblitérations artérielles des membres. Couer Med Interne 15:453, 1976
12. Wolfson RH, Kumpe DA, Rutherford RB: The role of intra-arterial streptokinase in the treatment of arterial thromboembolism. Arch Surg 119:697, 1984
13. Glover JL, Bendick PJ, Dilley RS, et al: Balloon catheter dilation for limb salvage. Arch Surg 118:557, 1983

14. Rush DS, Gewertz BL, Lu CT, et al: Limb salvage in poor risk patients using transluminal angioplasty. Arch Surg 118:1209, 1983

15. Graor RA, Young JR, McCandless M, et al: Percutaneous transluminal angioplasty: review of iliac and femoral dilations at the Cleveland Clinic. Cleveland Clin Quart 51:149, 1984

16. Lu CT, Zarins CK, Yang CF, et al: Percutaneous transluminal angioplasty for limb salvage. Radiology 142:337, 1982

17. Health & Public Policy Committee, American College of Physicians: Percutaneous transluminal angioplasty. Ann Intern Med 99:864, 1983

18. Knight RW, Kenney GJ, Lewis EE, et al: Percutaneous transluminal angioplasty: results and surgical implications. Am J Surg 147:578, 1984

19. Glover JL, Bendick PJ, Dilley RS, et al: Efficacy of balloon catheter dilatation for lower extremity atherosclerosis. Surgery 91:560, 1982

20. Zeitler E, Richter EI, Rother F, et al: Results of percutaneous transluminal angioplasty. Radiology 146:57, 1983

21. Schubart PJ, Porter JM: Arterial complications associated with the use of balloon catheters, in Bernhard VM, Towne JB (eds.): Complications in Vascular Surgery. Orlando, Grune & Stratton, 1985

22. Beinart C, Sos TA, Souheil S, et al: Arterial spasm following renal angioplasty. Radiology 149:97, 1983

23. Miller FM, Mineau DE: Transcatheter arterial embolization—major complications and their prevention. Cardiovas Intervent Radiol 6:141, 1983

24. Kumpe DA, Jones DN: Percutaneous transluminal angioplasty—radiological viewpoint. Vasc Diagnos Therapy 3:19, 1982

25. Sinning MA, Dixon GD, Pinkerton JA: Percutaneous transluminal angioplasty. J Kansas Med Soc 84:331, 1983

26. Campbell WB, Jeans WD, Cole SEA, et al: Percutaneous transluminal angioplasty for lower limb ischemia. Br J Surg 70:736, 1983

27. Johnston KE, Colapinto RF: Peripheral arterial transluminal dilatation: early results. Can J Surg 25:532, 1982

28. Jones BA, Maggisno R, Robbe A, et al: Transluminal angioplasty: results in high risk patients with advanced peripheral vascular disease. Can J Surg 28:150, 1985

29. Krepel VM, van Andel GJ, van Erp WFM, et al: Percutaneous transluminal angioplasty of the femoropopliteal artery: initial and long term results. Radiology 156:325, 1985

Giacomo A. DeLaria

Emergency Vascular Complications Following Intraaortic Balloon Pumping

Intraaortic balloon pumping is firmly established as a method to support patients with complications of ischemic heart disease or severely depressed left ventricular function. Access for such circulatory assistance is usually through the femoral artery. Direct exposure of the femoral artery was required for balloon insertion until the introduction of the percutaneous balloon pump by Bregman in 1980.[1] Now, influenced by either experience or clinical findings, either route, open exposure or percutaneous insertion can be selected.

In patients with atherosclerotic disease, routine cannulation of peripheral arteries with large bore (8 French or larger) catheters would be expected to cause arterial injury. Many past reports have documented these complications and a vascular complication incidence as high as 30 percent has been recorded.[2-7] Serry, in our institution, reported in 1983 a complication rate approaching 22 percent.[8] Increasing technical experience, along with improvements in *matériel,* should result in reduction of complications. Conversely, greater familiarity with any technique and increased application with liberalization of indications can result in more complications. For these reasons, no analysis of vascular complications of balloon pumping can rely on historical data but must begin by reviewing contemporary results.

CLINICAL REVIEW

Intraaortic balloon pumping has been regularly used at Rush-Presbyterian-St. Luke's Hospital and Medical Center since 1972. Initially, all balloon pumps were placed through femoral artery cut-downs by either a resident or attending cardiovascular surgeon. With the advent of the percutaneous device, cardiologists and their fellows took over a significant proportion of balloon insertions, especially in the medical intensive care unit and cardiac catheterization laboratory. Selection between percutaneous or cut-down insertion techniques was always made by the senior available physician. Since 1984, the cut-down approach has been reserved for those patients in whom percutaneous balloons could not be

Vascular Surgical Emergencies
ISBN 0-8089-1843-5

431

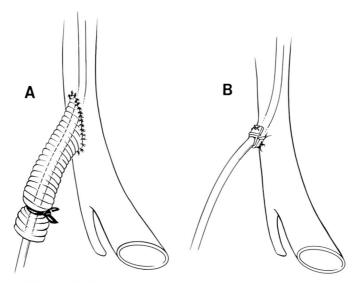

Fig. 1. Cutdown insertion of balloon pumps can be accomplished utilizing either side-arm grafts (A) or pledgets (B). The pledget technique is preferable because, when balloon assistance is discontinued, all fabric material can be removed, allowing primary arterial repair.

placed. When a cut-down was required, balloons were inserted through either a 10 mm Gore-Tex chimney sewn directly to the femoral artery or more recently through two pledgeted sutures[9] (Fig. 1). Until 1983, all balloon pumps on the surgical service, including percutaneous devices, were removed in the operating room to allow inspection and direct repair of punctured arteries. However, over the past 2 years, increasing experience with percutaneous devices has given us increased confidence to remove the balloon and rely on 30 minutes external pressure to control bleeding and prevent late false aneurysms.[10] Accordingly, that technique has now become routine and surgical exploration is reserved for specific indications. No special instruments for counter pressure have been required.[11] All vascular complications of balloon pumps inserted on either the medical or surgical service were managed by the cardiovascular surgical team; usually the same attending surgeon responsible for either the balloon insertion or the patient's subsequent cardiac operation.

CLINICAL EXPERIENCE

Between January 1, 1982 and December 31, 1985, 375 patients had successful insertion of intraaortic balloon pumps on either the medical or surgical service and survived long enough to either undergo balloon removal or sustain a vascular complication.

Medical Experience

Two hundred and forty-six patients were initially on the medical service. Eighty-one (33 percent) were female. As can be seen in Figure 2, percutaneous technique of insertion

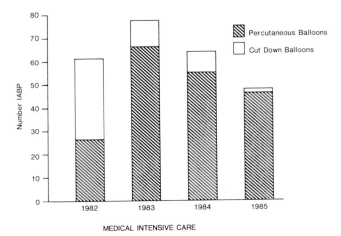

Fig. 2. Percutaneous balloon insertion technique has been used
with increasing frequency in our medical intensive care unit. More
patients arriving from community hospitals with balloon pumps in
place explains the recent decrease in balloon insertions.

was used with increasing frequency over this observation period. The declining number of
balloon insertions after 1983 reflects no real reduction in the use of the device but rather
the large numbers of patients arriving from community hospitals with balloon pumps
already in place.

Emergency vascular complications requiring either surgical repair or balloon removal
occurred in 25 medical patients (10 percent). Ischemia with threatened limb loss was the
most common complication and was noted in 20 patients. Fourteen were male and six
were female, a percentage comparable to the overall group. Eighteen (90 percent) occurred after percutaneous balloon pump insertion. Complications were severe and, despite
vigorous attempts at vascular reconstruction, 3 of 20 patients (15 percent) required later
amputation. Two patients developed bleeding and one a rapidly expanding false aneurysm. In one patient, the arterial injury was not by the percutaneous balloon pump but
rather by cannulation of the adjacent femoral vein that, in this case, also transversed the
superficial femoral artery. Two final patients experienced thoracic dissections. Both were
suspected during fluoroscopic insertion of the device and confirmed by the injection of
contrast into the false lumen.

Surgical Experience

One hundred and sixty-four patients underwent intraaortic balloon pump insertion in
either the surgical intensive care unit or operating room. One hundred and twenty-four (76
percent) survived long enough to either undergo balloon removal or sustain a vascular
complication. As in the medical group, proportionally more female patients required
balloon pumping than predicted from operative census. Thirty-eight percent of balloon
pump patients were female as compared to an 18 percent incidence of females requiring
coronary artery bypass grafting over the past 14 years.[12] Thirty-three (27 percent) were
percutaneous insertions. The remainder were inserted via femoral cut-down. The relatively lower frequency of percutaneous balloon insertions as compared to the medical
service may be explained in two ways. First, there remains a definite surgical bias against

percutaneous devices. Secondly, in many operating room patients experiencing low output with reduced pulse pressure, groin cannulation of the femoral artery can be difficult while direct surgical exposure is more expeditious. Over the past year, femoral artery monitoring catheters have enjoyed a renewed popularity on our service. When the catheter is included in the operative field, the arterial line can be used for guide wire insertion into the femoral artery and subsequent placement of the percutaneous device.

Vascular complications occurred in 7 surgical balloon patients (6 percent). Four patients experienced limb ischemia or thrombosis. All but one were percutaneous insertions and two patients were female. One patient required emergency axillofemoral bypass for aortoiliac thrombosis. Two patients bled; one from an associated femoral vein cannulation with passage of a Swan-Ganz catheter through the femoral artery. A second operative insertion patient bled from the suture line between the Gore-Tex tube and the femoral artery. The last patient, a percutaneous insertion, experienced a dissection of the profunda femoris artery that required urgent balloon removal.

OPERATIVE MANAGEMENT

Vascular complications of balloon pumping requiring emergency management fall into four typical categories: ischemia, hemorrhage, dissection, and infection. Complicating the vascular trauma, however, is the associated cardiac decompensation, which in many cases prevents balloon removal and straightforward arterial reconstruction. In extreme cases, a choice between life and limb may be necessary. Thus, a vascular surgeon called to repair a balloon pump injury must not lose sight of the whole patient or forget that open heart surgery and coronary bypass grafting could well be an integral part of the treatment of an ischemic limb.

Ischemia

Approximately 20 percent of all balloon pump insertions sustain a vascular complication and of these the majority are ischemic. This is particularly true with the percutaneous device. [13-16] This complication is reportedly more common in females.[17] Ischemia usually begins soon after balloon insertion but can occur later from progressive thrombosis. In our experience, ischemia has been more common with the percutaneous device and unrelated to duration of pumping. Although it could be assumed that the duration of pumping would influence the frequency of ischemic complications, that relationship has only been noted in two reports.[18-19]

When ischemia occurs, the patient first complains of leg numbness followed by leg pain. On examination, the foot is cool and pulseless. In severe cases, capillary refill is poor and Doppler ankle sounds are absent. Ideal treatment would include balloon removal, vessel inspection, thrombectomy, and intimal repair by direct suture or vein patch angioplasty. However, the patient's cardiac status influences management. If the patient underwent balloon insertion for cardiogenic shock, a period of observation, along with heparin to prevent thrombosis progression is in order if motor function and cutaneous sensation remain intact. Often, balloon pumping and fluid resuscitation increases cardiac output with improvement in peripheral circulation and vascular repair can be deferred until elective balloon removal. Conversely, the patient whose leg becomes ischemic while being treated for unstable angina is usually maximally vasodilated and has maximum cardiac output. In these patients, rapid progression of ischemia can be predicted and the balloon catheter must be removed. If coronary anatomy has already been defined angiographically and coronary bypass is planned, emergency coronary surgery along with femoral artery repair is appropriate. When angiography has not been done or in those cases with low cardiac output who develop neurologic changes, restoration of peripheral circulation or an alternative route for balloon pumping must be used.

Two solutions are possible: (1) Remove the balloon and replace it on the opposite side; (2) Perform a femoral-femoral cross-over graft. Of these two approaches, we prefer the former. Patients selected for percutaneous balloon insertion often have normal pulses. Occlusion typically occurs by fracture and displacement of an anterior flap in a firm but relatively patent vessel (Fig. 3). Run-off is impaired and thrombus build-up is rapid. This injury is best treated in the operating room. Both groins are prepared and infiltrated with local anesthetic and the patient is heparinized. Through a longitudinal incision, the uninvolved artery is exposed, and a new balloon is inserted up to the iliac bifurcation through a transverse arteriotomy buttressed with pledgeted sutures. The involved side is exposed through a similar incision leaving the introducer in position and the balloon functioning. Exposure of this vessel can be difficult, especially in those cases in which multiple "sticks" have resulted in periarterial hematoma or arterial puncture has been high, either under or through the inguinal ligament. Once control of the puncture site is obtained, the balloon is removed and vessels occluded with vascular clamps. Simultaneously, the new balloon is advanced to its proper location and balloon pumping resumed to provide continuous cardiac support. The new wound is irrigated with antibiotic solution and closed to the subcutaneous level. The injured artery can now be repaired. The edges are trimmed and the flap excised. Distal and proximal thrombectomy are accomplished through the opening and an adequate section of saphenous vein harvested and trimmed to size. A generous vein patch angioplasty utilizing continuous monofilament suture restores limb circulation. Repair with autogenous tissue is preferred but a small prosthetic patch can be used. Finally, the skin edges are approximated.

Occasionally, the opposite femoral vessel is unsuitable for cannulation and an attempt must be made to reinsert the device into the same artery. This can be accomplished in a balloon-dependent patient but requires assistance. It is necessary to watch the patient and optimize inotropic support during the period the intraaortic balloon pump is temporarily stopped. In this circumstance, after the first balloon has been removed and the vessel has been debrided and cleared of thrombus a new small caliber balloon, passed first through an 8 or 10 mm Gore-Tex tube, is reinserted into position. The balloon pump is turned on and the tube graft carefully sewn to the femoral artery as a generous patch. Another

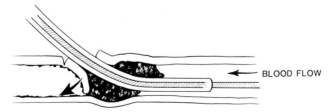

BLOOD FLOW

Fig. 3. Femoral artery thrombosis occurring after percutaneous balloon insertion often begins with fracture displacement of the anterior arterial wall into its lumen. Run-off is compromised producing stasis and eventually total arterial occlusion.

alternative could be insertion higher in undamaged artery followed by repair of the earlier and lower entry site. This has not proven to be feasible in our experience.

Femoral-femoral cross-over bypass has been recommended as treatment for limb ischemia associated with balloon pumping.[20] The major advantage of this method is the possibility of completing the vascular repair without interfering with balloon support or utilizing a new device on the contralateral side. In the past 14 years, we have used this technique only twice. In both cases, the initial balloon had been introduced via a tube conduit through a diseased femoral artery. As all angioplastic maneuvers had already been used, it was unlikely that balloon removal and repair would be successful. Accordingly, a cross-over graft originating from the contralateral side was fashioned. In both cases, limb ischemia was reversed but the patients ultimately died of complications of their underlying cardiac disease. Another patient who thrombosed her distal aorta shortly after returning from successful operative repair of a left ventricular aneurysm and ventricular septal defect, had the balloon removed and reconstruction accomplished utilizing an axillofemoral and cross-over femoral-femoral bypass. Our reluctance to greater utilization of femoral-femoral bypass to treat acute limb ischemia after balloon pumping is that most often a lesser procedure is successful and the opportunity to repair the injured artery without using prosthetic material is lost. The patient is at greater risk for infection, although reportedly that risk is low.[21] Our technique does require a second balloon but if successful leaves the patient with an anatomic circulation and no prosthetic material to serve as a later focus of infection.

Of course, in occasional patients with severe peripheral vascular disease, following median sternotomy intraaortic balloon pump insertion can be readily accomplished through a stab wound into the ascending aorta.[22] Limb ischemia is prevented, but unplanned cannulation of either the carotid or subclavian artery must be avoided.[23,24] Direct cannulation of the subclavian artery to access the descending thoracic aorta has recently been reported.[25] However, we as yet have not found a need to utilize this technique.

Hemmorhage

Hemorrhage that occurs in association with balloon pumping requires immediate treatment. As with ischemia, this complication is more common with the percutaneous device. If multiple entries into the artery have been made, or the vessel is unusually brittle or friable, arterial disruption can result in brisk bleeding.

If the patient is balloon-dependent, a new device must be inserted into the opposite limb, while pressure is being maintained on the bleeding side. That vessel can then be exposed following the sheath to its entry site. Proximal and distal control allows balloon removal and arterial repair, usually with a vein patch. Bleeding, which persists after balloon removal but stops with digital pressure, can often be controlled with a carefully applied pressure dressing (Fig. 4). This dressing is much more effective than the usual sandbag and bulky pad. In addition, it is more comfortable for the patient and allows greater mobility.

Another complication of balloon pumping is late development of a false aneurysm. Although the incidence is reportedly low, rapid expansion could require urgent operation.[10] We have thus far encountered only two patients with this complication. One occurred in the intensive care unit and was controlled by exposure and direct repair of the entry wound into the artery. A second case (Fig. 5) presented late after operative balloon

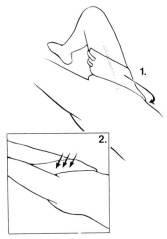

Fig. 4. An elastic adhesive bandage applied from the inner thigh to the outer buttocks, with the hip flexed, will tighten and effectively compress the femoral artery when the hip is extended.

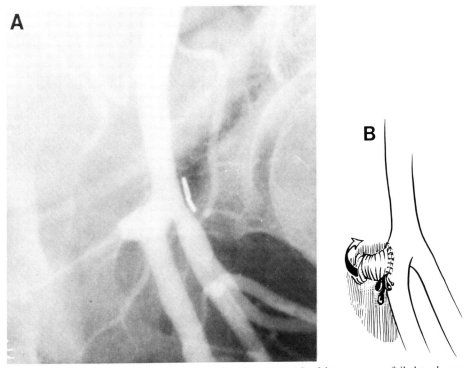

Fig. 5. (A) Arteriogram in a patient with clinical findings of a false aneurysm failed to demonstrate an abnormality in either the ligated side-arm graft or its attachment to the femoral artery. (B) At operation, a partial dehiscence with intermittent bleeding into surrounding tissue was found.

437

insertion. The patient came to the emergency room complaining of a groin mass and right leg pain. An acute incarcerated femoral hernia was diagnosed. Angiography failed to define an aneurysm. However, at operation the trimmed and amputated Gore-Tex tube had partially dehisced at the suture line, resulting in an adjacent expanding hematoma. Repair with a new patch was uncomplicated.

Infection

Arterial infection after balloon pumping has been described in several large reviews but has been the subject of a special report in only one instance.[26] Infection is rare after percutaneous balloon insertion. Local erythema and skin breakdown are possible but rarely involve the artery. Once the balloon and cannula have been removed, appropriate antibiotics and local care will suffice. In the presence of a prosthetic graft, the infection becomes difficult to manage. Repair with autogenous vein is required along with muscle flap reinforcement.[26] If this fails, arterial ligation to control hemorrhage can be necessary leaving the wound open for irrigation. In the absence of severe peripheral vascular disease, collateral flow can be expected to maintain limb viability. Threatened limb loss would require extraanatomic reconstruction, usually by obturator bypass. To help prevent late infections at the time of balloon removal, culture followed by routine irrigation with antibiotic solution is recommended. If a pathogen is grown from that culture, appropriate antibiotics are maintained for 4–6 weeks to minimize the possibility of future infection.

Dissection

In our series, dissection was identified in three patients. In two it was confirmed at fluoroscopy. Dissection was probably more frequent than recognized. Two reports confirm that adequate balloon pumping can be accomplished even in the presence of dissection.[27,28] Balloon dissection of the aorta has been reported to cause lower extremity paraplegia.[29] When dissection is recognized, treatment is generally balloon removal. In the absence of proximal intimal injury, the false channel will decompress and no additional therapy is required.

CONCLUSION

Balloon pumping will continue to be a useful technical adjunct in the treatment of patients with cardiac decompensation and ischemic heart disease. Vascular complications are frequent but the incidence, at least in our experience, is decreasing. Complications are more common and serious in females, a group requiring proportionally more balloon support. Nevertheless, treatment of vascular complications utilizing standard principles of repair and reconstruction should result in limb salvage, except in those cases in which underlying cardiac decompensation, along with extensive peripheral vascular obstructive disease so compromises the repair that thrombus recurs and reconstruction cannot be accomplished.

REFERENCES

1. Bregman D, Casarella WJ: Percutaneous intraaortic balloon pumping: initial clinical experience. Ann Thor Surg 29:153, 1980
2. Alpert J, Bhaktan EK, Gielchinsky I, et al: Vascular complications of intraaortic balloon pumping. Arch Surg 3:1190, 1986
3. Sutorius DJ, Majeski JA, Miller SF: Vascular complications as a result of intra-aortic balloon pumping. Amer Surg 45:512, 1979
4. Beckman CB, Geha AS, Hammon GL, et al: Results and complications of intraaortic balloon counterpulsation. Ann Thor Surg 24:550, 1977
5. Kozloff L, Rich NM, Brott WH, et al: Vascular trauma secondary to diagnostic and therapeutic procedures: Cardiopulmonary bypass and intraaortic balloon assist. Amer J Surg 140:302, 1980
6. Sanfelippo PM, Baker NH, Ewy HG, et al: Results and complications with intraaortic balloon counterpulsation. Chest 80(3):369, 1981
7. Perler B, McCabe CJ, Abbott WM, et al: Vascular complications of intra-aortic balloon counterpulsation. Arch Surg 118:957, 1983
8. Serry C: In discussion. Intraaortic balloon pump morbidity. Ann Thor Surg 36(6):651, 1983
9. Zada F, McCabe JC, Subramanian VA: Simplified technique for intraaortic balloon insertion. Ann Thor Surg 29(6):573, 1980
10. Vignola PA, Swaye PS, Gosselin AJ: Guidelines for effective and safe percutaneous intraaortic balloon pump insertion and removal. Amer J Cardiol 48:660, 1981
11. Rodigas PC, Finnegan JO: Technique for removal of percutaneously placed intraaortic balloons. Ann Thor Surg 40(1):80, 1985
12. DeLaria G, Najafi H: Coronary artery revascularization: A clinical review of 14 years' experience. Clinical Essays on the Heart 2:287, 1984
13. Harvey JC, Goldstein JE, McCabe JC, et al: Complications of percutaneous intraaortic balloon pumping. Circulation 64 (Suppl II):114, 1981
14. Grayzel J: Clinical evaluation of the Percor percutaneous intraaortic balloon: cooperative study of 722 cases. Circulation 66 (Suppl I):223, 1982
15. Hauser AM, Gordon S, Gangadharan V, et al: Percutaneous intraaortic balloon counterpulsation. Chest 22(4):422, 1982
16. Martin RS, Moncure AC, Buckley MJ, et al: Percutaneous intra-aortic balloon insertion. J Thorac Cardiovasc Surg 85:186, 1983
17. Shahian DM, Neptune WB, Ellis FH Jr, et al: Intraaortic balloon pump morbidity: A comparative analysis of risk factors between percutaneous and surgical techniques. Ann Thor Surg 36(6):644, 1983
18. McCabe JC, Abel RM, Subramanian VA, et al: Complications of intra-aortic balloon insertion and counterpulsation. Circulation 57(4):769, 1978
19. Pace PD, Tilney NL, Lesch M, et al: Peripheral arterial complications of intra-aortic balloon counterpulsation. Surgery 5:685, 1977
20. Alpert J, Parsonnet V, Goldenkranz RJ, et al: Limb ischemia during intraaortic balloon pumping: Indication for femorofemoral crossover graft. J Thorac Cardiovasc Surg 79(5):729, 1980
21. Gold JP, Cohen J, Shemin RJ, et al: Femorofemoral bypass to relieve acute leg ischemia during intra-aortic balloon pump cardiac support. J Vasc Surg 3(2):351, 1986
22. Gueldner TL, Lawrence GH: Intraaortic balloon assist through cannulation of the ascending aorta. Ann Thor Surg 19(1):88, 1975
23. Frazier OH, Crager GJ, Painvin GA, et al: Morbidity in balloon counterpulsation: Transfemoral versus transthoracic insertion. Trans Amer Soc Artif Intern Organs 30:108, 1984

24. Meldrum-Hanna WG, Deal CW, Ross DE: Complications of ascending aortic intraaortic balloon pump cannulation. Ann Thor Surg 40(3):241, 1985
25. Rubenstein RB, Karhade NV: Supraclavicular subclavian technique of intra-aortic balloon insertion. J Vasc Surg 1:577, 1984
26. Grantham RN, Munnell ER, Kanaly PJ: Femoral artery infection complicating intraaortic balloon pumping. Amer J Surg 146:811, 1983
27. Biddle TL, Stewart S, Stuard ID: Dissection of the aorta complicating intra-aortic balloon counterpulsation. Amer Heart J 92(6):781, 1976
28. Isner JM, Cohen SR, Virmani R, et al: Complications of the intraaortic balloon counterpulsation device: Clinical and morphologic observations in 45 necropsy patients. Amer J Cardiol: 45:260, 1980
29. Scott IR, Goiti JJ: Late paraplegia as a consequence of intraaortic balloon pump support. Ann Thor Surg 40(3):300, 1985

PART X

Venous Emergencies

W. Andrew Dale

Venous Gangrene

The panorama of deep venous thrombosis (DVT) includes "silent" events, which because of paucity of symptoms continue unrecognized until either embolism occurs or the process subsides, as well as thrombi accompanied by local signs of more or less severity. Some of these may be termed *phlegmasia alba dolens*—the extremity is swollen and tender. A few venous thromboses are so widespread that extreme swelling and cyanosis occur—"blue phlebitis" or *phlegmasia cerulea dolens* (PCD). If the arterial flow becomes impeded or absent, gangrene of venous origin results (Figs. 1 and 2). Venous thrombosis in its minor to moderate forms, without pulmonary embolism is relatively common. Fortunately its extreme forms are unusual. Although Haimovici's survey indicated that an average 6.4 percent of DVT cases had ischemic venous thrombosis[1] I think that figure is too high, probably because the several writers were referring to the more severe problems of DVT. My experience would indicate the figure to be about 1 percent of patients with venous thrombosis.

Of the extreme cases of PCD about a third exhibit arterial insufficiency with tissue necrosis. Many such patients have a severe underlying generalized disease process that itself requires extensive treatment, further complicating the problems of management. Approximately 40–50 percent of patients with venous gangrene of an extremity die of that or an associated disease process.[2]

Occasionally venous gangrene strikes the upper extremity. The 16 cases, including 3 of their own, recently collected from the literature by Smith and associates must represent a fraction, since most are not reported. I have treated approximately ten arms with severe venous thrombosis, PCD, but none with gangrene of the hand or arm.

PATHOLOGIC PHYSIOLOGY

Iliofemoral venous thrombosis usually begins proximally and extends distally. Abnormalities of the coagulation mechanism may underlie the lesion, abetted by local pressure upon the great pelvic veins. This may originate at the proximal end of the left

Vascular Surgical Emergencies
ISBN 0-8089-1843-5

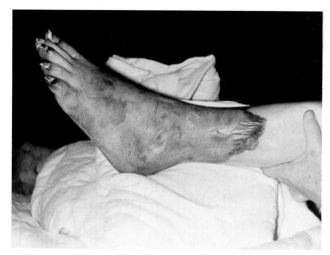

Fig. 1.   Phlegmasia cerulea dolens with gangrene of the feet.

common iliac vein where it is crossed by the right iliac artery, as well as underlaid by the vertebral bodies so that it is pinched. Also, small pelvic vein thromboses may extend to involve the iliac-femoral venous system.

Brockman and Vasko in 1966[3] reported their classic canine experiments, which clearly explain how complete venous occlusion with resultant venous hypertension leads to severe edema as fluid passes into the interstitial tissues. When the pressure exceeds the "critical closing pressure" level of the arterioles that side of the circulation also ceases, although the arteries remain patent. The entire process is mechanical; vasospasm has no significant role (Fig. 3).

The indicated treatment is to clear the venous system of clot, to prevent recurrent clotting by anticoagulant treatment, and to replace fluid losses. Unfortunately this plan

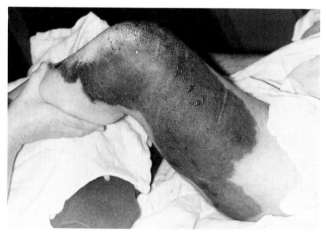

Fig. 2.   Same patient showing a higher level of skin gangrene. This patient eventually died.

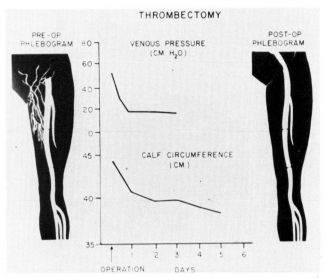

Fig. 3. Surgical thrombectomy reduced venous pressure and swelling of the limb. The preoperative iliofemoral venous occlusion with collateralization of venous drainage (left) was changed to normal (right) by the procedure.

does not always work successfully due to inability to perform a perfect clean-out and absolutely to prevent early recurrence (Fig. 4).

A rare cause of venous gangrene is heparin induced thrombocytopenia.[4] It is now generally recognized that platelet counts should be followed regularly in heparinized patients. A decreasing count, particularly when there appears to be resistance to heparin, indicates cessation for fear of platelet aggregation with arterial (and at times venous) clotting. Early recognition of the problem with immediate cessation of heparin usually allows spontaneous reversal of the process. Whether venous thrombectomy would be useful after the process had progressed to venous gangrene is unknown.

DIAGNOSIS

The clinical diagnosis of most DVT by history and physical examination is so unreliable that laboratory investigation is mandatory. The reliability and sensitivity indices of the several available noninvasive techniques are less than perfect, usually dependent upon the experience and dedication of the operator. Comerota, White, and Katz have discussed[5] these methods in relation to ascending phlebography, which is more reliable although more time-consuming and expensive.

Modern techniques of phlebography using less concentrated radiopaque material[6] and preinjection heparinization[7] combine safety with reliability so that it remains the definitive critical study of DVT (Fig. 5).

When DVT has progressed to the stage of PCD ("blue phlebitis") with threatened or actual venous gangrene the clinical diagnosis is fairly certain. Noninvasive methods may corroborate the diagnosis but add little of significance (except their cost). Phlebography

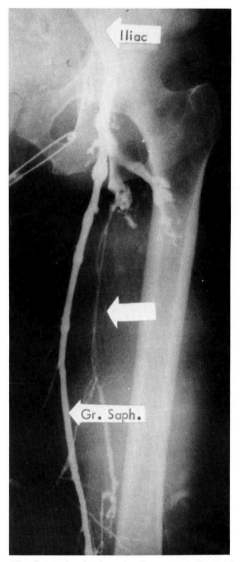

Fig. 4. The femoral vein thrombosis was not cleared by thrombectomy; the iliac segment was successfully opened.

may therefore not be required to corroborate an obvious diagnosis, particularly if nonoperative therapy is to be used.

If on the other hand thrombectomy is contemplated for further severe DVT it is
important to determine whether there is clot in the proximal veins (iliac in the lower and
subclavian for the upper extremity) because those are more available to surgical thrombectomy than is distal thrombosis, where the results of operation are poor.

Ascending phlebography may be difficult or impossible via a distal vein. The femoral
route for phlebography and arteriography may be considered if confirmation is deemed
essential.

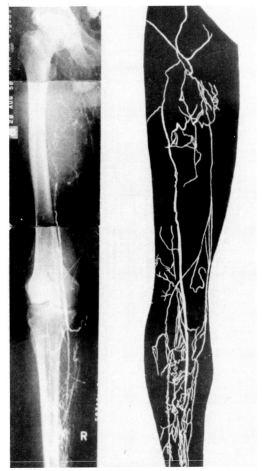

Fig. 5. Phlebogram shows widespread occlusion of the veins of the entire limb.

Angiography

An arteriogram is not usually needed to assess the situation, but can be obtained without added hazard if there is indecision regarding an acute arterial occlusion by thrombosis or embolism.

In clinical terms the presence or absence of pedal pulses is critical. If these pulses are absent, or detectable only by Doppler, early operative thrombectomy should be considered, to reverse the process and salvage threatened tissue. On the other hand, the presence of pedal pulses encourages nonoperative therapy.

The overall condition of many of these patients is serious, yet operation can be performed using local anesthesia, or low spinal block, so poor general condition is not a strict contraindication to venous thrombectomy.

TREATMENT

Anticoagulant therapy by heparin with warfarin follow-up has become recognized as the standard treatment of DVT with inferior vena caval control by clips or filters needed in some instances to prevent pulmonary embolism.

Early initiation of a 10–14 day course of intravenous heparin followed by 3–4 months of oral warfarin effectively protects most patients against pulmonary embolism, although later limb sequelae are common. It seems likely that shorter courses of heparin are less effective in terms of long-term vein damage, although that thesis is unproven.

Thrombolytic therapy using streptokinase or urokinase continues to attract advocates[8] who note the excellent results that sometimes occur more than the frequent failures and occasional tragic complications. Kakkar and Lawrence in 1985 concluded that thrombolytic therapy "can produce virtually complete thrombolysis in about a third of patients but is disappointing in the remainder." Their results were "no better" than conventional anticoagulation in 153 patients.[9] Available evidence to date does not suggest that thrombolytic therapy should replace prompt heparinization for most patients.

When the venous thrombotic process has progressed to the clinical stage of PCD, especially if tissue necrosis is threatened or established, the necessity for restoration of the arterial circulation becomes paramount and forces immediate consideration of any measures that will be effective at once (Fig. 6).

Surgeons in Europe first tried operative venous thrombectomy many years ago.[10] By the 1950s there were numerous examples. Howard Mahorner of New Orleans popularized the procedure in the United States.[11] In 1960 we,[12] in 1967 Haller,[13] and in 1970 Sawyers, Foster, and Edwards[14] reported further experiences with venous thrombectomy. The indications were not clear. In the 1960s operation was often advised by surgeons for any relatively new venous thrombosis with severe swelling. It became recognized in the 1970s that many of these limbs fared as well with anticoagulation therapy.[15] Operative indications were restricted to those with a brief 2–3 day history.

General opinion now has changed to limit operations to patients with compromised arterial circulation. In other words, if the tissues are well perfused arterially there is time for heparinization (or alternately, thrombolysis) and elevation to relieve the acute problem. If there is arterial failure this time is lacking and immediate venous thrombectomy is required.

The 1984 results of Roder's team illustrate the present situation. Among 46 venous thrombectomies (21 with impending venous gangrene) no limbs required amputation, there was no postoperative pulmonary embolism, and 5–13 years later 40 percent were asymptomatic. On the other hand the morbidity (22 percent infections) along with the 60 percent showing postphlebitic syndrome indicates that venous thrombectomy is a far from perfect therapy.[16]

The Stirnemann group's experience with 37 venous thrombectomies was even less optimistic. One amputation, 4 perioperative embolisms, and 53 percent failure to improve the phlebographic image also suggests caution in application of the operation, yet most patients did obtain "prompt relief of symptoms."[17]

Surgical Technique

1. Local or low spinal anesthesia may be used.
2. The common femoral vein along with its profunda, superficial and saphenous tributaries are exposed and looped for temporary vascular control.

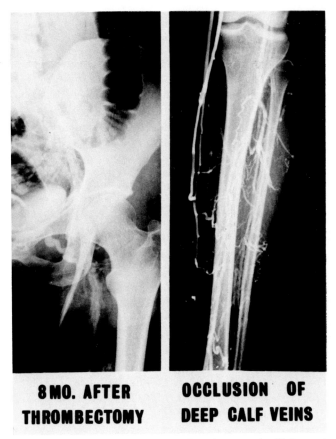

8 MO. AFTER THROMBECTOMY

OCCLUSION OF DEEP CALF VEINS

Fig. 6. Eight months after venous thrombectomy the iliofemoral system is patent while the calf veins are still occluded.

3. 5000 units of heparin are administered prior to clamping any vessel.

4. A short longitudinal incision is made on the anterior wall of the common femoral vein opposite the entry of its profunda component, to allow easy access to that. The lips of this opening are held apart by fine stay sutures to prevent repeated trauma by steel forceps.

5. The largest balloon catheter that will fit is passed proximally well into the inferior vena cava (by external measurement to above the level of the umbilicus), from which it is withdrawn with the balloon inflated. Whether a Valsalva maneuver by the patient during this withdrawal is really prophylactic against embolization is unknown. A well sedated patient may not be able to accomplish that.

6. Appropriately sized balloon catheters are passed distally into all branches. If the superficial femoral vein cannot be cleared from this approach a guide may be passed from the popliteal vein at the knee, tied onto the balloon catheter and thus achieve its distal passage.[18]

7. Wrapping a tight bandage about the distal limb may help to extrude clots.

8. Completion phlebography by injecting 25–40 cc of radiopaque material via a small needle into the proximal vein will furnish information regarding completion of the clean-out.

9. The vein wall is closed with a continuous 6–0 monofilament suture.
10. Wound closure should include a suction drain, since postoperative heparinization often leads to small leaks.

The fear of pulmonary embolism during balloon catheter removal of thrombus has led some to advocate placement of a temporary occluding balloon into the inferior vena cava via the contralateral femoral-iliac vein.[19] The actual incidence of embolization during thrombectomy is small. The only one observed personally was not fatal. Against the possible benefit of contralateral catheterization may be measured its disadvantages in terms of time, additional blood loss, and the potential for inciting thrombosis. In the absence of factual proof, good judgment lies on the side of simplicity; avoid complicating the procedure by a contralateral operation.

A-V Fistula

In an effort to improve the hemodynamics of blood flow within veins after vein repair or clean-out a number of surgeons have constructed temporary arteriovenous fistulas. Most of these efforts have occurred in Europe during the past decade.[20,21] Eklof, Einarsson, and Plate in 1985 described the results of creating a saphenous-superficial end femoral end-to-side fistula accompanying venous thrombectomy among 120 patients in Sweden and 20 in Kuwait. While operation was reported superior to nonoperative management (42 percent vs 7 percent of symptoms along with better phlebographic results for an unstated time of follow-up) the effect of addition of the fistula was not clarified. The complications, 10 percent trauma to the artery requiring repair, 11 percent wound hematomas and a 24 percent infection rate, serve as a warning for such procedures.[21]

A few American surgeons[22,23] have performed concomitant A-V fistulas, but most have hesitated to add an uncertain and potentially dangerous procedure that requires a second stage correction and whose merits are unproven.

The role of fasciotomy is not clear, particularly because either heparin or thrombolytic therapy is at least partly contraindicated by extensive wounds such as this causes. Here again the few instances of venous gangrene treated by any one person are too few to allow an authoritative opinion. If the choice is between fasciotomy and heparinization, I favor the anticoagulant.

POSTOPERATIVE CARE

Firm wrapping of the limb with an elastic bandage and elevation of the legs in the venous position are essential. The venous position requires that the feet and ankles be above the level of the heart. Elevation of the head therefore defeats simultaneous elevation of the feet. Properly fitted elastic hose are used thereafter for at least a year. Heparin anticoagulation is advised for 10–14 days after such a severe episode of venous thrombosis.

There is no factual evidence that bed rest prevents pulmonary embolism, so early ambulation is dependent on the general status of the patient.

Skin or deeper areas of necrosis are managed appropriately. Early removal of dead tissue (even amputation) is indicated to avoid absorption of toxic metabolites and of infection.

REFERENCES

1. Haimovici H: Treatment of ischemic deep venous thrombosis, in Bergan JJ, Yao JST (eds.): Surgery of the Veins, Orlando, FL, Grune & Stratton, 1985, p. 165
2. Smith BM, Shield GW, Riddell DH, et al: Venous gangrene of the upper extremity. Ann Surg 201:511, 1985
3. Brockman SK, Vasko JS: The pathologic physiology of phlegmasia cerulea dolens. Surgery 59:997, 1966
4. Battey PM, Salam AA: Venous gangrene associated with heparin-induced thrombocytopenia. Surgery 97:618, 1985
5. Comerota HA, White JB, Katz ML: Diagnostic methods for deep vein thrombosis: phleborheography, iodine-125, fibrinogen uptake and phlebography. Am J Surg 150(4A):14, 1985
6. Bettman MA, Salzman EW, Rosenthal D, et al: Reduction of venous thrombosis complicating phlebography. Am J Roentgenol 134:1169, 1985
7. Dale WA, Lewis MR: Heparin control of venous thromboembolism. Surgery 101:744, 1970
8. Persson AV, Persson CA: Thrombolytic therapy for deep vein thrombosis. Am J Surg 150(4A):50, 1985
9. Kakkar VV, Lawrence D: Hemodynamic and clinical assessment after therapy for acute deep vein thrombosis. Am J Surg 150(4A):50, 1985
10. Schepelmann E: Demonstration eines Patienten mit Thrombose der linken Vena subclavia seltener Actiologie. Munch Med Wochenschr 2:2444, 1940
11. Mahorner H: New method of management for thrombosis of deep veins of the extremities. Am Surg 20:487, 1954
12. DeWeese JA, Jones TI, Lyon J, et al: Evaluation of thrombectomy in the management of iliofemoral venous thrombosis. Surgery 47:140, 1960
13. Haller JA: Deep Thrombophlebitis, Pathophysiology and Treatment. Philadelphia, W. B. Saunders Co., 1967
14. Sawyers JL, Foster JH, Edwards WH: Iliofemoral venous thrombosis. Reappraisal of thrombectomy. Ann Surg 171:961, 1970
15. Lansing AM, Davis WM: Five year follow-up study of iliofemoral venous thrombectomy. Ann Surg 168:629, 1968
16. Roder OC, Lorentzen JE, Hanse HJ: Venous thrombectomy for iliofemoral thrombosis: Early and long-term results in 46 consecutive cases. Acta Chir Scand 150:31, 1984
17. Stirnemann P, Althaus U, Kirchhof B, et al: Early phlebographic results after iliofemoral venous thrombectomy. Thorac Cardiovasc Surg 32:299, 1984
18. Kiely PE: A new venous thrombectomy technique. Brit J Surg 60:850, 1973
19. Edwards WH: Iliofemoral venous thrombosis: the role of thrombectomy, in Rutherford RB (ed.): Vascular Surgery, Philadelphia, W. B. Saunders Co., 1977, p 1995
20. Vollmar JF, Hutschenreiter S: Temporary arteriovenous fistulas in pelvic and abdominal veins, in May R, Weber J (eds): Pelvic and Abdominal Veins: Progress in Diagnostics and Therapy. Princeton, Excerpta Medica, 1980
21. Eklof B, Einarsson E, Plate G: Role of thrombectomy and temporary arteriovenous fistula in acute iliofemoral venous thrombosis, in Bergan JJ, Yao JST (eds.): Surgery of the Veins, Orlando, FL, Grune & Stratton, 1985, p. 131
22. Edwards WS: Femoral AV fistula as a complementary or primary procedure for iliac venous occlusion, in Bergan JJ, Yao JST (eds.): Surgery of the Veins, Orlando, Grune & Stratton, 1975, p. 267
23. Husni EA: The postphlebitic limb. Hosp Med 7:73, 1971

Lazar J. Greenfield

Pulmonary Embolectomy and Vena Caval Interruption

An individual surgeon's experience with pulmonary thromboembolism is usually limited since the postoperative mortality rate in a general surgery practice is less than 0.4 percent.[1] However, pulmonary embolism remains the most frequent cause of death following cholecystectomy, herniorrhaphy, hysterectomy, and childbirth for a total of over 11,000 postsurgical deaths per year. Therefore, it hovers as an infrequent but potentially disastrous postoperative complication.

DIAGNOSIS

Faced with the unexpected sudden collapse of a patient, the surgeon must proceed through the differential diagnoses in order to provide the most effective therapy and improve the chances for a favorable outcome. The presence of distended neck veins helps to rule out hypovolemic causes of shock and a chest x-ray and electrocardiogram help to exclude pneumothorax and myocardial infarction. In this situation where one is dealing with the possibility of major embolism, verification of the diagnosis should be by pulmonary angiogram rather than by radionuclide perfusion scan, which is a more appropriate screening test for patients suspected of having minor pulmonary embolism. Further support for the diagnosis comes from measurement of arterial blood gases that can be expected to show both hypoxemia and hypocarbia with levels of $PaCO_2$ less than 30 torr. With these suggestive findings, it is appropriate to administer a therapeutic dose of heparin (150–200 units per kg body weight) and proceed to angiography. While the radiologist is inserting the catheter into the pulmonary artery, it is helpful to insert a radial artery line as well as a Swan-Ganz catheter for hemodynamic monitoring. Inotropic agents also may be necessary to support systemic blood pressure and we usually favor dopamine for this purpose.

Despite the presence of "classical" signs and symptoms of pulmonary embolism, more than 70 percent of the angiograms will be negative.[2] This is perhaps the best reason for obtaining the angiogram since it so often redirects the approach to a more appropriate

Vascular Surgical Emergencies
ISBN 0-8089-1843-5

Table 1
Classification of Pulmonary Thromboembolism

Class	Signs	Occlusion (%)	$\overline{PA}$ Pressure (mm Hg)	Management
I	None	< 20	Normal	Anticoagulation
II	Tachypnea	20–30	< 20	Anticoagulation
III	Collapse, Hypoxemia	30–50	> 20	Anticoagulation, filter
IV	Shock, hypoxemia	> 50	> 25–30	Embolectomy, filter
V	Cor pulmonale	> 50	> 40	Anticoagulation, filter

explanation for the problem, most often undetected sepsis or a primary pulmonary process. Pulmonary angiography itself carries minimal risk provided that the angiograms are performed selectively in one pulmonary artery and with a smaller amount of contrast medium. Should the angiography suite not be available, an alternative approach that we have found useful is to proceed directly to the operating room where a catheter can be positioned under fluoroscopy for hand injection to confirm the diagnosis. This is less desirable technically due to the lack of cut films, especially in patients with chronic lung disease whose pulmonary perfusion would already be abnormal. Once the diagnosis is confirmed, the severity of the problem can be assessed and the patient stratified on the basis of the classification shown in Table 1. This physiologic classification is based upon the hemodynamic effects of the embolic load in that particular patient.

We define major pulmonary embolism as that degree of acute pulmonary vascular occlusion sufficient to produce systemic hypotension, either transient (Class III) or sustained and requiring vasopressor support (Class IV). If the patient has chronic recurrent thromboembolism (Class V) that has obliterated a sufficient number of vessels to produce chronic pulmonary hypertension, the presentation may be similar but the situation is much more grave since most of the pathology is irreversible. Minor degrees of embolism in patients who are not hemodynamically compromised can be evaluated by perfusion lung scan, which is a sensitive test but not sufficiently specific to justify a course of anticoagulation without other objective signs of deep vein thrombosis. Both impedance plethysmography and Doppler venous examination can serve to verify the presence of deep vein thrombosis, which warrants a course of heparin followed by warfarin usually for a minimum of 4 months.

MANAGEMENT OF MASSIVE EMBOLISM

Patients who are in shock (Class IV) are managed by administration of heparin and after angiographic confirmation of the diagnosis with the patient remaining on the fluoroscopy table, a steerable cup-catheter is inserted under local anesthesia through either the right femoral or internal jugular vein (Fig. 1). The technique of catheter embolectomy has been described[3] and modified by more frequent use of the jugular rather than the femoral vein. Multiple passages of the catheter result in removal of the major emboli and reduction of the pulmonary artery pressures to normal. The procedure is completed by insertion of a Greenfield filter.[4]

Patients who are unable to maintain systemic pressure and require closed chest resuscitation should be taken to the operating room for placement on femorofemoral

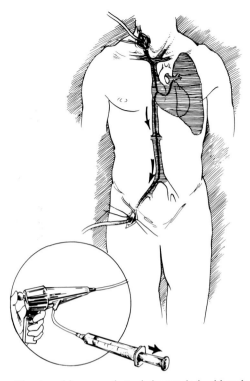

Fig. 1.   The steerable cup-catheter is inserted via either the femoral or jugular vein for positioning under fluoroscopy in contact with the embolus. Syringe suction captures the embolus in the cup for removal by withdrawing the catheter.

bypass prior to general anesthesia for open pulmonary embolectomy. Open embolectomy also remains an option for patients who fail to obtain adequate improvement by catheter embolectomy. Our present experience with these techniques consists of 29 patients who have had catheter pulmonary embolectomy since 1974. All but one of them were in Class IV or V, the exception being a Class III patient with congestive heart failure. Embolic material was extracted successfully in 26 of them (90 percent) but there were 7 postoperative deaths (24 percent). These included two patients who had cardiac arrest at the time of angiography before we recognized the importance of selective injection of a small amount of contrast medium in one pulmonary artery to minimize the insult of this procedure. Two other deaths were attributed to postoperative myocardial infarction and the remainder were associated with irreversible pulmonary hypertension. Two patients who had inadequate clearance of emboli by catheter underwent open embolectomy. Both were Class V patients with chronic pulmonary hypertension and neither survived. During this period, a total of 8 open pulmonary embolectomy procedures were performed with 4 deaths, for a 50 percent mortality rate. Successful catheter embolectomy has also been reported by others.[5]

In some institutions, it may be preferable for the radiologist to manipulate the embolectomy catheter for thrombus extraction, but the most important consideration is that a team of surgeon and radiologist be available, especially where there are no facilities for cardiopulmonary bypass. This approach under local anesthesia can be accomplished quickly and, if a balloon-tipped catheter has been left in the pulmonary artery, the effectiveness of sequential removal of emboli can be monitored. Even subtotal removal of emboli will often produce a dramatic increase in cardiac output and reduction in pulmonary arterial pressures.

In a recent review of pulmonary embolectomy, Del Campo reported on 651 procedures in patients with massive pulmonary embolism.[6] In 537 patients (82 percent) the operation was performed on extracorporeal circulation and in 26 percent of them, partial bypass was used prior to sternotomy. The remaining 114 patients were operated upon without circulatory support. The mortality rate was less in the patients who had cardiopulmonary bypass (41 percent vs. 52 percent). There was also information concerning selective thrombolytic therapy with streptokinase in 30 patients with 26 survivors (87 patients). However, only five of them were in shock before the procedure and the degree of fibrous organization of most emboli along with the time factor usually precludes the use of lytic therapy. The unstable Class IV patient tends to follow a progressive downhill course unless the obstruction to pulmonary blood flow can be relieved. In this situation, thrombolytic drugs cannot be expected to act rapidly enough to correct the problem.

MANAGEMENT OF SUBMASSIVE EMBOLISM

The management of Class III thromboembolism requires clinical assessment of the patient's risk for recurrent embolism. For patients who have significant underlying heart or pulmonary disease or who will require prolonged intensive care, filter placement is indicated along with standard anticoagulation. This approach evolved from a series of four Class III patients seen in one year who were managed in an intensive care unit with heparin anticoagulation alone. Two of them had recurrent embolism while in the therapeutic range of anticoagulation and died.

At present, the most common indications for vena caval filter placement are a contraindication to anticoagulation (37 percent) and recurrent embolism while on anticoagulants (30 percent). Other frequent indications include prophylaxis for a free-floating thrombus at the femoral level or above (17 percent) and a complication of anticoagulation forcing the treatment to be discontinued (17 percent). Least common indications included concurrent catheter embolectomy or previous device failure.

Access for filter placement can be obtained usually through the right jugular vein (Fig. 2). If it proves to be too small or if there is an open wound of the neck, the right common femoral vein can be used with a femoral carrier. If neither the jugular nor the femoral vein are suitable, the left jugular or axillary vein may be used although dilation of the latter will usually be required. When open pulmonary embolectomy has been performed, the filter may be inserted from the atrium but in the absence of fluoroscopy, no attempt should be made to discharge it below the renal veins. Instead, the distance to a level just below the hepatic veins should be marked and the filter discharged in a suprarenal location.

Suprarenal placement has been well tolerated and effective but carries the theoretical possibility of sudden occlusion by a massive embolus. Our experimental studies suggest that even this can be well tolerated in the normal dog with only a transient impairment in renal function.[7] Any patient with a filter can have sudden occlusion if the embolus is large enough, producing a sudden reduction in venous return and cardiac output. Tragic misin-

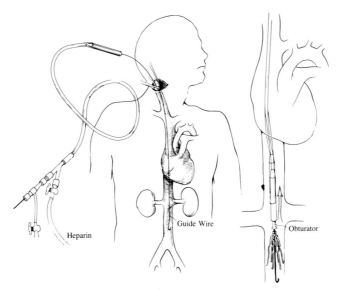

Fig. 2. Insertion of a flexible guide wire into the inferior vena cava facilitates passage of the carrier catheter through the heart. Heparin infusion prevents thrombus formation in the carrier. The filter is discharged over the guide wire which is then removed. (Reprinted from Greenfield LJ, Stewart JR, Crute S: Improved technique for Greenfield vena caval filer insertion. Surg Gynecol Obstet 156(2):217–219, 1983. By permission of Surgery, Gynecology & Obstetrics.)

terpretation of this as recurrent embolism rather than functional hypovolemia with treatment by vasopressor agents rather than volume repletion resulted in one death in our experience.

The majority of our patients (87 percent) have filters inserted at the infrarenal level of L3, which effectively controls embolism originating from the lower extremities. When venous thrombosis has propagated into the vena cava, the filter should be placed above its upper limit to prevent contact between propagating thrombus and the filter and allow unobstructed flow through it. Other indications for suprarenal placement include tumor invasion of the vena cava with adjacent thrombus and pregnancy or any possible source of pelvic vein thrombosis that requires gonadal vein protection.[8]

Errors in filter placement can occur under fluoroscopic control due to patient movement at the time of discharge, incorrect identification of the lumbar vertebrae, or angulation of the arm of a portable fluoroscopy unit. A technique for filter retrieval has been reported[9] and is possible for a period of about 7 days from insertion. The consequences of filter misplacement are not significant for the vein involved but the patient remains unprotected from recurrent embolism. The most significant misplacement in our experience has occurred in the tricuspid valve from which the filter was retrieved successfully. Misplacement at the atriocaval injunction is usually well tolerated and does not necessarily require filter removal.

Filter insertion has been simplified by the most recent adaptation of routine guide wire placement prior to filter discharge. Positioning of the guide wire in the inferior vena cava prior to insertion of the filter carrier-catheter not only makes passage through the right heart easier, but also makes misplacement unlikely and minimizes the time that the carrier remains in contact with blood. This reduces the possibility of a thrombus forming within the carrier. Intermittent or continuous infusion of heparinized saline also serves to retard thrombus formation. Once the filter has sprung open and the hooks are embedded in the wall of the vena cava, the guide wire, which has preserved axial orientation of the filter, can be withdrawn. The guide wire should be retracted before discharge of the filter when the femoral vein approach is used to avoid angling the filter. Since the hooks do penetrate the wall of the vena cava, further migration of the filter is unlikely but has been observed by others.[10]

Septic thromboembolism has not been considered a contraindication to filter placement since the stainless steel filter is inert. Optimal management requires control of the source of sepsis and appropriate antibiotics. The author's clinical experience in four patients has been satisfactory and this approach seems preferable to caval ligation, which produces intraluminal abscess in experimental studies.[11] We have also demonstrated that a trapped thrombus can become infected after bacteremia but then a course of antibiotics can resterilize the filter. Therefore, antibiotic prophylaxis may be indicated in some patients.

Minor pulmonary embolism producing the well-known signs and symptoms of dyspnea, tachycardia, and tachypnea (Class II) usually can be well managed by anticoagulation alone. When anticoagulation fails to prevent recurrent embolism, when it produces hemorrhagic complications, or when there is a contraindication to its use, mechanical protection by vena caval filter placement is needed. We have also used the filter for pulmonary hypertension,[12] regardless of the etiology since right ventricular failure predisposes these patients to venous thrombosis and they are unable to tolerate even a minor volume embolic event.

Long-term follow-up of our filter patients, which now exceeds 12 years in this institution, shows that the long-term patency rate exceeds 95 percent as has been reported by others.[10,13,14] Occlusion of the filter by massive embolism is a rare event (2 percent) and has occurred only within the first 2 weeks of insertion in our experience. Smaller volume embolism to the filter produces no symptoms and is found occasionally at routine follow-up study. Subsequent venacavograms show spontaneous resolution of the trapped embolus within 6 weeks, even in patients who are not anticoagulated. The need for long-term anticoagulation should be based on the activity of the venous thrombotic disorder rather than the presence of the filter. Many of these patients will develop recurrent venous thrombosis in spite of anticoagulation and require long-term care.

The incidence of recurrent pulmonary embolism in our filter patients is 5 percent and if it occurs, a contrast venacavogram should be obtained to determine whether there is thrombus propagating above the level of the filter. If this is found, the options for management include thrombolytic therapy[15] or a second filter placed at a higher level. The latter approach has been used where the length of the thrombus made lytic therapy a risk of further embolism. We have also combined filter placement with selective thrombolytic therapy by catheter for totally occluded vena cavas, especially in younger patients; and in 2 rare cases of uncontrolled subclavian vein thrombosis, the filter has been placed in the superior vena cava.

REFERENCES

1. Dalen JE, Alpert JS: Natural history of pulmonary embolism. Prog Cardiovasc Dis 17:257, 1975
2. Goodall RJR, Greenfield LJ: Clinical correlations in the diagnosis of pulmonary embolism. Ann Surg 191:219, 1980
3. Greenfield LJ: Pulmonary embolism: Diagnosis and management. Curr Probl Surg 13(4):1, 1976
4. Greenfield LJ: Complications of venous thrombosis and pulmonary embolism, in Greenfield LJ (ed.): Complications in Surgery and Trauma. Philadelphia, JB Lippincott Co., 1984, pp 406–421
5. Moore JH Jr, Koolpe HA, Carabasi RA, et al: Transvenous catheter pulmonary embolectomy. Arch Surg 120:1372, 1985
6. Del Campo C: Pulmonary embolectomy: a review. Canad J Surg 28:111, 1985
7. Greenfield LJ, Peyton JWR, Crute S: Hemodynamics and renal function following experimental suprarenal vena caval occlusion. Surg Gynecol Obstet 155:37, 1982
8. Stewart JR, Peyton JWR, Crute SL, et al: Clinical results of suprarenal placement of the Greenfield vena cava filter. Surgery 92(1):1, 1982
9. Greenfield LJ, Crute SL: Retrieval of the Greenfield vena caval filter. Surgery 88:719, 1980
10. Gomez GA, Cutler BS, Wheeler HB: Transvenous interruption of the inferior vena cava. Surgery 93:612, 1983
11. Peyton JWR, Hylemon MB, Greenfield LJ, et al: Comparison of Greenfield filter and vena caval ligation for experimental septic thromboembolism. Surgery 93(4):533, 1983
12. Greenfield LJ, Scher LA, Elkins RC: KMA-Greenfield filter placement for chronic pulmonary hypertension. Ann Surg 189:560, 1979
13. Cimochowski GE, Evans RH, Zarins CK, et al: Greenfield filter vs. Mobin-Uddin umbrella: The continuing quest for the ideal method of vena caval interruption. J Thorac Cardiovasc Surg 79:359, 1980
14. Wingerd M, Bernhard VM, Maddison F, et al: Comparison of caval filters in the management of venous thromboembolism. Arch Surg 113:1264, 1978
15. Greenfield LJ, Peyton R, Crute S, et al: Greenfield vena caval filter experience: Late results in 156 patients. Arch Surg 116:1451, 1981
16. Greenfield LJ, Stewart JR, Crute S: Improved technique for Greenfield vena caval filter insertion. Surg Gynecol Obstet 156(2):217, 1983

James S. T. Yao
William R. Flinn

Emergency Management of Superficial Venous Problems

Despite the abundance of superficial veins, vascular emergencies involving this system are relatively rare. Most reports on venous emergencies are centered on acute deep-vein thrombosis and pulmonary embolism or on penetrating injuries. There is little information available on emergency management of superficial venous problems. This chapter attempts to summarize the experience we have had in dealing with this unusual emergency.

The most common emergency problems related to the superficial veins involve (1) varicose veins, (2) superficial thrombophlebitis, (3) postsaphenectomy soft tissue infection, (4) intraoperative emergencies following vein stripping, and (5) after sclerotherapy.

VARICOSE VEINS

Varicose veins are common, and it has been stated that nearly 10 percent of the population has some degree of varicosities in the superficial veins. Most varicose veins are uncomplicated and may be present for years without symptoms. Invariably, most surgeons regard varicose veins as a benign condition, and it is true that it seldom presents a life-threatening emergency. Acute hemorrhage of varicose veins, therefore, is relatively unknown to most vascular surgeons. In the textbook on pathology and surgery of the veins of the lower limb, Dodd and Cockett have emphasized that bleeding from varicose veins may account for death in elderly patients with long-standing varicose veins.[1] Recently, Villavicencio and his coworkers have also found that acute hemorrhage from varicose veins, though uncommon, is a real vascular emergency.[2]

Bleeding may occur spontaneously, or it may occur as a result of trauma. Spontaneous bleeding is most dangerous, and it is seen commonly in elderly patients with long-standing varicose veins. In the last ten years, the authors have seen three patients admitted to the Northwestern University Medical Center because of spontaneous bleeding from varicose veins. At St. Thomas' Hospital in London, there are between six and ten emergency admissions per year due to severe spontaneous bleeding from varicose veins.[1]

The diagnosis is seldom difficult. Most of these patients have severe varicosities with numerous small dilated veins around the ankle covered by paper-thin skin. The cause of bleeding is often related to the presence of an incompetent ankle perforating vein, and the presence of high venous pressure in the erect position is responsible for the spontaneous bleeding. Most bleeding is brisk and occurs without warning, and the patient is always surprised and terrified by the extent of the bleeding. Standing in a pool of blood is often the story given by the patient. Unless pressure is applied immediately and followed by steep elevation, profuse and uncontrollable bleeding leading to hypotension may occur. In most instances, pressure dressings and elevation will stop the bleeding, and definitive treatment by urgent vein stripping will prevent recurrent bleeding.

Occasionally, bleeding from varicose veins is due to obvious trauma, which may cause subcutaneous rupture of the veins. A large hematoma may occur and require urgent evacuation.

SUPERFICIAL THROMBOPHLEBITIS

Superficial thrombophlebitis is common, and there are two types of thrombotic process that affect the superficial veins. These are (1) thrombophlebitis of the long or short saphenous vein and (2) suppurative phlebitis due to an indwelling catheter.

Thrombophlebitis of the Long or Short Saphenous Vein

Thrombophlebitis of the saphenous vein is easy to diagnose by the presence of a firm, palpable, tender cord corresponding to the course of the saphenous vein. In most instances, the superficial thrombophlebitis is self-limited and is seen in patients with varicose veins. In the absence of varicose veins, superficial thrombophlebitis may be part of the clinical picture of Buerger's disease or occult malignancy. Superficial thrombophlebitis involving the varicose saphenous vein may ascend cephalad, and the possibility of deep vein involvement with subsequent pulmonary embolism must be entertained. Superficial thrombophlebitis may spread into the deep veins in three ways: (1) into the femoral vein via the saphenofemoral junction and the groin (ascending saphenous thrombophlebitis), (2) into the popliteal vein at the junction of the short saphenous vein in the popliteal fossa (ascending short saphenous thrombophlebitis), or (3) into the deep calf veins (posterior tibial) via one of the ankle perforators.

The incidence of superficial thrombophlebitis in varicose veins is difficult to estimate because milder cases may escape the attention of the patient or the physician. In a report by Lofgren and Lofgren of the Mayo Clinic,[3] 163 of 3941 patients with varicose veins seen in a 10-year period had superficial thrombophlebitis. In a recent review, Husni and Williams[4] noted a higher incidence, however (221 of 779 patients). Fortunately, superficial thrombophlebitis extending into the deep veins is rather rare. With the exception of the report by Gjöres,[5] the incidence of deep vein involvement is less than 10 percent (Table 1). Diagnosis of deep vein involvement is aided by the use of noninvasive tests and venography.

Certainly, a major concern is pulmonary embolism. The incidence of pulmonary embolism in superficial thrombophlebitis is low, ranging from 2 to 4 percent in most reported series.[5-9] Recently, Husni and Williams have reported a 10 percent incidence.[4] In that series, most patients were bedridden, which probably accounts for the high incidence.

Table 1
Incidence of Superficial Thrombophlebitis Extending into Deep Veins

Author	No. Cases	Total Series	Percent Occurrence
Gervais[6]	4	64	6
Hafner, et al[7]	9	94	10
Gjöres[5]	13	40	32
Husni and Williams[4]	10	139	7
Plate, et al[21]	4	28	14

Emergency surgical intervention is needed when there is evidence of proximal propagation of the thrombotic process to the saphenofemoral junction. Some authors have called this "migratory thrombophlebitis."[10] Migratory thrombophlebitis, however, should not be confused with migrating phlebitis. The latter is often associated with Buerger's disease. Both clinical and Doppler ultrasound examination will help to determine the need for surgery. In general, when the thrombotic process is in the vicinity of the upper thigh, surgical treatment should be considered. Some authors even recommend surgery when the thrombus is above the knee.[1,4,11] Although some authors have advocated removal of the entire phlebitic vein,[3,5,7,12] we favor high ligation of the saphenous vein under local anesthesia. This approach avoids the use of heparin and prolonged hospitalization.

Suppurative Phlebitis of Indwelling Catheter

The use of indwelling catheters for administration of chemotherapeutic agents or for hyperalimentation is now a common practice. Many of these patients are immunoincompetent, and therefore, are susceptible to infection. Most infection can be treated by removal of the catheter, local heat, and appropriate antibiotic therapy. Because of a change in bacterial flora in hospital infections, gram-negative bacteria, notably the Klebsiella-enterobacter group,[13] may serve as the focus for continuing sepsis despite antibiotic therapy. In prolonged intravenous catheter placement, the possibility of Candidal suppurative thrombophlebitis must be kept in mind.[14] Fever, signs of sepsis, and a positive blood culture for Candida establish the diagnosis. In patients with septic nonsuppurative or Candidal suppurative thrombophlebitis, removal of the thrombosed vein may be needed to eliminate the focus of infection. This is often done by excision under local anesthesia. The involved vein should be excised to the point where the vein wall is normal and blood flows freely from the vein.

POSTSAPHENECTOMY SOFT TISSUE INFECTION

In 1984, Baddour and Bisno[15] called attention to a newly recognized complication following coronary artery bypass. The condition is characterized by recurrent cellulitis in the saphenous venectomy limb, with fever and chills. The condition is often mistaken for deep vein thrombosis. Not only coronary artery bypass patients are susceptible to this infection. Patients who have undergone femoropopliteal saphenous vein bypass may also develop this type of soft tissue infection. In recent years, we have encountered five patients who had cellulitis and lymphangiitis months after the removal of the saphenous vein for femorotibial bypass (Fig. 1). The characteristics of this infection are (1) redness of the skin with evidence of cellulitis or lymphangiitis, (2) the presence of beta-hemolytic Streptococci, (3) initial attacks often occur weeks to months post venectomy, and (4) the presence of fungal infection between the toes (tinea pedis). The pathogenesis of the infection is thought to be a combination of factors, such as impairment of the venous and lymphatic drainage, dermatophytosis, Streptococcal exotoxins, and immunologic status of the host.

Vascular surgeons must be aware of this newly recognized clinical problem and must not treat this condition as deep vein thrombosis. Treatment is by administration of penicillin. Prevention of recurrence is aided by eradication of the fungal infection.

INTRAOPERATIVE EMERGENCIES AFTER VEIN STRIPPING

Perhaps the most catastrophic complication related to varicose vein surgery is inadvertent stripping of the femoral artery instead of the saphenous vein. Recently, two reports have documented such occurrences, and personal communication with the author of one report uncovered several other unreported cases with limb loss.[16,17] In addition to lack of anatomical orientation, absence of pulsation in the femoral artery resulting from spasm following operative exposure obviously played a significant role in this grave error. Recognition of this injury should not be a problem, and prompt treatment with a vein graft from the contralateral limb or a prosthetic graft should restore arterial blood flow.

Another major emergency related to varicose vein surgery is accidental division of the femoral vein. Once again, lack of familiarity with the usual anatomical variation of the saphenofemoral junction accounts for the error. The injury, however, must be regarded as rare, probably one in 10,000 operations,[18] and it has been reported in the literature only sporadically.[18,19] Massive swelling is often noted in this injury. Treatment is by immediate restoration of femoral vein continuity. Because of the discrepancy of size between the femoral and saphenous veins, a spiral graft using the saphenous vein is needed for femoral vein replacement.

SCLEROTHERAPY

Recently, sclerotherapy for varicose veins has found renewed interest in the United States. If sclerotherapy is used to eliminate varicose veins, the operating surgeon should beware of accidental intraarterial injection. A serious complication occurs if the sclerosant is inadvertently injected into an artery instead of a vein.[20] The area in which injection is most likely to cause arterial damage is the medial aspect of the distal half of the leg, with the posterior tibial artery being most commonly involved. Gangrene of the foot with limb loss due to sclerotherapy has been reported.[1,20] Immediate treatment with heparin and low molecular weight dextran may be of value. However, once arterial damage is initiated, gangrene of the toes usually ensues, and amputation of toes or forefoot depends on the extent of injury. In extensive injury, a below-knee amputation is often needed. Other than intraarterial injection, serious complications of sclerotherapy include anaphylactic reaction and pulmonary embolism.

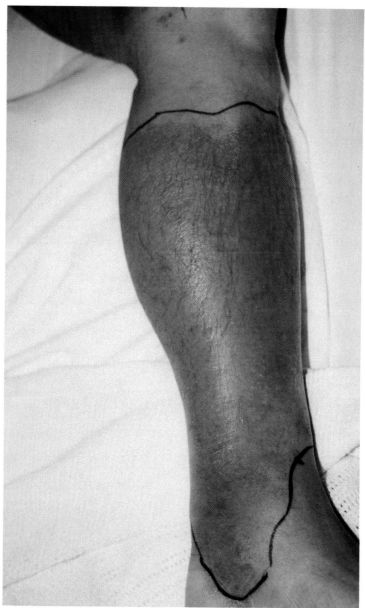

Fig. 1. Typical appearance of cellulitis and lymphangiitis following removal of saphenous vein for bypass grafting.

REFERENCES

1. Dodd H, Cockett FB: The Pathology and Surgery of the Veins of the Lower Limb. London, Churchill Livingstone, 1976
2. Villavicencio JL, Collins GJ Jr, Youkey JR, et al: Nonoperative management of lower extremity venous problems, in Bergan JJ, Yao JST, (eds.): Surgery of the Veins. Orlando, Grune & Stratton, 1985, pp. 323–345
3. Lofgren EP, Lofgren KA: The surgical treatment of superficial thrombophlebitis. Surgery 90:49, 1981
4. Husni EA, Williams WA: Superficial thrombophlebitis of lower limbs. Surgery 91:70, 1982
5. Gjöres JE: Surgical therapy of ascending thrombophlebitis in the saphenous system. Angiology 13:241, 1962
6. Gervais M: Les thromboses veineuses superficielles. Lyon Chir 52:89, 1956
7. Hafner CD, Cranley JJ, Krause RJ, et al: A method of managing superficial thrombophlebitis. Surgery 55:201, 1964
8. Ternberg JL, Bailes PM, Butcher HR Jr: Acute superficial saphenous thrombophlebitis. Amer J Surg 102:691, 1961
9. Williams RD, Zollinger RW: Surgical treatment of superficial thrombophlebitis. Surg Gynecol Obstet 118:745, 1964
10. Backman LE, Strömberg L: Some views on the acute, operative treatment of migratory thrombophlebitis in the great saphenous vein. Acta Chir Scand 137:511, 1971
11. Coffman JD: Diseases of the peripheral vessels, in Wyngaarden JB, Smith LM (ed.): Cecil's Textbook of Surgery. Philadelphia, WB Saunders, 1982, p. 316
12. Glover WJ, Vaughn AM, Annan CM, et al: Venous thrombectomy in the management of acute venous thrombosis of the saphenous system. Amer J Surg 93:798, 1957
13. Zinner MJ, Zuidema GD, Lowery BD: Septic nonsuppurative thrombophlebitis. Arch Surg 111:122, 1976
14. Torres-Rojas JR, Stratton CW, Sanders CV, et al: Candidal suppurative peripheral thrombophlebitis. Ann Intern Med 96:431, 1982
15. Baddour LM, Bisno AC: Recurrent cellulitis after coronary bypass surgery: Association with superficial fungal infection in saphenous venectomy limbs. JAMA 251:1049, 1984
16. Eger M, Goleman L, Torok G, et al: Inadvertent arterial stripping in the lower limb: Problems of management. Surgery 73:23, 1973
17. Liddicoat JE, Bekassy SM, Daniell MB, et al: Inadvertent femoral artery "stripping": Surgical management. Surgery 77:318, 1975
18. Tera H: Emergency repair of femoral vein accidentally divided at operation for varicose veins. Acta Chir Scand 133:283, 1967
19. Bevan PG, Green SH, Stammers FRR: Low termination of the internal saphenous vein. Br Med J 1:610, 1956
20. Fegan WG, Pegum JM: Accidental intra-arterial injection during sclerotherapy of varicose veins. Br J Surg 61:124, 1974
21. Plate G, Eklöf B, Jensen R, et al: Deep venous thrombosis, pulmonary embolism and acute surgery in thrombophlebitis of the long saphenous vein. Acta Chir Scand 151:241, 1985

PART X I

Acute Extremity Ischemia

James S. T. Yao
William R. Flinn

Emergencies in Upper Extremity Ischemia

Unlike vascular emergencies involving the lower extremity, acute ischemia of the upper extremity is relatively uncommon. Because of the richness of collateral circulation, gangrene of the hand is rare, and consequently, amputation is seldom performed for upper extremity ischemia. Even so, loss of dexterity of the hand as a result of arterial ischemia in a workman may result in prolonged loss of workdays and may eventually lead to a change of occupation. Early diagnosis and prompt treatment are needed to avoid this unpleasant result.

There are multiple causes for upper extremity ischemia. Of these, trauma, embolic occlusion, and iatrogenic injury account for most upper extremity ischemia.

ETIOLOGY

Table 1 outlines the etiology accounting for upper extremity ischemia. Trauma or iatrogenic injury is often self-evident, and the diagnosis is seldom difficult. In recent years, drug abuse has become common, and the surgeon must be aware of the deadly complications that can result from this injury.

DIAGNOSIS

In the absence of trauma or iatrogenic injury, a thorough history taking is necessary to establish the diagnosis. The history taking must include pharmacological, occupational, and medical aspects. Acute ischemia can occur in patients who are being treated for migraine headache with ergot derivatives or in patients who are receiving dopamine infusion. For embolic occlusion, the presence of atrial fibrillation or a history of myocardial infarction will help to establish the diagnosis. Arterial injury due to athletic activities is often subacute; however, acute thrombosis can occur as a result of sudden thrombosis due to the blunt force of the trauma.

Vascular Surgical Emergencies
ISBN 0-8089-1843-5

Table 1
Etiology of Acute Upper
Extremity Ischemia

Trauma
   Penetrating
      Gun shot
      Stabbing
Iatrogenic injury
   Cardiac catheterization
   Transaxillary or brachial arteriography
   Radial artery
      Arterial line
      Blood gas sampling
Athletic injury
   Baseball players
   Handball and frisbee players
Drug abuse
   Intraarterial injection
   Infected aneurysm
   Compartment syndrome
Pharmacologic-induced ischemia
   Ergot poisoning
   Dopamine
Embolic
Arterial graft complications
Infection
Thoracic outlet compression
Radiation injury

Physical examination must include careful examination of pulses and neurological function. Sensory and motor function of the hand must be assessed in all patients even when pulses are palpable. A loss of sensory function is indicative of severe ischemia, and emergency surgical intervention is needed. Swelling and tightness of the compartments of the forearm must be included in the examination. Auscultation of the subclavian artery or palpation of the supraclavicular space is essential to determine whether there is a proximal lesion. The presence of a loud bruit or palpable pulsatile mass should alert the surgeon to the possibility of vascular complication due to thoracic outlet syndrome, and various thoracic outlet maneuvers, in particular, the abduction-external rotation (AER) positional test, will help to confirm the diagnosis. Examination of the upper extremity is not complete unless an Allen test is performed.

NONINVASIVE TESTING

Noninvasive testing, in particular, the Doppler ultrasound flow detection technique, is helpful to confirm clinical findings. Of particular value is finger systolic pressure recording because of the difficulty in palpation of finger pulses. Also, the Doppler technique is more accurate than physical examination in the determination of patency of the palmar arch and is more sensitive in determination of patency of the ulnar artery at the wrist level. The latter is often inaccessible to pulse palpation. In addition to establishing the diagnosis, the level of systolic pressure, especially the forearm pressure, is helpful to ascertain the status of collateral circulation. In the absence of nerve dysfunction, a systolic pressure > 60 mm Hg may be sufficient to maintain viability so that surgical intervention may be deferred if the condition is not optimal for emergency intervention. Finally, noninvasive testing is helpful to assess the result of surgery or to monitor the development of collateral circulation.

Recently, the B-mode scan of peripheral arteries has been introduced, and this technique may offer an alternate test for diagnosis of acute upper extremity ischemia.

ARTERIOGRAPHY

Arteriography, if indicated, should be done by the retrograde femoral catheterization technique described by Seldinger in 1956. Brachial arteriography is no longer used because of the possibility of complications and also because the technique fails to reveal information on the arteries proximal to the puncture site. Arteriography, however, is not always needed in the emergency situation. In a typical case of embolic occlusion, the diagnosis can be made simply by physical examination with confirmation by noninvasive testing. Similarly, most iatrogenic injuries can be managed without arteriography. The recent introduction of the B-mode scan has provided an alternate technique to confirm the diagnosis. In combination with Doppler flow detection, the B-mode scan may be used to replace arteriography (Fig. 1). The B-mode scan is of particular value to determine the extent of injury, including proximal dissection by the catheter.

In addition to diagnostic use, arteriography yields information on anatomical variations. Unlike the lower extremity, there are many anatomical variations in the blood supply to the forearm and hand. In approximately 20 percent of cases, the radial or ulnar artery will arise high on the brachial artery. Also, the palmar arch is subject to a wide variety of anatomical configurations, and arteriography yields valuable information about the completeness of the palmar arch.

In selective instances, the additional use of a vasodilator may help to improve visualization of the digital arteries. The use of papaverine infusion may indeed be considered a useful adjunct in management of acute hand ischemia.

ACUTE ISCHEMIA CONDITIONS

Pharmacologically-induced Ischemia

Ergot Poisoning

Most of the patients are young working women, the ratio of women to men being five to one. This finding probably reflects the higher incidence of migraine headache in women. Since the introduction of ergot compounds in the treatment of migraine headache by Stoll, the most common cause of ergot poisoning has become an overdose of the drug.[1] Although ergotamine is an alpha-adrenergic blocker, in large doses it acts directly on vascular smooth muscle to cause vasoconstriction. Methysergide maleate, a semisynthetic amino alkaloid commonly used for migraine, may also cause ischemia.[2] The combination of heparin and dihydroergotamine in pharmacological prophylaxis for deep-vein thrombo-

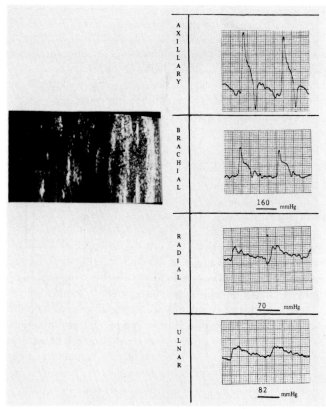

Fig. 1. The combination of B-mode scan and transcutaneous Doppler flow detection provided a comprehensive diagnostic technique in a patient who sustained acute embolic occlusion of the brachial artery.

sis, introduced recently, may also cause severe vasospasm, precipitating acute hand ischemia.[3]

The diagnosis should be suspected in all young adults who have a history of migraine headache. Careful history taking including drug intake will establish the diagnosis. Ergot poisoning presents with characteristic arteriographic findings. These are (1) generalized intense spasm of the artery, often in both limbs with symmetrical appearance, (2) a long string appearance of the brachial artery, and (3) the presence of rich collaterals (Fig. 2).

Treatment is by immediate withdrawal of the drug. Heparin, nitroprusside, dextran, nifedipine, and captopril have been reported to be helpful.[4-6] Once the ergot preparation is discontinued, relief of symptoms usually ensues within 24 to 48 hours, with dramatic return of pulses. The Doppler flow detection technique has been shown to be of value in monitoring the improvement.[7] Follow-up arteriography often demonstrates that the main artery has reverted to normal appearance, with loss of collateral pathways (Fig. 2).

Dopamine-induced Ischemia

Dopamine hydrochloride is now a commonly-used pharmaceutical agent in treatment of cardiogenic and septic shock because of its inotropic effect. At low dosages (10 μg/kg/min) in normal subjects, dopamine decreases total peripheral resistance while increasing

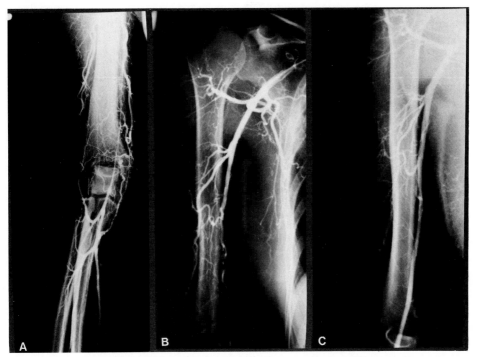

Fig. 2. Typical arteriographic findings in a patient with ergot poisoning who presented with acute ischemia of the hand. (A) Intense spasm of the brachial artery and richness of collateral pathways; (B) Long string appearance of the main (brachial) artery; (C) Normal appearance of the brachial artery one week after cessation of the ergot intake.

cardiac output. At higher doses, dopamine may cause vasoconstriction as a result of increased peripheral resistance due to alpha-adrenergic effect. Because of intense vasoconstriction, severe ischemia affecting the fingers can occur, and it may progress to gangrene if the condition is not recognized. Dopamine gangrene often occurs in patients with disseminated intravascular coagulation or with sepsis,[8] and it may occur even at low doses[9] or in neonates.[10] In general, when the dose is in excess of 10 μg/kg/min, vasoconstriction occurs, and acrocyanosis is the first sign of ischemia. Similar to all drug-induced ischemia, the treatment is immediate cessation of the drug. Administration of phentolamine (Regitine), an alpha-adrenergic antagonist, intravenously and into the skin of the involved area has been reported to be effective. The recommended dosage is 5 to 10 mg of phenotolamine intravenously, and it should be used with caution because phentolamine can precipitate hypotension.

Iatrogenic Injury

The placement of arterial lines and cardiac catheterization are the most common causes of iatrogenic injury to the brachial or radial artery. Diagnostic arteriography via the axillary or brachial route may also be responsible for arterial ischemia. Most of these injuries are self-evident, and diagnosis is readily made by clinical examination. The use of B-mode scan in combination with Doppler flow detection is helpful to establish the diagnosis without repeat arteriography. The B-mode scan may also help to detect arterio-venous communication and to locate the site of the fistula. Whether there is proximal dissection can also be determined by this technique.

The incidence of brachial artery injury following cardiac catheterization ranges from 0.3 percent to as high as 28 percent, and this wide range obviously is related to the expertise of the invasive cardiologist.[11-14] The basic pathology of catheter injury consists of denuded endothelium, fracture, and retraction of the intimal elastic lamina, with partial necrosis of the media of the arterial wall. In some instances, pressure necrosis of the entire posterior wall of the artery has been observed.[15] Such injury, if unrecognized, may proceed to complete thrombosis of the artery.

Percutaneous radial artery catheterization for monitoring of blood pressure or blood gas sampling has become a commonly used procedure in care of critically ill patients. Though uncommon, severe ischemia of the hand can occur after the placement of a catheter in the radial artery. Factors that predispose to this complication are an incomplete palmar arch (negative Allen test), prolonged placement of the catheter, and the hyper-coagulable state. The reported incidence of radial artery thrombosis following cannulation ranges from 10 to 25 percent.[16,17] Because of adequate collateral circulation, severe ischemia occurs in only 0.2 to 0.5 percent of patients.[17-19] Gangrene or necrosis of the forearm as a result of radial artery thrombosis has been reported.[18,20,21]

In addition to injury to the artery, compartment syndrome or hematoma around the puncture site could also cause nerve dysfunction. This is particularly true in arteriography using the axillary artery. Early recognition and prompt surgical intervention are needed to prevent sequelae of nerve injury. In general, drainage of the hematoma around the neuro-vascular bundle is all that is needed to accomplish the goal of decompression.

The treatment for iatrogenic injury is prompt surgical intervention. Once the diagnosis is established, intravenous heparin must be given to prevent propagation of the thrombotic process. Most brachial or radial artery injuries can be repaired under local anesthesia. Surgical repair usually consists of thrombectomy and repair of the intimal flap, with the arteriotomy closed with a vein patch. Occasionally, a short-segment interposed vein graft is needed to restore continuity because of extensive circumferential damage to the arterial wall.[22]

Occasionally, a false aneurysm may develop after catheterization of either the brachial or the radial artery. In addition to possible embolization to the digits, this expanding aneurysm may cause nerve compression and require surgical intervention. The treatment is rather simple. In most cases, lateral repair with vein patch is needed to restore arterial continuity.

Embolic Occlusion

Table 2 outlines the causes of embolic occlusion. Of these, the cardiac source is the most common. Of all emboli to the extremities, those to the upper extremity occur ten times less frequently than the lower extremity.[23] The most common source of cardiac emboli is atherosclerotic heart disease and atrial fibrillation.[24] The brachial artery accounts for the third most common site of lodgement of an embolus of cardiac origin. The treatment is immediate heparinization followed by catheter embolectomy (see chapter by Cranley).

Table 2

Cardiac Sources of Peripheral Emboli

Acute myocardial infarction
Atrial fibrillation associated with
    rheumatic heart disease
    thyrotoxicosis
Sinoatrial disease
Left ventricular aneurysm with mural thrombus
Mitral valve prolapse
Cardiac valvular prostheses
Atrial myxoma
Following cardioversion
Paradoxical emboli
Endocarditis

Trauma

Injury to the upper limb arteries due to penetrating wounds or orthopaedic trauma is discussed elsewhere in this volume and will not be repeated here.

Athletic Injury

Arterial injury due to blunt force can also cause acute arterial occlusion. One of the uncommon forms of blunt trauma is related to athletic activity. Of particular interest is arterial injury in baseball players. Although most such arterial injury is chronic in nature, acute thrombosis of the subclavian artery due to thoracic outlet compression in a major league pitcher has been reported.[25] In the report by Fields et al[25] the patient suffered a major stroke as a result of retrograde propagation of the thrombotic process to the origin of the right common carotid artery. Emergency thrombectomy was performed but failed to prevent subsequent arm ischemia.

Another form of injury is occlusion of the ulnar artery as a result of the impact of a baseball accidentally hitting the wrist (Fig. 3). Hand injury is also observed in frisbee players. Again, the impact of the frisbee hitting the palmar aspect of the hand during catching can result in sudden occlusion of the palmar arch (Fig. 4). Severe ischemia ensues as a result of the injury.

The treatment of hand injury due to athletic activity is conservative and expectant. Supportive treatment with Dextran-40 infusion and intraarterial infusion of a vasodilating agent during arteriography may also help to relieve spasm commonly associated with this type of injury (Fig. 5). Avoidance of athletic activity for 2 to 3 weeks is necessary to allow optimal development of collateral circulation.

Arterial Graft Complications

The axillofemoral bypass is now a commonly performed procedure, and the complications arising from such grafting can cause upper extremity ischemia. Upper extremity emboli secondary to axillofemoral graft thrombosis have recently been recognized as a cause of acute hand ischemia.[26] Disruption of the suture line probably is due to inappro-

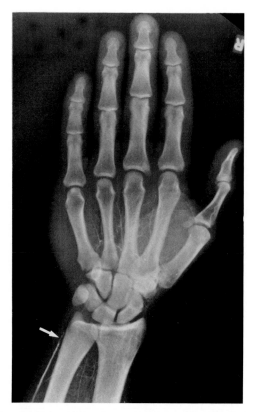

Fig. 3. Occlusion of the ulnar artery (arrow) in a baseball player.
Note the spasm of the ulnar artery.

priate placement of the anastomosis and may also present with acute ischemia. Avulsion of the graft from the axillary artery has been reported and is thought to be due to mechanical factors.[27] When the upper extremity is fully abducted, the graft pathway may increase in length up to 8.5 cm (range 4 to 12 cm). Failure to take into account this graft lengthening when the graft is placed may cause graft rupture, especially if the nonexpandable polytetrafluoroethylene (PTFE) graft is used.

For embolic occlusion, the treatment is embolectomy and thrombectomy of the graft. Rupture of the graft or of the proximal anastomosis requires restoration of flow to the distal artery and placement of a new graft to avoid further injury.

Drug Abuse

There is little doubt that this form of arterial ischemia will be seen with increasing frequency, and management of surgical emergencies due to drug abuse is discussed in the chapter by Berguer and Benitez. Because of easy accessibility of the brachial or radial artery, intraarterial injection of various substances by drug users has been known to cause

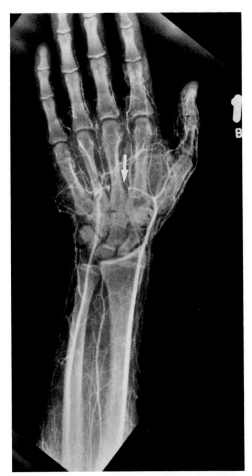

Fig. 4. Occlusion of the palmar arch (arrow) in a frisbee player.

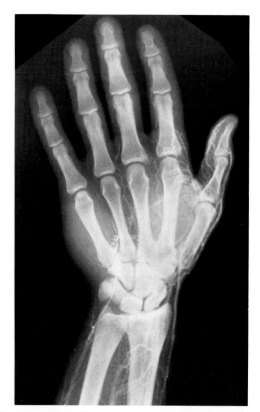

Fig. 5. Arteriogram of the same patient seen in Figure 3 after papaverine infusion. Relief of spasm by papaverine infusion improved filling of contrast media. Filling of digital arteries, however, remained poor.

catastrophic complications. Table 3 shows the various substances known to produce arterial damage. Once the damage is done, treatment is largely supportive. In cases with compartment syndrome, decompression of the compartment is often needed (see chapters by Schuler and Flanigan, Russell and Burns).

Infection

Arterial ischemia leading to gangrene of the fingers due to overwhelming sepsis associated with intravascular coagulation is uncommon but has been reported.[28] In patients with atypical pneumonia, such as mycoplasma pneumonia, the presence of cold agglutinins may be the responsible factor in development of ischemia of the hand or fingers.[29] Determination of cold agglutinin titer will help to establish the diagnosis. Arteriography often shows intense spasm. Not only are the main arteries involved, but the

Table 3
Drugs Known to Produce Gangrene

Generic Name	Trade Name
Thiopentone	Pentothal
Quinalbarbitone	Secobarbital, Seconal
Pentobarbitone	Nembutal, Prodormol
Amobarbital	Amytal
Promazine	Sparine
Chlorpromazine	Largactyl, Taroctyl, Thorazine
Mephenesin	Myanesin, Tolosate
Tubocurain	—
Meperidine	Pethidin, Dolestin, Demerol, Pro-Meperdan
Promethazine	Phenergan
Propoxyphene	Darvon
Hydroxyzine	Atarax
Heroin	—
Diazepam	Valium
Amphetamine	Benzedrine, Novydrine
Ether	—
Sulfobromophthalein	Bromsulphalein
Methylphenidate	Ritalin
Pentazocine	Talwin
Methohexitone	—
5-hydroxytryptamine	

From Goldberg I, Bahar A, Yosipovitch Z: Gangrene of the upper extremity following intraarterial injection of drugs: A case report and review of the literature. Clin Orthopaed 188:223, 1984. With permission.

branch arteries may be affected, with multiple segmental occlusions (Figs. 6 & 7). Unless the surgeon is familiar with this condition, treatment with appropriate antibiotics may be delayed. Even when the cause is identified, the result of this type of ischemia is often disappointing because of the magnitude of sepsis and associated disseminated intravascular coagulation.

Thoracic Outlet Compression

Vascular complications of thoracic outlet compression are due to bony abnormalities, such as a cervical rib. Most vascular presentations are subacute or chronic in nature. Acute ischemia, however, can develop when an unrecognized aneurysm develops acute thrombosis. Most such aneurysms also cause embolization, precipitating acute ischemia (Fig. 8). Failure to recognize this condition and to perform embolectomy could result in serious complications. Careful palpation of the supraclavicular space helps to establish the diagnosis. A plain x-ray showing a cervical rib is certainly diagnostic. Arteriography is needed to confirm the diagnosis. Surgical treatment consists of two incisions, one placed supraclavicularly and one infraclavicularly, to gain proximal and distal control. A saphenous vein graft is used for restoration of continuity.

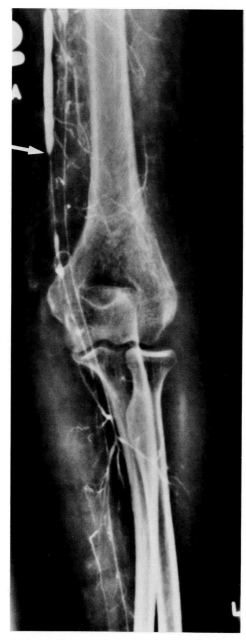

Fig. 6. Arteriogram in a patient with gangrene of the hand due to sepsis and intravascular coagulation. The brachial artery shows intense spasm (arrow).

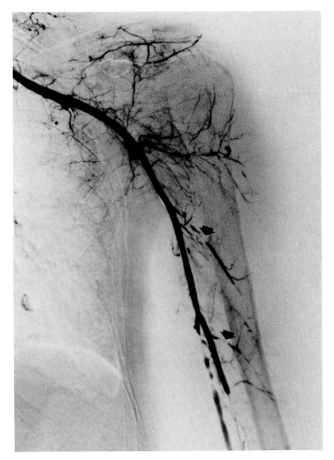

Fig. 7. Arteriogram in the same patient notes the segmental occlusion of all branches (arrows).

Radiation Injury

Irradiation may cause damage not only to small vessels but also to large arteries, such as the subclavian or iliac artery.[30-32] Most injuries to the arteries present with subacute symptoms or late manifestation due to stenosis as a result of fibrosis of the arterial wall. Acute presentation of ischemia, however, can occur, and it is commonly seen during the first interval. According to Butler et al,[33] there are three intervals following irradiation. The first interval is at 5 years following irradiation, when most patients present with mural thrombus. These patients can develop acute occlusion of the brachial and digital arteries due to embolization (Fig. 9). The second and third stages occur at 10 and 20 years, respectively, with most lesions related to fibrotic occlusion or accelerated atherosclerosis. Not infrequently, emergency treatment is needed because of hemorrhage due to severe damage to the artery.[32] In the acute thrombotic stage, thrombectomy and bypass grafting is the treatment of choice.

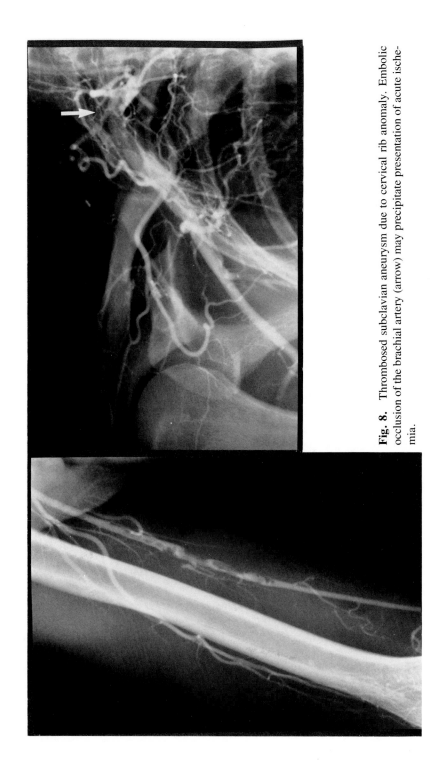

Fig. 8. Thrombosed subclavian aneurysm due to cervical rib anomaly. Embolic occlusion of the brachial artery (arrow) may precipitate presentation of acute ischemia.

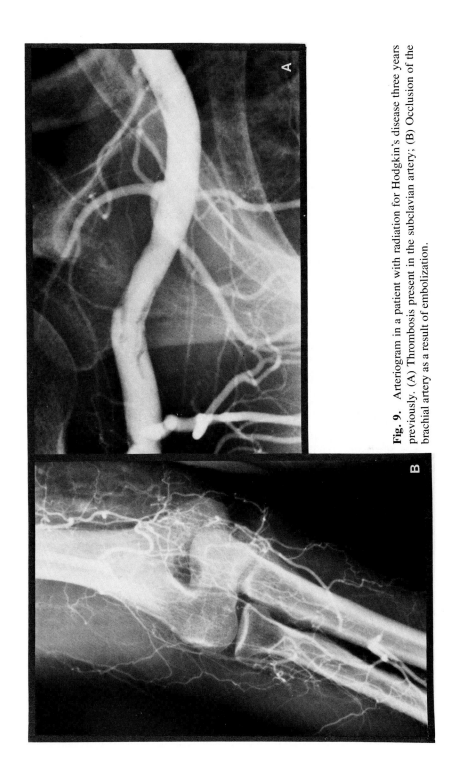

Fig. 9. Arteriogram in a patient with radiation for Hodgkin's disease three years previously. (A) Thrombosis present in the subclavian artery; (B) Occlusion of the brachial artery as a result of embolization.

483

REFERENCES

1. Stoll A: Recent investigations on ergot alkaloids. Chem Rev 47:197, 1950
2. Apesos J, Folse JR: Lower extremity arterial insufficiency after long term methysergide maleate therapy. Arch Surg 114:964, 1979
3. Cunningham M, de Torrente A, Ekoe JM, et al: Vascular spasm and gangrene during heparin-dihydro-ergotamine prophylaxis. Br J Surg 71:829, 1984
4. Zimran A, Ofek B, Hershko C: Treatment with captopril for peripheral ischaemia induced by ergotamine. Br Med J 288:364, 1984
5. Andersen PK, Christensen KN, Hole P, et al: Sodium nitroprusside and epidural blockade in the treatment of ergotism. N Engl J Med 296:1271, 1977
6. Dagher FJ, Pais SO, Richards W, et al: Severe unilateral ischemia of the lower extremity caused by ergotamine: Treatment with nifedipine. Surgery 97:369, 1985
7. Yao JST, Goodwin DP, Kenyon JR: Case of ergot poisoning. Br Med J 3:86, 1970
8. Winkler MJ, Trunkey DD: Dopamine gangrene. Association with disseminated intravascular coagulation. Am J Surg 142:588, 1981
9. Alexander CS, Sako Y, Mikulic E: Pedal gangrene associated with the use of dopamine. N Engl J Med 293:591, 1975
10. Maggi JC, Angelats J, Scott JP: Gangrene in a neonate following dopamine therapy. J Pediat 100:323, 1982
11. Menzoian JO, Corson JD, Bush HL Jr, et al: Management of the upper extremity with absent pulses after cardiac catheterization. Am J Surg 135:484, 1978
12. Rich NM, Hobson RW II, Fedde CW: Vascular trauma secondary to diagnostic and therapeutic procedures. Am J Surg 128:715, 1974
13. Kitzmiller JW, Hertzer NR, Beven EG: Routine surgical management of brachial artery occlusion after cardiac catheterization. Arch Surg 117:1066, 1982
14. Youkey JR, Clagett GP, Rich NM, et al: Vascular trauma secondary to diagnostic and therapeutic procedures: 1974 through 1982. A comparative review. Am J Surg 146:788, 1983
15. Karmody AM, Lempert N, Jarmolych J: The pathology of post-catheterization brachial artery occlusion. J Surg Res 20:601, 1976
16. Bedford RF, Wollman H: Complications of percutaneous radial artery cannulation. Anesthesiology 38:228, 1973
17. Evans PJD, Kerr JH: Arterial occlusion after cannulation. Br Med J 3:197, 1975
18. Baker RJ, Chunprapaph B, Nyhus LM: Severe ischemia of the hand following radial artery catheterization. Surgery 80:449, 1976
19. Mozersky DJ, Buckley CJ, Hagood CD, et al: Ultrasonic evaluation of the palmar circulation. Am J Surg 121:810, 1973
20. Johnson FE, Sumner DS, Strandness DE Jr: Extremity necrosis caused by indwelling arterial catheters. Am J Surg 131:375, 1976
21. Falor WH, Hansel JR, Williams GB: Gangrene of the hand: A complication of radial artery cannulation. J Trauma 16:713, 1976
22. McMillan I, Murie JA: Vascular injury following cardiac catheterization. Br J Surg 71:832, 1984
23. Elliott JP Jr, Hageman JH, Szilagyi DE, et al: Arterial embolization: Problems of source, multiplicity, recurrence, and delayed treatment. Surgery 88:833, 1980
24. Abbott WM, Maloney RD, McCabe CC, et al: Arterial embolism: A 44 year perspective. Am J Surg 143:460, 1982
25. Fields WS, Lemak NA, Ben-Menachem Y: Thoracic outlet syndrome: Review and reference to stroke in a major league pitcher. Am J Neuroradiol 7:73, 1986
26. Bandyk DF, Thiele BL, Radke HM: Upper-extremity emboli secondary to axillofemoral graft thrombosis. Arch Surg 116:393, 1981

27. Daar AS, Finch DRA: Graft avulsion: an unreported complication of axillofemoral bypass grafts. Br J Surg 65:442, 1978
28. Goodwin JN, Berne TV: Symmetrical peripheral gangrene. Arch Surg 108:780, 1974
29. Mackay D: A bizarre case of gangrene. Hospital Practice, Oct, 1977, pp 153–158
30. Mavor GE, Kasenally AT, Haper DR, et al: Thrombus of subclavian-axillary artery following radiotherapy for carcinoma of the breast. Br J Surg 60:983, 1973
31. Butler MS, Lane RHS, Webster JHH: Irradiation injury to large arteries. Br J Surg 67:341, 1980
32. Kretschmer G, Niederle B, Polterauer P, et al: Irradiation-induced changes in the subclavian and axillary arteries after radiotherapy for carcinoma of the breast. Surgery 99:658, 1986
33. Goldberg I, Bahar A, Yosipovitch Z: Gangrene of the upper extremity following intraarterial injection of drugs: A case report and review of literature. Clin Orthopaed 188:223, 1984

John J. Cranley

Acute Embolic Occlusion of Major Arteries

Historically, the management of arterial embolism can be divided into recognizable phases that reflect medical knowledge at a given point in time. First came recognition of the disease and a plan of treatment that, though logical, was not yet possible. The compelling appropriateness of surgical removal was apparent to John Hunter in 1768, according to Murray,[1] but 15 attempted embolectomies resulted in failure between Sabanejeff's first effort in 1895[2] and Labey's first successful removal of an embolus in 1910.[3] The second phase opened when Key performed the second embolectomy and reported it in the German literature in 1921 and in the English literature in 1923.[4] He readily appreciated the important role of distal propagating thrombosis in the poor outcome of arterial embolism and noted that extension did not always occur. He reported on 10 operations of his own and collected 51 cases from the literature. He noted that in no case was an operation fully successful if done more than 24 hours after lodgement of the embolus. This second phase, beginning with the first successful embolectomy, spans an indefinite period of time, but may be considered to have come to an end in the 1940s,[5,6] when anticoagulant therapy became available for the use of surgeons. Thereupon, both physicians and surgeons began to look upon embolectomy as the treatment of choice, inasmuch as there was the possibility of preventing recurrence of embolism by the use of anticoagulant agents. However, another obstacle remained to be overcome, namely, the misconception that autonomically controlled reflex arterial vasospasm existed distal to an embolus and that it could be released by vasodilating agents or sympathetic blocks.[7] Another highly logical but ineffective nonsurgical method of treatment was the use of intermittent positive–negative pressures in the belief that the negative pressure would stimulate collateral circulation by reducing peripheral resistance (PAEVEX).[8] In my opinion, the occasional successes by these methods of therapy were due to the fact that the thrombus does not always propagate.

On beginning private practice in 1952, I was convinced that embolectomy was indeed the treatment of choice and 10 years later reported[9] on what I believed to be the prime principles of management, which I still follow today with virtually no modifications. I fully realize that these concepts were not original with me, but were the algebraic

Vascular Surgical Emergencies
ISBN 0-8089-1843-5

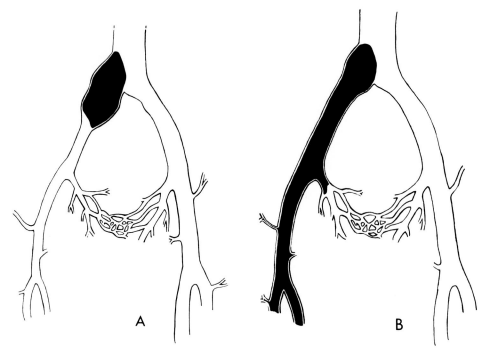

Fig. 1. (A) Prior to formation of a progagating thrombus the circulation distal to an embolic occlusion may be adequate because of numerous collateral arterial pathways. (B) Gangrene caused by progressive occlusion of all collateral arterial pathways by propagating thrombus.

sum of all I had been taught and had gathered from the literature. My personal mentor, F.A. Simeone, convinced me that "reflex spasm" of major arteries does not exist; R.L. Linton was a firm advocate of early embolectomy, the direct approach, and postoperative anticoagulant therapy; and L. G. Herrmann both baffled and deeply impressed me with his successful nonoperative management.[8] In addition, I profited greatly from reviewing the surgical literature, particularly the work of Key,[3] Murray,[5,6] Haimovici,[10] Warren,[11] Shaw,[12] Lord,[13] and Julian and Dye.[14]

PRINCIPLES AND CONCEPTS OF TREATMENT

1. Embolectomy is indicated in all patients, except those not expected to live and in those who have a gangrenous limb.
2. Since distal thrombosis is the major cause of havoc associated with arterial embolism (Fig. 1) heparin should be given as soon as the diagnosis is made whether it be by the family physician or the operating surgeon.
3. Lower pressure and normal vasomotor tone cause the small diameter of the artery distal to the thrombus (Fig. 2), erroneously thought to be secondary to "reflex arterial spasm," and therefore lumbar sympathetic blocks and vasodilating agents are of no value and are contraindicated because their use might interdict the use of heparin.
4. Contrary to our earlier belief, the indirect approach, using the balloon embolectomy catheter, is preferred. Fogarty's catheter, developed in our laboratory in 1962,[15]

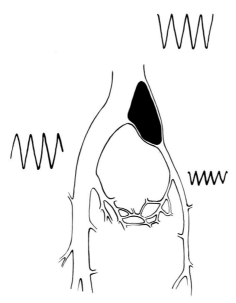

Fig. 2. Lower pressure and normal vasomotor tone cause the small diameter of the artery distal to the thrombus. (From Cranley JJ: Vascular Surgery, Vol. I. Peripheral Arterial Disease. Hagerstown, Harper & Row, 1972, pp 93–107. With permission.)

permits the removal of aortic and iliac artery emboli atraumatically from below through femoral incisions. In the preceding few years there had been numerous reports of successful embolectomies using the indirect approach through suction or other instruments. These methods worked well on younger patients with rheumatic heart disease whose arteries were good. However, fear of damage to the sclerotic arteries of patients with coronary artery disease had deterred me from using suction or manipulative measures. Since 1962, we have used the balloon catheter on all abdominal and all peripheral emboli (Fig. 3). When a common femoral artery embolus is removed, the catheter is used to ensure that the distal arterial tree is patent.

5. The time between lodgement and removal of the embolus no longer is the major determinant of operability. Influenced by Key,[3] many surgeons during the early years of embolectomy believed that the prime determinant of success was the length of time from the lodgement to removal of the embolus. Gradually, surgeons realized, as did we, that successful operation could be performed days and even weeks after lodgement. The reason for this fact, in our opinion, is that distal propagation has not taken place. Today, the status of the limb determines operability.

6. Distal discontinuous clot may be present despite excellent back bleeding because collateral arteries exist between the arteriotomy and the distal thrombi (Fig. 4). We detected this by extracting clot from the distal tree with the Fogarty catheter in patients with good back bleeding. It is of interest that we reported this phenomenon on the same program on the same day and immediately preceding Spencer and Eiseman's report[16] on their observation of distal discontinuous clot on intraoperative arteriograms.

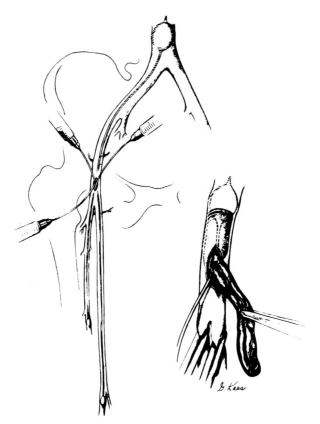

Fig. 3. Technique of balloon catheter embolectomy. (From
Cranley JJ: Vascular Surgery, Vol. I. Peripheral Arterial Disease.
Hagerstown, Harper & Row, 1972, pp 93–107. With permission.)

7. All patients should be on anticoagulant therapy for life after a major embolism. This
   is particularly true of patients with rheumatic heart disease, but includes all patients
   for as long as cardiac irregularity persists.

MATERIALS AND METHODS

Between 1952 and 1986, 631 patients underwent 689 operations for arterial embolism; 152 (22 percent) of the operations were done before 1962, when the Fogarty
embolectomy catheter was developed. The remaining 537 operations (78 percent) were
done using the catheter technique. Fifty-eight (9 percent) of the patients had more than 1
operation: 2 had 4 operations on the same artery (in 1 case, the external iliac; in the other,
the femoral); 5 patients had 3 operations on either the right or left femoral artery. The
remaining 51 patients had 2 embolectomies, either on the bilateral lower limbs or on 1
upper and 1 lower extremity.

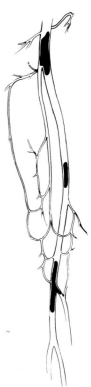

Fig. 4. Multiple areas of discontinuous thrombosis distal to the major arterial embolism. (From Cranley JJ: Vascular Surgery, Vol. I. Peripheral Arterial Disease. Hagerstown, Harper & Row, 1972, pp 93–107. With permission.)

Demographics

Gender and Age

It is of interest that 71 percent of the patients in the earlier series were female; in the last 5-year period, there is virtual sexual parity. Also in the earlier series, both the males and females were younger than those in the later series, average age being 66 for females and 67 for males. The median age was 67 for females and 60 for males. Patients in the later series averaged 71 years for females and 75 for males; the median age was 75 for females and 67 for males. The youngest patient was a female aged 21 and the oldest, a female aged 101. In the earlier series, 65 percent of the patients were over 60, and in the later series, 82 percent were over 60. This difference we think may in part be explained by the fact that in the earlier series, 27 percent of the patients had rheumatic heart disease and in the later series, the incidence was only 4 percent.

Cardiac Status

Concurrent cardiac conditions are tabulated in Table 1. In our earlier series, when we personally examined all patients,[9] we believed that atrial fibrillation was present in 95 percent of the cases. Since that time, with many associates working in many different hospitals, it has not been possible to keep such uniform records. Certainly one subset is clear, that patients with an embolus following myocardial infarction number 16 percent.

Table 1
Cardiac Status in 631 Patients
(689 Embolectomies)*

Coronary artery disease	85%
Myocardial infarction	16%
Rheumatic heart disease	7%
Atrial fibrillation:	
Early series	95%
Recent series	66%
Normal	1%
Unknown	5%

*Concurrent conditions tabulated

Patients with coronary artery disease may have periodic intermittent fibrillation; thus, a patient with an arterial embolus may have been fibrillating but not at the specific time of examination. In order to get some evidence of the current incidence, we reviewed the charts of the last 150 patients with arterial embolectomy, looking specifically for proof of atrial fibrillation at or near the time of lodgement of the embolus in the set of patients who had not had a recent myocardial infarction. Atrial fibrillation was reported in 66 percent of the patients.

Source of the Embolus

The heart was undoubtedly the source of the embolus in the majority of cases (Table 2). On clinical grounds, we considered that in 90 percent of the patients, the embolus originated in the heart. We recognized arteriogenic origin in 1 percent. In 7 percent, there was no evidence to suggest that the heart or the peripheral arteries were the source. These cases are listed as of unknown origin. However, with bi-plane arteriography we are finding an increasing incidence of arterial abnormalities as the source of these small emboli, but this is beyond the scope of this chapter. This was dealt with in an earlier report.[17]

Site of Lodgement of the Embolus

In the 34 years of our experience, there has literally been no variation in incidence of site of lodgement of the embolus: in the axillary-brachial area, 15 percent; aortoiliac, 25 percent; femoropopliteal, 60 percent; and tibial, less than 1 percent. Cerebral and visceral emboli were excluded from this tabulation.

RESULTS

Table 3 summarizes operative results related to site of lodgement in 537 embolectomies performed using the catheter technique. Results of our earlier series have been previously reported.[18,19]

Assessment of results is not without its difficulties and it is our belief that many of the differences may be explained by the method of reporting. This applies especially to limb necrosis at the time of death and early amputation but also has a bearing on operative

Table 2

Source of Arterial Embolus in 631 Patients
(689 Embolectomies) 1952–1986

I.	Heart		568 (90%)
II.	Aneurysm:		
	Abdominal aortic aneurysm: plaque	4	
	Resection of ruptured aneurysm	3	9 (1%)
	Resection of elective aneurysm	1	
	Femoral aneurysm*	1	
III.	Atherogenic:		8 (1%)
	Distal aorta:		
	Plaque	3	
	Atheromatous matter	1	
	Fibrin from wall	1	6
	Thoracic aorta:		
	Pseudocoarctation		
	2º ulcerative plaque†	1	
	Iliac: plaque	1	
	Femoral:		2
	Atheromatous matter‡	1	
IV.	Miscellaneous		
	Plastic valve		1
	Sepsis		3
	Unknown		43 (7%)

*Found at amputation
†Found at operation for coarctation
‡Propagated to tibial artery intra-common femoral endarterectomy

Table 3

Operative Results Related to Site of Lodgement
537 Embolectomies (Catheter Technique)

Artery	N	Survived, Improved N (%)	Amputation or Necrosis of Limb at Death N (%)	Early Death N (%)
Axillary	29	21 (72%)	1 (3%)	8 (28%)
Brachial	52	36 (69%)	4 (8%)	15 (29%)
Aorta	34	23 (67%)	1 (3%)	10 (29%)
Iliac	97	74 (76%)	2 (2%)	21 (22%)
Femoral	287	208 (72%)	28 (10%)	63 (22%)
Popliteal	35	31 (89%)	2 (6%)	2 (6%)
Tibial	3	2 (67%)	1 (33%)	0 (0%)
		396 (74%)	39 (7.6%)	119 (22%)

mortality. Early death is probably the clearest subset, but only if one includes every patient who died while still hospitalized or within 30 days of operation and does not consider extenuating circumstances. For example, a patient had a shower of emboli to his brain and an embolus to the bifurcation of his aorta. He was comatose. Clinically, it seemed certain that unless the aortic embolus was removed, he would either die or lose both lower extremities. The neurosurgeon thought that the patient might survive his cerebral embolism. Accordingly, aortic embolectomy was carried out successfully, with restoration of all pulses in his limbs. He lived approximately 8 weeks and then died in the hospital. We are reluctant to include this case as a successful embolectomy, since the strict criterion, death while hospitalized, was fulfilled. Nevertheless, it is clear that his death was not related to the embolectomy.

Amputation Rate

This would seem to be a definitive subset of patients, yet two problems may obscure the results. The first error is one of interpreting every unamputated limb as a successful outcome. Some patients die with an ischemic limb that would require amputation had the patient lived. Accordingly, we have reported not only the amputations but also the irreversibly ischemic extremities at the time of death as failures.

The second problem with using amputation as the criterion of failure is that it may be necessary even in a "successful" operation. For example, a 30-year-old parturient was seen 3 days following lodgement of an aortic embolus. At the time she was examined, both feet were gangrenous and her legs were mottled to the high-thigh area. She was transferred to our hospital and operation was performed to clear the aorta, the iliac, and femoral arteries with restoration of pulses down to the popliteals. It was then possible to do below-the-knee amputations, which healed. The patient was able to be rehabilitated with two prostheses. Certainly, this operation was successful in the sense that it may have saved her life and in any event, spared her bilateral high-thigh amputations. Nevertheless, she is a patient who has a double amputation following embolectomy. We have listed her in the category of patients surviving, improved (see below).

Survived, Improved

This is a clearcut category, if one is objective about improvement. Many patients whose embolus does not propagate will survive, as will their limbs, without treatment or despite postoperative thrombosis. Nevertheless, today, the presence of pulses and measurement of segmental pressures using the Doppler technique permit one to make an objective assessment of the success of the operation.

Operative Mortality

Table 4 shows the causes of death in 30 days of 165 (26 percent) of the patients. Cardiac disease accounts for 69 percent of the deaths; stroke, for 10 percent. As pointed out by Blaisdell,[19] operative mortality in most series has not changed significantly in this current phase of accepted operative treatment. Although our operative mortality improved following introduction of the Fogarty catheter, it remains high as reported by others, with the exception of Fogarty.

Table 4

Cause of Death in 30 Days of 165 (26%) of
631 Patients (689 Embolectomies)

Cardiac		114 (69%)
Congestive failure	96 (58%)	
Myocardial infarct	18 (11%)	
Cerebral vascular accident		16 (10%)
Visceral emboli		7 (4%)
Pulmonary embolism		4 (2%)
Acute respiratory distress		3 (2%)
Renal failure		3 (2%)
Carcinoma		4 (2%)
Lung		
Liver		
Miscellaneous		
Shock		8 (4%)
Ruptured abdominal aneurysm		
Dissecting aneurysm		
Septicemia		
Perforated viscus		
Unknown		7 (4%)

Life-Table Analysis of Survival After Embolectomy

Figure 5 presents the cumulative survival rate of 498 patients undergoing embolectomy with the catheter technique over a 24-year period. Late deaths numbered 93, 47 percent succumbing between 2 and 6 months postembolectomy. One patient survived 12½ years. Cardiac disease was the cause of death in 55 percent, malignancy in 13 percent, and stroke in 11 percent of the patients.

The life-table method of analysis does not reflect the late amputation rate. There were 10 late amputations. Five occurred in the first postoperative year and these might be considered to be possible complications of the embolic process. The other five occurred years later and possibly were secondary to progression of obliterative arterial disease. However, we recognize the possibility that the obliterative process itself may be compounded by multiple small emboli, particularly of the arteriogenic variety.

Operative Complications

By far the most common complication is anticoagulation hemorrhage postoperatively. This is a particular problem with which the surgeon has to struggle. It is highly tempting to continue the heparin in elderly patients from whose highly sclerotic arteries emboli have been removed in which thrombosis has been present for several hours or even days. Nevertheless, in our experience, if we maintain the heparin continuously there is a very high incidence of hemorrhage. Therefore, an effective policy is to delay the administration of further heparin after the operation for 6 to 12 hours, and then to use smaller doses for the first 24 hours. We today recommend longterm or permanent anticoagulant therapy

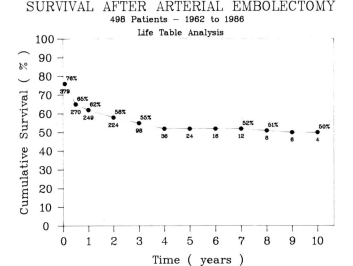

Fig. 5. Life-table analysis of survival after embolectomy, a 24-year followup of 498 patients undergoing 537 balloon catheter embolectomies.

for as long as the patient has an irregular cardiac rhythm. In patients who seem to have an arteriogenic source of the embolism, some of our associates use aspirin, others use full anticoagulation with sodium warfarin (Coumadin®).

Foot drop

This complication occurred in 4 patients in our recent series. Eight patients had post-embolectomy fasciotomy, 6 for anterior and 2 for posterior tibial compartment syndrome. Two patients had skin grafts in this area. In all instances, the foot drop improved.

One patient had a thrombosis after brachial artery embolectomy. He was treated by anticoagulant therapy. One month later, he had a cervical sympathectomy. His arm was good 10 months following embolectomy, but intermittent claudication was a sequela.

DIAGNOSIS

We are convinced that the history of the manner of onset is of critical importance. The usual categories of acute or sudden onset do not suffice. It is helpful to use the term "instantaneous," or "gradually," over a period of hours or days. Typically, the patient with a major embolus will be awakened from sleep or will be able to state precisely the moment of onset. The patient with arterial thrombosis, on the other hand, cannot do so. Rather, they state that they awakened, or rose from a chair, and found that the limb was numb. The large majority of patients report the instantaneous onset of pain and this is the best clue to arterial embolism. The onset may be described as very painful or as a sensation of numbness, then coldness, and then gradual loss of function of the limb. On physical examination, the color changes of the skin are striking. The Caucasian skin becomes lemon-yellow in color when there is a complete occlusion of the arterial system.

A good description of this color of the skin of all races is the appearance of the skin on the anterior aspect of the cadaver supine on the autopsy table. Depending on the lapse of time from lodgement of the embolism to examination, the affected extremity will be cooler than its opposite, and the pulses will be absent. It is helpful if the patient has had a previous examination and is known to have had palpable pulses, or if the pulses in the opposite limb are palpable. With common femoral emboli, one can almost always feel the common femoral artery. But as he moves his fingers down the superficial femoral artery, the pulse disappears. If one measures the segmental arterial pressures in the limb, they will be virtually zero and may be contrasted with those of the opposite limb. Only on rare occasion have we found it necessary or advisable to obtain an arteriogram for diagnosis.

CURRENT PLAN OF MANAGEMENT

As soon as the diagnosis is made, be it by the family physician or the operating surgeon, 5000 units of heparin are administered intravenously. If delay is unavoidable until operation, 10,000 units are given. The patient is taken to the operating room with the heparin not reversed; however, if there should be excessive bleeding during the procedure, one can always reverse the heparin with protamine. Today, virtually all emboli are removed in the lower extremity from the common femoral artery under local anesthesia. On occasion, we have opened the popliteal artery below the knee or the anterior or posterior tibial artery in the foot to remove thrombosis. Emboli in the shoulder area can be taken out through the brachial artery. If the embolism is in the forearm, we prefer to make an incision directly over the bifurcation of the brachial artery, so that a small catheter can be used on the radial and ulnar arteries.

Patients with very small arteries present a special problem. The surgeon may find it necessary to use a patch graft.

Postoperative Care

Normally, we do not reverse the heparin administered during or just prior to the operation. We recommend waiting 6 hours or more before giving additional heparin. As soon as the patient is able to take medication orally, warfarin sodium (Coumadin®) therapy is begun. When the prothrombin time has been within the therapeutic range for 2 days, the heparin is stopped. Longterm anticoagulant therapy is recommended as long as the patient has an irregular cardiac rhythm, and as well in some patients believed to have an arteriogenic source for the embolus.

EPILOGUE

The mortality rate for embolectomy is still high in all reported series. This fact suggests that the common denominator is not the technique, which has been standard for the past 20 years, but rather the nature of the disease, arterial emboli occurring in very high-risk patients. While further technical improvement is still possible, it is more likely that the next phase in the management of arterial embolism will emerge when safer and more predictable enzymatic agents are available.

REFERENCES

1. Murray DGW: Embolism in peripheral arteries. Canad Med Assoc J 35:61, 1936
2. Höpfner E: Ueber Gefässnäht, Gefässtransplantation and Replantation von amputirten Extremitäten. Arch Klin Chir 70:417, 1903
3. Labey, in Mosny DJ: Embolie fémorale au cours d'un rétrécissement mitral pur: Artériotomie; guérison. Bull Acad Med Paris 66:358, 1911
4. Key E: Embolectomy in the treatment of circulatory disturbances in the extremities. Surg Gynecol Obstet 36:309, 1923
5. Murray DGW: Heparin in thrombosis and embolism. Brit J Surg 27:567, 1940
6. Murray DGW: Anticoagulant therapy with heparin. Am J Med 3:468, 1947
7. Allen EV, Barker NW, Hines EA: Peripheral Vascular Diseases. Philadelphia, W.B. Saunders Company, 1962, p 394
8. Herrmann LG, Reid MR: Passive vascular exercises: Treatment of obliterative arterial diseases by rhythmic alternation of environmental pressure. Arch Surg 29:697, 1934
9. Cranley JJ, Krause RJ, Strasser ES, et al: Peripheral arterial embolism: Changing concepts. Surgery 55:57,71, 1964
10. Haimovici H: An evaluation of special problems in arterial embolism. Arch Surg 80:1, 1960
11. Warren R, Linton R: The treatment of arterial embolism. N Engl J Med 238:421, 1948
12. Shaw RS: A more aggressive approach toward the restoration of blood flow in acute arterial insufficiency. Surg Gynecol Obstet 103:279, 1956
13. Lord JW, Burke G: The comprehensive surgical management of aortic saddle emboli. Surgery 33:294, 1953
14. Olwin JH, Dye WS, Julian OC: Late arterial embolectomy. Arch Surg 66:480, 1953
15. Fogarty TJ, Cranley JJ, Krause RJ, et al: A method for extraction of arterial emboli and thrombi. Surg Gynecol Obstet 116:241, 1963
16. Spencer FC, Eiseman B: Delayed arterial embolectomy—a new concept. Surgery 55:64, 1964
17. Cranley JJ: Arterial Embolism, in Rob C (ed): Advances in Surgery. Vol. XI. Chicago, Year Book Med Publishers, 1977, pp 267–283
18. Cranley JJ, Krause RJ, Strasser ES, et al: Catheter technique for arterial embolectomy: A seven-year experience. J Cardiovas Surg 11:44, 1970
19. Stallone RJ, Blaisdell FW, Cafferata HT, et al: Analysis of morbidity and mortality from arterial embolectomy. Surgery 65:207, 1969

George H. Meier
David C. Brewster

Acute Arterial Thrombosis

Acute arterial occlusion, often resulting in sudden and severe ischemia, continues to present a challenging problem for the vascular surgeon. Despite numerous diagnostic and therapeutic advances, appropriate management of many patients in this diverse and heterogeneous group remains controversial and unsettled. Even recently reported experience emphasizes that the clinical outcome of acute limb ischemia is still associated with considerable morbidity, limb loss, and mortality.[1-3]

Acute arterial occlusion results, in almost all instances, from either trauma, embolus, or thrombosis in situ. While traumatic lesions are easily differentiated and managed by principles specific to injured vessels, separation of embolic and thrombotic causes of acute arterial ischemia is often considerably more difficult. For this reason, many authors choose to consider them together under the broad classification of acute arterial ischemia. The natural history, clinical implications, and optimal treatment of these two groups of patients are often substantially different, however, making it important to separate these causes as best possible. This chapter will focus on conditions causing acute arterial thrombosis, as distinct from arterial embolic occlusion that has been discussed in detail elsewhere. It should be acknowledged, however, that such conditions may indeed overlap, and that precise differentiation is often difficult and inexact. Once recognized as the cause of acute ischemia, subsequent therapy of arterial thrombosis is directed at prevention of further clot formation, determining the need for and timing of operation, and selection of a surgical procedure appropriate to the cause.

CAUSES OF ACUTE ARTERIAL THROMBOSIS

The acute onset of arterial thrombosis represents a heterogeneous group of patients with diseases that affect every level of the arterial circulation. Because there is no single etiology of thrombosis, it is the physician's task to differentiate between the myriad of possibilities and initiate treatment based on the most likely etiology of acute ischemia.

As indicated in Table 1, a large and diverse group of conditions may lead to acute arterial thrombosis.[4-7] Conceptually, these may be divided into intrinsic and extrinsic causes, based upon the location of the causative lesion or mechanism of occlusion.

By far the most common cause is thrombosis secondary to arteriosclerotic occlusive disease. This may occur as simply the terminal event in a vessel with a pre-existent severe stenosis due to slowly progressive chronic occlusive disease; in such cases, the thrombotic episode is unlikely to produce significant ischemia and clinical manifestations are apt to be relatively mild or even unrecognized. In other instances, however, arterial thrombosis may occur due to thrombus formation on a relatively nonocclusive atherosclerotic plaque, particularly if the surface of the plaque is ulcerated. Alternatively, sudden occlusion may be attributable to hemorrhage within or beneath a relatively nonocclusive plaque. Such a mechanism is widely accepted as a cause of sudden symptomatology or acute worsening of carotid occlusive lesions. If either of these two mechanisms is responsible, manifestations of acute ischemia may be much more severe, presumably due to the suddenness of the occlusion and lack of previously developed coliateral circulation.

Aneurysmal lesions of the arterial circulation often present with acute symptoms related to rupture; however, on occasion the initial manifestation of arterial aneurysms is acute thrombosis. Thrombosis of the aneurysm is more common the more peripherally the aneurysm is located anatomically. Thus, acute thrombosis is common for popliteal aneurysms, and often complicates femoral aneurysms.[8-11] Indeed, the frequency of acute thrombosis is one of the most compelling indications for elective repair of even small peripheral arterial aneurysms.[12,13] Acute thrombosis of aortic aneurysms is more unusual, but its occurrence often represents a catastrophic event and requires urgent surgical intervention.[14,15]

Previous arterial reconstructions, including both grafts and endarterectomy, clearly predispose the patient to acute thrombosis, not only secondary to post-surgical changes but also because previous surgery usually indicates the presence of diffuse arteriosclerotic occlusive disease. The diagnosis and management of acute ischemia resulting from thrombosis of prior arterial reconstructions is discussed in detail in other chapters and remains beyond the scope of the discussion here.

Several nonatherosclerotic arterial lesions may be responsible for acute thrombosis. Fibromuscular dysplasia, causing occlusion by either thrombosis in situ or local dissection, usually involves the carotid and renal arteries, but occasionally involves the iliac vessels or other peripheral arteries. Cystic adventitial disease may cause thrombosis of the

Table 1

Cause of Acute Arterial Thrombosis

Intrinsic	Extrinsic
Arteriosclerotic occlusive disease	Direct arterial injuries
Aneurysmal disease	Iatrogenic vascular injury
Failure of prior arterial reconstructions	Mechanical compression
Nonatherosclerotic vascular lesions	Hypercoagulable states
Aortic dissection	Metabolic and miscellaneous

popliteal artery, or rarely the femoral artery.[16] In the totally occluded vessel, diagnosis may be unsuspected preoperatively, although thrombosis of the popliteal artery in a young patient, without other risk factors, should certainly suggest the possibility of cystic disease or popliteal entrapment syndrome. Thromboangiitis obliterans usually involves relatively small vessels, but rarely may affect aortoiliac, femoral, or brachial vessels. Various arteritides, such as Takayasu's aortitis and giant cell arteritis, may result in arterial thrombosis. Obviously this represents a diverse group of diseases without clearly unifying features except for their predisposition to most often involve aortic arch branches, upper extremity vessels, or peripheral small arteries of the distal circulation.

A final intrinsic arterial lesion that may cause acute arterial thrombosis is arterial dissection. Although usually originating in the thoracic aorta, propagation of an aortic dissection and its false channel may compromise upper or lower extremity vessels as well as visceral branches of the aorta.[17] In some instances, acute extremity ischemia may be the first manifestation of an aortic dissection, particularly if the typical accompanying chest pain is minimal or absent, and mislead the unaware vascular surgeon into inappropriate efforts at embolectomy, et cetera.[18] On other occasions, arterial dissections may originate at diseased sites of the infrarenal aorta, iliac arteries, or similar peripheral locations, and be the cause of acute thrombosis.[19]

By far the most common extrinsic cause of acute arterial thrombosis is arterial injury, due to either blunt or penetrating trauma or iatrogenic causes. These problems are discussed in detail in other chapters. Less common conditions sometimes causing acute arterial thrombosis by extrinsic mechanisms include the thoracic outlet and popliteal entrapment syndromes. In each instance, sudden thrombosis may occur in an area of poststenotic aneurysm formation or due to intimal damage secondary to repeated compression and trauma.[20,21]

Various causes of hypercoagulability may cause acute arterial or venous thrombosis. Such conditions include heparin-induced thrombosis, anti-thrombin III deficiency, abnormalities of the fibrinolytic system, and abnormal platelet aggregation.[22] Many of these problems are difficult to recognize and incompletely understood, and diagnosis is often made only after excluding most other possible etiologies. Nonetheless, such conditions may be responsible for acute thrombosis occurring de novo in relatively normal arteries, or for unexplained postoperative occlusions.

Arterial thrombosis may occur secondary to various hematologic diseases, including polycythemia vera, thrombocytosis, or various types of dysproteinemias.[4] Again, these may often involve sudden thrombosis of relatively normal vessels, usually small vessels such as digital arteries. Hematologic consultation is often required for proper evaluation and therapy.

Finally, major arterial thrombosis may occur in a variety of miscellaneous conditions associated with abnormal physiologic states, even in the absence of intrinsic arterial disease. Various malignancies, particularly when advanced or highly undifferentiated, may be associated with acute arterial occlusion, presumably secondary to the existence of an ill-defined hypercoagulable state. Cardiac disease, septicemia, or other causes of a low output syndrome may result in arterial thrombosis due to flow reduction and vasoconstriction. Various medications associated with vasoconstriction, such as ergotism, have also been reported to cause ischemic symptoms and acute arterial thrombosis. Finally, intravascular effects of illegal substance abuse or vessel injury secondary to their intravascular injection may cause acute ischemia.[23,24]

INCIDENCE OF ACUTE ARTERIAL THROMBOSIS

The true incidence of acute arterial thrombosis is difficult to accurately determine, particularly for the diverse and more unusual causes. Some data are available regarding the most common form, acute thrombosis complicating arteriosclerotic occlusive disease. In general, acute arterial thrombosis accounts for one-third to one-half of all instances of acute arterial ischemia.[2,4] Haimovici summarized seven reports from the literature, comprising 1576 cases. An average of 43 percent of all acute arterial occlusions described in these reports were attributed to acute thrombotic causes.[25]

In a long term study of 1850 limbs, reported by Humphries and associates, sudden worsening of arterial insufficiency attributable to superimposed thrombosis occurred in 11 percent of patients with aortoiliac disease, 27 percent of patients with combined occlusive disease of both aortoiliac and femoropopliteal segments, and in 31 percent with femoropopliteal disease.[26] In the same study, sudden occlusion was the initial presentation of chronic occlusive disease in 6 percent of patients with aortoiliac disease, 8 percent with combined disease, and in 27 percent with femoropopliteal disease. Similar figures have been summarized by Spittell.[27] It must be remembered, however, that separation of thrombotic and embolic causes of acute arterial occlusion is often difficult, even at surgery or autopsy. In addition, the true incidence is difficult to ascertain as the patient often forgets exacerbations of symptoms if relatively mild or transient, or often fails to identify an acute event unless asked specifically about this.

PATHOPHYSIOLOGY

The overall effects of ischemia due to acute arterial thrombosis are, in general, similar to acute ischemia from any etiology. While acute embolic occlusion may often be somewhat more severe than thrombotic occlusion of atherosclerotic vessels, due to the existence of better collateral vessel formation in the latter category, the effects of equivalent degrees of ischemia are quite similar. The more active the cell's metabolism, the greater its susceptibility to anoxic damage. Because of differences in tolerance to ischemia and varying metabolic requirements, severe and sometimes irreversible anoxic injury appears to occur histologically in skeletal muscle or peripheral nerves at about 4 to 6 hours after the onset of profound and total ischemia, while other tissues such as skin may remain viable for longer periods.[28]

Several anatomic factors influence the extent of distal ischemia with thrombosis: location of the occlusion, size of the vessel involved, amount of clot present, and adequacy of collateral circulation. Quite obviously, occlusion of large vessels usually produces more dramatic manifestations. The amount of thrombus is of importance because of the greater likelihood that propagation of clot will compromise further branch vessels and interfere with critical collateral circulation. Quite clearly, however, the chief determinant of the effects of any acute arterial occlusion is the adequacy of collateral blood flow. If thrombosis occurs in relatively normal vessels or early in the course of an intrinsic arterial disease process, collateral formation may be poorly developed and resulting ischemia more severe. Alternatively, if thrombosis occurs late, collateral circulation may be well developed and significant distal ischemia minimal.

In the early stages of extremity ischemia, signs and symptoms are usually localized. If local ischemia is neglected, however, or if the ischemic process is more extensive,

systemic and secondary effects may soon follow. The toxic byproducts of tissue ischemia may have far reaching effects, and lead to systemic acidosis, hyperkalemia, myoglobinemia, renal failure, myocardial and/or CNS depression, and in late stages septicemia or superimposed associated deep venous thrombosis.[29] Many of these systemic effects are the cause of the high mortality associated with acute arterial ischemia, such as that seen in advanced thrombosis.[1]

Formerly, much emphasis was placed upon the necessity to intervene therapeutically within a 4 to 6 hour period, as it was felt that this usually represented the maximum period of tolerable ischemia. While this may be true in some instances, it is now well recognized that no arbitrary time limit can be applied to all cases, and that the physiologic state of the limb rather than elapsed time from the onset of occlusion best determines operability and salvageability. In many instances, enough collateral circulation may be present to allow survival of the ischemic limb although its function may be impaired. Indeed, in many instances of acute thrombosis, enough adequate collateral circulation may exist to allow heparinization and avoidance of emergency revascularization.

After revascularization, perfusion to the distal extremity may not return to normal for several hours. This "impaired reflow phenomenon" is most likely the result of cellular swelling after prolonged ischemia. Clearly, tissues lose membrane integrity with prolonged ischemia, possibly as a result of failure of the sodium pump.[30] Pretreatment with mannitol has been shown to be protective in these circumstances, suggesting that cellular swelling is involved in the prolongation of ischemia.[31] No matter what the etiology of delayed reperfusion, the end result of this process is prolonged distal ischemia. As a consequence, the actual length of tissue hypoperfusion is unpredictable and limb salvage uncertain no matter how rapidly revascularization is performed. Additionally, distal propagation of clot may occur and permanently impair distal collateral vessels and not be amenable to thrombectomy or other forms of management despite successful proximal revascularization. Such considerations reemphasize the importance of early therapeutic intervention in the acutely ischemic limb, and the importance of immediate administration of full doses of heparin as soon as the diagnosis of limb-threatening ischemia is confirmed.

DIFFERENTIAL DIAGNOSIS

Establishing the etiology of acute arterial occlusion is obviously important to appropriate management. Careful history and physical examination remain the mainstay of diagnosis. Many of the conditions causing acute arterial thrombosis have unique and characteristic features in the patient's history and examination that will allow their identification and guide therapy specific to each condition.

The major difficulty usually lies in distinguishing between the two major causes of acute arterial occlusion: embolic versus thrombotic. This separation may be difficult and sometimes inaccurate, even at the time of surgical exploration or autopsy. Nonetheless, distinguishing between these two major causes of the acutely ischemic limb is extremely important in selection of further therapy. Each condition has its own set of implications and associated problems that require recognition and treatment. Most importantly, the decision to proceed with surgical intervention is often substantially different, unless the limb is clearly nonviable. Thus, it is generally agreed that prompt surgical embolectomy, often without angiography and performed under local anesthesia, is the optimal treatment for acute arterial emboli. In contrast, attempts at simple thrombectomy for acute thrombosis in situ are often unsuccessful and indeed may worsen the degree and extent of ischemia. For arterial thrombosis, arterial reconstruction by grafting procedures or endarterectomy, often under general anesthesia, is generally necessary for a successful outcome. In such circumstances, avoiding emergency operation has several advantages, as outlined by Dale.[2] First, there may be uncertainty in the acute situation as to whether further thrombosis will occur, either proximally or distally, which might cause an arterial reconstruction to fail. Second, delay allows more complete evaluation and compensation of any associated disease processes. Third, further time is gained to obtain proper preoperative angiograms and the detailed anatomic information they offer. Fourth is the desirability of performing major arterial procedures with proper surgical and anesthetic personnel, appropriate instruments, et cetera, rather than with a partial team hastily assembled at odd hours. Finally, and perhaps most importantly, delay may allow development of improved collateral circulation. While this will rarely make elective reconstruction unnecessary, it may favorably influence the results of grafting procedures by improving runoff. Poor results of emergency graft procedures for acute ischemia have been reported by Couch and associates[32] and McPhail and colleagues[33] among others, and are well recognized by most experienced vascular surgeons. Presumably, poor results with emergency reconstructions reflect many of the factors above, and form the basis for the preference of most vascular surgeons to employ heparin and a nonoperative approach initially for acute thrombosis as long as the viability of the limb allows.

As shown in Table 2, several features of the history and physical examination may help make the distinction between acute embolic occlusion and acute arterial thrombosis. A history of prior claudication and findings of diminished pulses in other areas suggest the prior existence of occlusive disease and make thrombosis more likely. Although such symptoms have been found in over 80 percent of patients with acute thrombosis in some series,[33] other authors report that less than one-half of patients with acute thrombosis gave a history of prior occlusive symptoms.[3] In addition, embolic events may be superimposed on chronic occlusive disease, an event that is becoming increasingly common as the patient population with arterial emboli becomes more elderly and arteriosclerotic heart disease emerges as responsible for most cardiac conditions leading to arterial emboli.[34,35] A history or physical findings of a cardiac source of a peripheral arterial embolus certainly makes embolic occlusion more likely. In particular, the presence of atrial fibrillation makes an embolus highly probable, being found in 74 percent of patients with acutely

Table 2
Differentiation of Embolus from Thrombosis

	Embolus	Thrombosis
Identifiable source for embolus	Usual, particularly atrial fibrillation	Less common
History of claudication	Rare	Common
Physical findings suggestive of occlusive disease	Few; proximal and contralateral limb pulses normal	Often present; proximal or contralateral limb pulses diminished or absent
Arteriogram	Minimal atherosclerosis; sharp cutoff; few collaterals	Diffuse atherosclerosis; tapered, irregular cutoff; well-developed collaterals

ischemic limbs due to an embolus, as opposed to 4 percent felt to have acute thrombotic occlusion.[3]

Another finding felt classically to aid in differentiation of embolic and thrombotic etiologies is the temperature level demarcation. Typically, this is described as sharply demarcated in acute embolic occlusion, and less well defined in acute thrombosis due to better developed collateral networks. In reality, this finding is often inconclusive, however, and frequently not helpful in distinguishing embolus from thrombosis in limbs with equivalent severity of ischemia.

The anatomic location of an acute arterial occlusion may also be helpful. For example, acute brachial occlusion, without a history of trauma or other invasive procedures, is much more suggestive of embolic occlusion, as thrombosis in situ infrequently involves this area of the arterial tree.

Angiography may be extremely helpful. With acute thrombosis, evidence of occlusive disease will usually be noted in other vessels, and the site of occlusion will often be irregular with tapering and obvious plaquing evident above the occlusion. This is quite different from the classic findings in acute embolic occlusion, with nontapering normal vessels above the very sharply defined point of occlusion. With thrombosis, some contrast material may pass alongside the proximal portion of the clot; such "ghosting" is felt to suggest thrombosis in contrast to the sharp cutoff with a reversed meniscus typical of an acute embolic occlusion.

Several other angiographic features may help in differentiation. Obviously, the finding of multiple filling defects within several different arterial beds is almost certain to suggest an embolic etiology. The location of occlusion in an artery may also be helpful. For instance, occlusion noted in the mid to distal superficial femoral artery, centered about the adductor canal, would be typical of acute thrombotic occlusion, while an embolus typically lodges at arterial bifurcations. These findings may be obscured, however, by subsequent propagation of clot. For example, an acute popliteal embolus occluding the distal popliteal artery may develop secondary retrograde thrombus up the superficial femoral artery to the point of a large geniculate vessel, making determination of the exact point of occlusion less certain.

Perhaps the most helpful finding on angiography is the status of collateral vessels. A well developed network of collateral vessels clearly suggests acute thrombosis of a chronically diseased vessel, while scanty, poorly developed collateral vessels are much more typical of an acute embolic occlusion. With thrombosis, the distal arterial tree may often be reconstituted by collaterals and visualized on preoperative arteriography, whereas the absence of collaterals often makes it impossible to ascertain patency of the distal arterial bed with acute embolus and necessitates completion arteriography in the operating room when the clot is removed.

The advisability and usefulness of angiography for the acutely ischemic limb remains controversial. Our own feelings are that preoperative arteriography for embolic disease is rarely necessary or helpful. Indeed, the additional time taken often only prolongs the ischemia and increases the possibility of a poor outcome. In acute emboli, the distal outflow tract is often not visualized, and little useful information is gained.

In patients felt likely to have acute arterial thrombosis, however, preoperative arteriography is very important, both to delineate the site and extent of occlusion, evaluate alternative inflow sources for reconstruction, and ascertain patency of runoff vessels. In addition, the surgeon cannot be sure of the etiology of acute occlusion in many patients with an acutely ischemic limb, and in many of these instances angiography may be extremely helpful in deciding on the probable cause of occlusion. Therefore, it is our policy to utilize preoperative arteriographic study whenever uncertainty exists in the diagnosis. It is so often helpful and safe that its use should invariably be considered except in cases of clear-cut embolism.

MANAGEMENT

Management of acute ischemia involves reestablishment of distal circulation sufficient to avoid hypoxic damage to the tissues of the involved extremity. In most instances, surgical intervention is the mainstay of treatment of ischemia of any etiology. However, as already noted, emergency surgical procedures for acute thrombotic arterial occlusions may be associated with relatively poor results.[1,2] For this reason, immediate operation for acute thrombosis is avoided by many surgeons if possible, as determined by limb viability. In addition, problems with immediate operation for prolonged or severe ischemia have led some to suggest nonoperative treatment with high dose heparin alone, or initial management with thrombolytic therapy.

When a patient presents with acute ischemia, the initial management is similar, independent of the etiology. Prevention of further clot formation is of primary importance. Heparin should be administered immediately in any patient with compromised circulation, even prior to angiography, embolectomy, or acute reconstruction. The prevention of proximal and distal clot propagation is of critical importance and may provide the difference between a successful revascularization and amputation. This clot propagation can be largely prevented by early heparin administration, maintaining patent collaterals until such time as surgery may be undertaken. The normal dosage of heparin is 5000 units by intravenous bolus, followed by a drip of 1000 units/hour. If time allows, adjustment of dosage to maintain the partial thromboplastin time at 1.5 to 2 × control is optimal. Heparin is rarely a problem if everyone is aware of its use preoperatively; the one area where alteration of technique may be necessary is in anesthetic management, as epidural and spinal anesthetics are contraindicated in anticoagulated patients. If necessary, heparin is readily reversible with intravenous protamine on a milligram for milligram basis.

Concomitantly, initial history and physical examination should seek to identify the probable cause of the thrombotic occlusion and determine the necessity of immediate operative intervention. In acute arterial thrombosis, this later decision is generally based upon judgments of the degree of ischemia and limb viability. Advanced ischemia is characterized by diminished to absent motor and sensory function, reflecting ischemia to both muscles and nerves distal to the arterial occlusion.[34] The first modality of sensation lost is light touch; if this element is preserved, then the limb is likely viable. Paralysis and absence of light touch are grave signs that urgent revascularization is needed. With loss of sensation and motion preoperatively, the ultimate function of the involved limb may be permanently compromised and the ischemia may induce metabolic changes that can be systemic and occasionally life-threatening. If the limb is judged viable, further evaluation may be undertaken without the added risk of emergency intervention. Arterial reconstruction may be planned for a later time under more favorable circumstances. If, on the other hand, the limb is judged nonviable without immediate revascularization, emergency operation may be required for limb salvage and represent the only alternative to amputation.

Operative Therapy

Surgical therapy for limb-threatening acute arterial thrombosis remains the principal mode for restoration of distal circulation. Operative therapy begins with the choice of anesthesia for the procedure. While a localized procedure may be readily performed under local anesthesia, the patient and surgeon should be prepared for epidural or general anesthesia as the situation dictates. The operative field must be widely prepped so that extension of incisions can easily be accomplished or other dissections may be undertaken without further prepping or draping. Similarly, vertical incision should be utilized for easy extension.

Whereas embolic episodes are best treated by early embolectomy using a Fogarty catheter, thrombosis requires arterial reconstruction in nearly all situations to achieve maximum limb salvage.[2,3] If the surgeon is unsure of the diagnosis, it is reasonable to begin with attempted thromboembolectomy. However, the surgeon must be aware of the signs of atherosclerotic thrombosis and be prepared to move ahead with more definitive reconstructive surgery if indicated.

The type of reconstruction is dictated by the anatomy of the patient's disease, thus the importance of preoperative angiography. If the thrombosis is of a short segment and a good distal lumen is apparent, thrombectomy followed by endarterectomy may be an appropriate option. Patch closure of the endarterectomized segment may be useful if the arterial lumen appears narrow or closure might threaten patency. Conversely, if the thrombosis involves a long segment or distal disease precludes endarterectomy, then bypass is the mainstay of surgical therapy.

Emergency inflow procedures for aortic thrombosis carry a very high mortality and limb salvage rates are poor.[3] There are several explanations for the higher morbidity and mortality. First, extensive ischemia results from aortic occlusion, causing severe and diverse metabolic derangements. Second, in some patients with aortic thrombosis, extension of the thrombus proximally may impair renal function by occlusion of the orifices of the renal arteries.[15] In fact, in one series 6 of 12 patients who did not have surgery died secondary to renal failure from proximal extension of thrombus.[36] Bergan and Trippel suggested that aortic thrombosis extends to involve one or both renal arteries in 3 to 15 percent of patients with a distal aortic occlusion.[37] Proximal extension of thrombus may even cause occlusion of the superior mesenteric artery or celiac axis with resultant intestinal ischemia. In some instances, acute aortic thrombosis has also led to spinal cord ischemia, presumably from associated thrombosis of the spinal cord circulation.

If surgical management of an occluded aorta is necessary, this varies somewhat from the routine aortic operation.[15] Proximal dissection should extend to the suprarenal aorta and both renal arteries should be dissected free and controlled. The arteriotomy is initiated on the thrombosed segment of aorta and brought upward to about 2 centimeters distal to the renal arteries. Thrombectomy is then performed to remove the proximal clot, with the renal arteries clamped if jeopardized by this procedure. Initial digital control of the inflow may aid in performing the thromboembolectomy. The renal arteries are allowed to backbleed, clamp control of the aorta is obtained distal to the renal arteries and perfusion is restored to the renal arteries. From this point forward, standard aortic graft replacement is performed.

Extraanatomic bypass for acute aortic or iliac occlusions is a consideration in their management. With aortic occlusion, axillofemoral bypass is possible, but the risk of proximal clot propagation as discussed above is still present after revascularization. With unilateral iliac artery occlusion, femorofemoral bypass may be the easiest and best form of reconstruction in the emergency setting.

Acute thrombosis in the femoral and popliteal regions is often difficult to differentiate from embolic causes. The surgical approach in these areas often necessitates that exploration be undertaken, and surgical therapy be dictated by the findings at operation and intraoperative arteriography, as outlined above.

The metabolic derangements associated with revascularization of the acutely ischemic limb consist primarily of acidosis, hyperkalemia, myoglobin release, and byproducts of thrombus degeneration.[29] The acidosis, hyperkalemia, and myoglobin release can be adequately treated by intravenous administration of bicarbonate just prior to reperfusion. Similarly, mannitol should be given at the first sign of diminished urine output, as renal failure may be rapidly precipitated without antecedent changes. Some authors have gone so far as to advocate drainage of the initial venous outflow to avoid systemic effects from the byproducts present in the severely ischemic extremity.[7] In short, the period after initial reperfusion is critical, and anesthetic management of marked importance.

The operative success of revascularization is sometimes difficult to ascertain intraoperatively secondary to delayed reflow or slow reperfusion after surgical revascularization. However, it is essential that distal flow be assessed and adequate revascularization assured. There are several methods that are currently available for intraoperative assessment of success. Perhaps the most common and readily available technique is intraoperative completion arteriography. After completion of revascularization a single bolus of iodine-containing contrast (Renografin 60 or Conray 60, about 25 to 40 cc in the femoral location) is administered and a single x-ray plate is exposed in routine fashion. This resultant angiogram will produce a film of suitable quality for the detection of residual thrombus or incomplete revascularization. A second modality that may be employed is use of intraoperative Doppler flow probes for detection of distal flow beyond the reconstruction. The sound signal is qualitative, but normal arterial sounds are triphasic, extending into early diastole; with practice, one can insure flow representative of adequate revascularization. Finally, intraoperative plethysmography has been shown to be useful for objectively assessing adequacy of reconstruction.[38] This technique is useful in both intraoperative and postoperative evaluation of revascularization.

Postoperatively, heparin should not be routinely used; occasionally if the surgeon remains unsure as to the etiology of occlusion or if thrombectomy alone is performed, postoperative heparin therapy may be indicated. This will require careful monitoring to prevent an excessive incidence of hematomas or other bleeding problems in fresh operative wounds. Similarly, dextran may be useful in those cases where platelet thrombosis may be problematic or where small vessel spasm or thrombosis is involved. Endarterectomy or distal small vessel bypass may be appropriate situations where dextran is useful to prevent platelet aggregation and thrombus formation.

Fasciotomy is used to release lower extremity compartments to prevent swelling from impairing distal blood flow. While this has been applied commonly with arterial trauma or acute ischemia from venous causes, its use in acute arterial thrombosis is less well defined.[39] The arguments against performing fasciotomy center around the possibility of injuring peripheral nerves or vessels with resultant sensory deficits or bleeding, or of secondary wound problems involving the fasciotomy incisions themselves. Conversely, fasciotomy is easily performed, even at the bedside under local anesthesia. While some have advocated use of compartmental pressure measurements as a more objective indicator of the need for fasciotomy,[40,41] most surgeons have found them difficult and of

uncertain reliability. Final decisions regarding fasciotomy for acute thrombosis are often made based upon individual preferences and prior clinical experience. Fasciotomy, if used in these circumstances, is often best done as a delayed procedure if and when severe swelling develops following revascularization.

High Dose Heparin Therapy

Blaisdell[1] believes that the surgical results in acute arterial ischemia are suboptimal and that other treatment modalities may provide lower mortality and similar limb salvage. In an effort to improve results, he has adopted heparin anticoagulation as preferred therapy of the acutely ischemic extremity. He suggests a regimen of high dose anticoagulation as the primary treatment modality, with the use of surgery in conjunction with anticoagulation only if the patient is seen within 6 to 8 hours of the onset of ischemia. In his initial report, he and his associates selectively treated 29 acutely ischemic patients with high dose heparin therapy with a 20,000 unit bolus followed by 2,000 to 4,000 units/ hour. Seventeen additional patients underwent immediate thromboembolectomy, and six immediate amputation. His success is notable in that the overall mortality was only 7.5 percent and limb salvage was 67 percent.[1] This compares to historical controls where mortality is 25 to 29 percent and limb salvage is 60 to 70 percent. However, many criticisms have emerged to contradict the routine use of high dose heparin as the primary therapy for advanced ischemia. First, it has been noted that limb salvage rates in current series[42-44] are much better than previously reported, thereby lessening the impact of Blaisdell's data. Second, the dosage of heparin used in Blaisdell's series is much higher than that routinely used for systemic anticoagulation. Therefore the risk of bleeding complications with this therapy may be dramatically higher than that seen with routine doses. Third, there is no differentiation in Blaisdell's series among the various etiologies of acute, advanced ischemia. Differences in limb salvage are obviously influenced by the factors involved in causation. Finally, the definition of "advanced ischemia" is not clear among all observers, and results may vary accordingly.

Blaisdell's approach fits nicely in the management scheme of patients with acute arterial thrombosis who have viable limbs. In addition, this mode of treatment does not preclude operative therapy if the extremity worsens, but irreversible ischemic damage is a constant danger. We would take exception with its routine application to the patient with acute arterial thrombosis, as we believe greater limb salvage can be achieved by prompt operative therapy when necessary, at an acceptable mortality rate. His utilization of high dose heparin or immediate amputation may certainly have application, however, for the truly nonviable limb with advanced irreversible ischemia, in which revascularization has almost no hope of salvage and may be associated with devastating complications.

Thrombolytic Therapy

In recent years, another form of nonoperative therapy has become available for treatment of acute ischemia due to arterial thrombosis: use of intra-arterial thrombolytic therapy, sometimes combined with percutaneous transluminal angioplasty. With thrombolytic therapy, the body's intrinsic fibrinolytic system is activated with potential lysis of thrombus in acutely occluded vessels or arterial grafts as well as clots in distal vascular beds. In the late 1960s, a number of reports appeared regarding use of systemic therapy with streptokinase for the treatment of arterial occlusion. Systemic delivery of this agent resulted in a high incidence of hemorrhagic complications and only mediocre results of clot dissolution. Dotter et al in 1974 reported direct intra-arterial infusion of streptokinase in the treatment of acute and chronic arterial occlusion.[45] With this technique, clot lysis may be achieved with dosages far lower than that required by systemic infusion.

Two primary agents have been utilized for this mode of treatment, streptokinase and urokinase. Streptokinase was the first agent available for thrombolytic therapy and remains the least expensive. However, streptokinase may be difficult to regulate due to its antigenicity. Antibodies to streptokinase are found in a large percentage of patients due to previous exposure to B-hemolytic Streptococcus. After one course of treatment with streptokinase, essentially all patients develop antibodies in response to the agent. Such antibody titers may increase with streptokinase treatment and result in diminished effect with subsequent usage. Therefore the dose-response relationship is difficult to establish with any certainty. More recently, experience with urokinase as the fibrinolytic agent has accumulated. Urokinase, although more expensive, appears more controllable, quicker, and safer, perhaps due to its lack of antigenicity and direct conversion of plasminogen to plasmin. Selective intra-arterial infusion of either agent has the advantage of delivery of a higher concentration of the agent directly to the region of thrombosis, allowing a lower total infusion dose and potentially fewer side effects.

Recent reviews of thrombolytic therapy[46-49] suggest that low dose intra-arterial thrombolytic therapy may be an effective alternative in the treatment of acute thrombotic arterial occlusion. If angiography demonstrates a thrombotic occlusion and the patient's limb is viable, thrombolytic therapy offers the possibility of re-establishing blood flow, alleviating acute ischemia, and allowing definition of underlying arterial pathology. Subsequent elective revascularization, or even balloon angioplasty, may then be undertaken. Specific advantages of thrombolytic therapy may be its ability to provide a more accurate preoperative diagnosis, thereby allowing a simpler vascular reconstruction. In addition, thrombolytic therapy may open an occluded distal vascular bed, and make reconstruction feasible in what initially may appear to be a nonsalvageable situation. For example, the initial arteriogram of a patient presenting with acute thrombosis of a popliteal aneurysm may reveal only an occluded popliteal artery with poor or even no visualization of runoff vessels. Immediate selective intra-arterial thrombolytic therapy may open the popliteal artery, revealing a popliteal aneurysm as the cause of the occlusion and improving distal runoff. Less urgent and more limited reconstruction of the popliteal artery can then be carried out.

In a recent study, selective management with low-dose streptokinase allowed elective surgery for thrombosis in 37 percent and elective angioplasty in an additional 21 percent of patients.[46] Most authors, however, agree that the exact role of this mode of therapy has yet to be fully delineated and several questions remain.[50] First, since thrombolytic therapy often requires from 24 to 72 hours to achieve thrombolysis, it is clear that it is not appropriate for extremities with such advanced ischemia that immediate revascularization is required to preserve limb viability. Second, once successful, definitive therapy must still be undertaken to prevent rethrombosis, a situation where transluminal angioplasty may become more useful. Third, with partial dissolution of thrombus, peripheral embolization may occur that can be a serious problem, sometimes preventing any further therapy including surgery. Finally, a small but real risk exists for severe bleeding complications such as intracranial hemorrhage with the use of thrombolytic agents. A recently introduced agent, tissue plasminogen activator, may improve the specificity of thrombolysis and prevent bleeding complications while avoiding the hazards of intra-arterial therapy.[51] These questions must be more fully answered before the ultimate role of thrombolytic therapy in acute arterial ischemia is defined.

SMALL VESSEL THROMBOSIS

Acute arterial thrombosis occurs not only in large vessels but also in acral end arteries of the upper and lower extremities. Thrombotic events in small vessels are very different from those seen in large vessel occlusion and the etiology is more commonly related to systemic diseases other than atherosclerosis. A variety of causes contribute to small vessel thrombosis and many factors may interact to produce tissue ischemia. While some of these are applicable to large vessel thrombosis as well, most are unique to the arterial circulation and small vessels. Perhaps the factor most important in small vessels is vasospasm, a characteristic that compounds and prolongs any ischemic insult in the distribution of the artery involved.

Etiology

Without a doubt, the most significant risk factor for small vessel thrombosis is cigarette smoking. The vasospasm associated with small vessel disease of any cause is aggravated by the vasospastic effects of nicotine. Similarly, cold exposure may precipitate vasospasm even in normal arteries and therefore be a contributing factor in all but the most tropical of locales.

The causes of acute small vessel thrombosis are multiple and diverse and often difficult to establish conclusively.[52] The collagen vascular diseases are frequent offenders, with both scleroderma and systemic lupus erythematosus being the most common types. Other diseases may be more common in cold weather, such as frostbite, cryoglobuline-mia, and Raynaud's phenomenon of any cause. Pharmacologic therapy may give rise to arteriolar thrombosis when potent vasoconstrictors or ergot are administered. A variant of atherosclerosis seen in the end arteries is thromboangiitis obliterans, a disorder whose presenting symptoms often represent small vessel thrombosis.[53] Trauma to the hand vessels from chronic occupational injury can result in small artery aneurysms and thrombosis.[54] Polycythemia,[55] uremia,[56] and nonspecific arteritis all present commonly with small vessel thrombosis and digital ischemia or ulceration.

Management

The management of these diverse causes of small vessel thrombosis is made more difficult by the marked differences in pathophysiology among them. While specific therapy can be directed at the underlying etiology, the common thread at which therapy can be directed in all the disorders is vasospasm. There are two main approaches to treatment of vasospasm, pharmacologic manipulation and sympathectomy. In many patients, however, spontaneous resolution of the ischemia occurs for unknown reasons.[57]

Pharmacologic manipulations for the amelioration of vasospasm can follow any of several paths. Perhaps the simplest of approaches is oral administration of medication, either direct vasodilators or sympathetic blockers. While in theory these offer the most direct means of intervention in vasospasm, prediction of pharmacologic effect is impossible. Therefore sequential therapeutic trials are often necessary to find the most valuable medication in any individual's disease.

A second route of administration of medication is the intra-arterial path, often at the time of diagnostic angiography. The most common and perhaps most successful medication via this route is reserpine. Reserpine has effects of sympathetic blockade and vasodilatation for up to 6 months after a single administration. Recent concerns about possible tumor-genicity and commercial unprofitability have led to unavailability of parenteral reserpine currently. Other vasodilating agents such as nitroglycerine, calcium channel blockers, e.g., verapamil, tolazoline, or papaverine, may be utilized for intra-arterial infusion, but in general are short-acting and any benefits from vasodilatation short-lived. Although favorable reports on the use of various prostaglandins have appeared, mainly in the European literature, they remain of unproven value. The few randomized placebo-controlled studies with these agents have failed to show any consistent benefit.

Surgical sympathectomy has been proposed in the past as a mode of treatment in vasospastic disease. However, inconsistency in effect resulting from variation in surgical technique or variation in disease processes has limited the usefulness of this surgical adjunct. Current opinion is that sympathectomy has no utility in Raynaud's disease.[58] In those cases where no options exist for medical treatment or where tissue loss is not inevitable, sympathectomy may produce some relief of symptoms. However, the effects are often short-lived and tissue loss is sometimes unavoidable. Prior to surgery, sympathetic blockade using local anesthesia helps predict which patients might benefit from operation.

CONCLUSION

The diagnosis and treatment of acute atherosclerotic thrombosis is complex and difficult. However, several principles emerge that may be helpful in the management of this disorder. First, initial evaluation should attempt to differentiate thrombosis from embolus as the cause of ischemia. Although often difficult, separation may frequently be possible, particularly with liberal use of angiography. Second, while most embolic arterial occlusions are best treated by prompt operation, initial nonoperative management of acute arterial thrombosis is often best if viability of the limb allows. Third, all patients with acute ischemia should receive immediate full doses of intravenous heparin, irrespective of presumed diagnosis, while further evaluation proceeds. Fourth, immediate surgical reconstruction is still preferred for most patients with limbs judged nonviable without immediate revascularization, unless ischemia is very advanced and the limb clearly non-salvageable. The problems attendant to reperfusion must be recognized however. Fifth, thrombectomy alone is almost always inadequate for acute arterial thrombosis; some form of more definitive arterial reconstruction, most usually a bypass graft, is necessary. Sixth, several alternative forms of therapy are available for those patients with viable extremities. Finally, surgical therapy remains the standard of care in thrombotic occlusion and it is this form of therapy to which all alternative modalities must be compared.

Small vessel thrombosis is a potpourri of separate disease entities, each with nuances with regard to management. In most cases, the disease process is self-limiting if predisposing factors are corrected. In those patients whose disease progresses, however, it is often a matter of trial and error to find the most effective therapeutic intervention.

Ultimately, the treatment of each patient must be individualized, elected by the vascular surgeon after consideration of the events and features unique to each situation. While few universals exist in this area, successful management is possible in the majority of patients.

REFERENCES

1. Blaisdell FW, Steele M, Allen RE: Management of acute lower extremity arterial ischemia due to embolism and thrombosis. Surgery 84:822, 1978
2. Dale WA: Differential management of acute peripheral arterial ischemia. J Vasc Surg 1:269, 1984
3. Cambria RP, Abbott WM: Acute arterial thrombosis of the lower extremity. Arch Surg 119:784, 1984
4. Fairbairn JF, Joyce JW, Pairolero PC: Acute arterial occlusion of the extremities, in Juergens JL, Spittell JA Jr, Fairbairn JF II (eds): Peripheral Vascular Diseases. Philadelphia, WB Saunders Co., 1980, pp 381–401
5. Zimmerman JJ, Fogarty TJ: Acute arterial occlusions, in Moore WS (ed): Vascular Surgery: A Comprehensive Review. New York, Grune & Stratton, 1983, pp 693–711
6. Haimovici H: Acute arterial thrombosis, in Haimovici H (ed): Vascular Surgery: Principles and Techniques, 2nd edition. Norwalk, Appleton-Century-Crofts, 1984, pp 379–387
7. Perry MO: Acute arterial insufficiency of the extremities, in Rutherford RB (ed): Vascular Surgery, 2nd edition. Philadelphia, WB Saunders Co, 1984, pp 440–448
8. Vermilion BD, Kimmins SA, Pace WG, et al: A review of one hundred forty-seven popliteal aneurysms with long-term follow-up. Surgery 90:1009, 1981
9. Szilagyi DE, Schwartz RL, Reddy DJ: Popliteal arterial aneurysms: Their natural history and management. Arch Surg 116:724, 1981
10. Cutler BS, Darling RC: Surgical management of arteriosclerotic femoral aneurysm. Surgery 74:764, 1973
11. Graham LM, Zelenock GB, Whitehouse WM Jr, et al: Clinical significance of femoral artery aneurysms. Arch Surg 115:502, 1980
12. Reilly KM, Abbott WM, Darling RC: Aggressive surgical management of popliteal artery aneurysms. Am J Surg 145:498, 1983
13. Connolly JE: True aneurysms of the peripheral arteries, in Moore WS (ed): Vascular Surgery: A Comprehensive Review. New York, Grune & Stratton, 1983, pp 335–349
14. Johnson JM, Gaspar MR, Movius HJ, et al: Sudden complete thrombosis of aortic and iliac aneurysms. Arch Surg 108:792, 1974
15. Corson JD, Brewster DC, Darling RC: The surgical management of infrarenal aortic occlusion. Surg Gynecol Obstet 155:369, 1982
16. Flanigan DP, Burnham SJ, Goodreau JJ, et al: Summary of cases of adventitial cystic disease of the popliteal artery. Ann Surg 189:165, 1979
17. Hunter JA, Dye WS, Javid H, et al: Abdominal aortic resection in thoracic dissection. Arch Surg 111:1258, 1976
18. Amer NC, Schaeffer HC, Domengo RT, et al: Aortic dissection presenting as iliac-artery occlusion: an aid to early diagnosis. N Engl J Med 266:1040, 1962
19. Wychulis AR, Kincaid OW, Wallace RB: Primary dissecting aneurysms of peripheral arteries. Mayo Clin Proc 44:804, 1969
20. Dorazio RA, Ezzet F: Arterial complications of the thoracic outlet syndrome. Am J Surg 138:246, 1979
21. Rich NM, Collins GJ, McDonald PT, et al: Popliteal vascular entrapment: Its increasing interest. Arch Surg 114:1377, 1979

22. Towne JB: Hypercoagulable states and unexplained vascular thrombosis, in Bernhard VM, Towne JB (eds): Complications in Vascular Surgery, 2nd edition. Orlando, Grune & Stratton, 1985, pp 381–404

23. Wright CB, Geelhoed GW, Hobson RW, et al: Acute vascular insufficiency due to abuse of drugs, in Rutherford RB (ed): Vascular Surgery, 2nd edition. Philadelphia, WB Saunders Co, 1984, pp 501–512

24. Gaspar MR: Acute arterial lesions due to drug abuse, in Haimovici H (ed): Vascular Emergencies. New York, Appleton-Century-Crofts, 1982, pp 241–250

25. Haimovici H: Acute atherosclerotic thrombosis, in Haimovici H (ed): Vascular Emergencies. New York, Appleton-Century-Crofts, 1982, pp 213–223

26. Humphries AW, Young JR: The severely ischemic leg. Curr Probl Surg, June 1970, pp 1–59

27. Spittell JS Jr: Acute aortic and peripheral arterial occlusion: Incidence, and significance of thromboemboli, in Sherry S, Brinkhaus KM, Genton E, Stengle JM (eds): Washington D.C., National Academy of Sciences, 1969, p. 171

28. Malan E, Tattoni G: Physio- and anatomo-pathology of acute ischemia of the extremities. J Cardiovasc Surg 4:212, 1963

29. Haimovici H: Muscular, renal and metabolic complications of acute arterial occlusions. Myonephropathic-metabolic syndrome. Surgery 85:461, 1979

30. Krug A, de Rochemont W, Korb G: Blood supply of the myocardium after temporary coronary occlusion. Circ Res 19:57, 1966

31. Willerson JT, Powell WJ, Guiney TE, et al: Improvement in myocardial function and coronary blood flow in ischemic myocardium after mannitol. J Clin Invest 51:2989, 1972

32. Couch NP, Wheeler HB, Hyatt DF, et al: Factors influencing limb survival after femoropopliteal reconstruction. Arch Surg 95:163, 1967

33. McPhail NV, Fratesi SJ, Barber GG, et al: Management of acute thromboembolic limb ischemia. Surgery 93:381, 1983

34. Brewster DC: Arterial embolism: Diagnosis and management, in Coodley EL (ed): Geriatric Heart Disease. Littleton, Massachusetts, PSG Publishing Co., Inc., 1985, pp 239–247

35. Abbott WM, Maloney RD, McCabe CC, et al: Arterial embolism: A 44 year perspective. Am J Surg 143:460, 1982

36. Starrett RW, Stoney RJ: Juxtarenal aortic occlusion. Surgery 76:890, 1974

37. Bergan JJ, Trippel OH: Management of juxta-renal aortic occlusions. Arch Surg 87:60, 1963

38. O'Hara PJ, Brewster DC, Darling RC, et al: The value of intraoperative monitoring using the pulse volume recorder during peripheral vascular surgery. Surg Gynecol Obstet 152:275, 1981

39. Patman RD: Fasciotomy: indications and technique, in Rutherford RB (ed): Vascular Surgery, 2nd edition. Philadelphia, WB Saunders Co., 1984, pp 513–523

40. Whitesides TE, Haney TC, Harada H, et al: A simple method of tissue pressure determination. Arch Surg 110:1311, 1975

41. Matsen FA, Winquist RA, Krugmire RB: Diagnosis and management of compartment syndromes. J Bone Joint Surg (Am) 62:286, 1980

42. Plecha FR: Discussion of Blaisdell FW, Steele M, Allen RE: Management of acute lower extremity arterial ischemia due to embolism and thrombosis. Surgery 84:822, 1978

43. Fogarty TJ: Discussion of Blaisdell FW, Steele M, Allen RE: Management of acute lower extremity arterial ischemia due to embolism and thrombosis. Surgery 84:822, 1978

44. Tawes RL, Harris EJ, Brown WH, et al: Arterial thromboembolism. Arch Surg 120:595, 1985

45. Dotter CT, Rosch J, Seaman AJ: Selective clot lysis with low-dose streptokinase. Radiology 111:31, 1974

46. Rodriguez RL, Short DH, Puyau FA, et al: Selective management of arterial occlusion with low-dose streptokinase. Am J Surg 151:343, 1986

47. Berkowitz HD, Hargrove WC III, Roberts B: Thrombolytic therapy for arterial occlusion, in Kempczinski RF (ed): The Ischemic Leg. Chicago, Year Book Medical Publishers, Inc., 1985, pp 255–268

48. Katzen BT, Edwards KC, Albert AS, et al: Low-dose direct fibrinolysis in peripheral vascular disease. J Vasc Surg 1:718, 1984
49. Sicard GA, Schier JJ, Totty WG, et al: Thrombolytic therapy for acute arterial occlusion. J Vasc Surg 2:65, 1985
50. Porter JM, Taylor LM Jr: Current status of thrombolytic therapy. J Vasc Surg 2:239, 1985
51. Topol E, Ciuffo AA, Pearson TA, et al: Thrombolysis with recombinant tissue plasminogen activator in atherosclerotic thrombotic occlusion. J Am Coll Cardiol 5:85, 1985
52. McNamara MF, Takaki HS, Yao JST, et al: A systematic approach to severe hand ischemia. Surgery 83:1, 1978
53. Spittell JA: Some uncommon types of occlusive peripheral arterial disease. Curr Prob Cardiol 8:1, 1983
54. May JW, Grossman JA, Costas B: Cyanotic painful index and long fingers associated with an asymptomatic ulnar artery aneurysm: Case report. J Hand Surg 7:622, 1982
55. Barabas AP, Offen DN, Meinhard EA: The arterial complications of polycythemia vera. Br J Surg 60:183, 1973
56. Gipstein RM, Coburn JW, Adams DA, et al: Calciphylaxis in man. A syndrome of tissue necrosis and vascular calcification in 11 patients with chronic renal failure. Arch Intern Med 136:1273, 1976
57. Baur GM, Porter JM, Bardana EJ, et al: Rapid onset of hand ischemia of unknown etiology. Ann Surg 186:184, 1977
58. Dale WA: Thoracic sympathectomy, in Dale WA (ed): Management of Vascular Surgical Problems. New York, McGraw-Hill, 1985, pp 310–322

Paul Collier, Enrico Ascer
Frank J. Veith, Sushil K. Gupta
Anselmo A. Nunez

Acute Thrombosis of Arterial Grafts

Acute thrombosis of arterial bypass grafts can occur at any time after their insertion. Early graft thrombosis (within the first postoperative month) may be due to transient hypotension, an imperfectly chosen or performed operative procedure or an unusually elevated resistance in the outflow bed.[1-4] Late graft thrombosis (more than 1 month postoperatively) may be due to anastomotic intimal hyperplasia, intrinsic disease in the vein graft, or progression of proximal or distal atherosclerosis, although some prosthetic grafts can thrombose without any apparent explanation.[1,2,5] Intimal hyperplasia usually causes graft failure 2–18 months postoperatively, whereas disease progression usually produces graft thrombosis after the first postoperative year.[1,2]

The signs and symptoms of acute graft thrombosis are highly variable. Some patients present with loss of palpable pulses in their graft or distal arteries and are otherwise asymptomatic except possibly for redevelopment of their intermittent claudication. These patients need not be subjected to arteriography or reoperation. However, other patients develop acute symptoms when their grafts close. These symptoms range from pain in the distal limb to severe ischemia with loss of sensory and motor function and varying degrees of myonecrosis. It is these latter patients with threatened extremities who require urgent evaluation by arteriography and reoperation.

GRAFT SURVEILLANCE AND THE FAILING
GRAFT CONCEPT

Close follow-up of arterial bypasses with physical examination and noninvasive studies is essential to detect stenotic, flow reducing lesions prior to graft thrombosis. Intimal hyperplasia, proximal or distal disease progression or lesions within the graft itself can produce signs and symptoms of hemodynamic deterioration in patients with a prior arterial reconstruction without concomitant thrombosis of the bypass graft.[6-9] We have referred to this condition as a "failing graft" because, if the lesion is not corrected rapidly, graft thrombosis will occur.[6] The importance of this "failing graft" concept lies in the fact

Vascular Surgical Emergencies
ISBN 0-8089-1843-5

that many difficult lower extremity revascularizations can be salvaged by relatively simple interventions for protracted periods if the lesion responsible for the altered blood flow can be detected before graft thrombosis occurs.

Two years ago we added Duplex scanning to our follow-up protocol. Although graft insonation by Doppler techniques without direct visualization of infrainguinal bypass grafts has been reported to be predictive of imminent failure,[10] we have found that Duplex scanning is more accurate and can locate with precision the lesion responsible for a "failing graft." Great care is taken to assess the inflow and outflow vessels and the entire length of the bypass graft. The proximal and distal graft anastomoses are directly visualized and the midstream flow is sampled for the presence of hemodynamic disturbances. The technique for examining the distal graft anastomosis is variable and depends upon the condition of the outflow vessel. Grafts to the anterior tibial and posterior tibial arteries are best imaged with anterior and medial approaches respectively, while bypasses to the below-knee popliteal artery and tibio-peroneal trunk are best visualized from a posterior approach with the patient in the prone position. Anastomoses to the peroneal artery are difficult to visualize because the artery is in a deep position and is obscured by bony structures. We have found, however, that with the patient in the prone position and with the ankle supported, the peroneal artery can be easily visualized if the probe is placed one fingerbreadth medial to the posterior ridge of the fibula.

Duplex scanning is performed in the early postoperative period, 1, 3 and 6 months postoperatively and then every 6 months thereafter. Normally functioning grafts have well visualized anastomoses without changes in Doppler flow velocities throughout the course of the arterial reconstruction. Vein graft walls are indistinct from the surrounding tissues and normal PTFE grafts have a residual lumen diameter at least 95 percent of that present at insertion. Normal graft peak systolic velocities vary greatly, from 10.8 to 106 cm/sec (mean 70.7 $\pm$ 48.5 cm/sec). The anterior and posterior tibial arteries distal to the graft can be visualized to below the ankle, while the peroneal artery can be evaluated to its bifurcation above the ankle. Peak systolic velocities in the distal arteries are similar to those found in the distal graft segment. Failing grafts that have hemodynamically significant, flow reducing lesions also have decreased luminal diameters (≤ 1.9 mm), thickened graft walls and peak systolic flow velocities of < 30 cm/sec distal to the stenotic area. In some instances Duplex scanning has detected hemodynamically significant, flow reducing lesions before any evidence of impending graft failure was detected by other means. In one distal posterior tibial bypass graft, a routine Duplex scan revealed the presence of a 90 percent flow reducing stenosis that was not detected by bifemoral arteriography performed for ischemic symptoms of the contralateral extremity.

In 51 of our 68 failing grafts (75 percent) a percutaneous transluminal angioplasty corrected the lesion and prevented graft failure for prolonged periods; in the remaining cases a simple proximal graft extension (2 cases), distal graft extension (12 cases) or patch angioplasty (3 cases) were required.[2,6] For these reasons, we believe carefully performed and frequent follow-up examinations are essential for patients with infrainguinal and other limb salvage bypasses. Any change in pulse examination, return of symptoms or deterioration of function as determined by noninvasive laboratory parameters is an indication for urgent arteriography and appropriate correction of new or progressive lesions.[6] Failure to treat the failing graft aggressively will result in a higher incidence of acute graft thrombosis and increase the need for more complicated reoperations which do not achieve the same high rates of continued patency and limb salvage.

Table 1

Timing of Failure of PTFE Bypasses

Type of Bypass	Total Cases	Early Failure ($<$ 1 mo)	Late Failure ($>$ 1 mo)
Fem-AK Pop	228	11	32
Fem-BK Pop	199	7	26
Fem-distal	207	35	17
Fem-fem	96	2	7
Ax-fem	92	6	22
Total	822	61	104

THROMBOSIS OF POLYTETRAFLUOROETHYLENE (PTFE) BYPASS GRAFTS

Between January 1979 and December 1984, 165* of our 822 PTFE bypass grafts thrombosed and required reoperation for limb threatening ischemia (Table 1).[11] Distribution of local and systemic risk factors, techniques of initial operative and postoperative management, methods for patient observation and determination of graft patency, and life table patency rates for this group of patients have been previously reported.[12-16] This reoperated group included 43 femoral-to-above-knee popliteal (Fem-AK Pop), 33 femoral-to-below-knee popliteal (Fem-BK Pop), 52 femoral-to-distal (Fem-dist), 9 femoral-to-femoral (Fem-fem), and 28 axillary-to-femoral (Ax-fem) bypasses.[11] Of the 165 failed PTFE bypass grafts, 61 occluded within the first postoperative month and 104 occluded late, from 1 to 70 months after the initial operation. The results for reoperations on extra-anatomic bypasses (Ax-fem and Fem-fem) have been combined in this study because the results achieved for each were virtually identical. Thirty day operative mortality was 3 percent for all reoperative procedures. Patency rates were calculated from the time of first reoperation by the life table method.[17]

PLAN OF MANAGEMENT FOR EARLY PTFE GRAFT OCCLUSION

Early graft occlusion with recurrent, limb threatening ischemia occurred in 61 patients (Table 2). Repeat angiography was not performed preoperatively. Intravenous heparin was usually administered, and reoperation was undertaken as expeditiously as possible after graft occlusion.

Under regional or general anesthesia, the distal incision was opened and the distal anastomosis and adjacent artery were visualized and controlled. A 1.5 cm, longitudinal incision was made in the hood of the graft to within 1 or 2 mm of the tip of its beveled end (Fig. 1). Through this incision the graft was thrombectomized proximally, and the adjacent artery was gently thrombectomized proximally and distally using balloon catheters with only partial inflation of the balloon (Fig. 2). The distal anastomosis was completely inspected from within for intimal flaps or narrowing. The opening in the graft was closed

---

* This number does not include those patients with thrombosed grafts that did not require reoperation.

Table 2

Causes of Early (< 1 month) PTFE Bypass Graft
Occlusion, Appropriate Operative Treatment and
Incidence in 61 Failed Grafts

Cause	Treatment	Number	Incidence
None Found	Thrombectomy alone	34	56%
Hypotension	Thrombectomy alone	2	3%
Embolus	Thrombectomy alone	2	3%
Technical*	Patch graft	1	2%
Inflow Stenosis	Proximal extension	3	5%
Distal Disease	Distal extension	19	31%

*Unrecognized stenotic lesion just beyond distal anastomosis.

with continuous 6-0 polypropylene sutures, and an arteriogram of the distal anastomosis and outflow tract was obtained through a needle inserted in the graft. If there was any question about the adequacy of the inflow, pressure measurements were performed using the same needle.

In 34 cases, no anastomotic defect or distal stenosis was identified, and the reoperation was terminated (Table 2). Four grafts closed because of hypotensive episodes or emboli that originated from the heart. These 38 grafts were salvaged with thrombectomy alone. In one case a previously unrecognized stenosis was identified at the distal anastomosis and was corrected with a patch angioplasty (Fig. 3). In three cases, a stenotic lesion was identified in the inflow tract and a proximal graft extension was performed. In 19 cases, a hemodynamically significant stenosis was identified distal to the graft insertion,

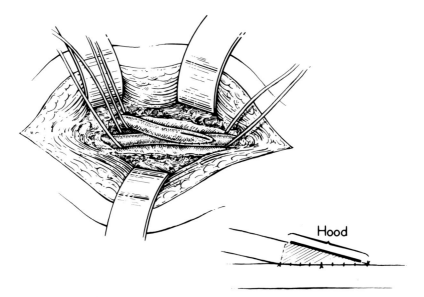

Fig. 1. Operative exposure of the distal anastomosis. The incision in the hood of the graft is made to within 1 mm of the distal end of the graft. This provides optimal exposure of the distal anastomosis and facilitates thrombectomy. (From Ascer E, Collier PE, Gupta SK, Veith FJ: Reoperation for PTFE bypass failure: The importance of distal outflow site and operative technique in determining outcome. J Vasc Surg (in press). By permission of the Journal of Vascular Surgery.)

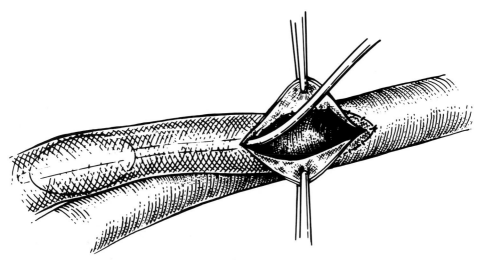

Fig. 2. Thrombectomy alone is performed through the distal graft incision when no cause for graft failure is identified. Clot is removed from the graft and, if needed, from the artery both proximally and distally. (From Ascer E, Collier PE, Gupta SK, Veith FJ: Reoperation for PTFE bypass failure: The importance of distal outflow site and operative technique in determining outcome. J Vasc Surg (in press). By permission of the Journal of Vascular Surgery.)

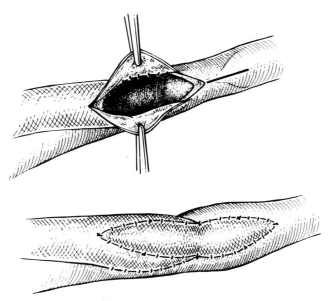

Fig. 3. A stenosis caused by intimal hyperplasia or an unrecognized atherosclerotic lesion is corrected by extending the graft incision distally across its apex and down the recipient artery until its lumen is no longer narrowed. A patch of PTFE or vein is then inserted across the stenosis to widen the lumen. (From Ascer E, Collier PE, Gupta SK, Veith FJ: Reoperation for PTFE bypass failure: The importance of distal outflow site and operative technique in determining outcome. J Vasc Surg (in press). By permission of the Journal of Vascular Surgery.)

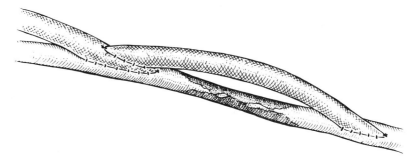

Fig. 4. When graft failure is due to progression of atherosclerosis, a short graft extension is inserted from the graft incision to the artery distal to the atherosclerotic narrowing. (From Ascer E, Collier PE, Gupta SK, Veith FJ: Reoperation for PTFE bypass failure: The importance of distal outflow site and operative technique in determining outcome. J Vasc Surg (in press). By permission of the Journal of Vascular Surgery.)

and a segment of autologous vein or a PTFE graft was used to extend the bypass from the opening in the graft to a patent artery distal to the stenosis (Fig. 4). No postoperative anticoagulation was administered although all patients received 0.6–0.9 g of aspirin and 100–375 mg of dipyridamole daily thereafter. Observation of graft patency by previously described objective methods has been complete in 60 of the 61 patients. One patient was lost to follow-up, with a patent Fem-distal graft, 29 months after reoperation. Twenty-six of these 61 patients (43 percent) required more than one reoperation.

PLAN OF MANAGEMENT FOR LATE PTFE GRAFT OCCLUSION

In 104 patients in whom PTFE graft occlusion occurred from 1 to 37 months after the original operation, limb threatening ischemia again developed. Once limb survival was deemed unlikely, preoperative femoral angiography was performed with visualization of the arterial tree from the aorta to the forefoot. In this way inflow problems proximal to the graft origin could be assessed and the character and patency of arteries distal to the graft insertion could be determined.

Under regional or general anesthesia, the distal incision was reopened. The graft was identified and traced distally until the anastomotic sutures could be seen. The proximal and distal artery was dissected beyond the area of perianastomotic scarring. Heparin was administered, and a longitudinal incision was made in the hood of the graft (Fig. 1) to permit thrombectomy of the graft and arterial tree and to provide visualization of the interior of the distal anastomosis and arterial lumen (Fig. 2). In 91 of 104 cases (88 percent) it was possible to restore unimpeded proximal flow by this approach, while in 10 cases it was necessary to open the proximal incision to remove adherent clot or fibrin from the proximal graft with or without revision of the proximal anastomosis. In 3 of these reoperations a totally new bypass was constructed because all fibrin and debris could not be removed from the graft.

In all but the last 3 cases, after all clot was removed and proximal flow was reestablished, attention was directed to the distal anastomosis to determine the cause of graft occlusion so that appropriate corrective measures could be taken (Table 3). If intimal

Table 3
Causes of Late PTFE Bypass Graft Occlusion, Incidence* and Surgical Treatment

Cause of Failure	Number of Cases	Incidence*	Treatment
Intimal Hyperplasia	22	21%	Thrombectomy, Incision and Patch Graft
Progression of Distal Disease	39	37%	Thrombectomy and Distal Graft Extension or New Bypass to more Distal Artery
Progression of Proximal Disease	12	12%	Thrombectomy and Proximal Graft Extension
None Found	29	28%	Thrombectomy Alone
Hypotension/Technical	2	2%	Thrombectomy Alone

*104 PTFE bypass grafts failed out of a total of 882 PTFE bypasses performed. The incidence of cause of failure is reported in this table as a percentage of the 104 PTFE grafts that failed and required reoperation.

hyperplasia narrowed the recipient artery at or near the distal graft insertion (22 cases), the graft incision was extended distally across its apex and down the recipient artery until its lumen was no longer narrowed. A PTFE or vein patch was inserted across the stenosis to widen the lumen (Fig. 3), and an arteriogram was obtained to assure adequacy of the repair and outflow. If no intimal hyperplasia was present at or beyond the distal anastomosis, the graft incision was closed and operative arteriography and pressure measurements were performed. If these assessments revealed any stenotic or occlusive lesion due to distal disease progression (39 cases), a segment of vein or PTFE graft was inserted side-to-end into the old graft to extend the bypass to a patent artery below the stenotic lesion (Fig. 4) or a new bypass to the same artery more distally was constructed when the original graft could not be effectively reopened. Often the preoperative arteriogram was helpful in identifying progressive atherosclerotic lesions responsible for graft thrombosis. If graft failure was due to proximal disease progression (12 cases), a segment of PTFE was inserted to extend the bypass proximal to the lesion. Recently we have also utilized Duplex scanning to assess the physiologic significance of distal or proximal disease and, therefore, to plan the most appropriate operation. If no cause of late graft closure could be identified (29 cases), the operation consisted of thrombectomy alone. Two other cases in which thrombosis was thought to be secondary to hypotensive episodes were similarly managed. Postoperative management and patency evaluation were as described for early graft occlusion. Fifty-two of these 104 patients (50 percent) required more than one reoperation to prolong patency of their grafts. Five patients (4.8 percent) were lost to follow-up between 12 and 29 months after their first reoperation. All had patent grafts at the time of their last examination.

RESULTS

The results of our management plans for PTFE graft closures were highly dependent upon the location and status of the outflow site. Those grafts that terminated at the femoral or above-knee popliteal level fared much better than those grafts which inserted into vessels below the knee joint (Fig. 5).

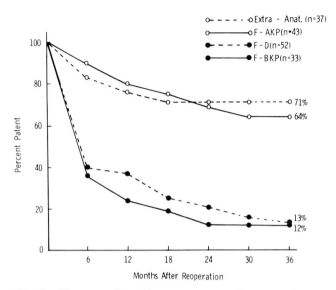

Fig. 5. Three year life-table patency rates after reoperation on 37 extra-anatomic, 43 Fem-AK Pop, 33 Fem-BK Pop and 52 Fem-distal PTFE bypasses. There is a statistically significant difference by the log rank test[17] between the 80 grafts that terminated above the knee and the 85 grafts that terminated below the knee (p < 0.001). (From Ascer E, Collier PE, Gupta SK, Veith FJ: Reoperation for PTFE bypass failure: The importance of distal outflow site and operative technique in determining outcome. J Vas Surg (in press). By permission of the Journal of Vascular Surgery.)

In no subset of patients was any significant difference noted between grafts occluding early or late (Table 4-A). The results of reoperation on PTFE grafts terminating at the femoral or above knee popliteal arteries were not influenced by the status of the runoff, while those terminating below the knee were (Table 4-B). For extra-anatomic and Fem-AK Pop grafts, when the cause of graft failure could be identified and treated specifically by patch angioplasty or graft extension, the results were not statistically different than if no cause of failure was found and thrombectomy alone was performed (Table 4-C). However, the patency rates for grafts to the below-knee popliteal or infrapopliteal arteries were significantly improved if a cause of failure was identified and either a patch angioplasty or graft extension was performed (Table 4-C).

NEW SECONDARY BYPASS

Although we previously attempted to salvage all thrombosed PTFE bypasses by the techniques described above, we have been influenced by the relatively poor late patency rates of reoperations for failed bypasses inserting below the knee. Accordingly, we have recently altered our management of failed below knee popliteal and infrapopliteal PTFE grafts and have generally performed entirely new bypasses using either vein or PTFE grafts anastomosed to virginal inflow and outflow arteries. Originally we used this approach only when the original PTFE bypass was complicated by infection or was per-

Table 4

Factors Potentially Influencing Graft Patency in
165 Failed PTFE Bypasses

(A) Timing of Failure After Primary Operation		
	3-year Patency Rate After Reoperation	
Graft Location	Early Failure (< 1 mo)	Late Failure (> 1 mo)
Extra-Anatomic	58%	75%
Fem-AK Pop	48%	61%
Fem-BK Pop	14%	10%
Fem-Distal	12%	25%

(B) Runoff*		
	Good	Poor
Extra-Anatomic	77%	55%
Fem-AK Pop	62%	34%
Fem-BK Pop	16%	0%[†]
Fem-Distal	31%	4%[†]

(C) Identified Cause of Failure		
	Yes	No
Extra-Anatomic	73%	56%
Fem-AK Pop	61%	44%
Fem-BK Pop	21%	0%[†]
Fem-Distal	33%	8%[†]

*"Good Runoff" for bypasses to the popliteal or infrapopliteal arteries was
defined as at least one outflow vessel that was continuously patent to the
pedal arch; "Poor Runoff" was defined as the absence of any such patent
vessel. For extra-anatomic bypasses "Good Runoff" was defined as the
presence of a patent superficial and deep femoral artery; "Poor Runoff"
was defined as the absence of a patent superficial femoral artery.
[†]Statistically significant difference ($P < 0.01$).

formed at another institution and the technical details of the primary operation could not
be ascertained. For the last 3 years we have also performed entirely new bypass grafts
when a Fem-BK Pop or Fem-distal bypass failed and no cause of failure could be detected
or failed for a second time. Although accurate and conclusive comparisons are not
possible at present, this modified approach has resulted in 3 year patency rates of 48
percent and 39 percent for secondary operation after failure of previous Fem-BK Pop and
Fem-distal PTFE bypasses, respectively.

THROMBOSIS OF REVERSED SAPHENOUS VEIN BYPASS GRAFTS

The outlook for restoring patency to an autologous saphenous vein Fem-Pop or Fem-
distal bypass that fails after the immediate postoperative period has generally been poor. A

completely new secondary bypass is probably the best option for reversing ischemia[18] although some success with vein thrombectomy and graft revision has been reported by Whittemore and his associates,[8] and this has been our experience. If reoperation is conducted within 24 hours after occlusion of the vein graft, simple thrombectomy with correction of defects in the vein or the inflow and/or outflow tracts is a method that can restore patency.[8] Only when such defects are identified and repaired (ideally, before they cause graft thrombosis) can simple reoperative correction be performed with uniformly good results.[6-9] We have performed thrombectomy of vein grafts in 5 cases and have achieved prolonged graft patency in 4 of them.

Often, thrombosed saphenous vein grafts require the creation of a new bypass using virginal vessels for inflow and outflow and ectopically harvested autologous vein from the arms or contralateral leg, or PTFE. Preoperative arteriography is essential and often preoperative venography is helpful in determining whether the ipsilateral saphenous vein or other veins are available and useful.[19] We have achieved 3 year patency rates of 52 percent and 48 percent, respectively, in a group of 19 secondary femoropopliteal and 25 infrapopliteal vein grafts that required reoperation because of a primary vein graft failure. Thirty-five of these new bypasses were constructed of PTFE alone, 5 were composite, sequential (PTFE and vein) bypasses, and 4 of the new bypasses were constructed completely with autologous vein.

DISCUSSION

These results show that PTFE Fem-AK Pop and Extra-anatomic bypasses that occlude can be effectively treated by aggressive reoperation with salvage of the original graft. If the reoperation is appropriately performed and monitored by intraoperative angiography and pressure measurements, long-term graft patency can result. These results are not significantly affected by the length of primary graft patency, the status of the runoff vessels, whether or not an exact cause is identified for the graft thrombosis, or the nature of the operation required for graft failure. Importantly, if this surgical approach to graft failure for PTFE reconstructions terminating above the knee is followed, recurrent thromboses as well as initial thrombosis of these grafts can be effectively managed by similar techniques.

Similar reoperative techniques applied to PTFE bypasses terminating below the knee have not been as rewarding. We now only use this approach with reoperation directly on the old failed below-knee graft if the preoperative arteriogram shows a good quality artery with continuous runoff to the foot. In all other circumstances, when a Fem-BK Pop or Fem-distal PTFE graft thromboses, we now construct a totally new bypass to a virginal outflow vessel. This approach greatly simplifies the reoperation since dissection of arteries in surgically scarred areas is not required, the risk of wound infection is decreased, and it is often possible to replace the thrombosed PTFE graft with autologous vein. Most importantly, this change from preserving the original graft to creating a totally new bypass appears to have improved the patency rates achieved with reoperation for thrombosed Fem-BK Pop and Fem-distal PTFE bypasses.

Our good results for reoperations on above-knee PTFE grafts also contrast sharply with the results of autologous saphenous vein femoropopliteal bypasses that require early reoperation for thrombosis. Craver and his associates[20] reported the results of 66 patients with failed femoropopliteal bypasses, the majority of which were constructed of autologous vein. Only 28 percent of these patients had a patent graft after 1 year. In their series, simple thrombectomy of a graft when no cause of failure could be identified and corrected was always followed by rethrombosis.[20] More recent results with reoperation for failed femoropopliteal vein grafts confirm the general ineffectiveness of simple thrombectomy, but indicate that some thrombectomized vein grafts may remain patent if a technical defect is recognized and corrected appropriately.[8] However, an occasional vein graft will remain patent following simple thrombectomy if no defect is present to account for the thrombosis. Thus PTFE bypasses that terminate above the knee appear to be unusual in that thrombectomy alone can often restore long-term patency after graft thrombosis.

We have previously noted that intimal hyperplasia at or just beyond the distal anastomosis is a major cause of PTFE graft closures that occur 2 months or more after reoperation.[13] Echave and his associates have also noted that intimal hyperplasia causes failure of tapered femoropopliteal PTFE grafts, and this group has recommended treatment by graft thrombectomy and extension to a distal artery.[21] Our findings and management concepts concerning this lesion differ in some ways from those of Echave and his colleagues. We have observed intimal hyperplasia as a cause of PTFE graft failure even when uniform tubes 6 mm in diameter were employed. In addition, we have not found intimal hyperplasia to be a prominent cause of late PTFE femoropopliteal bypass failure (Table 3). Furthermore, we believe that incision and patch grafting is a better technique than graft extension for managing this lesion, since it leaves the maximal amount of undisturbed distal artery should subsequent reoperation be required. However, O'Donnell and his colleagues have not had equally good results with patch grafting for intimal hyperplasia.[22]

ACKNOWLEDGMENT

This work was supported in part by the James Hilton Manning and Emma Austin Manning Foundation.

REFERENCES

1. Veith FJ, Gupta SK, Daly V: Management of early and late thrombosis of expanded polytetrafluoroethylene (PTFE) femoropopliteal bypass grafts: Favorable prognosis with appropriate reoperation. Surgery 87:581, 1980
2. Veith FJ, Gupta SK: Expanded polytetrafluoroethylene vascular grafts, in Rutherford RB (ed): Vascular Surgery. Philadelphia, WB Saunders, 1984, pp 394–404
3. Ascer E, Veith FJ, Morin L, et al: Quantitative assessment of outflow resistance in lower extremity arterial reconstruction. J Surg Res 37:8, 1984
4. Ascer E, Veith FJ, Morin L, et al: Components of outflow resistance and their correlation with graft patency in lower extremity arterial reconstructions. J Vasc Surg 1:817, 1984
5. Ascer E, Veith FJ, Gupta SK, et al: Comparison of axillounifemoral and axillobifemoral bypass operations. Surgery 97:169, 1985
6. Veith FJ, Weiser RK, Gupta SK, et al: Diagnosis and management of failing lower extremity arterial reconstructions. J Cardiovasc Surg 25:381, 1984
7. O'Mara CS, Flinn WR, Johnson ND, et al: Recognition and surgical management of patent but hemodynamically failed arterial grafts. Ann Surg 193:467, 1981
8. Whittemore AD, Clowes AW, Couch NP, et al: Secondary femoro-popliteal reconstruction. Ann Surg 193:35, 1981

9. Berkowitz HD, Hobbs CL, Roberts B, et al: Value of routine vascular laboratory studies to identify vein graft stenosis. Surgery 90:971, 1981

10. Bandyk DF, Cato RF, Towne JB: A low flow velocity predicts failure of femoropopliteal and femorotibial grafts. Surgery 98:799, 1985

11. Ascer E, Collier PE, Gupta SK, Veith FJ: Reoperation for PTFE bypass failure: The importance of distal outflow site and operative technique in determining outcome. J Vasc Surg (in press)

12. Veith FJ, Moss CM, Fell SC, et al: Comparison of expanded polytetrafluoroethylene and autologous saphenous vein grafts in high risk arterial reconstructions for limb salvage. Surg Gynecol Obstet 147:749, 1978

13. Veith FJ, Moss C, Daly V, et al: New approaches to limb salvage by extended extra-anatomic bypasses and prosthetic reconstructions to foot arteries. Surgery 84:764, 1978

14. Bergan JJ, Veith FJ, Bernhard VM, et al: Randomization of autogenous vein and polytetrafluoroethylene grafts in femoral-distal reconstruction. Surgery 157:437, 1982

15. Veith FJ, Gupta SK, Ascer E, et al: Six-year prospective multicenter randomized comparison of autologous saphenous vein and expanded polytetrafluoroethylene grafts in infrainguinal arterial reconstructions. J Vasc Surg 3:104, 1986

16. Ascer E, Veith FJ, Gupta SK, et al: Six year experience with expanded polytetrafluoroethylene arterial grafts for limb salvage. J Cardiovasc Surg 26:468, 1985

17. Colton T: Statistics in Medicine. Boston, Little Brown, 1974, p 237

18. Szilagyi DE, Elliot JP, Smith RF, et al: Secondary arterial repair: The management of late failures in reconstructive arterial surgery. Arch Surg 110:485, 1975

19. Veith F, Moss CM, Sprayregen S, et al: Preoperative saphenous venography in arterial reconstructive surgery of the lower extremity. Surgery 85:253, 1979

20. Craver JM, Ottinger LW, Darling C, et al: Hemorrhage and thrombosis as early complications of femoropopliteal bypass grafts: Causes, treatment, and prognostic implications. Surgery 74:839, 1973

21. Echave V, Kornick A, Haimov M, Jacobson JH: Intimal hyperplasia as a complication of the use of the polytetrafluoroethylene graft for femoral-popliteal bypass. Surgery 86:791, 1979

22. O'Donnell TF Jr, Mackey W, McCullough JL Jr, et al: Correlation of operative findings with angiographic and noninvasive hemodynamic factors associated with failure of polytetrafluoroethylene grafts. J Vasc Surg 1:136, 1984

C. William Cole
Wesley S. Moore

Emergency Amputation

Emergency amputation of an injured limb was one of the earliest surgical procedures to be recognized as a life-saving measure in some circumstances and until very recent times represented the optimal treatment for patients with an extremity affected by profound ischemia and/or at high risk for septic complications. Today, with modern anesthesia and sophisticated vascular, orthopedic, and plastic reconstructive procedures, it is possible to salvage a large proportion of limbs that would have been managed by immediate amputation only 50 years ago. Despite the remarkable advances in all fields of medicine and surgery that allow for the salvage of the large majority of injured limbs, some are beyond our capabilities because of the extent of the injury while others become threats to life because of systemic complications that appear as a result of sepsis or necrosis. It is this category of affected extremities, those that actively threaten the life of the patient, that will be addressed in this chapter.

With few exceptions, largely due to trauma,[1] the indications for emergency amputation of a compromised extremity fall into two specific groups: (1) extensive myonecrosis and (2) uncontrolled sepsis. Prompt amputation in these circumstances may be life-saving and delay lethal complications.

MYONECROSIS

Historical Aspects

Physicians first recognized the potential for severe systemic toxic effects due to the breakdown products of ischemic skeletal muscle during the early part of this century, but the first reported cases to receive widespread notice came during World War II. During the bombing of London many victims were trapped under rubble causing severe ischemic muscle injury. When the casualties were freed and the circulation to the ischemic muscle mass was restored a significant number developed a syndrome of oliguria, anuria and death that became known as the "crush" syndrome.[2-7] There are occasional instances of a similar mechanism causing this syndrome in peacetime, usually as a result of natural disaster or industrial accident, but the most frequently observed clinical correlate in present-day surgical practice is prolonged ischemia as a result of acute arterial occlusion due to embolus or thrombosis.[8] Both clinical and experimental evidence suggests that the ischemic muscle injury that accompanies acute arterial occlusion is a major factor in the high mortality rate seen in the surgical treatment of these patients.

Pathophysiology

The pathophysiology of the "crush" syndrome is incompletely understood, but is generally considered to be due to the systemic effects of metabolic breakdown products resulting from ischemic necrosis of skeletal muscle that are released when circulation to the limb is restored.[9,10] The metabolic complications that result from restoration of the circulation will clearly depend upon the degree and duration of the ischemic period and the rapidity with which the metabolites are released into the systemic circulation.

Observations from experimental animal models[11-17] and from studies of human muscle[18] and blood[19] during and after periods of ischemia necessitated by operative procedures, have plotted the course of the metabolic changes that occur in acutely ischemic skeletal muscle and the systemic effects following reperfusion. Ischemic skeletal muscle produces lactate and pyruvate by anaerobic glycolysis via the Embden-Myerhoff pathway; tissue pH and bicarbonate fall as a result. As energy requirements exceed the needs of the ischemic cell, the sodium pump fails and sodium leaks into the cell drawing water with it, which causes cell swelling. Intracellular potassium exits the cell as the pH falls and seeks to equilibrate with the surrounding interstitial fluid. ATP required for muscle contraction and nerve function is depleted[20] and the enzyme and reparative functions of all cells that depend upon this energy source are unable to maintain their integrity, resulting in the breakdown of structural and functional proteins. Myosin and actin (rhabdomyolysis), enzymes (SGOT, SGPT, CPK) as well as the products of erythrocyte lysis (hemoglobin) are released into the extracellular milieu.

When severely ischemic skeletal muscle has its circulation restored the potential for profound systemic effects is apparent. The influx of large concentrations of potassium and acid metabolites into the systemic circulation may cause cardiac arrest within minutes of restoration of blood flow due to hyperkalemia and acidosis. Acidosis is usually corrected within minutes of reestablishing blood flow,[21] but the serum potassium concentration may continue to rise as it continues to be released from the compromised muscle. Cardiac arrest that occurs a few hours following a surgical procedure to reestablish the arterial circulation to an ischemic limb may be the result of the insidious rise in serum potassium being "washed out" of the reperfused limb. The serum BUN rises following reperfusion and frequently has begun to do so before the flow of blood has been restored to the ischemic limb. Myoglobinuria appears early in the course of severe ischemic compromise to a large muscle mass and may also begin to appear before blood flow is reestablished. Myoglobin may precipitate in renal tubules causing renal failure and there is some evidence that myoglobin has a direct toxic effect upon renal tubular cells in addition to mechanical obstruction.

The venous outflow from a previously severely ischemic extremity may carry microthrombi, which can embolize to the pulmonary circulation and may account for part of the "toxic" effect of reperfusion frequently manifest clinically as shock.[22] Prolonged ischemic insult may cause stasis and thrombosis in the venous circulation, occluding the egress of blood from the limb and further compromising the chances for successful outcome.

The ischemic limb frequently develops massive edema following reperfusion due to muscle swelling and may require extensive fasciotomy to avoid further muscle necrosis and to relieve the venous and capillary network of the occlusive pressure. Pain resulting from ischemia may be exacerbated by the restoration of blood flow and is often relieved by fasciotomy.

Acute Arterial Occlusion

Despite improved surgical ability to deal with ischemic limbs, it was alarming to discover during the 1960s that attempts to salvage limbs that were severely ischemic resulted in a mortality rate between 25 percent and 35 percent. This high mortality rate is probably due to the age of the population presenting with these problems and the frequency of concomitant cardiac disease.[23] This observation prompted many surgeons to reassess their approach to patients with acute ischemia[24] and to take a more scientific approach to the problems of ischemic muscle injury and the systemic effects of reperfusion. Limbs made ischemic by the acute occlusive process, either by embolus or thrombosis, depend entirely upon collateral circulation, which is sufficient in the majority of cases to prevent the severe ischemic changes indicative of an unsalvable extremity. Immediate embolectomy, when indicated, may restore the normal circulation without systemic effects. When the clinical situation suggests thrombosis as the etiology, or when embolectomy has been delayed because of other considerations, heparin therapy will prevent propagation of thrombus distal to the point of occlusion and keep the capillary network within the limb patent while the collateral circulation develops.[25] In patients with an unstable cardiac status, streptokinase may offer a suitable alternative to embolectomy,[26,27] since the procedure has been reported to carry a 40 percent mortality rate among patients whose emboli came from an infarcted myocardium.[28] The limb must be continuously reassessed and while it remains viable, complete investigation including arteriography can be completed and reconstruction carried out electively if indicated.

Diagnosis of the Nonviable Extremity

The best indicator of limb viability is the history of the event and the clinical appearance of the ischemic limb. The most apparent symptom of severe ischemia is *pain*, which is exacerbated by passive motion of the limb and muscle tenderness to palpation. This is followed in quick succession (in *complete* ischemia not more than 2 to 3 hours) by paralysis and loss of sensation and the development of a woody consistency to the normally soft muscle mass. Swelling develops gradually and may be massive after 12 hours and involves the entire limb in most cases when the occlusion is at the level of the femoral artery. The ischemic insult to the muscles of a limb as a result of these mechanisms is invariably abetted by clamps applied to the major arteries during reconstructive vascular procedures and the ischemic damage will be more severe if thrombosis occurs in a graft previously placed for symptomatic ischemia where collateral network is poorly developed. Patients with collateral circulation adequate to provide even minimal blood flow to the ischemic limb usually will not develop the full range of profound signs and symptoms described here unless treatment is delayed.

In most instances, limbs that are not viable at the time of presentation should be amputated urgently. Limbs that are only marginally viable as a result of profound and lengthy ischemia must be carefully considered before revascularization is carried out because the heavy influx of potassium and acid metabolites of skeletal muscle necrosis that occurs at the time when blood flow is restored may reach lethal proportions, particularly in the elderly and those with a compromised myocardium. Emergency amputation should be considered when there is evidence of these metabolites already in the systemic circulation. Important signs of systemic toxic effects due to myonecrosis are (1) acidosis, (2) hyperkalemia, (3) myoglobinuria or renal failure, (4) hypotension, (5) cardiac arrhythmia, and (6) elevation of serum CPK. Patients with systemic evidence of the toxic effects of myonecrosis by these criteria should not have immediate restoration of the circulation to the affected extremity. Emergency measures to control these effects should be undertaken in an intensive care unit with constant monitoring of the cardiac status. They include administration of sodium bicarbonate to control hyperkalemia and acidosis and to alkalinize the urine in an effort to prevent the precipitation of myoglobin in the renal tubules; cation exchange resins may be administered to lower the serum potassium, but levels approaching 7 mEq per liter must be treated immediately with intravenous glucose and insulin and with dialysis if these measures fail to have the desired effect. In patients in whom continuing systemic influx of toxic metabolites is apparent, emergency amputation must be considered. In situations where even mild toxic systemic effects would be potentially hazardous, amputation of a nonviable extremity should be carried out without delay as an urgent procedure. When amputation cannot be safely carried out immediately, freezing the limb has been suggested as an alternative temporary solution to limit the toxic systemic effects of the gangrenous extremity and spare the patient the anesthetic and surgical risks associated with the procedure.[29]

SEPSIS

Uncontrolled sepsis continues to be a major indication for emergency amputation that, in the nontrauma patient population, is almost always in diabetics,[30] where a gangrenous extremity may represent a major threat to life.[31]

Pathophysiology

Diabetic patients have two principle causes for foot sepsis: (1) ischemia and (2) sensory neuropathy. Diabetes has a deleterious effect on the small arterial capillary network and for the most part spares the medium and large sized vessels affected by atherosclerosis. While ischemia may play a significant role once sepsis has become established, most foot ulcers in diabetic patients are due to trauma that goes unrecognized by the patient with an insensitive foot. Chronic ulceration eventually leads to sepsis, frequently deep and involving bony structures of the foot. Local debridement, digit, or ray amputation is sufficient to manage the majority of these lesions. Occasionally the septic process affects a closed space in the mid portion of the foot and may lead to fulminant sepsis with systemic manifestations.

Bacteriology

The most common organism found in the septic foot lesions of diabetics is *Staphylococcus aureus Proteus* and other enteric pathogens such as *Escherichia coli, Bacteroides* and *Klebsiella* are often mixed. *Clostridium welchii* is a relatively infrequent pathogen in septic foot lesions of diabetic patients, but can be one of the most devastating forms of sepsis when present.

Diagnosis

Sepsis in a diabetic foot is invariably associated with a neuropathic ulcer, which occurs at characteristic sites at pressure points over the metatarsal heads or the heel, or with an ischemic digit. More significant, deep septic processes are to be suspected when diabetes has become uncontrollable with the usual hypoglycemic regimen or there is an elevation in the white blood cell count or fever. X-ray studies may demonstrate osteomyelitis or the presence of gas within the soft tissues of the foot. The presence of gas in the subcutaneous tissues of a gangrenous extremity of a diabetic is usually the result of nonclostridial organisms,[32] although occasionally clostridial organisms are the principal ones and must not be forgotten. When open drainage of the septic process exists the systemic manifestations will usually be minimal. However, when confined to a closed space such as the forefoot, more systemic manifestations are usually present although diabetic patients frequently do not manifest generalized signs of sepsis until the process is far advanced.

Treatment

Immediate drainage and excision of all necrotic tissue is essential as well as the identification of the infective organism(s) and the administration of appropriate intravenous antibiotics. Amputation under these circumstances is usually the best form of surgical drainage and may require excision of a part (ray or transmetatarsal) or the whole extremity (usually below-knee) and should be carried out as a guillotine amputation of the distal portion of the extremity[33] unless proximal clean tissue planes are clearly defined.[34]

AMPUTATION LEVEL SELECTION AND TECHNIQUE

Myonecrosis

Myonecrosis sufficient to require emergency amputation will invariably require that it be carried out at a level above the knee. This amputation is best performed at the high thigh level. A circular skin incision is made and is then carried down through the fascia. If the muscle is necrotic at this level, a hip disarticulation may be required to achieve closure in healthy tissue. If the muscle is viable the surgeon may proceed with amputation at that level. The skin and fascia are retracted cephalad and the muscle is incised approximately one inch proximal to the line of the skin incision. The femoral artery and vein are identified, clamped, divided, and ligated. The sciatic nerve is mobilized, clamped, divided, and ligated as far proximal as possible. The femur is divided sufficiently proximal to the line of muscle division in order to permit adequate soft tissue for closure of the skin and fascia, in a transverse manner, without tension.

Sepsis

When amputation is performed for infection in a diabetic patient, the circulation of the extremity may be good enough to permit a conservative amputation of the affected area, provided that sepsis is controlled by this procedure. Usually the septic process will involve the forefoot together with fascial-tendon spaces. There may be evidence of lymphangitis extending proximal to the ankle joint. In spite of this, amputation at the below knee level will be feasible provided that the septic process is controlled and the blood supply is adequate. A debridement guillotine amputation at the level of the malleoli will remove the septic focus and permit clearing of the proximal infection by drainage and antibiotic therapy. A circular skin incision is made at the malleoli and carried down to the bone. A reciprocating saw is used to divide the distal tibia and fibula cleanly. The end of the amputation stump is dressed open after hemostasis has been achieved and high dose, organism-specific antibiotic therapy is continued for the next 2 to 3 days. As soon as it becomes evident that local sepsis is controlled by inspection of the extremity as well as confirmation that systemic sepsis is not present, a definitive, below-knee amputation may be carried out in the usual fashion.

It is unusual to perform amputation successfully at more conservative levels in the presence of infection in diabetic patients. Nonetheless, a Syme's or transmetatarsal amputation may be feasible if carried out in a two-stage manner.

REFERENCES

1. Stewart RD, Young JC, Kenney DA, et al: Field surgical intervention: An unusual case. J Trauma 19:780, 1979
2. Bywaters EGL: Ischemic muscle necrosis. JAMA 124:1103, 1944
3. Bywaters EGL, Beall D: Crush injuries with impairment of renal function. Brit Med J 1:427, 1941
4. Bywaters EGL, Belsey AHR, Miles JAR: A case of crush injury with renal failure. Brit Med J 1:432, 1941
5. Mayon-White R, Solandt OM: A case of limb compression ending fatally in uraemia. Brit Med J 1:434, 1941
6. Bywaters EGL, Delory GE: Myohaemoglobinuria. Lancet 1:648, 1941
7. Bywaters EGL, Delory GE, Remington C, et al: Myohaemoglobin in the urine of air raid casualties with crushing injury. Biochem J 35:1164, 1941
8. Haimovici H: Metabolic syndrome secondary to acute arterial occlusions, in Haimovici H (ed): Vascular Emergencies. New York, Appleton-Centrury-Crofts, 1982, pp 267–289
9. Green HN: Shock-producing factor(s) from striated muscle. Lancet 2:147, 1943
10. Haimovici H: Muscular, renal and metabolic complications of acute arterial occlusions: Myonephropathic-metabolic syndrome. Surgery 85:461, 1979
11. Trazzi R, Pannacciulli E, Biasi G, et al: Experimental metabolic modifications in acute ischemia. J Cardiovasc Sug 14:635, 1973
12. Zamecnick RC, Aub JC, Brues AM, et al: The toxic factors in experimental shock, V: Chemical and enzymatic properties of muscle exudate. J Clin Invest 24:850, 1945

13. Montagnani CA, Simeone FA: Observations on the liberation and elimination of myohemoglobin and of hemoglobin after release of muscle ischemia. Surgery 34:169, 1953

14. Dunant J, Nosbaum J, Waibel P: Metabolic changes during induced ischemia of the leg. J Cardiovasc Surg 14:586, 1973

15. Chiu D, Wang HH, Blumenthal MR: Creatine phosphokinase release as a measure of tourniquet effect of skeletal muscle. Arch Surg 111:71, 1976

16. Snyder DD, Campbell GS: Humoral effects of experimental crush syndrome. Surgery 47:217, 1960

17. Thompson WW, Campbell GS: Studies on myoglobin and hemoglobin in experimental crush syndrome in dogs. Ann Surg 149:235, 1959

18. Haljamäe H, Enger E: Human skeletal muscle energy metabolism during and after complete tourniquet ischemia. Ann Surg 182:9, 1975

19. Fisher DR, Fogarty TJ, Morrow AG: Clinical and biochemical observations of the effect of transient femoral artery occlusion in man. Surgery 68:323, 1979

20. Keaveny TV, O'Boyle A, Fitzgerald PA: Effect of surgical procedure on muscle ATP. J Cardiovasc Surg 14:601, 1973

21. Fisher RD, Fogarty TJ, Morrow AG: Clinical and biochemical observations of the effect of transient femoral artery occlusion in man. Surgery 68:323, 1970

22. Dexter L: Cardiovascular responses to experimental pulmonary embolism, in: Sasahara AA, Stein M (eds): Pulmonary Embolic Disease. New York, Grune & Stratton, 1965

23. Palmberg S, Hirsjärvi: Mortality in geriatric surgery. Gerontology 25:103, 1979

24. Blaisdell FW, Steele M, Allen RE: Management of acute lower extremity arterial ischemia due to embolism and thrombosis. Surgery 84:822, 1978

25. Gregg RO, Chamberlain BE, Myers JK, et al: Embolectomy or heparin therapy for arterial emboli? Surgery 93:377, 1983

26. Berni GA, Bankyk DF, Zierler RE, et al: Streptokinase treatment of acute arterial occlusion. Ann Surg 198:185, 1983

27. Hess H, Ingrisch H, Mietaschk A, et al: Local low-dose thrombolytic therapy of peripheral arterial occlusions. N Eng J Med 307:1627, 1982

28. Gregg RO, Chamberlain BE, Myers JK, et al: Embolectomy or heparin therapy for arterial emboli? Surgery 93:377, 1983

29. Harbrecht PJ, Nethery H, Ahmad W, et al: A technic for freezing an extremity in preparation for amputation. Am J Surg 135:859, 1978

30. Fierer J, Daniel D, Davis C: The fetid foot: Lower-extremity infections in patients with diabetes mellitus. Rev Inf Dis 1:210, 1979

31. Kahn O, Wagner W, Bessman AN: Mortality of diabetic patients treated surgically for lower limb infection and/or gangrene. Diabetes 23:287, 1974

32. Bessman AN, Wagner W: Nonclostridial gas gangrene. JAMA 233:958, 1975

33. McIntyre KE, Bailey SA, Malone JM, et al: Guillotine amputation in the treatment of non-salvageable lower-extremity infections. Arch Surg 119:450, 1984

34. Fearon J, Campbell DR, Hoar CS, et al: Improved results with diabetic below-knee amputations. Arch Surg 120:777, 1985

Index